CARDIOVASCULAR RISK FACTORS

Edited by **Armen Yuri Gasparyan**

Cardiovascular Risk Factors
Edited by Armen Yuri Gasparyan

Published by InTech
Janeza Trdine 9, 51000 Rijeka, Croatia

Publishing Process Manager Silvia Vlase

Technical Editor Teodora Smiljanic

Cover Designer InTech Design Team

Edition 2014

Additional hard copies can be obtained from orders@intechopen.com

Cardiovascular Risk Factors, Edited by Armen Yuri Gasparyan
p. cm.
ISBN 978-953-51-0240-3

For EU product safety concerns:
IN TECH d.o.o., Prolaz Marije Krucifikse Kozulić 3, 51000 Rijeka, Croatia,
info@intechopen.com or visit our website at intechopen.com.

Meet the editor

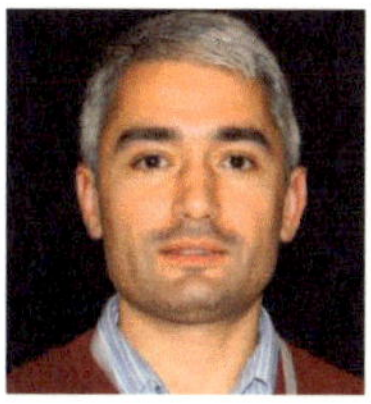

Dr Armen Yuri Gasparyan has been involved in clinical research on cardiovascular issues in inflammatory disorders since 1994, and got his PhD degree in 2002. In 2006 he was awarded an academic title of Associate Professor of medicine. Since 2007, he has been a post-doctoral research fellow in thrombosis and cardiovascular rheumatology in the UK, supported by the European Society of Cardiology and the European League Against Rheumatism. Over the past four years, Dr A.Y. Gasparyan has also organized international seminars on science editing. He is a reviewer at The Lancet, Thrombosis Research, Rheumatology (Oxford), Seminars in Arthritis and Rheumatism, Current Pharmaceutical Design, Rheumatology International, Academic Medicine and other journals. In 2007-2010, Dr Gasparyan served as the executive editor of Archives of Medical Science (Poland), and joined the World Association of Medical Editors and the European Association of Science Editors. Since 2011, he is a chief editor of European Science Editing and council member of the European Association of Science Editors. A.Y. Gasparyan published numerous papers, reviews and editorials.

Contents

Preface

An Insight on Cardiovascular Risk Factors: Challenges and Opportunities

Our understanding of the implications of cardiovascular risk factors has greatly improved over the past two decades. It has been postulated that numerous risk factors and markers of inflammation and immune response trigger pathologic changes in the vascular wall from early life, leading to atherosclerotic cardiovascular disease in later life [1]. It has also been widely recognized that no single risk factor causes atherosclerotic disease, and that the likelihood of the disease depends on a multifactorial genetic and environmental background. The complex nature of risk factors and their interdependence implies the need of multidirectional preventive measures, which should be monitored and assessed with the use of multiple demographic, clinical, genetic and laboratory parameters.

Over the past decades, the dominating concept of cardiovascular prevention has been based on the initial results of the landmark Framingham Heart Study, which linked the burden of cardiovascular disease with a combination of traditional risk factors, such as age, sex, arterial hypertension, hyperlipidemia, smoking, obesity, diabetes, and sedentary lifestyle. The study led to the validation and wide-spread use of the Framingham Risk Score, which is an indispensable tool for stratifying cardiovascular risk and treatment by clinicians and deploying strategies for community-based primary preventive measures by health administrators [2, 3].

The decades-long application of the Framingham Risk Score in different populations worldwide has also revealed its inherent limitations and led to the development of several alternative tools (e.g., SCORE [Systematic Coronary Risk Evaluation], Reynolds Risk Score, QRISK [QRESEARCH Cardiovascular Risk Algorithm]) [4]. Though the new tools have addressed some problems, none of these has been universally accepted, raising concerns over ethnicity, psychosocial background, comorbidities, drug therapies, and validity of biomarkers incorporated in the risk scores. For example, a recent large study showed that currently available risk scores do not provide precise estimates of cardiovascular risk in patients with rheumatoid arthritis [5], leaving the issue of risk-score-based cardiovascular prevention in this particular population uncertain. The guidance based on cardiovascular risk scores in patients with inflammatory disorders may either underestimate, which is more likely, or overestimate the real risk. Given the results of statistical analyses in large cohorts, an attempt was made to correct values of risk scores in patients with rheumatoid arthritis by using a 1.5 multiplier [6]. In practice, however, the latter approach was not regarded as realistic [7], necessitating more research into cardiovascular pathophysiology and therapies in inflammatory disorders.

There are still many uncertainties over the interaction between traditional and novel risk factors leading to premature cardiovascular morbidity and mortality in the general population and in patients with diseases predisposing to vascular damage and accelerated atherothrombosis. Systemic inflammation has long been regarded as a crucial factor of premature cardiovascular disease. Initial evidence for this stems from the Physicians' Health Study [8], which highlighted the significance of subclinical inflammation and slight elevation of C-reactive protein (CRP) level undetectable by conventional laboratory tests. A more recent large trial, the Justification for Use of statins in Prevention: an Intervention Trial Evaluating Rosuvastatin (JUPITER), reaffirmed that the suppression of low-grade inflammation (CRP just above 2 mg/l) can bring benefits in terms of primary cardiovascular prevention in the general population [9]. The JUPITER study also proved that the greatest cardiovascular risk reduction as a result of antiinflammatory therapy with rosuvastatin is expected in subjects with the highest levels of CRP. Whether the same or even greater risk reduction can be derived in high- and low-grade inflammatory disorders and whether statins can occupy their niche in the combined treatment of the patients are still a matter of debate, which may be resolved once the results of specifically designed and powered trials become available [10-12].

Several lines of evidence, mainly derived from retrospective cohort studies, suggest that systemic inflammation drives atherogenesis in cohorts of patients with systemic lupus erythematosus (SLE) and rheumatoid arthritis (RA). The exposure to high-grade inflammation is a crucial pathogenic factor in these patients, justifying aggressive antiinflammatory treatment, which, in turn, proved to reduce atherosclerotic burden among other disease-modifying effects [13-15]. The link between inflammation and atherosclerotic cardiovascular disease, however, is not universally evident across cohorts of patients with inflammatory disorders [16]. A recent systematic review on vascular function in RA revealed discrepancies across numerous cross-sectional and longitudinal studies, and questioned the direct link between rheumatoid inflammation and vasculopathy [17]. Moreover, numerous studies of varying levels of evidence suggested the lack of association between persistent low-grade inflammation and atherosclerotic vascular disease in patients with systemic vasculitides, including those with Wegener granulomatosis [18] and Behçet disease (BD) [19], the latter viewed as a model of venous thrombosis [20]. Obviously, the reported discrepancies indicate the complexity of atherogenic pathways and warrant further research into novel cardiovascular risk markers.

Over the past decade, several promising markers of inflammation-mediated atherosclerosis have emerged. Of these, markers of activated platelets, such as platelet-bound P-selectin, CD40 ligand, beta-thromboglobulin, platelet factor 4, platelet-derived microparticles, as well as platelet count and size have been tested in the general population, in cohorts of patients with RA and some other inflammatory disorders in association with cardiovascular risk factors and vascular end-points [21-23]. Mean platelet volume was shown to be a readily available, well-standardized marker of inflammation and thrombosis predictive of atherosclerotic vascular end-points in some well-designed retrospective and prospective cohort studies [24]. Furthermore, a suggestion was made to routinely assess mean platelet volume and a set of other markers of platelet activation and their genetic variability to guide antiplatelet therapies and overall cardiovascular prevention [25].

With the advent of noninvasive vascular imaging tools, our understanding of the mechanisms of accelerated atherosclerosis has further deepened. The availability of standardized ultrasound techniques for assessing flow-mediated dilation of the brachial artery, intimal-medial thickness (IMT) and atherosclerotic plaques in the common carotid artery holds particular promise for instrumental diagnostics of macrovascular pathology and prediction of vascular events across populations of healthy subjects and patients [26, 27]. Most notably, the largest ARIC (Atherosclerosis Risk in Communities) study involving 13,145 subjects proposed a new model for prediction of 10-year coronary heart disease risk, best assessed when carotid IMT and plaques added to the traditional cardiovascular risk factors model [28]. A recent meta-analysis, based on 22 retrospective cohort studies, proved the increase of carotid IMT in RA patients and affirmed the use of IMT for evaluation of cardiovascular burden in this population of patients [29]. Finally, the latest prospective cohort study with 64 RA patients, followed up for a mean of 3.6 years, revealed an association of traditional cardiovascular risk factors and low-dose corticosteroids, but not systemic inflammation with plaque formation [30]. These data coupled with a comparative study of IMT and atherosclerotic plaques in patients with SLE or familial Mediterranean fever [31], shed light on the interactions of cardiovascular and inflammation-mediated risk factors in the process of atherogenesis, and may suggest the use of noninvasive markers of carotid alterations for modelling cardiovascular risk across populations of healthy subjects and those with low- and high-grade inflammatory disorders.

Some other tools for cardiovascular risk prediction are now under evaluation. Of these, coronary artery calcium score assessed by multi-detector computed tomography seems particularly useful for primary cardiovascular predictive models and for stratifying patients in the emergency setting [32]. Another promising technique is intravascular ultrasound employed by invasive cardiologists for detecting vulnerable atherosclerotic plaques and guiding pharmacotherapy and invasive procedures in cardiovascular disease [33]. Though these techniques allow more precise evaluation of atherosclerotic burden, their wide-spread use for community-based cardiovascular prevention is limited owing to the narrow scope of implications, financial concerns, and invasive nature.

Overall, recent advances in understanding of sophisticated pathways of atherogenesis and the emergence of a multitude of laboratory and instrumental markers of atherosclerosis are seemingly shifting preventive and therapeutic strategies toward multi-dimentional and more personalized approaches. Better equipped and well supplied by old and new cardiovascular drugs communities as well as cardiological and general internal medicine units are now required to comprehensively evaluate cardiovascular risk and closely monitor efficiency of cardiovascular prevention. As a prime example, the efficiency of preventive use of an old drug, acetyl salicylic acid, is now known to be dependent on the physicians and patients' adherence to its administration as well as on the correction of low-grade inflammation and comorbid conditions which may attenuate the clinical implications of the therapy [34, 35]. In addition, the elucidation of a wide range of pleiotropic effects of statins and the strong evidence favoring their use for primary and secondary prevention, particularly in conditions associated with systemic inflammation (based on the data from the JUPITER trial), have reserved a place for this class of drugs next to acetyl salicylic acid, angiotensin-converting enzyme (ACE) inhibitors, angiotensin II receptor blockers, and beta-blockers in the schemes of combined therapies of cardiovascular disease. More recent studies, however, tapered some of the enthusiasm with the universal applicability of statins, owing to the lack of benefit and risk of adverse effects, such as liver and kidney dysfunction, myopathy, and cataract, particularly in high-risk groups of patients, such as those with heart failure and kidney disease [36, 37]. Finally, the rationale for a more differentiated approach to cardiovascular prevention by different drugs of the same class has recently been appreciated thanks to the evidence from the landmark HOPE (Heart Outcomes Prevention Evaluation) and ONTARGET (The Ongoing Telmisartan Alone and in Combination with Ramipril Global Endpoint Trial) trials suggesting that among numerous ACE inhibitors and angiotensin II receptor blockers only ramipril and telmisartan bring most benefits of cardiovascular protection in high-risk populations of patients [38].

Undoubtedly, knowledge of cardiovascular risk factors has greatly advanced over the past decades. Old dogmas over cholesterol as the only target of cardiovascular prevention have been replaced by theories supporting the diversity of atherosclerotic pathways and the need for combined and personalized interventions. The modern armamentarium of cardiovascular prevention is enriched with the abundance of efficacious nonpharmacological and pharmacological means. Many more are still subject of large-scale research studies, and initiatives are underway to bring more benefits and better care for the population-at-large.

Armen Yuri Gasparyan and
George D. Kitas

Department of Rheumatology, Clinical Research Unit,
Dudley Group NHS Foundation Trust
(A Teaching Trust of University of Birmingham),
Russell's Hall Hospital,
Dudley, West Midlands DY1 2HQ,
United Kingdom

References

[1] Kelishadi R. Inflammation-induced atherosclerosis as a target for prevention of cardiovascular diseases from early life. Open Cardiovasc Med J 2010;4:24-29.

[2] Borden WB, Davidson MH. Updating the assessment of cardiac risk: beyond Framingham. Rev Cardiovasc Med 2009;10(2):63-71.

[3] Hobbs FD, Jukema JW, Da Silva PM, McCormack T, Catapano AL. Barriers to cardiovascular disease risk scoring and primary prevention in Europe. QJM 2010;103(10):727-739.

[4] Berger JS, Jordan CO, Lloyd-Jones D, Blumenthal RS. Screening for cardiovascular risk in asymptomatic patients. J Am Coll Cardiol 2010;55(12):1169-1177.

[5] Toms TE, Panoulas VF, Douglas KM, Griffiths H, Sattar N, Smith JP, Symmons DP, Nightingale P, Metsios GS, Kitas GD. Statin use in rheumatoid arthritis in relation to actual cardiovascular risk: evidence for substantial undertreatment of lipid-associated cardiovascular risk? Ann Rheum Dis 2010;69(4):683-688.

[6] Peters MJ, Symmons DP, McCarey D, Dijkmans BA, Nicola P, Kvien TK, McInnes IB, Haentzschel H, Gonzalez-Gay MA, Provan S, Semb A, Sidiropoulos P, Kitas G, Smulders YM, Soubrier M, Szekanecz Z, Sattar N, Nurmohamed MT. EULAR evidence-based recommendations for cardiovascular risk management in patients with rheumatoid arthritis and other forms of inflammatory arthritis. Ann Rheum Dis 2010;69(2):325-331.

[7] Crowson CS, Gabriel SE. Towards improving cardiovascular risk management in patients with rheumatoid arthritis: the need for accurate risk assessment. Ann Rheum Dis 2011;70(5):719-721.

[8] Ridker PM, Cushman M, Stampfer MJ, Tracy RP, Hennekens CH. Inflammation, aspirin, and the risk of cardiovascular disease in apparently healthy men. N Engl J Med 1997;336(14):973-979.

[9] Ridker PM, MacFadyen J, Libby P, Glynn RJ. Relation of baseline high-sensitivity C-reactive protein level to cardiovascular outcomes with rosuvastatin in the Justification for Use of statins in Prevention: an Intervention Trial Evaluating Rosuvastatin (JUPITER). Am J Cardiol 2010;106(2):204-209.

[10] Lodi S, Evans SJ, Egger P, Carpenter J. Is there an anti-inflammatory effect of statins in rheumatoid arthritis? Analysis of a large routinely collected claims database. Br J Clin Pharmacol 2010;69(1):85-94.

[11] Semb AG, Holme I, Kvien TK, Pedersen TR. Intensive lipid lowering in patients with rheumatoid arthritis and previous myocardial infarction: an explorative analysis from the incremental decrease in endpoints through aggressive lipid lowering (IDEAL) trial. Rheumatology (Oxford) 2011;50(2):324-329.

[12] El-Barbary AM, Hussein MS, Rageh EM, Hamouda HE, Wagih AA, Ismail RG. Effect of atorvastatin on inflammation and modification of vascular risk factors in rheumatoid arthritis. J Rheumatol 2011;38(2):229-235.

[13] Pahor A, Hojs R, Gorenjak M, Rozman B. Accelerated atherosclerosis in pre-menopausal female patients with rheumatoid arthritis. Rheumatol Int 2006;27(2):119-123.

[14] Kitas GD, Gabriel SE. Cardiovascular disease in rheumatoid arthritis: state of the art and future perspectives. Ann Rheum Dis 2011;70(1):8-14.

[15] Miller AM, McInnes IB. Cytokines as therapeutic targets to reduce cardiovascular risk in chronic inflammation. Curr Pharm Des 2011;17(1):1-8.

[16] Gasparyan AY, Stavropoulos-Kalinoglou A, Mikhailidis DP, Toms TE, Douglas KM, Kitas GD. The rationale for comparative studies of accelerated atherosclerosis in rheumatic diseases. Curr Vasc Pharmacol 2010;8(4):437-449.

[17] Sandoo A, Veldhuijzen van Zanten JJ, Metsios GS, Carroll D, Kitas GD. Vascular function and morphology in rheumatoid arthritis: a systematic review. Rheumatology (Oxford) 2011;50(11):2125-2139.

[18] Cocco G, Gasparyan AY. Myocardial ischemia in Wegener's granulomatosis: coronary atherosclerosis versus vasculitis. Open Cardiovasc Med J 2010;4:57-62.

[19] Seyahi E, Ugurlu S, Cumali R, Balci H, Ozdemir O, Melikoglu M, Hatemi G, Fresko I, Hamuryudan V, Yurdakul S, Yazici H. Atherosclerosis in Behçet's Syndrome. Semin Arthritis Rheum 2008;38(1):1-12.

[20] La Regina M, Gasparyan AY, Orlandini F, Prisco D. Behçet's Disease as a Model of Venous Thrombosis. Open Cardiovasc Med J 2010;4:71-77.

[21] Gasparyan AY, Stavropoulos-Kalinoglou A, Mikhailidis DP, Douglas KM, Kitas GD. Platelet function in rheumatoid arthritis: arthritic and cardiovascular implications. Rheumatol Int. 2011;31(2):153-164.

[22] Sharma G, Berger JS. Platelet activity and cardiovascular risk in apparently healthy individuals: a review of the data. J Thromb Thrombolysis 2011;32(2):201-208.

[23] Sari I, Bozkaya G, Kirbiyik H, Alacacioglu A, Ates H, Sop G, Can G, Taylan A, Piskin O, Yildiz Y, Akkoc N. Evaluation of circulating endothelial and platelet microparticles in men with ankylosing spondylitis. J Rheumatol 2012;39(3):594-599.

[24] Gasparyan AY, Ayvazyan L, Mikhailidis DP, Kitas GD. Mean platelet volume: a link between thrombosis and inflammation? Curr Pharm Des 2011;17(1):47-58.

[25] Shanker J, Gasparyan AY, Kitas GD, Kakkar VV. Platelet function and antiplatelet therapy in cardiovascular disease: implications of genetic polymorphisms. Curr Vasc Pharmacol 2011;9(4):479-489.

[26] Gasparyan AY. The use of carotid artery ultrasonography in different clinical conditions. Open Cardiovasc Med J 2009;3:78-80.

[27] Sandoo A, van Zanten JJ, Metsios GS, Carroll D, Kitas GD. The endothelium and its role in regulating vascular tone. Open Cardiovasc Med J 2010;4:302-312.

[28] Nambi V, Chambless L, Folsom AR, He M, Hu Y, Mosley T, Volcik K, Boerwinkle E, Ballantyne CM. Carotid intima-media thickness and presence or absence of plaque improves prediction of coronary heart disease risk: the ARIC (Atherosclerosis Risk In Communities) study. J Am Coll Cardiol 2010;55(15):1600-1607.

[29] van Sijl AM, Peters MJ, Knol DK, de Vet HC, Gonzalez-Gay MA, Smulders YM, Dijkmans BA, Nurmohamed MT. Carotid intima media thickness in rheumatoid arthritis as compared to control subjects: a meta-analysis. Semin Arthritis Rheum 2011;40(5):389-397.

[30] Zampeli E, Protogerou A, Stamatelopoulos K, Fragiadaki K, Katsiari CG, Kyrkou K, Papamichael CM, Mavrikakis M, Nightingale P, Kitas GD, Sfikakis PP. Predictors of new atherosclerotic carotid plaque development in patients with rheumatoid arthritis: a longitudinal study. Arthritis Res Ther 2012;14(2):R44.

[31] Ugurlu S, Seyahi E, Cetinkaya F, Ozbakir F, Balci H, Ozdogan H. Intima-media thickening in patients with familial Mediterranean fever. Rheumatology (Oxford) 2009;48(8):911-915.
[32] Sharma RK, Sharma RK, Voelker DJ, Singh VN, Pahuja D, Nash T, Reddy HK. Cardiac risk stratification: role of the coronary calcium score. Vasc Health Risk Manag 2010;6:603-611.
[33] Garcia-Garcia HM, Costa MA, Serruys PW. Imaging of coronary atherosclerosis: intravascular ultrasound. Eur Heart J 2010;31(20):2456-2469.
[34] Gasparyan AY, Watson T, Lip GY. The role of aspirin in cardiovascular prevention: implications of aspirin resistance. J Am Coll Cardiol 2008;51(19):1829-1843.
[35] Gasparyan AY. Aspirin and clopidogrel resistance: methodological challenges and opportunities. Vasc Health Risk Manag 2010;6:109-112.
[36] Hippisley-Cox J, Coupland C. Unintended effects of statins in men and women in England and Wales: population based cohort study using the QResearch database. BMJ 2010;340:c2197.
[37] Antonopoulos AS, Margaritis M, Lee R, Channon K, Antoniades C. Statins as Anti-Inflammatory Agents in Atherogenesis: Molecular Mechanisms and Lessons from the Recent Clinical Trials. Curr Pharm Des 2012;18(11):1519-1530.
[38] Volpe M. Should all patients at high cardiovascular risk receive renin-angiotensin system blockers? QJM 2012;105(1):11-27.

1

Cardiovascular Risk Investigation: When Should It Start?

Anabel Nunes Rodrigues[1],
Gláucia Rodrigues de Abreu[2] and Sônia Alves Gouvêa[2]
[1]*School of Medicine, University Center of Espírito Santo, Colatina,*
[2]*Postgraduate Program in Physiological Sciences,*
Federal University of Espírito Santo, Vitória,
Brazil

1. Introduction

Childhood can be considered the period of structuring of life, where patterns such as diet and lifestyle are built. Although atherosclerotic disease (AD) becomes symptomatic at a later period of life, early identification and modification of risk factors may further reduce their incidence (Kelishadi et al., 2002). Thus, several studies demonstrate the importance of investigating the presence of risk factors for atherosclerotic disease at this stage as it may result from profound implications for the risk of developing diseases in adulthood (Lenfant & Savage, 1995; Purath et al., 1995; Gerber & Zielinsky, 1997; Akerblom et al., 1999).

This chapter presents the main studies that describe the importance of investigating the childhood risk factors for diseases cardiovascular that may emerge in adult life. Thus, the studies involving analysis of cardiovascular risk factors should always register the prevalence and their correlations in childhood, as an essential to identify a population at risk. Thus, beyond the direct benefits on children evaluated such studies could point out other family members carrying from such risks.

Therefore the detection of the risk factors in asymptomatic children can contribute to a decrease in cardiovascular disease, preventing those diseases such as hypertension, obesity and dyslipidemia becomes the epidemic of this new century.

2. Cardiovascular risk factors

Atherosclerosis begins early in life. Thus, it is critical to detect cardiovascular disease risk factors during childhood and adolescence in order to prevent future complications. Monitoring these factors helps to identify previous signs that, once modified, can either decrease or even reverse the progression of the dysfunction. Figure 1 shows that a range of risk factors, such as genetic factors, hypertension, dyslipidemia, obesity, metabolic syndrome, atherogenic diet and physical inactivity, are associated with cardiovascular disease. The same figure shows an increase in the prevalence of cardiovascular disease among children and adolescents (Hedley et al., 2004; Eckel et al., 2005; Rodrigues et al., 2006a; Rodrigues et al., 2009).

Lifestyle and eating habits are risk factors considered to be critical for protection from, the appearance of and the progression of atherosclerotic disease (AD), which is considered the main factor in the genesis of cardiovascular disease (Berlin, 1996, Esrey et al., 1996). For these reasons, a healthy lifestyle and eating habits should be part of heart disease prevention programs (Guedes & Guedes, 2001). Hypercholesterolemia, hypertriglyceridemia, being overweight, hyperglycemia, hypertension and physical inactivity stand out among these factors (Austin, 1999). Correlation with plasma cholesterol levels and both reductions and delay in the progression of AD through diet and lifestyle changes have been documented (Coelho et al., 1999). Some studies have also suggested that the degree of atherosclerosis in childhood and young adulthood might be correlated with the same risk factors identified in adults. Therefore, an increase in the incidence of cardiovascular disease is likely to occur when today's adolescents enter adulthood. Thus, it is important to either eliminate or reduce risk factors in young people and other age groups (Williams et al., 2002)

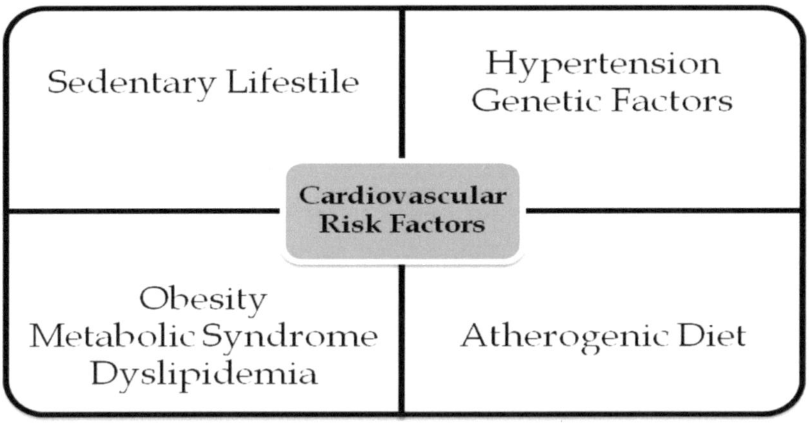

Fig. 1. Factors associated with cardiovascular risk in children and adolescents.

2.1 Atherosclerosis

Although AD becomes symptomatic at a later period of life, identifying risk factors early and changing them as soon as possible may further reduce the incidence of AD (Kelishadi et al., 2002). Such diseases currently stand out as the most frequent causes of death. Coronary atherosclerosis is the most evident pathology, and it can affect even young people (Puska, 1986). Studies have suggested that the atherosclerotic process, a disease as old as the human species (Lotufo 1999), begins in childhood. Therefore, its prevention should begin early in life because at this stage, the disease is considered reversible. High levels of lipoproteins present in the blood are critical for the generation of atherosclerosis (Massin et al., 2002). Michaelsen et al. (2002) revealed that children usually do not develop atherosclerosis; however, they develop fatty streaks in the aorta that are reversible. These researchers focused on the fact that a high-fat diet influences blood lipid levels from the first years of life, as do other traditional vascular risk factors.

The variety of criteria for defining optimal lipid levels in adolescence makes it difficult to compare the results in the global literature. However, studies have shown, for example, the presence of atheromatosis in the aortic intima of patients with cholesterol levels between 140 to 170 mg%. Therefore, the epidemiological goal for children should be, on average, 150 mg% for plasma cholesterol (Srinivasan, 1991). In a review of studies conducted in 26 countries (1975 to 1996) involving 60,494 children and adolescents aged 2 to 19 years, Brotons (1998) reported an average of 165 mg / dL for cholesterol, 60 mg / dL for HDL-cholesterol and 67 mg / dL for triglycerides.

Studies conducted in Brazil have shown higher levels of cholesterol in adolescents from private schools than in adolescents from public schools (Gerber, 1997; Giuliano, 2005). This trend was corroborated by other studies (Guimarães, 1998 e 2005; Rodrigues et al., 2006a) wherein individuals with lower family income and adolescents from public schools presented lower cholesterol levels than those from higher income families and private schools. These data lead us to agree with the suggestions made by Guimarães (2005) that families with higher socioeconomic status do not necessarily have a better diet or lifestyle. Therefore, children from the lowest income families in developing countries may have less access to the high calories that come from large amounts of saturated fatty acids and a diet with high cholesterol. In addition, students from public schools tend to expend more energy daily because they have to walk to school or walk to get to public transportation.

Regardless of the methodological limitations to calculating LDLc as part of the lipid profile, its determination is widely considered to be the "gold standard" for both risk assessment and for intervention programs for cardiovascular disease (Srinivasan, 2002b). Previous studies by Schrott et al. (1982) and Moll et al. (1983) showed that children and adolescents with elevated LDL-cholesterol often come from families with a high incidence of coronary heart disease. This fact reinforces the importance of LDL-cholesterol determination in adolescence and of autopsy studies performed in children and young people (Newman, 1986), which have indicated that the fatty streaks in the aorta are also directly related to this part of the lipid profile. Thus, by determining the levels of LDLc, it is possible to detect family risks early, and interventions can be implemented before the occurrence of coronary events. It is known that total cholesterol and LDLc can penetrate, produce endothelial injury and stimulate the proliferation of smooth muscle cells, whereas HDL-C is involved in the removal of cholesterol (Reed, 1989). High-density lipoprotein (HDL-cholesterol) carries approximately a quarter of serum cholesterol. Some studies have shown that high levels of HDL-cholesterol are correlated with a lower risk of developing atherosclerosis (Salomen, 1991; Gordon, 1986).

Triglycerides are strongly associated with the risk of developing atherosclerotic disease because they can deposit on the vessel wall and then start the process of low-density lipoprotein accumulation. High levels of triglycerides are a key component of so-called metabolic syndrome (MS). (Johnson, et al. 1999; Santos et al. 2008; Cobayashi et al. 2010).

It is important to emphasize that when dyslipidemia begins in childhood, it tends to remain during growth, and that studies describe a direct relationship between total cholesterol levels in children and cardiovascular disease in adults (Forti, 1996). Studies conducted in Brazil (Rodrigues, 2006; Giuliano & Caramelli, 2005) have shown that cholesterol levels in childhood may explain 87% of deaths from cardiovascular disease in adulthood in this country.

The association of inflammatory processes with the development of atherosclerosis provides important links between underlying mechanisms of atherogenesis and risk factors. Several studies have examined different circulating markers of inflammations, such as cytokines and adhesion molecules, as potential predictors of the present and the future risk of cardiovascular diseases. Moreover,functional and structural changes are documented in arteries of children with a familial predisposition to atherosclerotic diseases; these changes are associated with clusters of inflammatory factors and markers of oxidation. In addition to the development of atheromatous plaques, inflammation also plays an essential role in the destabilization of artery plaques, and in turn in the occurrence of acute thrombo-embolic disorders . As lifestyle modification trials have been successful in decreasing endothelial dysfunction and the level of markers of inflammation among children and adolescents it is suggested that in addition to expanding pharmacological therapies considered for secondary prevention of atherosclerotic diseases aiming to control the inflammatory process and prevention of atherosclerosis (Kelishadi, 2010).

2.2 Obesity

Obesity, which is defined as excessive body fat accumulation, is a heterogeneous disorder with a final common pathway in which energy intake chronically exceeds energy expenditure, and genetic and environmental factors overlap in this disorder (Sorensen, 1995). The energy imbalance frequently begins in childhood, and if it occurs in children that are in the higher percentiles for body fat, it may increase their probability of obesity in adult life. Obesity among youth has increased in recent years (Kelishadi, 2007).

Obesity represents the most common chronic disorder, and it has especially increased prevalence among poor children and minorities (Troiano & Flegal, 1998). Excessive adiposity in childhood represents a greater risk to the health of an adult than adulthood obesity. The risk of disease in adulthood is greater for overweight children and adolescents than those of normal weight (Gunnell et al., 1998; VanHorn & Greenland, 1997). Obesity results from a complex interaction of metabolic, physiological, environmental, genetic, social and behavioral factors. The Bogalusa Heart Study, conducted in children and adolescents in Louisiana (USA), showed that obesity, lipoprotein levels (especially LDL) and insulinemia are all significantly correlated with the risk of cardiovascular disease (Srinivasan et al., 1976, Newman et al., 1983, Kikuchi et al., 1992).

Although studies have shown a clear association between severe obesity and increased mortality, there is controversy about the actual damages caused by being overweight. However, its importance as a risk factor for cardiovascular disease is becoming more evident every day (Zanella, 1999). Obesity has received special attention together with two other well-known risk factors: diabetes and hypertension. Therefore, it is important to control obesity during childhood, because obesity acquired in this period of life tends to persist into adulthood (Gerber & Zielinsky, 1997). Studies have reported a significant increase of overweight children and adolescents in the last decades, which has been associated with an increased risk of hypertension, lipid disorders, type II diabetes, early atherosclerotic lesions and risk of adult obesity and mortality in young adults (Williams et al., 2002; Coronelli & Moura, 2003, Daniels et al., 2005). Preventing childhood obesity is the best opportunity to make changes in lifestyle and to reduce cardiovascular morbidity and mortality (Buiten & Metzger, 2000). Diagnosing someone as overweight or obese is difficult because there are questions that remain about the best criteria to be used in order to determine these conditions in this age group. One of the areas of disagreement refers to the cutoff for identifying overweight and obese individuals. However, the body mass index (BMI), which is based on international standards, has been useful, inexpensive and reproducible (Giugliano, 2004). Recently, the term obesity has been defined as body mass index ≥ 95th percentile in children and adolescents (Daniels, 2005), as shown Table 1.

Statistics on childhood and adolescent obesity worldwide are still limited. A lack of consistency in definitions and age groups studied complicates comparing between prevalences. It is well established that obesity in children and adolescents has increased significantly, including in developing countries (Mello, 2004). Whereas in the United States, obesity affects mainly the social classes with lower purchasing power (Dietz, 1986), in Brazil (for example), the most affected children belong to the wealthiest social classes. Data estimate that childhood obesity affects 16% of children in Brazil (Giugliano, 2004), and that the prevalence of overweight and obesity is higher in families with higher incomes, (Abrantes, 2002; Moura, 2004). The National Health and Nutrition Examination Survey estimated a prevalence of 30% for overweight and/or obesity (≥ 85th percentile) and 15% for obesity (≥ 95th percentile) between the ages of 6 and 19 years (O'Brien, 2004).

2.3 Metabolic syndrome

Metabolic syndrome (MS) is currently characterized by the combination of a number of risk factors for cardiovascular diseases, including dyslipidemia (hypertriglyceridemia, low HDLc and increased LDLc), high blood pressure, disorders of carbohydrate metabolism and obesity (Reaven, 1988, (Kelishadi, 2007). It has also been demonstrated in children that a direct association between obesity and insulin resistance syndrome is a major precursor of atherosclerotic cardiovascular disease and type II diabetes (Williams et al., 2002).

Although a worldwide consensus on the definition and diagnosis of MS in adults and children does not exist, it is known that MS is associated with a 1.5-fold increase in general mortality and a 2.5-fold increase in cardiovascular mortality (Lakka et al., 2002). Given its importance, many organizations have proposed criteria for the definition and treatment of MS; among them are the World Health Organization (WHO) (Alberti et al., 1998), the National Cholesterol Education Programme Adult Treatment Panel III - NCEP ATP III (NCEP, 2001), European Group for the Study of Insulin Resistance-EGIR (Balkau et al., 1999) and the International Diabetes Federation.

To determine the prevalence of MS in children and adolescents, criteria applied to adults have been modified and used either as pediatric reference values (Cook et al., 2003) or as specific cutoff points (Csabi et al., 2000, Srinivasan et al., 2002). Some studies have suggested that the cutoff points corresponding to the 95th percentile of each variable by gender and age be combined with the height percentile when dealing with blood pressure (NHBPEP, 2004; CDCDM, 1999). However, the lack of consensus results in a markedly different prevalence of this syndrome as reported in many studies (Isomaa et al., 2001, Kelishadi, 2007). Table 1 shows values for lipids, blood pressure and body mass index that characterize children and adolescents that are not considered cardiovascular risk factors.

Prospective studies have shown that obesity appears many years before the onset of insulin resistance (Taskinen, 2003), and insulin resistance is mainly responsible for the hemodynamic and metabolic disturbances of this syndrome (Morton et al., 2001). It is believed that MS is due to a combination of genetic and environmental factors wherein obesity plays a primary role, leading to excessive insulin production, which is associated with increased blood pressure and dyslipidemia (Daniels et al, 2005). It is estimated that one million North American adolescents already meet the criteria for MS (Daniels et al., 2005), with a prevalence of 4% between 12 and 19 years. In addition, MS is present in 30 to 50% of overweight children (Cook et al., 2003 and Weiss et al., 2004).

	Acceptable
Lipids (mg/dL)	
Total Cholesterol	<150
LDL-c	<100
HDL-c	≥45
Triglycerides	<100
Systolic blood pressure (mmHg)	<90th Percentile ≤130
Fasting glucose (mg/dL)	≤100
Waist circumference or Body mass index (Kg/m^{2})	<90th percentile <95th percentile

Table 1. Reference values proposed for children and adolescents.

2.4 Hypertension

Arterial hypertension (AH) has been identified as one of the most potent antecedents of coronary heart disease. It is usually asymptomatic. Prevention is the most efficient way to combat HA, thus avoiding the high social cost of its treatment and complications. Therefore, it is necessary to identify individuals with high blood pressure and control it. The worldwide prevalence of AH is extremely variable (2-13%), and it is dependent on the methodology employed. In Brazil, for example, it is estimated that the prevalence of hypertension in children and adolescents is 4% (Ministry of Health, 2006), and it is considered imperative to measure blood pressure starting at age 3. It is known that blood pressure (BP) usually increases with age, and that elevated values in young people are a predictor of AH in adulthood (Williams et al., 2002; Falkner et al., 2008). It is worth noting that increasing BP with age is not normal physiological behavior.

BP should be understood as a result of environmental influences on the expression of several genes that, in turn, also have their own regulatory genes (Bartosh & Aronson, 1999; Berenson et al., 1998). Several factors known to be related to BP in adults are also associated with the behavior of BP in children and adolescents, with an emphasis on sex, age, family history of AH and the presence of either excess weight or obesity. Although AH contributes to the development of cardiovascular complications per se, its association with multiple risk factors increases the risk of major cardiovascular events even more (Kavey et al., 2003, Chobanian et al., 2003; Lieberman, 2002).

It has been accepted that a diagnosis of AH is confirmed when the values of systolic blood pressure (SBP) and/or diastolic blood pressure (DBP) are greater or equal to the 95th percentile for sex, age and height percentile plus 5 mmHg on three separate occasions. A range called pre-hypertension should be identified and assessed for the purpose of adopting strict preventive measures. BP values ≥ 90th percentile and <95th percentile characterize pre-hypertension. According to a recommendation proposed by the JNC 7, values that are included in this range and exceeding the limits of 120/80 mmHg should also be considered pre-hypertension for adults (Chobanian et al., 2003).

It is estimated that 30% of overweight/obese children and adolescents have AH (Sorof & Daniels 2002). Thus, the presence of overweight/obesity appears to be one of the most important factors related to AH in children and adolescents worldwide (Chobanian et al., 2003, Campana et al., 2009; European Society of Hypertension 2003). Several studies have shown that the presence of overweight/obesity is associated positively with the occurrence of pre-hypertension in children and adolescents, and when combined they increase the risk of developing AH in adulthood (JAMA, 1992, Monteiro et al., 2003, Rosa et al., 2006, Srinivasan et al., 2006). There are also factors associated predominantly with arterial hypertension in adolescence such as smoking, contraception and drugs: cocaine, amphetamines, alcohol, anabolic steroids, phenylpropanolamine and pseudoephedrine (nasal decongestants).

Thus, changes in lifestyle such as weight control, reducing sodium intake and physical exercise are crucial to preventing hypertension. Although the threshold for blood pressure is not yet well defined, its effects on target organs probably occur in children as well as in adults. Dietary intervention, weight monitoring and regular physical activity should be encouraged at this stage as a primary prevention method (Massin et al., 2002). Studying the stiffness of large arteries, a condition attributed to the aging of blood vessels, Rodrigues et al. (2011) demonstrated that chronic hypotension is the only factor studied able to explain why blood vessel aging did not occur in the study group. In addition to the disturbing reality of the existence of old risk factors in a young population, the presence of these factors not only in isolation, but also in association, has been acknowledged.

2.5 Sedentary lifestyle

It has been shown that the mortality rate for cardiovascular disease is lower in individuals who exercise regularly and that the quality of life achieved through a physical fitness program is unquestionably superior. However, this improvement in quality of life depends on a proper exercise prescription wherein the intensity, duration and modality are key elements in achieving a satisfactory outcome. Prescribing physical activities that are performed between the ventilatory threshold and the respiratory compensation point for adults is recommended to obtain beneficial effects on cardiopulmonary capacity (Rondon et al., 1998).

In children, the beneficial effects associated with physical activity include weight control; reductions in cholesterol, insulin resistance and low blood pressure; psychological well-being; and an increased predisposition to perform physical activities as a young adult (Williams, et al., 2002).

A major challenge for public health authorities has been to increase the cardiorespiratory capacity of the population. Therefore, childhood and adolescence seem to be the optimal periods for promoting good exercise habits and preventing sedentary behavior in adulthood, which turns preventing cardiovascular disease into a pediatric challenge (Massin et al., 2002). In recent decades, children have become less physically active, with a decrease of 600 kcal/day of energy expenditure when compared to children 50 years ago (Boreham & Riddoch, 2001). Physical inactivity is recognized as an important determinant of chronic diseases, and an increase in its prevalence during childhood has been reported (Twisk, 2001).

Alerts have been issued about the need for physical education programs in schools and for community recreation centers. However, few empirical studies have been conducted to assess the impacts of such facilities and programs on the levels of physical activity and inactivity in adolescents (Gordon-Larsen et al., 2000).

Freedman et al. (1997) report that a sedentary lifestyle is a growing problem; there is a tendency among adolescents to be less engaged in physical activities offered by schools and other vigorous activities, and they spend more time watching television. These behavioral changes may impact future health problems. On the other hand, better physical fitness has been related to a lower risk of cardiovascular compromise in children and adolescents (Al-Hazaa, 2002) and lower levels of blood pressure in both boys and girls (Fraser et al., 1983, Hofman et al., 1987, Gutin et al., 1990, Hansen et al., 1989, Shears et al., 1986)

It is known that identifying maximal oxygen uptake values (VO2max) supports studies performed attempting to correlate physical aptitude with cardiovascular risk. It is also important to note that VO_{2max} is used to guide exercise prescription and to analyze the effects of training programs (Obert et al., 2003, Armstrong et al., 1994). The aerobic capacity measured by VO_{2max} depends on cardiovascular, respiratory and hematological components and on oxidative mechanisms of muscles during physical activity. It is measured by cardiopulmonary exercise testing, which allows the functions of the cardiovascular and respiratory systems (for instance, gas exchange) to be evaluated simultaneously, (Armstrong et al., 1994). Gas exchange measurements are important to help reveal mechanisms that restrict exercise, because physical activity requires an integrated cardiopulmonary response to compensate for the increase in the metabolic needs of muscle. The fact that cardiorespiratory capacity has been determined by different methods (directly versus indirectly) may explain the variable predictive power of this important physiological variable, and it may also explain the fact that several studies have found that cardiorespiratory capacity is not an independent predictor of blood lipids in children (Tolfrey, 1999).

Adolescence is a period of transition to adulthood in which there are many structural, hormonal, physiological and biochemical changes. Many of these changes interfere with maximum oxygen consumption (Tourinho Filho et al., 1998). Thus, it is necessary to establish VO_{2max} values for each age group. The international literature presents reference values for healthy children and adolescents (Armstrong et al., 1994, Turley et al., 1997; Stanganelli et al., 1991; Rodrigues et al., 2006b).

Described as a behavior, physical activity includes any type of muscle activity in which there is a significant increase in energy expenditure. Physical aptitude is described as a quality, and it usually refers to the ability to perform physical work. It is considered to be an adaptive state and it is (to some extent) genetically determined (Thomas, 2003). It has been suggested that physical aptitude testing should be performed instead of physical activity due to its greater objectivity and reduced possibility of errors. Furthermore, aerobic fitness has been shown to correlate better with cardiovascular disease, which is not true for physical activity. Thus, efforts should be intensified to identify the starting point for daily physical activity to elevate the physical aptitude of young people (Bouchard, 1992; McMurray, 1998; Thomas, 2003). However, the assessment of this variable is not yet a global reality, and empirical evaluations have been performed. The use of cardiopulmonary exercise testing enables cardiorespiratory and metabolic capacity to be precisely determined by direct measurement of maximum oxygen consumption (VO_{2max}), which is the most important physiological measure for the definition of aerobic capacity. It also accurately determines physical aptitude level and thus the correct exercise intensity such that a fitness program will only have healthy consequences (Rondon et al., 1998; Rodrigues, 2006).

3. Conclusion

Although the manifestations of coronary heart disease occur in adulthood, detecting risk factors during childhood/adolescence is crucial for establishing a prognosis and preventing target organ damage in adults. Thus, initiating disease detection and prevention at this stage of life and introducing changes in lifestyle can reduce the incidence and severity of cardiovascular diseases.

Risk factors are more meaningful when they are integrated. Hence, studies of cardiovascular risk factors in a region, city or country should always report their prevalence and correlations in childhood as a fundamental step toward identifying the population at risk.

The facts reported here highlight a serious public health problem that must be addressed. There is an urgent need to discuss health promotion issues and the prevention of future diseases that result from the risk factors mentioned herein.

Finally, this chapter demonstrates that risk factors for coronary heart disease begin in childhood, and therefore prevention should start early in life. This increases the need for pediatric care in this age group in order to make early diagnoses and offer preventive advice. Dyslipidemia, for example, is the most well known risk factor, and it can be altered by a moderate restriction of fat without compromising the growth or development of children older than 2. Thus, in the future, a major decrease in cardiovascular diseases could be obtained by assessing asymptomatic children and adolescents.

Thus, social awareness is necessary at all levels, as are studies with planned actions and programs for the control of dyslipidemia, obesity, arterial hypertension and physical inactivity in this age group in order to prevent these risk factors from becoming the epidemic of this new century.

4. Acknowledgment

This study was supported by a grant from CEPEG-UNESC-ES.

5. References

Abrantes, M.M., Lamounier, J.A. & Colosimo, E.A. (2002). Prevalência de sobrepeso e obesidade em crianças e adolescentes das regiões Sudeste e Nordeste. *Journal of Pediatrics*, Vol.78, No.4, pp. 335-340.

Al-Hazaa, H.M. (2002). Physical activity, fitness and fatness among Saudi children and adolescents: implications for cardiovascular health. *Saudi Medical Journal*, Vol.23, pp. 144-150.

Alberti, K.G. & Zimmet, P.Z. (1998). Definition, diagnosis and classification of diabetes mellitus and its complications: Part 1. Diagnosis and classification of diabetes mellitus provisional report of a WHO consultation. *Diabetic Medicine*, Vol.15, pp. 539-553.

Akerblom, H.K., Viikari, J., Raitakari, O.T. & Uhari, M. (1999). Cardiovascular risk in Young Finns Study: general outline and recent developments. *Annals of Medicine*, Vol.31, pp. 45-54.

Armstrong, N. & Welsman, J.R. (1994). Assessment and interpretation of aerobic fitness in children and adolescents. *Exercise and Sport Sciences Reviews*, Vol.22, pp. 435-476.

Austin, M.A. (1999). Epidemiology of hypertriglyceridemia and cardiovascular disease. *American Journal of Cardiology* , Vol.83, No.9, pp. 13-16.

Balkau, B. & Charles, M.A. (1999). Comment on the provisional report from the WHO consultation. European Group for the Study of Insulin Resistence (EGIR). *Diabetic Medicine*, Vol.16, pp. 442-443.

Bartosh, S.M. & Aronson, A.J. (1999). Childhood hypertension: an update on etiology, diagnosis and treatment. *Pediatric Clinics of North America*, Vol.46, pp.235-252.

Berenson, G.S., Srinivisan S.R., Bao, W., Newman III, W.P., Tracy, R.E. & Wattigney, W.A. for the Bogalusa Heart Study (1998). Association between multiple cardiovascular risk factors and atherosclerosis in children and young adults. *The New England Journal of Medicine*, Vol.338, pp. 1650-1656.

Berlin, J.A. & Colditz, G.A. (1996). A meta-analysis of physical in the prevention of coronary heart disease. *American Journal of Epidemiology*, Vol.132, pp. 612-628.

Boreham, C. & Riddoch C. (2001). The physical activity, fitness and health of children. *Journal of Sports Sciences* , Vol.19, No.12, pp. 915-929.

Bouchard, C., Dionne, F.T., Simoneau, J.A. & Boulay, M.R. (1992). Genetics of aerobic and anaerobic performances. *Exercise and Sport Sciences Reviews*, Vol.20, pp. 27-58.

Brotons, C., Ribera, A., Perich, R.M., Abrodos, D., Magana, P., Pablo, S., Terradas, D., Fernadez, F. & Permanyer, G. (1998). Worldwide distribution of blood lipidis and lipoproteins in childhood and adolescence: a review study. *Atherosclerosis*, Vol.139, pp. 1-9.

Buiten, C. & Metzger, B. (2000). Childhood besity and risk of cardiovascular disease: a review of the science. *Pediatric Nursing*, Vol.26, No.1, pp. 13-18.

Campana, E.M.G., Brandão, A.A., Magalhães, M.E.C., Freitas, E.V., Pozzan, R. & Brandão, A.P. (2009). Pré-hipertensão em crianças e adolescentes. *Revista Brasileira de Hipertensão*, Vol.16, No.2, pp. 92-102.

Chobanian, A.V., Bakris, G.L., Black, H.R., Cushman, W.C., Green, L.A., Izzo, J.L.Jr., Jones, D.W., Materson, B.J., Oparil, S., Wright, J.T.Jr. & Roccella, E.J. (2003). The Seventh Report of the Joint National Committee on Prevention, Detection, Evaluation, and Treatment of High Blood Pressure. *The seventh report of the Joint National Committee (JNC 7 Report) JAMA*, Vol.289, No.19, pp. 2560-2572.

Cobayashi, F., Oliveira, F.L.C., Escrivão, M.A.M.S., Silveira, D. & Taddei, J.A.A.C. (2010). Obesity and Cardiovascular Risk Factors in Adolescents Attending Public Schools. *Arquivos Brasileiros de Cardiologia*, Vol.95, No.2, pp. 200-206.

Coelho, O.R., Ueti, O.M. & Almeida, A. (1999). Lípides como Fator de Risco. In: Mion Jr. D, Nobre F, (Eds). *Risco Cardiovascular Global.* São Paulo: Lemos Editorial, p.45-64.

Cook, S., Weitzman, M., Auinger, P., Nguyen, M. & Dietz, W.H. (2003). Prevalence of a metabolic syndrome phenotype in adolescents: findings from the third National Health and Nutrition Examination Survey, 1988-1994. *Archives of Pediatrics & Adolescent Medicine,* Vol.157, No.8, pp. 821-827.

Coronelli, C.L.S. & Moura, E.C. (2003). Hipercolesterolemia em escolares e seus fatores de risco. *Saúde Pública,* Vol.37, No.1, pp. 24-31.

Csabi, G., Torok, K., Jeges S. & Molnar, D. (2000). Presence of metabolic cardiovascular syndrome in obese children. *European Journal of Pediatrics,* Vol.159, pp. 91-94.

Daniels, S.R., Arnett, D.K., Eckel, R.H., Gidding, S.S., Hayman, L.L., Kumanyika, S., Robinson, T.N., Scott, B.J., St Jeor, S. & Williams, C.L. (2005). Overweight in children and adolescents: pathophysiology, consequences, prevention, and treatment. *Circulation,* Vol.111, No.15, pp. 1999-2012.

Dietz, W.H. (1986). Prevention of childhood obesity. *Pediatric Clinics of North,* Vol.33, pp. 823-833.

Eckel, R.H., Daniels, S.R., Jacobs, A.K. & Robertson, R.M. (2005). America's children: a critical time for prevention. *Circulation,* Vol.111, pp.1866–1868.

Esrey, K.L., Joseph, L. & Grover, S.A. (1996). Relationship between dietary intake and coronary heart disease mortality: lipid research clinics prevalence follow-up study. *Journal of Clinical Epidemiology,* Vol.49, pp. 211-216.

European Society of Hypertension. 2003 European Society of Hypertension–European Society of Cardiology guidelines for the management of arterial hypertension. *Journal of Hypertension,* Vol.21, pp. 1011-1053.

Executive summary of the third report of the National Cholesterol Education Program (NCEP) expert panel on detection, evaluation, and treatment of high blood cholesterol in adults (adult treatment panel III) (2001). *JAMA,* Vol.285, pp. 2486-2497.

Falkner, B., Gidding, S.S., Portman, R. & Rosner, B. (2008). Blood pressure variability and classification of prehypertension and hypertension in adolescence. *Pediatrics, Vol.*122, No.2, pp. 238-242.

Forti, N., Diogo Giannini, S., Diament, J., Issa, J., Fukushima, J., Dal Bó, C. & Pereira Barretto A.C. (1996). Fatores de risco para aterosclerose em filhos de pacientes com doença coronariana precoce. *Arquivos Brasileiros de Cardiologia,* Vol.66, No.3, pp. 119-123.

Fraser, G.E, Phillips, R.L. & Harris, R. (1983). Physical fitness and blood pressure in school children. *Circulation,* Vol.67, No.2, pp. 405-412.

Freedman, D.S., Srinivasan, S.R., Valdez, R.A., Williamson, D.F. & Berenson, G.S. (1997). Secular increases in relative weight and adiposity among children over two decades: The Bogalusa Heart Study. *Pediatrics,* Vol.99, pp. 420-426.

Gerber, Z.R.S. & Zielinsky, P. (1997). Fatores de Risco de Aterosclerose na infância. Um Estudo Epidemiológico. *Arquivos Brasileiros de Cardiologia,* Vol.69, No.4, pp. 231-236.

Giugliano, R. & Melo, A.L.P. (2004). Diagnóstico de sobrepeso e obesidade em escolares: utilização do índice de massa corporal segundo padrão internacional. *Journal of Pediatrics,* Vol.80, No.2, pp. 129-134.

Giuliano, I.C.B. & Caramelli, B. (2005). Dislipidemias em Crianças e Adolescentes. *Revista da Sociedade de Cardiologia do Estado de São Paulo,* Vol.6, pp. 535-543.

Giuliano, I.C.B., Coutinho, M.S.S.A., Freitas, S.F.T., Pires, M.M.S., Zunino, J.N. & Ribeiro, R.Q.C. (2005). Lípides sérico em crianças e adolescentes de Florianópolis, SC - Estudo Floripa Saudável 2040. *Arquivos Brasileiros de Cardiologia*, Vol.85, No.2, pp. 85-91.

Gordon, D.J., Knoke, J., Probstfield, J.L., Superko, R. & Tyroler, H.A. (1986). High-density lipoprotein cholesterol and coronary heart disease in hypercholesterolemic men: the Lipid Research Clinics Coronary Primary Prevention Trial. *Circulation*, Vol.74, No.6, pp. 1217-1225.

Gordon-Larsen P., McMurray, R.G. & Popkin, B.M. (2000). Determinants of Adolescent Physical Activity and Inactivity Patterns. *Pediatrics,* Vol.105, No.6, pp. 1-8.

Guedes, D.P. & Guedes, J.E.R.P. (2001). Atividade física, aptidão cardiorrespiratória, composição da dieta e fatores de risco predisponentes às doenças cardiovasculares. *Arquivos Brasileiros de Cardiologia,* Vol.77, No.3, pp. 243-250.

Guimarães, A.C., Lima, A., Mota, E., Lima, J.C., Martinez, T. & Conti, A.F. (1998).The cholesterol level of a selected brazilian salaried population: biological and socioeconomic influences. *CVD Prevention,* Vol.1, pp. 306-317.

Guimarães, I.C.B. & Guimarães, A.C. (2005). Prevalence of cardiovascular risk factors in selected samples of schoolchildren - socioeconomic influence. *Preventive Cardiology,* Vol.8, pp. 23-28.

Gunnell, D.J., Frankel, S.J., Nanchahal, K., Peters, T.J. & Davey Smith, G. (1998). Childhood obesity and adult cardiovascular mortality: a 57-y follow- up study based on the boyd orr cohort. *American Journal of Clinical Nutrition*, Vol.67, No.6, pp. 1111-1118.

Gutin, B., Basch, C., Shea, S., Contento, I., DeLozier, M., Rips, J., Irigoyen, M. & Zybert, P. (1990). Blood pressure, fitness and fatness in 5- and 6- year-old children. *JAMA,* Vol.264, No.9, pp. 1123-1127.

Hansen, H.S., Hyldebrandt, N., Froberg, K. & Nielsen, J.R. (1989). Blood pressure and physical fitness in school children. The Odense School Children Study. *Scandinavian Journal of Clinical & Laboratory Investigation Supplement*, Vol.192, pp. 42-46.

Hedley, A.A., Ogden, C.L., Johnson, C.L., Carroll, M.D., Curtin, L.R. & Flegal, K.M. (2004). Prevalence of overweight and obesity among US children, adolescents, and adults, 1999–2002. *JAMA,*Vol.291, pp. 2847–2850.

Hofman, A., Walter, H.J., Connelly, P.A. & Vaughan, R.D. (1987). Blood pressure and physical fitness in children. *Hypertension,* Vol.9, pp. 188-191.

Isomaa, B., Almgren, P., Tuomi, T., Forsén, B., Lahti, K., Nissén, M., Taskinem, M. & Groop, L. (2001). Cardiovascular morbidity and mortality associated with the metabolic syndrome. *Diabetes Care*, Vol.24, No.4, pp. 683-689.

Johnson, W.D., Kroon, J.J.M., Greenway, F.L., Bouchard, C., Ryan, D. & Katzmarzyk, P.T. (2009). Prevalence of risk factors for metabolic syndrome in adolescents national health and nutrition examination survey (NHANES), 2001-2006. *Archives of Pediatrics & Adolescent Medicine,* Vol.163, No.4, pp. 371-377.

Kavey, R.W., Daniels, S.R., Lauer, R.M., Atkins, D.L., Hayman, L.L. & Taubert, K. (2003). American Heart Association Guidelines for Primary Prevention of Atherosclerotic Cardiovascular Disease Beginning in Childhood. *Circulation,* Vol.107, pp. 1562-1566.

Kelishadi, R. (2010). Inflammation-induced atherosclerosis as a target for prevention of cardiovascular diseases from early life. *Open Cardiovascular Medicine Journal*, Vol.4, pp. 24-29.

Kelishadi, R. (2007). Childhood overweight, obesity, and the metabolic syndrome in developing countries. *Epidemiologic Reviews*,Vol.29, pp. 62-76.

Kelishadi, R., Zadegan, N.S., Naderi, G.A., Asgary, S. & Bashardoust, N. (2002). Atherosclerosis risk factors in children and adolescents with or without family history of premature coronary artery disease. *Medical Science Monitor*, Vol.8, No.6, pp. 425-429.

Kikuchi, D.A., Srinivasan, S.R., Harsha, D.W., Webber, L.S., Sellers, T.A. & Berenson, G.S. (1992). Relation of serum lipoprotein lipids and apolipoproteins to obesity in children: the Bogalusa heart study. *Preventive Medicine*, Vol.21, No.2, pp. 177-190.

Lakka, H.M., Laaksonen, D.E., Lakka, T.A., Niskanen, L.K., Kumpusalo, E., Tuomilehto, J. & Salonen, J.T. (2002). The metabolic syndrome and total cardiovascular disease mortality in middle-aged men. *JAMA*, Vol.288, No.21, pp. 709-716.

Lenfant, C. & Savage, P.J. (1995). The early natural history of atherosclerosis and hypertension in the young: National Institutes of Health perspectives. *American Journal of the Medical Sciences*, Vol.310, No.1, pp. 3-7.

Lieberman, E. (2002). Hypertension in childhood and adolescence, In: *Kaplan*, N.M. Clinical Hypertension (Ed.8), 512-526, Baltimore, Williams & Wilkins, Philadelphia, New York.

Lotufo, P.A. (1999). Novos conceitos sobre uma velha realidade. In: *Mion* Jr. D, Nobre, F., (Eds), 31-43, Risco Cardiovascular Global, Lemos Editorial, São Paulo.

Massin, M., Coremans, C. & Palumbo, L. (2002). Preventive cardiology: the role of the pediatrician. *Italian Journal of Pediatrics*, Vol.28, pp. 98-104.

McMurray, R.G., Ainsworth, B.E., Harrell, J.S., Griggs, T.R. & Williams, O.D. (1998). Is physical activity or aerobic power more influential at reducing cardiovascular disease risk factors? *Medicine & Science in Sports & Exercise*, Vol.30, No.10, pp. 1521-1529.

Mello, E.D., Luft, V.C. & Meyer, F. (2004). Obesidade infantil: como podemos ser eficazes? *Journal of Pediatrics*, Vol.80, No.3, pp. 173-182.

Michaelsen, K.F., Dyerberg, J., Falk, E., (2002). Children, fat and cardiovascular diseases. *Ugeskr Laeger*, Vol.164, No.10, pp. 1334-1338.

Ministério da Saúde (2006). Hipertensão arterial sistêmica, sáude da familia. *Cadernos de Atenção Básica*, No.15, Brasília, Distrito Federal.

Moll, P.P., Sing, C.F., Weidman, W.H., Gordon, H., Ellefson, R.D., Hodgson, P.A. & Kottke, B.A. (1983). Total cholesterol and lipoproteins in school children: prediction of coronary heart disease in adult relatives. *Circulation*, Vol.6, pp. 127-134.

Monteiro, C.A., Conde, W.L. & Castro I.R. (2003). The changing relationship between education and risk of obesity in Brazil: 1975-1997. *Cadernos de Saúde Pública*, Vol.19, No.1, pp. 67-75.

Morton, N.M., Holmes, M.C., Fiévet, C., Staels, B., Tailleux, A., Mullins, J.J. & Seckl, J.R. (2001). Improved lipid and lipoprotein profile, hepatic insulin sensitivity and glucose tolerance in 11 beta hydroxyesteroid dehydrogenase type 1 null mice. *The Journal of Biological Chemistry*, Vol.276, No.44, pp. 41293-41300.

Moura, A.A., Silva, M.A.M., Ferraz, M.R.M.T. & Rivera, I.R. (2004). Prevalência de pressão arterial elevada em escolares e adolescentes de Maceió. *Jornal de Pediatria*, Vol.80, No.1, pp. 35-40.

National High Blood Pressure Education Program Working Group on High Blood Pressure in Children and Adolescents (2004). The Fourth report on the Diagnosis, Evaluation, and treatment of High Blood Pressure in Children and Adolescents. *Pediatrics*, Vol.114, pp. 555-576.

Newman, W.P., Freedman, D.S., Voors, A.W., Gard, P.D, Srinivasan, S.R., Cresanta, J.L.,Williamson, D., Webber, L.S. & Berenson, G.S. (1986). Relation of serum lipoprotein levels and systolic blood pressure to early atherosclerosis. *New England Journal of Medicine*, Vol.314, pp. 138-144.

Obert, P., Mandigouts, S., Notin, S., Vinet, A., N'Guyen, L.D. & Lecoq, A.M. (2003). Cardiovascular responses to endurance training in children: effect of gender. *European Journal of Clinical Investigation*, Vol.33, pp. 199-208.

O'Brien, S.H., Holubkoy, R. & Reis, E.C. (2004). Identification, evaluation, and management of obesity in an academic primary care center. *Pediatrics*, Vol.114, pp. 154-159.

Puska, P. (1986). Possibilities of a preventive approach to coronary heart disease strating in childhood. *Acta paediatrica scandinavica*, Vol.318, pp. 229-233.

Purath, J., Lancinger, T. & Ragheb, C. (1995). Cardiac risk evaluation for elementary school children. *Public Health Nursing*, Vol.12, pp. 189-195.

Reaven, G.M. (1988). Role of insulin resistance in human disease. *Diabetes*, Vol.37, pp. 1595-1607.

Reed, D.M., Strong, J.P., Resch, J. & Hayashi, T. (1989). Serum Lipids and Lipoproteins as Predictors of Atherosclerosis. An Autopsy Study. *Arteriosclerosis*, Vol.9, pp. 560-564.

Rodrigues, A.N. (2006). Perfil Cardiorrespiratório e Metabólico de Escolares da Rede Pública do Município de Vitória. Xiii, 112p., *Tese de Doutorado*, Universidade Federal do Espírito Santo.

Rodrigues, A.N., Moyses, M.R., Bissoli, N.S., Pires, J.G. & Abreu, G.R. (2006a). Cardiovascular risk factor in a population of Brazilian schoolchildren. *Brazilian Journal of Medical and Biological Research*, Vol.39, No.12, pp. 1637-1642.

Rodrigues, A.N., Perez, A.J., Carletti L., Bissoli, N.S. & Abreu, G.R. (2006b). Maximum oxygen uptake in adolescents as measured by cardiopulmonary exercise testing- a classification proposal. *Jornal de Pediatria*, Vol.82, No.6, pp. 426-430.

Rodrigues, A.N., Perez, A.J., Pires, J.G., Carletti, L., Araújo, M.T., Moyses, M.R., Bissoli, N.S. & Abreu, G.R. (2009). Cardiovascular risk factors, their associations and presence of metabolic syndrome in adolescents. *Jornal de Pediatria*, Vol.85, No.1, pp. 55-60.

Rodrigues, A.N., Coelho, L.C., Goncalves, W.L., Gouvea, S.A., Vasconcellos, M.J., Cunha, R.S. & Abreu, G.R. (2011). Stiffness of the large arteries in individuals with and without Down syndrome. *Vascular Health and Risk Management*, Vol.7, pp. 375–381.

Rondom, M.U.P.B., Forjaz, C.L.M., Nunes, N., Amaral, S.L., Barretto, A.C.P. & Negrão, C.E. (1998). Comparação entre a Prescrição de Intensidade de Treinamento Físico Baseada na Avaliação Ergométrica Convencional e na Ergoespirometria. *Arquivos Brasileiros de Cardio*logia, Vol.70, No.3, pp. 159-166.

Rosa, M.L., Fonseca,V.M., Oigman, G. & Mesquita, E.T. (2006). Arterial prehypertension and elevated pulse pressure in adolescents: prevalence and associated factors. *Arquivos Brasileiros de Cardiologia*, Vol.87, No.1, pp. 46-53.

Salomen, J. (1991). HDL, HDL2 and HDL3, subfractions and the risk of acute myocardial infarction. *Circulation*, Vol.84, pp.129-139.

Santos, M.G., Pegoraro, M., Sandrini, F. & Macuco, E.C. (2008). Fatores de Risco no Desenvolvimento da Aterosclerose na Infância e Adolescência. *Arquivos Brasileiros de Cardiologia*, Vol.90, No.4, pp. 301-308.

Schrott, H.G., Clarke, W.R., Abrahams, P., Wiebe, D.A. & Lauer, R.M. (1982). Coronary artery disease mortality in relatives of hypertriglyceridemic school children: the Muscatine study. *Circulation*, Vol.65, pp. 300-305.

Shears, C.S., Burke, G.L., Freedman, D.S. & Berenson, G.S. (1986). Values of childhood blood pressure measurements and family history in predicting future blood pressure status: results from 8 years of follow-up in the Bogalusa heart study. *Pediatrics*, Vol.77, pp. 862-869.

Sorensen, T.I.A. (1995). The genetics of obesity. *Metabolism*, Vol.44, No.3, pp. 4-6.

Sorof, J. & Daniels, S. (2002). Obesity hypertension: a problem of epidemic proportions. *Hypertension*, Vol.40, pp. 441-447.

Srinivasan, S.R., Frerichs, R.R., Webber, L.S. & Berenson, G.S. (1976). Serum lipoprotein profile in children from a biracial community: the Bogalusa Heart Study. *Circulation*, Vol.54, No.2, pp. 309-318.

Srinivasan, S.R. (1991). Racial (black-white) differences in serum lipoprotein (a)- distribution ant its relation to parental myocardial infarction in children: the Bogalusa Heart Study. *Circulation*, Vol.84, pp. 160-167.

Srinivasan, S.R., Myers, L. & Berenson, G.S. (2006). Changes in metabolic syndrome variables since childhood in prehypertensive and hypertensive subjects: the Bogalusa Heart Study. *Hypertension*, Vol.48, No.1, pp. 33-39.

Srinivasan, S.R., Myers, L. & Berenson, G.S. (2002). Distribution and correlates of non-high-density lipoprotein cholesterol in children: the Bogalusa Heart Study. *Pediatrics*, Vol.110, No.3, pp. 29-32.

Stanganelli, L.C.R. (1991). Mudanças no VO_2 máx e limiar anaeróbico em crianças pré-púberes ocorridas após treinamento de resistência aeróbia. *Festur*, Vol.3, No.2, pp. 42-45.

Taskinen, M.R. (2003). Diabetic dyslipidemia: from basic research to clinical practice. *Diabetologia*, Vol.46, pp. 733-749.

The Trials of Hypertension Prevention Collaborative Research Group (1992). The effects of nonpharmacologic interventions on blood pressure of persons with high normal levels: results of the trials of hypertension prevention, phase I. *JAMA*, Vol.267, pp. 1213-1220.

Thomas, N.E., Baker, J.S. & Davies, B. (2003). Established and recently identified coronary heart disease risk factors in young people: the influence of physical activity and physical fitness. *Sports Medicine*, Vol.33, No.9, pp. 633-650.

Tolfrey, K., Campbell, I.G. & Jone, A.M. (1999). Selected predictor variables and the lipid-lipoprotein profile of prepubertal girls and boys. *Medical Sciences and Sports Exercise*, Vol.31, pp. 1550-1557.

Tourinho Filho, H. & Tourinho, L.S.P.R. (1998). Crianças, adolescentes e atividade física: aspectos maturacionais e funcionais. *Revista Paulista de Educação Física*, Vol.12, pp.71-84.

Troiano, R.P. & Flegal, K.M. (1998). Overweight children and adolescents: descriptions, epidemiology, and demographics. *Pediatrics*, Vol.101, pp. 497.

Turley, K.R. & Wilmore, J.H. (1997). Cardiovascular responses to treadmill and cycle ergometer exercise in children and adults. J Appl Physiol Vol.83, No.3, pp. 948-957.

Twisk, J.W. (2001). Physical activity guidelines for children and adolescents: a critical review. *Sports Medicine,* Vol.31, No.8, pp. 617-627.

VanHorn, L. & Greenland, P. (1997). Prevention of coronary artery disease is a pediatric problem. *JAMA*, Vol.278, pp. 1779.

Weiss R., Dziura J., Burgert, T.S., Tamborlane,W.V., Taksali, S.E., Yeckel, C.W., Allen, K., Lopes, M., Savoye, M., Morrison, J., Sherwin, R.S. & Caprio, S. (2004). Obesity and the metabolic syndrome in children and adolescents. *New England Journal of Medicine*, Vol.350, pp. 2362-2374.

Williams, C.L., Hayman, L.L., Daniels, S.R., Robinson, T.N., Steinberger, J., Paridon, S. & Bazzarre, T. (2002). Cardiovascular health in childhood: a statement for health professionals from the committee on atherosclerosis, hypertension, and obesity in the young (AHOY) of the council on cardiovascular disease in the young, American Heart Association. *Circulation,* Vol.106, pp. 143-160.

Zanella, M.T. (1999). Obesidade. In: Mion Jr. D, Nobre F., (Eds). *Risco Cardiovascular Global,* São Paulo: Lemos Editorial, p. 103-114.

2

Early Identification of Cardiovascular Risk Factors in Adolescents and Follow-Up Intervention Strategies

Heather Lee Kilty and Dawn Prentice
Brock University, Nursing Department, Faculty of Applied Health Sciences, Canada

1. Introduction

This chapter will explore the strong case being made world-wide for the development and implementation of well designed research and intervention approaches with adolescents to help stem the tide of rising cardiovascular risk factors, and thus to reduce cardiovascular disease in adulthood. It is well established that atherosclerosis begins in childhood and adolescence and that cardiovascular risk in early years can be tracked into adulthood cardiovascular disease (CVD) (Berenson et al., 2010; McCrindle et al., 2010; McCusker, et al., 2004; Yoshinga et al., 2008) .

Research into adolescent cardiovascular (CV) risk factors provides evidence that the development of possible large-scale interventions may hold great promise if conducted before family history repeats itself and before lifestyle choices are entrenched. The more research guides us to identify risk factors and how to measure them accurately, the clearer the path we can follow to identify those adolescents at risk and engage them in reducing risks earlier. It is the hope of the authors that the information presented will serve as a resource to those researchers who provide valuable data and evidence to shape policies and programs to reduce CV risk. The information is also intended for clinicians who work directly with adolescents in the assessment and management of cardiovascular risk, as well as health educators who engage in primary, secondary and tertiary health promotion.

This chapter is dedicated to exploring aspects of adolescent heart health and risk factors:

1. Research on the prevalence, incidence and concurrence of cardiovascular disease risk factors in adolescents.
2. Research on associations and connections between adolescent CV risk factors, adult risk factors and the development of CVD.
3. Research methods and instruments used to study, screen, measure and test for cardiovascular risk factors in adolescents at the population health level and at the individual program research level.
4. Current approaches to adolescent heart health awareness, health promotion, screening, prevention, risk reduction, education, referral and treatment.

Examples of adolescent cardiovascular research studies, initiatives and projects in parts of the world and their results or evaluations will be described. Recommendations for researchers, health promotion educators, parents and treatment health practitioners working with adolescents on cardiovascular prevention and reduction will be presented. A suggested comprehensive model of cardiovascular adolescent heart health screening, education, consultation and treatment will be presented.

Adolescence is a particular stage in the lifespan that is characterized as being between childhood and adulthood. While adolescents vary in their experiences world-wide and in their degree of independence, adult responsibility, and access to education, it is a common experience that they begin the tasks of establishing their own identity within the wider culture and society within which they live. Their emerging independence includes beginning to exercise their own choices of food, physical activity or inactivity, smoking behaviours, sexual experiences, and social relationships. They carry out degrees of independence within the context of examples set by diverse parenting models, family histories, cultural contexts and societal influences. In many cultures, the majority of adolescents are still in school and this provides an ideal milieu for cardiovascular research, screening and health promotion. Parental and family influences, peers, educators and media all play a role in shaping adolescent health beliefs and lifestyle behaviours that are often carried into adulthood.

2. The status of cardiovascular disease and the need for earlier research and prevention

2.1 Cardiovascular disease: An area of needed research and intervention in the world

Cardiovascular diseases are a major cause of morbidity and premature mortality in men and women in the industrialized world and many developing countries (Hayman et al., 2004). The WHO (2009) indicates the leading global risks for mortality in the world are high blood pressure (13% of global deaths), tobacco use (9%), high blood glucose (6%), physical inactivity (6%) and overweight or obesity. These risks are responsible for raising the risk of chronic diseases such as heart disease and cancers. The WHO conference (2009) on a "second wave" epidemic of cardiovascular disease connected with arterial sclerosis, predicted that by the year 2020, cardiovascular diseases will be the leading cause of death in the entire world (Chmiel-Polec, & Cybulska, 2008).

Heart attacks and coronary heart disease (CHD) are primarily caused by atherosclerosis, where a narrowing and hardening of the arteries result from an accumulation of fat and cholesterol deposits called plaque. This narrowing, or blockage of the arteries stops the supply of blood to the heart and can cause a heart attack, heart failure or even cardiac arrest. "Atherosclerosis also occurs in other blood vessels, such as the carotid artery, which carries blood to the brain, or the arteries that provide blood to the legs, and can lead to similar problems. Significant atheroslerosis in the arteries supplying the brain may cause transient ischemic attacks (TIAs) or strokes, while peripheral arterial blood vessel disease, with intermittent claudication (pain on walking or similar activity) occurs when there is a significant atherosclerosis in the arteries in the legs" (Wong, 2000, p. 23).

Heart disease, which encompasses coronary heart disease and stroke, is estimated to cause one third of all deaths world-wide. Cardiovascular disease (CVD) is estimated to be the leading cause of death and loss of disability-adjusted life years (Yusuf et al., 2004). Although age-adjusted cardiovascular death rates have declined in several developed countries in the past decades, rates of CVD have risen greatly in the low-income and middle-income countries. Yusuf et al., (2001) outlined the global burden of cardiovascular diseases. These researchers from Canada and India describe the epidemiological transition in the world from the major causes of death from a predominance of infectious diseases and nutritional deficiencies to those classified as degenerative diseases such as CVD. Although many cardiovascular diseases can be treated or prevented, an estimated millions of people die worldwide each year.

Atherosclerotic cardiovascular disease (CVD) is described as a multi-factorial condition reflecting a lifelong pathological process that begins in childhood (Stary, 1989). Chronic disease and illness are commonly caused by exposure to risk factors many years prior to the onset of the condition. Dietary/ nutritional intake, consumption of alcohol and other substances, smoking, and inactivity are all behaviour patterns established during adolescence and have been linked to obesity and a number of illnesses that develop later in life (Hennekens & Bering (1987).

Yusef et al. (2004) make the case for a global strategy of cardiovascular research for the prevention of CVD: "Effective prevention needs a global strategy based on knowledge of the importance of risk factors for cardiovascular disease in different geographical regions and amongst various ethnic groups" (p. 937). The bulk of the research to date has been on European and North American, populations, but studies related to CVD in the general adult population and risk factors that begin in childhood and adolescence are adding to the cumulative body of research, theory and knowledge from many countries around the world. "Although more than 80% of the global burden of cardio-vascular disease occurs in low-income and middle-income countries, knowledge of the importance of risk factors is largely derived from developed countries. Therefore, the effect of such factors on risk of coronary heart disease in most regions of the world is unknown" (Yusuf et al, 2004, p. 937).

Yusuf et al. (2004) conducted a standardized case-control study of myocardial infarction in 52 countries, involving 262 centers representing every inhabited continent. This study was part of INTERHEART, a large international, standardized coronary heart disease case-control study designed as an initial step to assess the importance of risk factors for CVD. The study enrolled 15,152 cases and 14,820 controls. Nine easily measured and potentially modifiable risk factors accounted for an overwhelmingly large (over 90%) proportion of the risk of an initial acute myocardial infarction (MI). The research reported on the relationship of smoking, history of hypertension or diabetes, waist/hip ratio, dietary patterns, physical activity, consumption of alcohol, blood apoliproteins (Apoli), and psychosocial factors related to MI. The presence of multiple risk factors, hypertension and diabetes were found to increase the odds for acute MI. Obesity rates were found to vary in different parts of the world.

Each country is struggling to research the impact of CVD on their population, as well as the resultant impact on health services and finances. In Canada, as in many nations, CVD is the major cause of death, disability, and illness that has a significant impact on the health care system, accounting for more discharges from hospital than any other major disease group. The costs of hospitalization, medical care, drugs, and research related to CVD present a substantial cost burden to most countries (Yusef et al., 2004).

The Canadian Heart and Stroke Foundation's Annual Report (2010) warns that young Canadian adults are increasingly at risk for heart disease: And that "a perfect storm of risk factors and demographic changes are converging to create an unprecedented burden on Canada's fragmented system of cardiovascular care, and no Canadian young or old will be left unaffected" (p. 2). The report points out that "Young people are beginning their adult lives with multiple risk factors for heart disease." The report states that people used to think that heart disease and stroke, type 2 diabetes and high blood pressure were 'diseases of aging.' The report sounds a warning that these increases (in overweight and obesity, high blood pressure and diabetes) "will translate into an explosion of heart disease in the next generation" (p.2).

According to the *Canadian Community Health Survey* data 2007/2008, many heart health risk factors are already present in 20 to 34 year olds with health behaviours that began earlier in childhood and adolescence. Of the participants sampled, 47.0% were physically inactive, 40.5% were overweight or obese; 29.0% were smokers; 2.5% had high blood pressure and; 1% had diabetes. By ages 45-64, those numbers are: 52.8% reporting physical inactivity; 58.2% were overweight or obese; 23.1% were smokers; 22.9% had high blood pressure and; 8.3% had diabetes. For women and the aboriginal population, the numbers are even greater. CVD is the number one cause of death and disease in Canadian women.

While associations are being determined in the research between and among identified risk factors, the prevalence of each respective factor may vary in different populations. This phenomenon is referred to as *population attributable risk* (PAR) (Yusuf et al.2004). For example, lipids have not been found to be associated with heart disease disorders in South Asians; increases in blood pressure might be more important in Chinese people; serum cholesterol might be lower in the Chinese population; and diabetes and high blood pressure may be more prevalent in the North American Aboriginal population. The differences found in risk levels may be a result of cultural health habits, or they could be attributed to differences in the research design, analysis, information obtained and sample sizes. Cross-cultural research for adolescents and adult populations should examine their findings carefully in regard to making inferences about risk factors in varying populations and cultural contexts.

The WHO (2009) identified eight risk factors that account for 61% of cardiovascular deaths in the world: high blood pressure, high body mass index, high cholesterol, high blood glucose, low fruit and vegetable intake, alcohol use, and physical inactivity. Combined, these same risks factors "account for three quarters of ischaemic heart disease: the leading cause of death world-wide" (p. v). Many of these risk factors begin in childhood and adolescence.

3. Adolescence as an important target stage for research on the identification and modification of cardiac risk factors

3.1 The case for earlier intervention and the search for where to begin

Adolescent years are marked by many physical, social and emotional changes that take place within the cultural and political social and economic contexts within which adolescents begin to transition into adulthood and more habitual behaviours (Mathers, 1998). Nutritional intake, physical activity or inactivity and smoking attitudes and behaviours begin in childhood. These patterns get more established in adolescence and can transition into entrenched lifestyle habits in adulthood. Research on adolescents is valuable at this stage of lifespan development to identify those risk factors and their prevalence, so that individuals and societies can make decisions about where to put their health promotion and risk reduction efforts, based on the evidence.

Erikson (1950, 1977) described the lifespan developmental stages and the struggles, strengths and tasks of each period of development. He called the adolescent period of puberty and teenage times from age 12 to 18 years of age as a time of *identity vs role confusion*. He stated that up until this time, development depended mostly on what is done to us, whereas from that point on, development depended more on what the individual does. It is a time to find an identity separate from the family of origin, to struggle with social interactions, and to grapple with moral issues.

Many CV risk factors are adopted by adolescents without awareness of their present and long-term impacts on health or the potential development of heart disease. Adolescents are still shaping, re-shaping and creating their identities. Most writers acknowledge that heart health education and screening can and should be initiated in childhood before adolescence begins. However, adolescence is a key point of entry, where risk factors can be made known not only to families, health practitioners, and educators, but to the individual adolescent directly so he or she can be potentially informed, empowered and motivated to make their own changes.

It is generally postulated that CVD, including heart disease and stroke is largely preventable (apart from age and heredity) through adopting a healthy lifestyle that includes no smoking, healthy food choices, physical activity, the management of stress and the maintenance of healthy weight (Health Canada, 2011). Preventive care is appropriate to control blood pressure, blood cholesterol and other lipids. Flouris et al. (2007), in their study of CV disease risk factors in Ontario adolescents state that: "Within the limitations of the study adolescents, especially those with low cardiovascular fitness appear to be at an increased risk for developing CVD at a later life stage. These findings highlight the necessity of placing adolescents in the forefront of preventive cardiovascular disease programs and should receive particular attention by healthcare authorities in order to minimize future CVD attributed mortality rates" (p. 523). They caution that risk and gender findings could also be influenced by pubertal influences.

Adolescents of many nations are dealing with additional health threatening conditions of famine, war, and natural disasters that further complicate the process of moving through adolescence to adulthood. Regardless, adolescents of all cultures are often in that childhood to adulthood, in between stage where the health behaviours of childhood and family teachings shape some of their health behaviours and choices mixed along with some emerging independent choices of young adulthood. Eating, physical activity, smoking and substance using behaviours of youth have long been areas of study that have relevance to future heart health outcomes. Genetic, aging, cultural, societal, peer and family trends also have an impact on heart risks and CVD.

In many populations, adolescents tend to have a lower incidence and prevalence of psychosocial and medical disorders and are often the healthiest subgroup of the general population (Mathers, 1998). Despite this good news, the general health status of adolescents has not improved over the last 30 years (Stanton et al., 2000). The study of adolescent health and early established healthy and unhealthy behaviours is warranted if we wish to understand childhood and adolescent influences and intervene earlier in the development of CVD at an opportune time when the adolescent is beginning to make their own choices.

Adolescence is a life stage where the individual is still influenced by the family, but beginning to make independent choices in many areas to establish their own lifestyle habits, behaviours, values and beliefs. That in-between place makes working with adolescents on health promotion a very promising and challenging endeavour. In the case of the adolescent who has smoking parents, a physically inactive household and poor nutritional intake historically, and he or she begins to exercise, eat well and not smoke - these are positive changes in the right direction. For the adolescent who comes from healthy beginnings and begins to smoke, eat poorly and not exercise, - the choices may have a negative impact on heart health and the development of cardiovascular disease. For certain, the adolescent period is a period of influences from family, peers, education and media mixed with opportunities for change, for better or worse in regards to health.

4. Risk factors and research particularly related to adolescents

4.1 Categories of risk factors

A cardiovascular risk factor is a condition that is associated with an increased risk of developing cardiovascular disease. Cardiovascular (CV) risk factors fall into two distinct categories: those that cannot be changed and those that can be modified, treated or controlled (American Heart Association [AHA], 2007).

The major risk factors that cannot be changed are:

- *Increasing age* ... The risk of cardiovascular events increases as we get older. Many epidemiological studies have indicated that age is one of the strongest predictors of disease. Over half of those even up to 83% of people who die of coronary heart disease are 65 and older. At older ages, women who have heart attacks are more likely to die from them within a few weeks.
- *Gender* ... Men have a greater risk of heart attack than women and they have attacks earlier in life. Even after menopause, when women's death rates from heart disease increase, they are still not as great as the rates for men. We are not certain if male hormones (androgens) increase risks or female hormones (estrogens) protect against atherosclerosis. This gender difference could also be attributed to past smoking patterns where men smoked more than women. These patterns are changing and women could be losing their advantage in this area as smoking in women rises.
- *Heredity (including race)* ... Children who have parents or siblings who have heart disease are more likely to develop it themselves. They have a significantly greater likelihood of having a heart attack or stroke. Familial hypercholesterolemia and its accompanying biological defects are well characterized as a known risk for CVD. Individuals who have a family history of heart disease that occurred early (before 55) especially should be more vigilant and adopt modifiable healthy behaviours. People with a strong family history of heart disease often have one or more risk factors. African Americans have been found to have more severe high blood pressure than Caucasians, and a higher risk of heart disease. Heart disease risk is higher in the U.S. among

Mexican Americans, Native Americans, native Hawaiians and some Asian Americans; this is partially due to higher rates of obesity and diabetes (Adapted from AHA, 2007).

The major modifiable predisposing risk factors that can be prevented, treated or controlled:

- *Risk behaviours* ... tobacco smoking, physical inactivity, and poor eating habits
- *Risk signs* ... high blood cholesterol and related lipids, and high blood pressure,
- *Resulting conditions* ... obesity and overweightness, and the development of diabetes mellitus.

Other risk factors that have been identified with heart disease in the research are: individual stress response, depression, drinking too much alcohol, sleep patterns, and socio-economic status (SES).

Simply having a risk factor associated with heart failure does not mean that an individual will develop heart failure. Many of the factors are controllable and involve healthy heart lifestyle awareness and changes. Black, (in Wong et al. 2000) states that "The association is a statistical one, and so the fact that a particular person has a particular factor merely increases the probability of developing a certain type of cardiovascular disease, it does not mean that he or she is certain to develop heart or blood vessel disease. Conversely, the fact that an individual does not have a particular cardiovascular risk factor (or for that matter, any known cardiovascular risk factors) does not guarantee protection against heart disease" (p. 33).

Black suggests there are also certain *protective factors* that we need to understand more about and how they impact positively on cardiovascular disease. He includes the following in his list of identified protective factors: HDL cholesterol, exercise, estrogen, and the moderate intake of alcohol.

Example research studies related to the prevalence, co-occurrence or clustered presence of primary risk factors in adolescents will be discussed later in the chapter (smoking, blood pressure, cholesterol, BMI, physical activity, nutrition and obesity). Additional risk factors are also present in the adolescent stage that influence overall health and heart health that include: substance abuse, socio-economic status (SES), suicide, depression, drinking and driving, and sexually transmitted diseases. Several studies have explored the presence of individual risk factors and the presence of multiple factors and the associations between them. Several risk factors will be reviewed here, along with sample studies and approaches used to study and measure that particular risk factor in adolescents.

4.2 Research on the co-occurrence (clustering) of cardiovascular risk factors

It is well known that an increase or decrease in the number of CV risk factors is strongly associated with the improvement or worsening of individual risk factors (Nakumura et al., 2001; Yoshinaga et al., 2008; Yoshinaga et al., 2010).

Yoshinaga et al. (2010) stated that little is known about the impact of having one CV risk factor on the other levels of other CV factors in the general adolescent population. The researchers hypothesized that when adolescents have one risk factor, the level of the other CV risk factors worsens simultaneously. A sample of 1,257 healthy adolescents (549 males and 708 females) aged 15-18 years were assessed using: risk factors of abdominal obesity, hypertension, raised triglyceride levels, decreased HDL cholesterol levels and hyperglycemia. Homeostatic assessment of insulin resistance (HOMA-IR) was used as a surrogate marker of insulin resistance. The levels of all CV risk factors and HOMA-IR significantly and simultaneously worsened when adolescents had one risk factor, in both genders. Having one risk factor indicated the development of other risk factors in adolescents, especially the development of abdominal obesity in male subjects was found to have a harmful effect on other CV risk factors. They concluded that it is important to determine the presence or absence of CV risk factors before and/or during adolescence, because having one CV risk factor can indicate the start of an accumulation of CV risk factors in the general adolescent population.

Lobelo et al., (2010) in a cross-sectional study of 1,247 youth 12-19 years of age in the U.S. using data from the 1999-2002 *National Health and Nutrition Examination Survey* (NHANES), examined the association between cardiovascular fitness (CRF) distribution and CVD risk measured as continuous scores for individual and clustered CVD risk factors to explore the potential effect modification of the association exerted by weight status among adolescents. They used a treadmill test and categorized age and sex specific quintiles and researched five established risk factors with an adiposity index that included the sum of triceps and subscapular skinfolds; the homeostatic model assessment of insulin resistance; systolic blood pressure; triglycerides and total cholesterol/high density lipoprotein cholesterol, standardized for age and gender A clustered score was calculated as their average. The mean clustered risk score decreased with increasing CRF in both males and females. Most of the clustered CVD risk was found among adolescents within the lowest quintile of CRF distribution.

A cross-sectional study was conducted by McCrindle et al. (2010) with 20,719 beginning high school students in the Niagara Region of Ontario, Canada with data reported over a seven year period. The aim of a study conducted from 2002 to 2008 was to examine population trends of increasing cardiovascular risk factors in 14 to 15 year old students participating in the Niagara Schools Healthy Heart Program (NSHHP). The program provides identification of cardiovascular risk factors for teens enrolled in a grade nine physical education program in secondary schools in Niagara.

Through an assessment, adolescents were identified and referred to their family physician for further follow-up. The physical assessment measures included height and weight, capillary sample for non-fasting total cholesterol level, and blood pressure measurement. A family cardiovascular risk history assessment questionnaire was completed that asked about first degree family members who had hyperlipidemia, hypertension or diabetes. A lifestyle questionnaire completed by the students assessed the amount of physical activity over a week, amount of television watched, the amount of time spent on videogames and the amount of time spent on the computer. A self-reported nutritional questionnaire asked students about consumption of fruits and vegetables, fast-food intake, amount of soda and caffeine intake and whether or not the students ate breakfast. The McCrindle et al., (2010) study used the student's electoral district as a substitute marker to determine the socio-economic status.

Almost 20% of the students had one cardiovascular disease risk factor. The investigators reported that during the study period, the percentage of obese teens' body mass index (BMI) increased significantly, and non-fasting total high cholesterol levels also significantly increased. Additionally, the percentage of students with borderline high total cholesterol increased. The authors reported that "family history, low levels of physical activity, sedentary behaviours, poor nutrition and lower socioeconomic status were all independently and negatively associated with all aspects of cardiovascular risk" (p. 837). Findings from this study supported the need for continued surveillance to provide early identification and follow-up of students with cardiovascular risk factors.

Two sub-studies were conducted as part of the Niagara Schools Healthy Heart Program. (NSHHP) Data for the years 2002, 2003 and 2005 were analyzed by Prentice, Kilty, Stearne and Dobbin (2006). Over 10, 000 students from thirty schools participated in the NSSHP during that time frame. Trends indicated that more female students reported smoking; more male students reported being active for 30 minutes per days as compared to female students; and the amount of self-reported television watching and video game use decreased over the three years. The referrals of those identified with risk factors (higher blood pressure/ or cholesterol) to family health practitioners remained fairly constant at almost 5%. The researchers concluded that collaborative programs such as the NSHHP are challenging to implement within a school system, yet early assessment, education and identification of risk factors are essential in cardiovascular disease prevention.

A previous sub-study was conducted by Prentice, Kilty, Stearne and Dobbin (2008) with 3,639 grade nine students in 30 secondary schools in the Niagara Region. The study was part of an evaluation of the Niagara Schools Healthy Heart Program (NSHHP), a primary prevention program that was in effect since 1987. The Program has multiple components: a one hour educational session on heart health, CPR training, a self- assessment component which includes a self-rated questionnaire on dietary intake, caffeine intake, level of physical activity and smoking. A questionnaire on family history of cardiovascular disease is sent home to be completed in conjunction with parents. Registered public health school nurses measured height, weight to calculate the Body Mass Index (BMI). Blood pressure and non-fasting total cholesterol screening were also tested. If any abnormalities are detected, the students were referred to their primary health care provider for follow-up. Data were analyzed for the school year 2006. The researchers reported that 14% of the participants had one or more cardiovascular risk factors. The most common risk factor was BMI (13.7%). Of the sample, 5.0% had an elevated random total cholesterol >5.2 (6.2% females and 3.8% males); and 5.8% of the sample had a blood pressure systolic reading greater than 135mmHg and a diastolic reading of 85mmHg or greater. In terms of gender differences, female students reported smoking more and had higher cholesterol levels. Male students were more likely to have an increased BMI. There were no gender differences in the prevalence rates of elevated blood pressure. The findings suggest that cardiovascular risks are already present in adolescents. It was recommended that this group be followed up in the future and retested in grade twelve and that an additional focus should be on earlier prevention program initiatives with younger children.

Shatoor et al. (2010) conducted a cross-sectional study in Saudi Arabia on a stratified sample of 1,249 adolescent secondary school boys. More than 25% did not practice regular exercise and there was a high parental history of hypertension, diabetes and high blood pressure. They called for a national program to prevent cardiovascular risk factors among adolescents.

Andersen et al. (2003) conducted a study exploring biological cardiovascular risk factor clusters in Danish children and adolescents as part of the larger European Youth Heart Study. The aim of the study was to determine whether the number of participants with multiple coronary heart disease (CHD) risk factors exceeded the number expected from random distribution. The cross-sectional study included 1,020 randomly selected boys and girls, aged 9 and 15 years. The risk factors studied were: total cholesterol, HDL cholesterol, triglyceride, serum insulin, and blood pressure. Physical fitness was assessed from a maximal cycle test and body fat sum of four skinfolds taken. More participants than expected had four or five CHD risk factors. Four risk factors were found in 3.03 times as many participants as expected from random distribution and five risk factors were found in 8.70 times as many participants as expected. Fifty (5.4%) had 4 or 5 risk factors and in these individuals, physical fitness was 1.2 standard deviation lower and BMI was 1.6 SD higher than the mean values for the population. A clustering of risk factors was found for children and adolescents, where when one was present, several factors were also present.

Bouziotas and Koutedakis (2003) examined the prevalence of 14 modifiable CHD risk factors in a sample of 210 provincial Greek children as they progressed from 12 to 14 years of age. It was found that 46.2% of boys and 49.5% of girls had three or more risk factors at their 12th year; 42% boys and 51.1% girls in their 13th year and; 29.4% boys and 55% girls in their 14th year. Males had more physical activity and less body fat; girls had an elevated percentage of body fat, percentage of intake of saturated fat, and total cholesterol. They concluded that a high percentage of Greek boys and girls exhibit three or more modifiable CHD risk factors and as they progress from 12-13 years of age, gender differences start to emerge in the prevalence and development of CHD risk factors.

4.3 Research on the main cardiovascular risk factors for adolescents and their measurement

For each risk factor included in this review there will be:

- An introduction describing available information on that risk factor;
- Sample research studies on adolescent prevalence and data related to that risk factor;
- Measurement standards and approaches;
- World Health Organization results of the School-Aged Study conducted in regions around the world (2008) and;
- Suggested advice for this risk factor.

4.3.1 Smoking as a CV risk factor in adolescents

Introduction …

Cigarette smoking among adults primarily starts in adolescence and continues to be a major public health problem world-wide. Tobacco use is considered the number one individually preventable and modifiable cause of cancer and cardiovascular disease (Elders, 1994; United States of America (USA) Dept of Health and Human Services in Greenlund et al., 1996).

Known psychosocial risk factors for smoking among adolescents include the presence of other smokers in the family unit, smoking among friends, peer acceptance of smoking, age and socio-economic factors (Wang, Fitzbugh, Westerfield, & Eddy, 2003; Barber, Bolitho, & Berrand, 1999; Fied 1994 in Winter, de Guia, Ferrence & Cohen, 2002).

Sample studies …

Greenlund et al. (1996) studied trends in cigarette smoking among children in a U.S. southern community from 1976-1994 as part of the *Bogalusa Heart Study*, which conducted a long-term investigation of cardiovascular disease beginning in childhood with studies up to age 40 years. Smoking trends from 1976-1977 and 1992-1994 were examined to investigate cardiovascular disease risk factors among black and white; male and female adolescents. Age-race-sex specific tests for trends over five survey periods were conducted. In almost every age group, black boys and girls had sharp decreases and were less likely to be a current smoker than their white counterparts. These substantial decreases were not observed in white children.

Shields (2005) summarized the results from *National Population Health Survey (NPHS)* and the *Canadian Community Health Survey (CCHS)* in 2003 and reported that for those 12 and over 10.5% were exposed to second hand smoke at home; and 88.9% were not. According to the CCHS, (2003), one in ten (10%) of those 12-17 years old smoked cigarettes; more than half (50%) of those smoked daily; boys and girls were almost equally likely to report smoking (10% of boys and 11% of girls). The 2007/2008 CCHS reported that 29.0% of those 20-34 years smoked; 25.6% of those 35-44 years smoked; and 23.1% of those 45-64 years smoked.

Winter et al., (2002) examined the relationship between body weight perceptions, weight control behaviours and smoking status among adolescents. Although there is some evidence that smoking affects body weight, the direction of the causality is not clear, and the relationship appears to interact with age. Adult smokers have a lower BMI than non smokers; although the physiological mechanism responsible for this difference is still unclear. In adolescent populations, smokers tend to weigh more than non-smokers. This study used a major Canadian provincial database, the 1997 Ontario Students' Drug Use Survey (OSDUS) to examine the independent effects of body weight perception and both moderate and extreme weight control behaviours on smoking status among both male and female students. A 37% response rate surveyed a sample of 3,990 public and Catholic school students enrolled in grades 7, 9, 11 and 13 from 168 schools in Ontario, Canada were surveyed. This biannual survey was carried out by the Centre for Addiction and Mental Health (formerly, the Addiction Research Foundation) since 1977. Based on unadjusted analyses, females who believed they were overweight had more than 50% greater odds of being smokers compared to those who believed themselves to be of average weight or too thin. Weight perceptions were not associated with smoking among males.

SUGGESTED ADVICE REGARDING SMOKING
Quit smoking
Use effective smoking cessation strategies

4.3.2 Poor nutrition and eating habits as CV risk factors in adolescents

Introduction …

According to the U.S. National High Blood Pressure Education Program Working Group (2004), "Despite the lack of firm evidence about dietary intervention in children, it is generally accepted that hypertensive individuals can benefit from a dietary increase in fresh vegetables, fresh fruits, fiber, and nonfat dairy as well as a reduction of sodium" (p. 566).

Eating a healthy breakfast each day has been suggested. Siega-Riz et al. (1998) studied trends in breakfast consumption for children 1-10 years of age and adolescents 11-18 years from 1965-1991 and found a decline in breakfast consumption, especially for 15-18 year olds from 89.7% to 74.9% in boys and from 84.4% to 64.7% in girls. Results suggested that the decline was because of behavioural changes. They conclude that given the association of obesity with less frequent breakfast consumption, and the rise of obesity in this group, a renewed emphasis on the importance of breakfast is warranted. Smith et al. (2010) explored longitudinal associations with cardiometabolic factors in the childhood determinants of health in a sample of 9-15 year olds in Australia. They found that skipping breakfast over a long period may have detrimental effects on cardiometabolic health and that "Promoting the benefits of eating breakfast could be a simple and important public health message (p. 1316).

Sample studies …

In what has been referred to as the *Cardiovascular Risk in Young Finns Study* (Aatola et al., 2010) a cohort of 1,622 subjects was followed up for 27 years. The baseline data collected in 1980 for 3-18 year olds with lifetime data available since childhood. Arterial adult pulse wave velocity (PWV) was measured in 2007 by a whole-body impedance cardiography device. Vegetable consumption in childhood was found to be inversely associated with adulthood PWV. Vegetable consumption was also an independent predictor of PWV in adulthood. Persistently high consumption of both fruits and vegetables from childhood to adulthood was associated with lower PWV, compared to persistently low consumption. The number of risk factors in childhood was also directly associated with PWV in adulthood. Those findings suggest that lifetime lifestyle risk factors with low consumption of fruits and vegetables in particular are related to arterial stiffness in young adulthood.

Cardiologists and health specialists have long been concerned about dietary fat and added sugars. From 1970 to 2000 in adults, the prevalence of obesity tripled while the intake of energy from fat decreased significantly. During that time, sugar-sweetened beverages increased dramatically. Kavey (2010) reported on the analysis of the data from the *National Health and Nutrition Examination Survey (NHANES)* from 2007 to 2008. In children and adolescents, an analysis of the 1989-1991 *Continuing Survey of Food Intakes by Individuals* revealed that 2-18 year olds in the U.S. consumed 6.5% of their energy from sugar-sweetened beverages. From a Reedy and Krebs-Smith's study (2010), an analysis of the recall from children and adolescents revealed a per capita consumption of sugar-sweetened beverages and 100% fruit juice drinks went up from a mean of 242 kcal/day in the first day to 270 kcal/day in the second day. Combined, they account for 10-15% of total energy intake. High added sugar consumption in the form of sugar-sweetened beverages is associated with cardiovascular risk factors, both independently and through the development of obesity.

Consumption of added sugars and indicators of cardiovascular disease was studied by Welsh et al. (2010) in the United States. A cross-sectional study of 2,157 adolescents in the National Health and Nutrition Examination Survey (NHANES) from 1999-2004 collected and analyzed dietary data from one 24-hour recall along with sugar content data from the

U.S. Department of Agriculture MyPyramid Equivalents databases. Measures of CVD risk were estimated by the added sugar consumption levels. Added sugar consumption levels were positively correlated with low density lipoprotein cholesterol levels (mmol/L) which were 1.40 among the lowest consumers and 1.28 among the highest. Added sugars were found to be positively correlated with low intensity lipoproteins. Among the lowest and highest consumers, respectively, low-density lipoproteins were 2.24 (mmol/L) and 2.44 and triglycerides were 0.81 (mmol/L) and 0.89. Among those who were overweight or obese, added sugars were positively correlated with the homeostasis assessment model. Researchers concluded that consumption of added sugars among U.S. adolescents is positively associated with multiple measures known to increase cardiovascular disease risk.

World Health Organization (WHO, 2008): Health behavior in school-aged children international report from the 2005/2006 survey in 41 countries for 11, 13 and 15 year olds.
Eating habits - Daily fruit consumption varies between countries, is highest for 11 year olds and declines with age. Boys are less likely than girls to report eating fruit, as are those from less affluent families in almost all countries. The daily consumption of soft drinks also varies cross-nationally and tends to be higher among older adolescents. Consumption of soft drinks is associated with low family affluence in a majority of the countries, except in eastern Europe and the Baltic states where the reverse is found. Eating breakfast on school days decreases with age. Those from less affluent families, particularly in northern and western Europe are less likely to eat breakfast every school day.

Measurement …

Studies related to adolescents have measured dietary intake and eating habits in several ways:

- Recall of intake of fruits and vegetable and how much and how many servings per day; recall of sugar intake and how many added sugar drinks or foods and amounts were consumed daily; sodium and potassium intake daily; eating of breakfast; eating fats foods; and eating at home or in restaurants have been used in adolescent studies of risk factors. Recall is often recorded in a survey taken at one point in time, but requiring recall and reflection on daily or weekly intakes. Sometimes. participants are asked to choose from described levels of intake on a pre-determined Likert scale to describe their dietary habits.
- Daily diaries have also been used in studies, where the adolescent records and tracks what they eat and when.
- Studies related more to obesity management and weight control have given a suggested diet to participants and they record levels of adherence to the protocol for food intake. In some cases, an established diet that has been approved such as a special heart and diabetic diet or the Canada Food Guide (Health Canada, 2011) and other respective nationally accepted standards are part of the intervention and the evaluation.

A report on *Dietary Reference Intakes for energy, carbohydrate, fiber, fat, fatty acids, cholesterol, protein and amino acids* (2002/2005) was produced by the Institute of Medicine of the National Academies, with input from Canadian scientists. It presents a comprehensive set of reference values for nutrient intakes for healthy U.S. and Canadian individuals and populations (by age and risk characterization).

SUGGESTED DIETARY ADVICE
5 servings of fruits and vegetables per day
Low sodium intake
Reduce added sugars
Eat breakfast daily
Increase sources of fiber

4.3.3 Physical activity/inactivity as cardiovascular risk factors in adolescents

Introduction …

Regular physical activity has cardiovascular benefits. Increasing regular activity and decreasing sedentary activities such as watching television and playing video or electronic games have been found to be important components of paediatric obesity prevention and therefore, important to lowering of a CV risk factors (Robinson, 1999; Williams et al. 2002;). Physical activity has also been a included in the treatment protocol for obesity and weight-reduction trials to combat obesity (Kreb et al., 2003; Gutin & Owens, 1999). Researchers have found that inactivity, particularly television watching is an important factor in the development of obesity, one of the main factors associated with cardiovascular risk (Andersen et al., 1998; Gordon-Larsen et al., 2002; Gortmaker et al., 1996). Sedentary activity also involves the use of computer, cell phone or other electronic devices for texting, communication or entertainment.

Sample studies …

Maggio et al., (2010) studied long-term follow-up of CV risk factors after exercise training in obese children in Switzerland. The beneficial effects of physical activity on CV risk factors and BMI was previously demonstrated in their research. This study was to determine if those changes were maintained 2 years later. They involved 20 of the 38 from the previous study in the follow-up study. The mean 24-hour diastolic blood pressure significantly decreased; while systolic blood pressure was slightly reduced. BP changes were greater in children who diminished their BMI compared with ones who did not. In addition, the arterial intima-media thickness, BMI, body fat, and physical count remained stable two years after to indicate that the positive effects remained for that period after the exercise training was initiated.

Buchan et al. (2011), in Scotland studied the effects of time and intensity of exercise on novel and established markers of CVD in adolescents. Brief, intense exercise, compared to traditional endurance exercise was studied in 47 boys and 10 girls, 16.4 (+/- 0.7) years of age. Three weekly sessions were conducted over 7 weeks for three groups: moderate exercise (MOD), high intensity exercise (HIT) or the control group. They engaged in 4-6 repeats of maximal sprint running or 20 minutes continuous running. Significant improvements were found in systolic blood pressure, aerobic fitness and BMI in the HIT group. Significant improvements were found in aerobic fitness, percentage of body fat (%BF), BMI, fibrinogen (Fg), plasminogen inhibitor-1, and insulin concentrations in the MOD group. They concluded that exercise is beneficial, but brief intense exercise may be a time-efficient means for improving CVD risk factors in adolescents

In a U. S. study of a nationally representative sample of 12,759 participants in the *National Study of Adolescent Health* Gordon-Larsen et al (2002) collected data on moderate to vigorous and low-intensity physical activity (TV/video viewing, and videogame/computer use) by questionnaire. Multivariate analysis assessed the association of overweight by BMI, with initial and one year changes in activity and inactivity levels, controlling for age, ethnicity, socioeconomic status, urban residence, cigarette smoking, and region of residence. Overweight prevalence was found to be positively correlated with high levels of TV/video viewing among white boys and girls. The odds of being overweight decreased with high levels of moderate to vigorous physical activity among white, non-Hispanic black boys and girls, and Hispanic boys and girls.

In the next cycle of the same survey, an increase in physical activity was found to be associated with decreasing relative BMI in girls and overweight boys. An increase in inactivity (daily TV/videos/video games) was associated with increasing BMI in girls (Berkey et al. 2003). Activities that were found to be accessible and beneficial to most children were aerobic dancing and walking.

World Health Organization (WHO, 2008): Health behavior in school-aged children international report from the 2005/2006 survey in 41 countries for 11, 13 and 15 year olds.
Physical activity - Young people should participate one hour or more of at least moderate physical activity every day. Less than half of young people do so in almost every country and region. Slovakian boys and girls are most likely to meet the guidelines in every age group. Across countries and regions and all age groups, girls are less active than boys and the gender gap increases with age. Fifteen year olds are less likely (average 16%) to report meeting the guidelines than 11 year olds (average 26%) in the majority of the countries. In under half of the countries, those from more affluent families are more likely to meet guidelines.

Measurement …

Measurement of sedentary activity has primarily been conducted by self-report recall of number of hours estimated of video game/computer use, TV/video/DVD viewing, and cell phone use and texting, daily or weekly. Most studies have the individual estimate times in a one-time administered survey; however the use of a diary over a period of time to record daily activities has also proven to be effective. For exercise, both self report and actual testing have been used and quantified. Self-report surveys ask questions about types of exercise the adolescent engages in (cycling, running, swimming, walking), how often, at what level of intensity, and for what time duration. In addition, physical exercise testing has also been used with adolescents completing activity tests in a school setting such as the shuttle test (Flouris et al. 2008) or being observed and tested in a laboratory setting. In a study by Buchan et al. (2011), a group engaged in moderate level activity, and one in high level activity and a control group and correlated the time and intensity data with established markers of CVD in participating adolescents.

SUGGESTIONS FOR PHYSICAL ACTIVITY
Regular aerobic activity (30-60 minutes of moderate physical activity on most days) Limit sedentary activities (under 2 hours per day)

4.3.4 Hypertension, high blood pressure as a CV risk factor in adolescents

Introduction …

Hypertension has been linked to cardiovascular diseases, stroke and kidney disease (Chobanian et al, 2003). The medical management or control of blood pressure is thought to reduce the risk of serious cardiovascular disease. In obese or overweight adolescents, and the known early development of atherosclerosis in children, identification and treatment of blood pressure in children is essential (Luma & Spiotta, 2006).

Sample studies …

Rafraf et al. (2010) conducted a cross-sectional study in Iran to determine the blood pressure status and its relationship to BMI in 985 girls attending high school. Blood pressure, BMI (weight and height) was calculated and blood pressure measured as normal, pre-hypertension or hypertension was calculated using the 2004, Fourth Report blood pressure screening recommendations. Overweight and obesity were defined according to International BMI cutoff points for adolescents. The prevalence of pre-hypertension was 13.9% and hypertension was 19.4% in the sample. Overweight and obesity rates were 2.8% and 16.4% of the subjects respectively. The prevalence rates of hypertension and pre-hypertension increased with increasing BMI. The prevalence of high blood pressure in adolescent girls was higher than in other countries, despite a lower prevalence of obesity. They suggested taking blood pressure readings during at least 3 visits for increased accuracy in future studies.

Measurement of blood pressure in children and adolescents …

Measurement of blood pressure is a component of an assessment of cardiovascular risk. Identification of pre-hypertension and then continued monitoring of blood pressure is one method identified to decrease the risk of further cardiovascular disease. The Fourth Report on the diagnosis, evaluation, and treatment of high blood pressure in children and adolescents (2004) was prepared by the *National High Blood Pressure Education Working Group*. "Considerable advances have been made in detection, evaluation, and management of high blood pressure (BP), or hypertension, in children and adolescents. Because of the development of a large national database on normative BP levels throughout childhood, the ability to identify children who have abnormally elevated BP improved. On the basis of developing evidence, it is now apparent that primary hypertension is detectable in the young and it occurs commonly" (p. 555). The long-term health risks can be substantial and it is important that clinical measures be taken to reduce these risks and optimize health outcomes. The report reviews appropriate and specific approaches, including the administration of pharmacologic therapy for childhood hypertension (p. 567).

Current standards adopted for the identification of pre-hypertension and hypertension in children were outlined in The National High Blood Pressure Education Program Working Group on High Blood Pressure in Children and Adolescents (2004). In this document, the authors outlined the definition of hypertension particularly as it relates to children and adolescents:

- Hypertension is defined as systolic blood pressure (SBP), average SPB and/or diastolic BP (DBP) that is ≥ 95 percentile for gender, age, and height on ≥ 3 occasions.

- Pre-hypertension in children is defined as average SBP or DBP levels that are ≥90 percentile but < 95th percentile.
- As with adults, adolescents with blood pressure readings ≥ 120/80 mm Hg should be considered pre-hypertensive.

A patient with BP levels >95th percentile in a physician's office or clinic, who is normotensive outside a clinical setting, has "white-coat hypertension." Ambulatory BP monitoring (ABPM) is usually required to make a diagnosis. (National High Blood Pressure Education Working Group on High Blood Pressure in Children and Adolescents, 2004, p. 556).

SUGGESTED ADVICE FOR HIGH BLOOD PRESSURE
Be aware of family history and parents and siblings with high blood pressure
Have blood pressure tested earlier in childhood and adolescence and into adulthood
Monitor blood pressure regularly if there are signs of hypertension
Exercise
Eat well
Lower sodium intake

4.3.5 Cholesterol as a CV cardiovascular risk factor for adolescents

Introduction …

Cholesterol screening is also important for children and adolescents as hypderlipidemia is a known risk factor for the development of cardiovascular disease (McCrindle, 2000). Furthermore, the atherosclerotic process has been shown to begin in childhood (McGill et al., 1997; Newman et al., 1986).Treatment of high cholesterol has been proven effective in reducing cardiovascular disease and death in adults (McCrindle, 2000). Early detection and treatment of hypderlipidemia in children is indicated.

Sample studies …

Manios et al. (2003) conducted a twenty-year study of the dynamics in adiposity and blood lipids of Greek boys 12.2 (+/- 2.3) years of age. They recruited 277 in 1982 and 251 in 2002. They calculated height and weight for BMI, as well as plasma lipid concentrations to compare across cohorts for the 2 years. Significant changes in total cholesterol (TC) were observed for urban, but not rural boys. Regional differences reported that urban boys were taller, heavier and had higher BMI values and higher LDC-C concentrations. They found changes in anthropometric changes and lipids and suggest a national strategy to monitor and address some of these risk factors.

In order to obtain information about the concentrations of LDL cholesterol and total cholesterol in children and adolescents in the United States, Ford et al. (2009) conducted a study of children ages 6-17 years age. Using data from the *National Health and Nutrition Examination Survey* (NHANES) 1999- 2006, measurements for total cholesterol and fasting LDL cholesterol were examined. Of the 2,724 LDL cholesterol levels examined for participants aged 12-17, the mean concentration was 90.2 mg/dL and for total cholesterol the mean concentration for participants aged 6-17 years was 163.0 mg/dL. The researchers noted that approximately 0.8% of the 12-17 years olds would most likely be eligible for pharmacological interventions for their elevated LDL cholesterol levels.

Measurement ...

Standards for a cholesterol screening program for children were developed from the National Cholesterol Education Program (NCEP) of the National Heart, Lung and Blood Institute in the United States in 1992. Their approach includes screening children who have a family history of premature cardiovascular diseases or a family history of high cholesterol levels. They further recommend that children who have no known family history, or have other risk factors for cardiovascular disease should also be screened (Daniels, Greer & The Committee on Nutrition, 2008). Acceptable levels include a total cholesterol < 170 mg/dL, borderline 170-199 mg/dL and elevated > 200 mg/dL/. Acceptable levels for low density lipoprotein are, 100 mg/dL borderline 110-129 mg/dL, and elevated > 130 mg/dL.

SUGGESTED ADVICE FOR CHOLESTEROL
Be aware of family history
Get tested and monitor levels
Eat well and avoid certain fats in the diet

4.3.6 Obesity as a CV risk factor in adolescents

Introduction ...

The prevalence of overweight and obesity in children is increasing rapidly and the ongoing obesity epidemic represents a major public health burden world-wide (Ebbeling et al., 2002; Daniels et al., 2009). Obesity is thought to pose a major risk of morbidity and premature mortality in adulthood for those affected by cardiovascular disease. Obesity is identified as an independent risk factor for cardiovascular diseases and it significantly increases risks of morbidity and mortality. Childhood obesity is a global phenomenon affecting all socio-economic groups. "Aetiopathogenesis of childhood obesity is multi-factorial and includes genetic, neuroendocrine, metabolic, psychological, environmental and socio-cultural factors" (Raj & Kumar, 2010, p. 598).

The treatment and prevention of obesity often requires an interdisciplinary and holistic approach that includes: dietary management, increases in physical activity, restriction of sedentary behaviours, and psychotherapy and counseling. Pharmocology and bariatric surgery have also been included in the approaches used to deal with this pervasive and urgent health issue that often begins in youth. Doak et al. (2006) conducted an international review of interventions and programs in the prevention of obesity in children and adolescents. Flynn et al. (2006) did a synthesis of the evidence available on reducing obesity and related chronic disease risk in children and youth and summarized best practices and recommendations for improved approaches. They created an algorithm to guide the research process and the study of obesity with children and youth.

Sample studies ...

A U.S study examined the importance of age in the relationship of childhood obesity and cardiovascular disease risk factors in adulthood as part of the *Bogalusa Heart Study*. Freedman et al., 2001). They assessed the longitudinal relationship of childhood BMI to all levels of lipids, insulin and blood pressure among 2,617 participants. All participants were initially examined at ages 2 to 17 years and were re-examined at ages 18 to 37 years; the mean follow-up was 17 years. Of the overweight children initially identified, 77% remained obese as adults. Childhood overweight was related to adverse risk factor levels in adults, but the associations were weak. Although obese adults had adverse levels of lipids, insulin and blood pressure, levels of these did not vary with childhood weight status, or with age. The need for primary and secondary prevention was suggested.

A study by Barnabe et al (2010) in Brazil included 4,138 high school students (14-19 years) selected by cluster sampling in two stages. They obtained data using the *Global School-based Health Survey*, and anthropometric measurements were taken for determination of overweight and abdominal obesity. The identification of cases of abdominal obesity was performed by waist circumference analysis, using age and gender-related cutoff points as reference. Logistic regression was used for analysis of behavioural factors associated with the occurrence of abdominal obesity. They found the prevalence of abdominal obesity to be 6%, slightly higher for girls and lower than international estimates. Physical activity was significantly associated with the occurrence of obesity.

World Health Organization (WHO, 2008): Health behavior in school-aged children international report from the 2005/2006 survey in 41 countries for 11, 13 and 15 year olds.
Overweight - The data presented on overweight and obesity are derived from self-reported height and weight information used to calculate body mass index (BMI), not from actual measurements, and so need to be treated with some caution. The general term 'overweight' included two groups: those who are considered obese and those who are considered overweight, but not obese. The proportions of 13 to 15 year old boys and girls who are overweight range from 4% to 35% across countries and regions. Canada, Greenland, Malta and the United States have among the highest rates. Boys, and those from less affluent families report higher levels of overweight and obesity, particularly in North America and western Europe.

Measurements…

Body Mass Index measurement and levels in children and adolescents

Given the increasing focus on the prevalence of obesity in children and the health care risks associated with obesity including cardiovascular disease risk, close assessment and monitoring of children's growth is key to awareness and primary prevention. One common measurement that has been used to measure overweight in adults is the body mass index (BMI) (weight/height) (Cole et al. 2000). Although a cutoff point of 30kg/m has been suggested as an international reference for overweight adults (World Health Organization, 1995) currently no consistent standard cut- off point exists for children. In fact, several BMI reference standards: the Centre for Disease Control (CDC) in the United States; The World Health Organization Child Growth Standards; the United Kingdom 1990 BMI; and the standard definitions developed by the International Obesity Task Force are available for use with children (Flegal & Ogden, 2011). When using BMI cutoffs with children, the age, height, weight and sex of the youth must be considered. Monitoring children's growth and development is a key assessment factor.

Waist Circumference

Waist circumference is another common screening measurement used in tandem with the BMI. Waist circumference is an indicator for central adiposity (World Health Organization,

2011) and has been used as a predictor for the development of cardiovascular disease (Lee, Huxley, Wildman & Woodward, 2008) and diabetes (Huxley et al., 2010). Similar to the BMI, there is no one standard criteria percentile for waist to hip circumference for children and adolescents due to differences in growth rates and patterns among different population groups (Ma et al., 2010).

SUGGESTED ADVICE
Increased, regular physical exercise Dietary management Restrict and reduce sedentary activity Weight monitoring, control and reduction

4.3.7 Family history as a CV risk factor

Introduction ...

It has been well established that the family is the primary context in which health behaviours are learned, performed and developed over time (Allen & Warner, 2002; Laudenbauch & Ford-Gilboe, 2004). It has also been well established that family history of heart disease increases an offspring's chances of developing CV risk factors and CHD (McCusker, et al. 2004; Michos et al., 2004). This is true, particularly if a first degree family member (father, mother, or sibling) had a heart attack (O'Donnell, 2004). Parental history of CVD has been studied well and the coronary artery calcification sibling history has also been found to be more strongly associated than parental history (Nasir et al., 2004).

"Health work is positively influenced by the health potential of the family - the strengths, motivation and resources of the family unit and its members - as well as the extent to which nurses and other health professionals can use a strength-based, situation-responsive approach when working with families" (Laudenbach & Ford-Gilboe, 2004, p. 125). How heredity and genes play a part is still being studied, but the connections are clear. It is suggested that those with a family history of heart disease start early with reducing lifestyle risk factors. If family history indicates a genetic predisposition to heart attack, individuals are vulnerable to developing other contributing risk factors such as diabetes, obesity or high blood pressure.

Sample studies ...

Murabito, in the Framingham Offspring Study (2004) studied 2,475 participants and over eight years compared the occurrence of heart disease in people with or without siblings. They found participants who had a brother or sister with cardiovascular disease had higher levels of risk factors than those without the disease. This association had a 45% increased risk for the disease.

A cross-sectional study of families was conducted with nearly 8,500 adults in Ohio, U.S.A. with half older than 52 and half younger than 52 (Nasir et al., 2004). Family history of heart disease in the study was defined as a sibling or parent experienced fatal, or non-fatal heart attack or underwent some form of coronary revascularization, including bypass surgery by age 55. Signs of calcification and plaque build-up were observed in all groups, regardless of family history, but the burden was greatest among those who had a parental or sibling history of early heart disease, ranging from 36% to 78% for both men and women. These data support rigorous preventive measures should be taken by individuals with a history of premature heart disease.

Sdringola, Patel and Gould (2001) hypothesized that asymptomatic persons with coronary artery disease (CAD) had myocardial perfusion defects on positron emission tomography (PET) as markers of early CAD. After medical and family histories were taken and tests were conducted. This study documented the presence of quantitative, statistically significant, dipyridamole- induced myocardial perfusion abnormalities on PET in 50% of asymptomatic persons with a parent or sibling with CAD, independent of risk factors, to indicate preclinical coronary atherosclerosis.

Measurement ...

The *Health Options Scale* (HOS) is a 21 item version that has been used in studies of families who varied in structure, stage of the life cycle, socioeconomic status (SES) and the study of types of health challenges they face (Ford-Gilboe, 2002; Ford-Gilboe, 1997; Laudenbach & Ford-Gilboe, 2004). It has been used as a valid and reliable measure of health with mothers and preadolescent children, with adolescents and with women as sources of information about families and their health. Schuener (2004) summarized the clinical application of genetic risk assessment strategies for coronary heart disease involving both genotypes and primary care approaches.

SUGGESTED ADVICE FOR THOSE WITH A FAMILY HISTORY OF CVD

Assess family history of CVD and risk factors
Have family dialogue for awareness
Health check-ups and regular surveillance
Test risk factors such as blood pressure and cholesterol earlier
Quit smoking
Cut back on fatty foods
Increase exercise
Know your past - act in the present - Protect your future (The Chronic Disease Genomics Project)-
Explore use of medications with a healthcare professional

4.3.8 Sample studies of other cardiovascular risk factors and their associations with CVD in adolescents

Diabetes ...Type I Diabetes (TID) is a common disease of childhood and is increasing world-wide (Onkamo et al., 1999). Cardiovascular disease has been found to occur at a higher frequency and at a younger age in patients with TID compared to the general population (Laing et al., 1999; Libby et al., 2005).

A cross-sectional study by Krishnan et al.,(2011) examined the presence of cardiovascular risk factors in normal and overweight children, with and without TID in a sample of 66 children 16-22 years of age. A fasting blood sample was analyzed for a lipid profile (triglyceride cholesterol, high density lipoprotein cholesterol), and low-density cholesterol, apolilipidprotein B (apoB), and apolipoprotein C-III (apoC-III) levels. Body composition was measured by dual energy x-ray absorptiometry and vascular elasticity by HDI/Pulsewave CR-2000. Statistical analysis examined the effect of TID and body weight status and their interaction on cardiovascular risk factors. The study was unable to demonstrate an additive effect of body weight and TID on cardiovascular risk profiles with well-controlled children and adolescents with TID. However, there was a direct relationship of small artery elasticity to body weight that indicated further investigation was warranted.

Park et al., (2007) explored family history of diabetes and risk of atherosclerotic cardiovascular disease (ASCVD) in a cohort of 1,005,230 Koreans aged 30-95 years who were insured by the National Health Insurance Corporation who had a biennial medical evaluation during 1992-1995. The risk of ischemic heart disease (IHD) increased significantly in men, but not in women. Men with both diabetes and IHD were at significantly increased risk of developing IHD, ASCVD and cerebrovascular disease. This study demonstrated that risk of ASCVD is increased among those who have diabetes and a family history of diabetes, suggesting that genetic factors may increase the risk of ASCVD.

Depressive symptoms …

A study on depressive symptoms and subclinical markers of cardiovascular disease in adolescents was conducted by Dietz and Matthews (2011) with 157 black and white adolescents 16-21 years of age. The study was of psychosocial stress and cardiovascular risk factors with measurements of arterial stiffness as tested by pulse wave velocity (PWV) and intima media thickening (IMT). The Center for Epidemiological Studies *Depressive Scale* and the *Cook-Medley Hostility Inventory* subscales were used and described (Dietz & Matthews, 2011). Linear regression controlled for socio-demographic variables, health behaviours, blood pressure, BMI and heart rate. More severe depressive symptoms were found to be associated with higher levels of PWV, but not with IMT. Adolescent depression remained a significant predictor of PWV when controlling for adolescent hostility. More study is indicated regarding depressive symptoms and the pathogenesis of CVD.

Socio-economic status (SES) …

A Canadian study conducted by Schreier and Chen (2010) examined socio-economic status in one's childhood as a predictor of offspring cardiovascular risk. The literature was reviewed in the Canadian study that demonstrated living in a low socioeconomic status (SES) is linked to poorer health (Adler & Newman, 2002). A strong relationship has been demonstrated between low SES and increased mortality (Andersen et al 1997); between low SES and specific risk factors for diseases such as cancer (Conway et al, 2008; Shakley & Clark 2005); and diabetes (Eversen et al, 2002). One of the most consistent associations has been found between SES and cardiovascular disease (Kaplan & Keil, 1993; Pollitt et al, 2005) and stroke (Cox et al, 2006). Low SES and specific risk factors of blood pressure, cholesterol and subclinical CVD have also been studied (Appel et al., 2002; Colhoun et al., 1998; Grotto et al, 2008).

The Schreier and Chen study tested whether effects of socio-economic environments (as reported in 4 quintiles) persist across generations by examining the parents' childhood and if SES of the parents could predict blood pressure trajectories in their youth offspring. A sample of 88 healthy youth whose mean age was 13 (+/- 2.4 years) were involved in a 12 month study period including 3 study visits, each 6 months apart. If the parents' childhood SES was lower, children displayed increasing SBP and CRP and if it was higher, the reverse was found to be true. The study pointed out that intergenerational histories are important and SES is important. Improving overall socio-economic levels for all by a population health approach might have a positive effect on adolescent and adult cardiovascular disease.

Hormonal contraception …

Du et al. (2011) in a German study of hormonal contraceptive (HC) use in 2, 285 girls, 13-17 years of age. They compared users of HC and nonusers with the prevalence of cardiovascular risk factors, including systolic and diastolic blood pressure and serum concentrations of lipids, lipoproteins, high-sensitivity C-reactive protein (hs-CRP) and homocysteine. Users were more likely than nonusers to combine several behaviour-based health risks independent of socio-demographic factors. In particular, HC was strongly associated with current smoking. HC use and behavioural factors showed an additive effect on biological cardiovascular risk factors, explaining between 6% and 30% of the population variance. It is suggested that physicians, when prescribing HC, should systematically assess avoidable cardiovascular risk factors and provide counseling tailored to the risk profile of the individual patient.

Sleep apnea and deprivation and cardiovascular risk in children and youth…

In obese children, obstructive sleep apnea (OSA) has been linked to the early onset of cardiovascular morbidity and metabolic morbidity (Spicuzza, et al., 2008). The potential association between children with obstructive sleep apnea syndrome and blood pressure elevation has been explored; however, further investigation of this association is warranted (Bhattacharjee et al., 2009). Similarly, non-obese children with OSA have been shown to be at risk for endothelial dysfunction, necessitating further longitudinal studies of children with OSA and its impact on cardiovascular disease (Gozal et al., 2007). Studies in adults indicate that too little or too much sleep is associated with stroke and risk of CVD.

Cappuccio et al. (2011) from the University of Naples conducted a systematic global review and meta-analysis to assess the relationship between duration of sleep and later development of coronary heart disease (CHD) or stroke, as well as death from those diseases. They included studies where participants were free from disease at baseline. *Normal sleep* was classified as 7-8 hours; *short sleep* as less than, or equal to 5-6 hours; and *long sleep* as more than 8-9 hours. They pooled the risk figures for the associations between sleep duration and cardiovascular disease development, or death. The review included 15 studies on 24 cohorts covering 474,684 adults from eight countries. The duration of the follow-up was 6.9 to 25 years. They studied 16,067 cases of fatal and non-fatal cardiovascular events: 4,169 cases of CHD; 3,478 strokes; and 8,420 other CV events. They found that *short sleep,* compared to *normal sleep* was associated with increased risk of developing or dying from stroke, as was long sleep. For studies examining total CVD, researchers found that compared with *normal sleep, long sleep* was associated with increased risk of CVD. Both short and long sleep durations were found to be potential predictive markers of CVD outcomes.

Oureshi et al. (1997) explored the association between sleep duration and daytime somnolence (most always taking naps) with the incidence of stroke and CVD in a U.S.

national cohort of 7, 844 adults from the 1st National Health and Nutrition Examination Survey Epidemiological Follow-up Study over a 10 year follow-up period. After adjusting for age, race, gender, education, smoking and some of the other risk factors, the risk of stroke was increased for those who sleep more than 8 hours a day, compared to 6-8 hours. Similar results were found for the risk of CVD, although not found to be statistically significant.

5. Research and the study of adolescent cardiovascular health and risk

5.1 Research methodology

A majority of the research studies regarding adolescent cardiovascular risk factors reported in this chapter have been quantitative in nature. Quantitative research design can be non-experimental or experimental. Many epidemiological studies trending the prevalence of risk factors have been conducted using non-experimental cross-sectional survey data with various age groups and cohort sample populations. Trends have been reported with accompanying statistical analysis and tests to determine correlations or associations between and among the risk data. A few studies have been conducted with the same cohort in longitudinal designs, many over several years in studies conducted at the international, national and smaller community sampling levels. The variation apparent in the methods used; population sample age representation and selection process; and the approaches used for analysis and reporting make it difficult to have a truly accurate and comparable picture of cardiovascular risks from childhood, adolescence into adulthood. Even with all the challenges, the body of evidence is mounting and sounding an alarm. Regularly scheduled and reliable surveillance and mandatory staged testing of CV risks at several age points is beginning to make sense.

Studies are evident that include an evaluation of risk factors before and after specific interventions are introduced to reduce the risk factors with adolescents (i. e. the impact of physical activity or improved nutrition and the resultant impact on other risk factors). Only a few studies have used experimental designs and control group approaches to compare results.

Most studies have been conducted through schools or clinics with convenience samples, with only a few national strategies using random or stratified sampling approaches. Research Instruments and measurement standards have been developed over time and the reliability and validity of questions, surveys tools and designs have been tested. Measurements and standards relating to blood pressure, cholesterol testing and some activity testing have been developed or adapted specifically to the paediatric and adolescent populations.

Few qualitative studies have been conducted of a phenomenological nature to explore the lived experience of cardiovascular risks (such as obesity) in adolescents. We need to know more about what life is like for adolescents and what the meaning of the phenomenon is to those who live it. (i.e. smoking or not being active) so that our interventions are more effective. Ethnographic studies might help us to also understand the patterns and experiences of specifically defined cultural groups. This may help us to understand what the numbers really mean when they indicate there are differences in risk factors in different regions of the world, in different schools, in different ethno-racial adolescent groupings and in different age groups for adolescents. We might understand more about why exercise decreases or smoking increases in certain subsets of adolescents and be able to target our efforts more effectively..

5.2 Research instruments used in the study of adolescent cardiovascular risk factors

A variety of tools and scales have been tested in many of the studies described herein. A summary of the types of research tools used in the study of adolescent cardiovascular health are:

- *Self-reported survey questionnaires of lifestyle behaviours* are mostly collected by paper and pen survey or questionnaire administered in person, in group settings, over the telephone, through the internet or through a guided health interview.
- *Physical assessment tests* often include tests or measurements to determine blood pressure; cholesterol fasting and non-fasting levels; height and weight to calculate BMI; waist circumference; physical activity levels; and stress responses. Many of these tests require specialized equipment, processes and protocols so they are measured and interpreted in the same way. Some tests require trained staff to conduct the test, read the results and work with clients for feedback, consultation and follow-up. Some tests are best conducted in laboratory, clinical or school settings.
- *Self monitored and recorded diary entries* have been used as effective research tools in some studies for adolescents to track their own nutrition, smoking and physical exercise, daily and weekly over established periods of time. Diaries are handed in for quantification and analysis. Diaries can also be used to collect qualitative data about inner reflections, perceptions, attitudes and experiential information for analysis to establish core themes or to develop theories or models to guide practice from the data through grounded theory approaches,.
- *Use of existing reliable and valid instruments to assess stress, depression, self esteem, or hostility.* Many studies related to adolescent cardiovascular disease have also added existing social science instruments that have been developed to measure a wide range of topics from assertiveness, self-esteem, and hope. This information has been used to correlate with CV risk factors in the search for possible associations that impact on CV risk or have a mediating or protective effect.
- *Use of family history data.* Only a few adolescent studies used a family history of heart disease or health survey. Few also included a process by which the adolescent and parent were encouraged to have a dialogue about exploring family history and health data related to heart health, cardiovascular disease, diabetes, high blood pressure or cholesterol abnormalities in parents, siblings or grandparents as part of the research or as part of the awareness strategy.
- *Mortality and autopsy data.* Studies of adolescent cardiovascular risk data have involved autopsy data and mortality statistics. The collection and reporting of this data has been included in studies related to family history and parental and sibling data or in longitudinal tracking studies such as the Framingham study. Should some of the cross-sectional cohort studies track the same individuals over time, we could have more data on the final outcomes of the early identification of CV risk factors and morbidity and mortality outcomes. The case for genetic testing, counseling and intervention earlier for

high risk cases is emerging in many areas of health risk and heart disease certainly is an area of high risk.

Sample instrument ...

Many instruments have been developed about health and lifestyle factors related to youth in many of the projects reviewed in this chapter and there are many more in existence around the world. Only a few sample ones will be presented here. Surveys related to health and lifestyle have been developed by research collaborators and used in 52 countries called the *Health Behaviours in School-aged Children* (HBSC) (Yusef et al., 2001, 2008; WHO 2008). The *CATCH* instruments have been developed and used in many school projects in the U.S. along with surveys used in the Bogalusa studies. In Canada, the instruments used in the Census, Canadian Community Health Survey elicit and trend information about aspects of health and lifestyle for adolescents. The lifestyle survey components of the Niagara Healthy Heart School's Program has been adapted and widely used for almost a decade. Reed et al. (2007) developed and tested an instrument that measures and calculates the number and severity of cardiovascular risks in children and adolescents to determine an overall *Healthy Heart Score* (from 1-18) that could be used in develop a risk profile to be used in the identification of those at risk for intervention.

Stanton, Willis and Balanda (2000) conducted a study in a project in Australia to develop a survey to be used with secondary school students to monitor relevant health-related behaviours and the inter-relationship between them, with an emphasis on identifying clustering behaviours of negative outcomes with 12 to 18 year olds. They included a compendium of existing surveys. They described the stages to develop and test a survey for use with adolescents: draft stage, pilot testing, and formal and informal evaluation of the instrument. They included 308 juniors and 223 seniors in high school, of which 10% took part in testing the instrument for reliability and giving input to the researchers. They suggest further analysis and testing of a hopelessness scale be included.

5.3 Research limitations to date in the study of adolescent cardiovascular risk factors

A few of the major limitations in adolescent cardiovascular risk research will be reviewed.

5.3.1 There are few studies about adolescent CV risk factors using the same measurements and instruments and methodology to make comparisons possible ...

Sample studies ...

Three countries; England, Finland and Norway participated in the 1st *Health Behaviours in School-aged Children (HBSC) in 1982.* By 1985, 11 countries were involved and the WHO Regional Office for Europe began to play a coordinating role. Canada was invited as an associate member to participate in the 1993-4 and 1997-98 cycles. Twenty eight countries participated for the 2001-02 school year. Fifty two (52) countries are now involved. The HBSC is representative of the population health approach used in Canada and incorporates the determinants of health that include the home, school, social environment, individual health practices and gender.

The advantage of HBSC is to be able to compare and contrast youth responses to the same questions country to country. Combined data and individual country data are developed into national reports to guide health promotion in their area (i. e. The Health of Canada's Youth Report (King & Coles, 1992) was published by Health Canada; the 2nd report the Health of Youth (King et al. 1996) .

The HBSC was administered in classrooms in grades 6, 8 and 10 and grade equivalents in Quebec. Questions were developed by HBSC collaborators in an attempt to create a developmental perspective in order to examine changes in attitudes and behaviours from the onset of puberty to the middle years of adolescence. The research identifies health indicators and the factors that may influence them (smoking, alcohol use, level of physical activity, psychosocial states such as happiness and loneliness; and physical problems such as headaches and backaches). It also explores health influencing factors or determinants of health that include the school, parents, peers, and individual characteristics. Additional items regarding bullying were added in 1998.

Canada's study was based on a systematic single cluster procedure being the school class. They identified the potential number of grade 6, 8, 10 classes listed with 25 per class. A sample of 80 classes per grade was randomly selected to reach a sample size of 2000 per grade level. Other countries used a variety of sampling procedures. Ideally, it is suggested that surveys should be conducted at the same time each year. Ten countries were selected from the 23 to compare with Canada in the second survey that had structural factors in common or had policies and programs in place of interest. Five composite measures compared student relationships to parents; adjustment to school; self-esteem; social integration and; diet. The study also reported on relationships between the data (i.e. use of marijuana and smoking; and marihuana use and how you feel about school).

5.3.2 There are few longitudinal studies to track cardiovascular risk factors over the lifespan to track the development of CVD into adulthood

Sample longitudinal studies ...

Kavey (2010) reported on the analysis of the data from the *National Health and Nutrition Examination Survey* (NHANES) from 2007 to 2008 (Ogden et al., 2002) that indicated that 16.9% of children and adolescents had a BMI greater than the 95th percentile. There was a significant increase in boys 6-19 years of age. The community screening of 5-17 years olds in The *Bogalusa Heart Study* revealed that the prevalence of obesity increased more than five-fold from 5.6% in 1973-1974 to 30.8% in 2008-2009. Information from these longitudinal studies indicates that children with high BMI have a strong chance of becoming obese and developing serious conditions such as hyperinsulinemia/type 2 diabetes, hypertension and dylipidemia beginning in childhood and premature heart disease in adulthood.

A longitudinal tracking of adolescent health behaviours in two *Minnesota Heart Health Program* communities in the United States was conducted. Beginning in sixth grade, (1983) seven annual waves of behavioural measurements were taken (baseline n=2376). Self-reported data included smoking, physical activity and food preferences. The results showed a progressive change in weekly smoking status; as they began to experiment with smoking, they were more likely to remain a regular smoker. In physical activity and eating good foods, those who measured high at baseline, were more likely to remain high. This study reported some evidence of the early consolidation of habits in these three risk factor areas.

Intervention before grade six and before behaviour patterns become resistant to change is indicated. A cessation program is offered to those having trouble quitting.

5.3.3 There are few qualitative studies on adolescent cardiovascular risk factors

Qualitative studies can explore the experiences, perceptions, feelings and meanings as lived by the adolescent regarding a variety of phenomenon associated with heart risks and healthy behaviours. We have increasing alarming numbers and trends clearly in evidence before us. We need to know and understand more about what this means to adolescents and why and how they think and feel and change or don't change. The voices, thoughts and meanings of adolescents can add much to our understanding and planning of more effective health promotion or risk reduction approaches.

5.3.4 There are few studies on adolescents and their follow-up and use of health care providers when identified as having CV risk factors: what works and doesn't for referral, testing, follow-up and lifestyle counseling and change

There are few follow-up studies about whether adolescents, after being screened or having an awareness of risk and family history actually seek advice, further testing or consultation with a physician or health care provider.

Sample study ...

A qualitative study entitled, *Adolescent cardiovascular risk factors: A follow-up study* (Kilty & Prentice, 2010) examined the outcomes of grade nine students who were referred to their physician as a result of having an elevated cholesterol level or elevated blood pressure during a screening by Heart Niagara and a school nurse. The screening assessment was part of the Niagara Schools Healthy Heart Program which is comprised of an educational session on heart health, a screening assessment of blood pressure, height, weight, Body Mass Index (BMI), non-fasting total cholesterol level and a self-reported lifestyle assessment. CPR training is also a component of this program.

Telephone interviews were conducted with 304 participants over a three month period. The interviews included: 126 parent-teen dyads from the same family, 37 parents-only and 15 teens-only. Information on what happened as a result of the referral was queried including: actual attendance with follow-up referrals, medications prescribed, further tests conducted, and referrals to other specialists. Additionally, queries about changes in lifestyle as a result of the screening, awareness and follow-up were also explored.

Fifty percent of those who were referred to their physician for follow-up participated in the qualitative interviews. According to the parents, 63% of teens went for a follow-up appointment with their health care practitioner. The teens themselves reported that 58% had gone for follow-up. The reasons given for not following up with the referral were that it was not seen as 'urgent or necessary' or the teen appeared to be fine or was already seeing the physician for other reasons. Given that some adolescent behaviours may contribute to the development of diseases including cardiovascular disease in the future (Kilty & Prentice, 2010), it is important to understand why adolescents may or may not follow-up with referrals and the potential outcomes of follow-up consultation with a physician when identified as having potential CV risk factors. Early identification and follow-up in community settings can potentially ameliorate risk factors, if identified and treated early.

A review of information on adolescent help seeking behaviours and barriers to seeking health advice is included along with features of an adolescent friendly health care service delivery.

5.4 Settings for adolescent research on CV risk factors

Community settings for making contact with adolescents for research, health promotion and intervention have primarily been through the schools or health clinics and physicians' offices.

The school can be viewed as one of the most important settings in which social and psychological development occurs and it is likely that health and health behaviours may be associated with a relationship to school (Bond & Compas, 1989). Large numbers of adolescents can be reached for research and health education purposes through schools. Adolescents still have an affiliation with family and varying degrees of independence related to health issues. Researchers have to be aware that in some regions, consent can be completed by the adolescent to participate in research studies, and in other regions, the parent also has to give consent. The school system officials may have to review the research proposal and the attention paid to ethical issues, privacy and confidentiality before proceeding. Since schools are a good place to gather valuable information about adolescent health, efforts to coordinate studies are needed so that the schools and adolescents are not inundated with requests for participation. The school is also an ideal venue for health promotion and education about cardiovascular risk. Most schools have curriculum related well to health, health promotion and heart health. They also have teachers of science, health, sociology and physical education where content about cardiovascular health and risks are well suited.

Clinics and doctors' offices can also be viewed as potential places to conduct research. The only routine health intervention occurrences may be around immunization times that take place in teen years in some cultures.

6. Interventions, programs and strategies to reduce cardiovascular disease and risk factors in adolescents

6.1 Intervention approaches to reduce cardiovascular risk factors in adolescents

Conducting primary prevention of CVD, beginning in early childhood and sustained through adolescence has been well supported by the extensive evidence from epidemiological, clinical, and laboratory studies conducted world-wide and the examples reviewed in this chapter. Approaches to reduce and prevent cardiovascular disease can include *primary prevention* and health promotion for the general population before CVD occurs; *secondary prevention* to identify those at risk and provide opportunities for change; and *tertiary prevention* to identify those with CVD and associated risks such as diabetes and obesity and intervene. Some of the approaches used for adolescent heart health are:

- *Education and health promotion strategies* that include information on heart health, holistic health and well-being. These strategies can target, individuals, groups and populations.
- *Risk awareness programs* include overall surveillance data given to the adolescent, family, physician or community to raise awareness to stimulate readiness and change.

- *Risk assessment, testing and screening* methods that include testing and monitoring of blood pressure, cholesterol, BMI calculations, waist circumference and physical activity.
- *Specific lifestyle behaviour change* strategies that may include introducing specific interventions to reduce smoking, increase physical activity, improve nutrition, stop smoking; and reduce overweight and obesity. These approaches involve developing skills and behavioural changes.
- *Consultation, treatment and health counseling interventions* for those who are identified with cardiovascular risks include retesting, monitoring, consultation, counseling or treatment provided in adolescent friendly environments. These approaches require using effective referral, counseling, monitoring and treatment approaches that work best with adolescents.
- *Comprehensive, overall adolescent heart health programs* that include all aspects: health promotion; risk awareness and education; assessment, testing and screening; consultation, referral, counseling and treatment.

It is generally believed that *awareness* is the first step in an individual, a community or a society to be able to take action and adopt health promoting behaviours, especially with modifiable risk factors. Studies show mixed results on the connection between knowledge of CV risk factors and the adoption of healthier behaviours. The Canadian Heart Health Initiative, 1988-2005 reported that Canadians have a low awareness of the causes of CVD. A full 30% could not even name one of the major risks factors for heart disease (smoking, high blood pressure, elevated blood cholesterol, sedentary lifestyle, diabetes).

Smalley (2004) in a United States study assessed the *attitudes* of adolescents regarding CVD risk factors and determined their potential influence on reported health habits including exercise, smoking diet and BMI. This study included 141 males and 207 female adolescents at 2 clinic sites serving mostly Medicaid or uninsured populations using self-report scales. The majority of participants agreed that obesity, smoking and high fat diets may lead to heart disease. In the sample, 50% exercised 3 times or less a week. The occurrence of obesity was higher than national averages; smokers were 1.9 times as likely to be overweight or obese; and if they had parents or grandparents with a history of heart attacks, the adolescents were 2.7 times as likely to smoke. They concluded that adolescents possess knowledge of CV risk factors as reflected in their attitude assessments; however, their lifestyle choices contradict these beliefs.

6.2 Sample adolescent cardiovascular risk projects: Research, assessment, identification, education and intervention

This chapter has reviewed many research projects and initiatives related to aspects of cardiovascular risk in adolescents. Along with the research descriptions the health promotion, awareness and prevention interventions have been described that were part of the study or evaluation. Many programs involved specific or combined lifestyle behaviour change interventions or risk factor testing. Few programs were comprehensive in nature and included: family history and engagement, assessment and testing of risk factors; education and health promotion; and a defined or researched process for referral, follow-up, assessment and treatment with adolescents. Few were specifically designed for adolescents with both a research and comprehensive educational assessment or referral intervention component. Two comprehensive programs with many of the components will be described here: a Canadian overall heart health program and a Dutch school program for the prevention of obesity.

6.2.1 Niagara Schools Healthy Heart Program (NSHHP)

The Niagara Schools Healthy Heart Program (NSHHP) in Ontario, Canada is a primary prevention program developed for adolescents continuing over 24 years since 1987 by Heart Niagara, a community organization dedicated to the prevention of CVD and heart health education for all age groups. The adolescent program initially was delivered in collaboration with public health school nurses and teachers with each respective high school. In more recent years, it was delivered by a nurse practitioner and health promotion staff of Heart Niagara along with teachers. Research collaboration over the twenty four years has developed between Heart Niagara and the Brock University Nursing Department from 2002 to present. In 2007, the Division of Cardiology of the Labatt Family Heart Center, Department of Pediatrics, and The Hospital for Sick Children in Toronto also became a research partner.

The NSHHP is a comprehensive heart health program offered to all grade nine students enrolled in a physical education course in any of the 30+ secondary schools in Niagara Region, Ontario, Canada. The Program is a comprehensive heart health initiative targeted at adolescents who are mostly 14 -15 years of age. It has the following components:

- **Family history and involvement ...** the parent/guardian is engaged to review the program and sign permission for student involvement in the research, education and screening aspects of the program. The student and the parent/guardian also complete a questionnaire on *Family History of Cardiovascular Disease* that is sent home with the students. The family is encouraged to discuss the health history, particularly of cardiovascular disease in parents, siblings and grandparents, to begin the awareness process. If the student is identified through the screening to warrant a suggested referral for follow-up to their physician, parents are informed and are often engaged in this part of the process and dialogue.
- **Screening assessment and testing ...** Height and weight are measured to calculate Body Mass Index (BMI). Blood pressure and non-fasting total cholesterol screening is also conducted by a registered nurse at the school site. If some of the testing results are over the standards established, students are referred to their primary health care provider/physician for follow-up and a letter goes to the student, parent/guardian and physician.
- **Lifestyle assessment ...** Students complete a self-rated, paper and pen survey which includes questions about dietary intake, caffeine intake, level of physical activity, sleeping habits, smoking, and other lifestyle behaviours. This data forms part *of the student's heart awar*eness of their individual lifestyle risk factors and is collected for research purposes to trend heart risk factors for this age group.
- **Health promotion educational presentations ...** A one hour heart health promotion presentation is given in the classroom by Heart Niagara staff or volunteers along with teachers in the classroom. Students are taught about heart disease risk factors, and that heart disease begins in adolescence. They are also taught that heart disease can be prevented by knowledge of family history, awareness of personal health profiles and behaviours and adopting healthy choices in nutrition, activity and choosing not to smoke. *CPR training* is also offered by staff and volunteers of HN for all students in the

classroom. This part of the program builds the capacity for the community to engage in life saving, beginning early in adolescence.

- **Referral and follow up ...** Students whose questionnaire or individual assessment indicate any of the following are referred to their family physician to discuss the results: positive family histories; non-fasting total cholesterol above 95th percentile or non-fasting total cholesterol/high density lipoprotein ratios above 5.71; body mass index above 95th percentile; smokers who request help with cessation. Students and parents are informed that while the assessment is not definitive, they should follow-up with their family doctor or paediatrician. A diagrammatic referral process has been outlined. This program has developed several helpful process charts related to referral and follow-up.

Since the inception of the NSHHP in 1987, the questionnaires and process steps have been revised, improved and updated for effectiveness and enhanced awareness research capacities. Detailed descriptions of the program and protocols have been developed; training has been conducted for those doing the screening and testing to ensure consistency in equipment and measurements; and the use of standardized criteria for blood pressure and non-fasting total cholesterol readings have been implemented. Alogorithms have been developed regarding the referral and follow-up process and alogorithms have been developed to assist physicians regarding assessment and treatment of paediatric lipids; assessment, diagnosis and treatment of paediatric hypertension; assessment and treatment of overweight and obesity; and smoking cessation (Heart Niagara, 2007).

6.2.2 The Dutch Obesity Intervention in Teenagers (NRG-DOiT) (Singh et al. 2006)

This initiative applied the Intervention Mapping (IM) protocol in the systematic development, implementation and evaluation of their school-based intervention program aimed at the prevention of excessive weight gain. The program focused on the reduction of the consumption of sugar-sweetened beverages; reduction of energy intake derives from snacks; decreased levels of sedentary behavior; and increased levels of physical activity (i. e. active transport behaviour and sports participation). Steps in the development and implementation process of bringing this program to teens are well described and outlined.

7. Conclusion

7.1 Epidemiological and surveillance data should be collected to trend and monitor CV risk factors at a population health level for planning purposes

Global and national research surveillance and population health data about CV risk factors and their associations have been collected in the last three decades. Each nation has developed research tools and methodology for this task. More sharing of research methods and findings is occurring to improve the research and to improve health. Some examples will be presented here. The lack of comparable data and consistent criteria limits cross-country and cross national research to some degree has been limited up to now, but the capacity to collaborate in interdisciplinary and global research on adolescent health holds exciting potential. Initiatives regarding the prevention of disease for different age population, including adolescents have been developed and many of them are being evaluated for their impact on reducing specific or overall risks. We are beginning to have some best practices developing to improve our practice of health promotion and risk prevention with adolescents.

World-wide, the INTERHEART (Yusef et al., 2004) project of the World Health organization is a population health based surveillance approach operating in 52 countries world-wide to monitor changes in youth health and reporting on global, national and regional trends regarding many of the CV risk factors. This project uses a common methodology and survey tool and target ages with some variations in how the research samples are selected in each country.

In the United States, there are several large, ongoing long-term studies beginning in childhood and extending through adolescence, young adulthood and to middle age. The Framington Offspring study and the Bogalusa Heart Study (BHS) examine the predisposing characteristics, risk factors, and lifestyle behaviours related to future CVD, hypertension, and diabetes. A strong and highly significant correlation has been found between the acceleration and severity of coronary and aorta atherosclerosis and the increasing numbers of risk factors. Studies show that early onset of smoking, alcohol use, poor diets, and poor lifestyles are linked with clinical cardiovascular risk and beginning cardiovascular disease (Berenson et al., 2010, p. 272).

The Pathologic Determinants of Arteriosclerosis in Youth (PDAY) has shown a strong correlation between risk factors and actual lesions in the CV system (Wissler et al, 1998).

The American Heart Association's report from the Children's Heart Health Conference - *Improving Children's Heart Health* (1994 in Chicago) focused on public health, lifestyle and behaviour and outlined recommendations in the areas of physical activity, nutrition and tobacco. The AHA (1997) statement on integrated cardiovascular health promotion in children addressed the health professional's role in adolescent heart health.

In Canada, the Canadian Community Health Survey is conducted every 4 years with the population over 15 years of age and the census is conducted every 4 years with those over 18 years of age. Data on health and lifestyle behaviours are reported for the nation, the province and the region that can be used in planning.

Risk factors change throughout age and maturation; they are different by race and gender. "In childhood just as in adulthood – risk factors ocurr in a constellation - a condition called metabolic syndrome" (Berenson et al., 2010, p. 5). Obesity and insulin are driving factors of the myriad variables associated with body fatness. Long-term studies show that obesity precedes hyperinsulimemia/ insulin resistance. Obesity in childhood is the most consistent factor predictive of adult CV system changes - cardiac enlargement and evidence of vascular stiffness (Toprak et al., 2008 in Berenson, 2010).

7.2 Education and health promotion interventions for adolescents should be integrated into school-based, community-based and family-based health promotion approaches

A call to action is required for societies, communities, schools, families, physicians and individuals armed with information to take positive action for health changes. With current, reliable, valid and comparable data and evidence, we can better identify when and where to intervene and the specific and effective nature of the intervention: how it can be specified, shaped, targeted and evaluated. If we believe that interventions can change risk factors and therefore, reduce cardiovascular disease, then research on adolescent heart health should have several important health awareness target groups for overall effectiveness outcomes:

- *Awareness for parents to* understand the power of history, modeling and their health examples to continue to improve the health of family units as a social and influential target of improved lifestyle behaviours.
- *Awareness for health practitioners* armed with evidence should lead us to how to better promote health through our programs and individual efforts working directly with adolescents. Adolescent friendly and remove barriers ..
- *Awareness for educators* to play an increased role in health teaching, education and identification of CV risks.
- *Increased awareness for the adolescent* of their heart risk factors could provide an opportune time to make positive personal changes for their health such as exercising or stopping smoking.
- *Awareness for researchers* that there is some urgency to conduct reliable and valid research on adolescent cardiovascular health and risks and to make their results available in knowledge transfer approaches to individuals, the public and health planners and policy makers.
- *Awareness for health planners, policy makers and decision makers* of the importance of health promotion and disease prevention research and education that needs to be adopted on a large-scale and at an earlier age that is well planned, funded, delivered and evaluated.

Two sample international research reviews have been conducted to assess and guide intervention development, implementation and evaluation. Flynn et al. (2006) did a synthesis of the evidence related to reducing obesity and related chronic disease risk in children and youth and described best practices and recommendations that resulted from the review. They reviewed 982 reports, of which 500 were selected for critical appraisal. Appraisal scores on program development and evaluation were used. As a result of the review, they identified best practices and made recommendations to guide researchers, educators and care providers for increased effectiveness, This review process can be applied well in adolescent cardiovascular risk research and intervention to identify best practices.

Doak et al. (2006) conducted a review of interventions and programs for the prevention of overweight and obesity in children; one of the major CV risk factors, They assessed existing interventions qualitatively and quantitatively. The review focused on school-based programs with a quantitative evaluation using athropometric outcomes and those that intervene on diet and activity related behaviours. They found that 67% (17 of 25) were "effective" based on a statistically significant reductions in BMI, as well as skinfold measures. Physical activities in schools and the reduction of television viewing are two examples of interventions that were particularly effective. They observed that programs for sub-groups (such as immigrants) are not particularly well developed or effective This study has relevance for how to conduct a systematic review of interventions for other CV risk factors.

In 2004, the American Heart Association (AHA) issued a statement on cardiovascular health promotion in the schools. They reviewed the evidence regarding the efficacy and potential of such an approach. The collective results of school-based recommendations outlined in the AHA's *Guide for improving cardiovascular health at the community level* indicated that schools are an important component of a population-based health promotion and risk reduction approach. A majority of the school-based studies reviewed in this chapter are from school initiatives and the systematic reviews prepared by Resnicow et al (1996) and Meininger (2000) supported this direction. The AHA issued specific recommendations related to heart health education and health behaviours including goals and *recommendations for school policies, and school and community linkages*.

In Australia, the *Report on health goals and targets for Australian children and youth* (1992 in Stanton, Willis & Balanda, 2000) was to reduce the frequency of preventable premature mortality; to reduce the impact of disability (new or developed); to reduce the incidence of vaccine-preventable disease; to reduce the impact on conditions occurring in adulthood which have their origins in early manifestations in childhood or adolescence and; enhance family and social functioning (p. 182). *Better health* outcomes for Australians (CDHSH, 1994) is a document addressing the issue of youth health with a particular focus on cardiovascular disease, cancer, mental health and injury.

The report from the American Heart Association's Children's Heart Health Conference - Improving Children's Heart Health that had a focus on public health, lifestyle and behaviour developed recommendations in the areas of physical activity, nutrition and tobacco. An AHA (1997) statement on integrated cardiovascular health promotion in children oultined the health professional's role in adolescent heart health.

7.3 Treatment and clinical interventions

To merely identify those adolescents at risk is not enough. There also needs to be well trained primary care providers who are aware and knowledgeable about heart disease and skilled at working with adolescents, families, schools and communities in motivation, consultation and delivering adolescent friendly care. Laudenbach (2004) suggests we also offer family strengths-based interventions to help the entire family to get fit and heart healthy. The same is true of adopting a strengths-based approach where health care providers work with the community to build the capacity for health for all. Building a wider healthy community with good eating and physical activity habits would also positively affect adolescent cardiovascular health.

Treatment of cardiovascular risk factors is considered a challenging and evolving aspect of preventive medicine, especially with adolescents and young adults. Lule et al. (2006) suggest that efforts to improve the health of young people may be even more complex and challenging than for other age groups because many of their health issues are behaviour-based and actual symptoms of CVD may not be evident, or seen as serious yet. Walker et al. (2002) found few published reports of screening and health promotion in family practice settings and Walker and Townsend (1998) reported that according to 200 health care providers in 200 U. S. cities, youth are at a point when health intervention could make a difference, but that preventive, primary reproductive, and behavioural health care is not well matched to adolescent needs and preferences. The Canadian Task Force on Preventive Health care (2000) suggested that an adolescent friendly atmosphere is needed and teens reported that issues of confidentiality and access to telephone and good written information is needed. Access to computer health information and dialogue has become important. The

WHO (2002) described the features of adolescent friendly health services and called for appropriate changes to create them

7.4 A comprehensive model

The evidence is strong that cardiovascular risk factors begin and can be identified in childhood and adolescence that influence the development of CVD in adulthood. Evidence is growing that some effective best practices are developing about both individual approaches and holistic approaches in health promotion, early screening, and health care interventions that may have some positive potential for prevention and intervention. Interdisciplinary and interprofessional teams of researchers, clinicians, educators, parents and care providers are working together on this health issue and informing each other of their outcomes. Programs and policies are emerging from the information to guide practice to improve health and reduce risk. The time to act is now.

A comprehensive model for cardiovascular risk assessment, identification, education, health promotion, referral and treatment for adolescents (Kilty &Prentice, 2011)

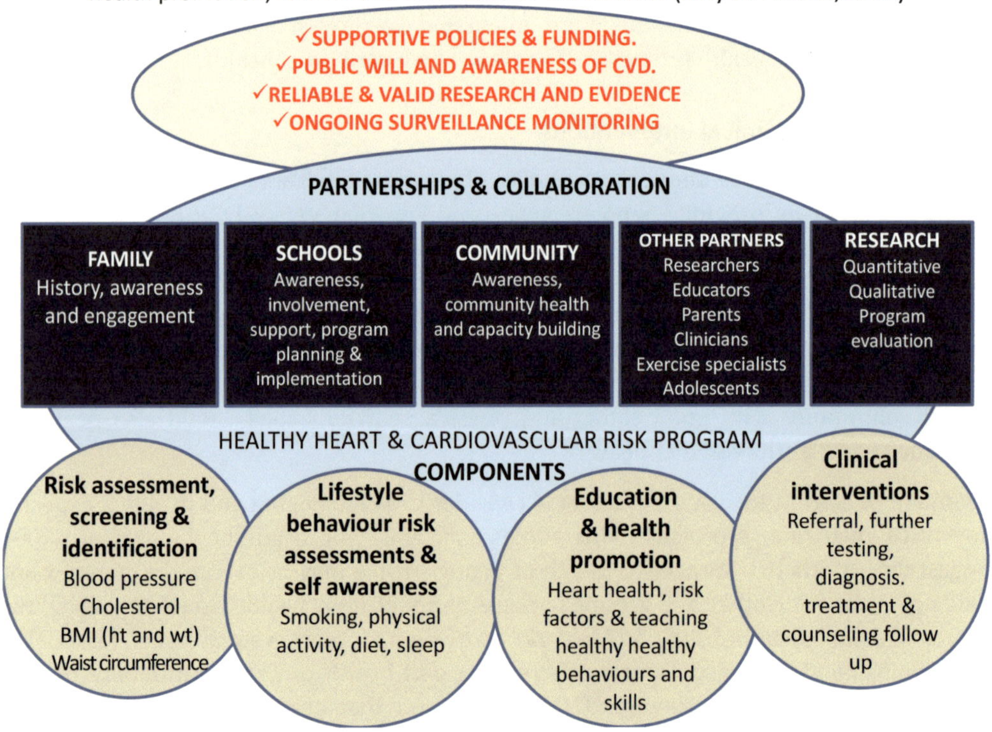

"Unlike treatment for problems that produce symptoms, preventive medicine is optional"

(Kamerow, 2008, p. 23)

"Knowing is not enough; we must apply. Willing is not enough; we must do."

Goethe

8. References

Aatola, H., Koivistoinen, T., Hutri-Kahonen, N., Juonala, M. et al. (2010). Lifetime fruit and vegetable consumption and arterial pulse wave velocity in adulthood: The cardiovascular risk in young Finns study. *Circulation, 122,* 2521-2528.

Adler, N. E., & Newman, K. (2002). Socioeconomic disparities in health: Pathways and policies. *Health Affairs, 21,* 60-76.

Allen, M., & Warner, M. (2002). A developmental model of health and nursing. *Journal of Family Nursing, 8*(2), 96-135.

American Heart Association (2007). *Risk factors and coronary heart disease.* Retrieved May 31, 2007 from http://www.americanheart.org/presneter.jhtml?indentifier=4726.

Andersen, R. T., Sorlie, P., Backlund, E., Johnson, N., & Kaplan, G. A. (1997). Mortality effects of community socioeconomic status. *Epidemiology, 8,* 42-47.

Andersen, L. B., Wedderkopp, N., Hansen, H. S. Cooper, A. R., & Froberg, K. (2003). Biological cardiovascular risk factors in Danish children and adolescents: The European Youth Heart Study. *Preventive Medicine, 37*(4), 363-367.

Andersen, R. C., Crespo, C. S., Bartlett, S. J., & Pratt, M. (1998). Relationship of physical activity and television watching with body weight and level of fatness in children. *Journal of the American Medical Association, 179,* 938-942.

Appel, S. J., Harrell, J. S., 7Deng, S. (2002). Racial and socioeconomic differences in risk factors for cardiovascular disease among southern rural women. *Nursing Research, 51,* 140-

Barker, J. G., Bolitho, F., & Bertrand, L. D. (1999). The predictors of adolescent smoking. Journal of Social Service Research, *26*(1), 51-66.

Berenson, G. S., S. R., Srinivasan, Fernandez, C., & Xu, J. (2010). Can adult cardiologists play a role in the prevention of heart disease beginning in childhood? *MDCVI, 4,* 4-9.

Berkey, C. S., Rockett, R. H., Gillman, M. W. & Colditz, G. A. (2003). One-year changes in activity and inactivity among 10-15 year old boys and girls: Relationship to body mass index. *Pediatrics, 111,* 836-843.

Bhattacharjee, R., Kheirandish-Gozal, Pillar, G., & Gozal, D. (2009). Cardiovascular complications of sleep apnea syndrome: Evidence from children, *Progress in Cardiovascular Diseases, 51* (5), 416-433.

Bond, L. A., & Compas, B. E. (Eds.). (1989). *Primary prevention and promotion in schools.* Beverley Hills, CA: Sage.

Bouziotas, C., & Koutedakis, Y. (2003). A three year study of coronary heart disease risk factors in Greek adolescents. *Pediatric Exercise Science, 15*(1), 9-18.

Brotons, C., Ribera, A., Perich, R. M., Abrodos, D., Magana, P., Pablo, S., et al. (1998). Worldwide distribution of blood lipids and lipoproteins in childhood and adolescence: a review study. *Atherosclerosis, 139*(1), 1-9.

Buchan, D. S., Ollis, S., Young, J. D. Thomas, N. E., Cooper, S. M., Tong, T. K., Nie, J., Malina, R. M., & Baker, J. S. (2011). The effects of time and intensity of exercise on novel and established markers of CVD in adolescent youth. *American Journal of Human Biology, 23*(4), 517-526.

Canadian Community Health Survey (2004/2005; 2007/2008). Statistics Canada.

Canadian Heart and Stroke Foundation (2010) A perfect storm of heart disease looming on our horizon. *Annual Report. Canadian Heart Health Initiative* 1988-2003

Cappuccio, F. P., Cooper, D., D'Elia, L. et al. (2011). Sleep duration predicts cardiovascular outcomes: A systematic review and meta-analysis of prospective studies. *European Heart Journal, 32*(12), 1484-1492.

Chmiel-Polec, Z., & Cybulska, J. (2008). Smoking and other risk factors of cardiovascular disease, connected with arteriosclerosis among youth. *Przegl Lek, 65,* 437-445.

Chobanian, A.V., Bakris, G.L., Black, H.R., Cushman, W.C., Green, L.A.,& Izzo Jr., J. L. (2003). National High Blood Pressure Education Program Coordinating Committee. *JAMA, 289* (19), 2560-2572.

Chronic Disease Genomics Project. Cardiovascular disease and family history. Minnesota Department of Health. http://www.health.mn.us/divs/hpcd/genomics/resources/fs/cv.html Retrieved May, 2007.

Cole, T.J., Bellizzi, M.C. Flegal, Flegal, K.M., & Dietz, W.H. (2000). Establishing a standard definition for child overweight and obesity worldwide international survey. *BMJ, 320,* 1-6.

Colhoun, H. M., Hemingway, H., & Poulter, N. R. (1998). Socio-economic status and blood pressure: an overview analysis. *Hypertension, 12,* 91-110.

Cox, A.M., McKevitt, C., Rudd, A. G., & Wolfe, C. D. A. (2006). Socioeconomic status and strole. Lancet Neurology, 5, 181-188.

Daniels, S.R., Greer, F.R., and the Committee on Nutrition. (2008). Lipid Screening and cardiovascular health in childhood. *Pediatrics, 122* (1), 198-208.

Daniels, S. R., Jacobson, M. S., & McCrindle, B. W., Eckel, R. H., & Sanner, B. M., (2009). American Heart Association childhood obesity research summit: Executive summary. *Circulation, 119,* 2114-2123.

Dietz, L. J., & Matthews, K. A. (2011). Depressive Symptoms and subclinical markers of cardiovascular disease in adolescents. *Journal of Adolescent Health, 48,* 579-584.

Doak, C. M., Visscher, L. S., Renders, C. M. & Seidell, J. C. (2006). The prevention of overweight and obesity in children: A review of interventions and programmes. International Life Sciences Institute, 7, 111-136.

dos Santos Cavalcanti, C. B., de Barros, M. V., Meneses, A. L., Santos, C. M., Azevedo, M. P., & Guimaraes, J. (2010). Abdominal obesity in adolescents: Prevalenece and association with physical activity and eating habits. *Arq. Bras. Cardiology, 94* (3),

Du, Y., Rosner, B. M., Knopf, H., Schwarz, S., Doren, M., & Scheidt-Nave, C. (2011). Hormonal contraceptive use among adolescent girls in Germany in relation to health behavior and biological cardiovascular risk factors. *Journal of Adolescent Health, 48,* 331-337.

Erikson, E. H. (1950). *Childhood and society.* New York, NY: Norton (1950); Triad/Paladin (1977), p.242.

Eversen, S. A., Maty, S. C., Lynch, J. W., & Kaplan, G. A. (2002). Epidemiological evidence for the relation between socioeconomic status and depression, obesity and diabetes. *Journal Psychosomatic Research, 53,* 891-895.

Ebbeling, C. B., Pawlak, D. B., & Ludwig, D. S. (2002). Childhood obesity: Public-health crisis, common sense cure. *Lancet, 360,* 473-482.

Flegal, K.M. & Ogden, C.L. (2011). Childhood obesity: Are we all speaking the same language? *Advances in Nutrition,* 2, 1595-1665.

Flouris, A. D., Canham, C. H., Faught, B. E., & Klentrou, P. (2007). Prevalence of cardiovascular disease risk in Ontario adolescents. *Arch. Dis. Child, 92*, 521-523.

Flynn, M. A., McNeil, D. A., Maloff, B., Mutasingwa, D., Wu, M., Ford, C., & Tough, S. C. (2006). Reducing obesity and related chronic disease risk in children and youth: A synthesis of evidence with "best practice" recommendations. *The International Association for the Study of Obesity, 7*, 7-66.

Ford-Gilboe, M. (2002). *Development and testing a measure of family health promotion behavior: The Health Options Scale.* Unpublished manuscript, Wayne State University, Detroit, Michigan.

Ford-Gilboe, M. (1997). Family strengths, motivation, and resources as predictors of health promotion in single-parent, and two-parent families. *Research in Nursing and Health, 20*, 205-217.

Ford, E.S., Li, C., Zhao, G., & Mokdad, A. H. (2009). Concentrations of low-density lipoprotein cholesterol and total cholesterol among children and adolescents in the United States. *Circulation, 119*, 1108-1115.

Freedman, D. S., Khan, L., Dietz, W. H., Srinivasan, S. R., & Berenson, G. S. (2001).Relationship of childhood obesity to coronary heart disuse risk factors in adulthood: The Bogalus Heart Study. *Pediatrics, 108*(3), 712-718.

Gidding, S.S., Deckelbaum, R. J., Strong, W., & Moller, J. H. (1995). Improving children's heart health: A report from the American Heart Association's Children's Heart Health Conference. (1995). *The Journal of School Health, 65*(4), 129-132.

Gordon-Larsen, P., McMurray, R. G., & Popkin, B. M. Determinants of adolescent physical activity and inactivity patterns, *Pediatrics, 105*(6).

Gortmaker,S. L., Must, A., Sobol, A. M., Peterson, K., Colditz, G. A. & Dietz, W. H. (1996). Television viewing as a cause of increasing obesity among children in the United States, 1986-1990. *Arch Pediatric Adolescent Medicine, 150*, 356-362.

Gozal, D., Kheirandish-Gozal,L.,Serpero,L.D., Sans Capdevila,O., & Dayyat, E. (2007). Obstructive sleep apnea and endothelial function in school-aged nonobese children: Effect of adenotonsillectomy, *Circulation, 116*, 2307-2314.

Grotto, I., Huerta, M., & Sharbi, Y. (2008). Hypertension and socioeconomic status. *Curr. Opin. Cardio., 23*, 335-339.

Greenlund, K. J., Johnson, C., Wattigney, W., Bao, W., Webber, L. S., & Berenson, G. S. (1996). Trends in cigarette smoking among children in a southern community 1976-1994: The Bogalusa Heart Study. *American Journal of Pediatric Obesity, 89*(8), 1345-1348.

Gutin, B., & Owens, S. (1999). Role of exercise interventions in improving body fat distribution and risk profile in children. American *Journal of Human Biology, 11*(2), 237-247.

Hayman, L. L., Williams, C. L., Daniels, S. R., Steinberger,J., Paridon, S., Dennison, B. A., & McCrindle, B. W. (2004). Cardiovascular health promotion in the schools: a statement for health and education professionals and child health advocates from the Committee on Atherosclerosis, hypertension, and obesity in Youth (AHOY) of the Council on Cardiovascular Disease in the Young. *Circulation,110*(5), 2266-2275.

Health Canada (2011) *Canada Food Guide.* Ottawa, ON.

Health Canada. (2011). *Trends in the health of Canadian youth: Youth health behaviours in school-aged children.* Ottawa, ON.

Heart Niagara. (2008). *Identifying and managing adolescent cardiovascular risk.* Niagara Falls, ON: Heart Niagara.

Hemmings, S., Connor, A., Maffulli, N., & Morrissey, D. (2011). Cardiovascular disease risk factors in adolescent British South Asians and whites: A pilot study. *Postgraduate Medicine, The Royal London Hospital, 123*(2), 104-111.

Hennekens & Bering (1987) p. 3

Huxley, R., Mendis, S., Zheleznyakov, E., Reddy, S. & Chan, C. (2010). Body mass index, waist circumference and waist: hip ratio as predictors of cardiovascular risk- a review of the literature. *European Journal of Clinical Nutrition, 64,* 16-22.

Institute of Medicine. (2002/2005). *Dietary reference intakes for energy, carbohydrates, fiber, fat, fatty acids, cholesterol, protein, and amino acids.* Washington, DC: The National Academies Press.

Kamerow, D. (2008). Should we screen for and treat childhood dyslipidaemia? *BMJ, 337,* a886.

Kaplan, G. A., & Keil, J. E. (1993). Socioeconomic factors and cardiovascular disease: A review of the literature. *Circulation, 88,* 1973-1998.

Kavey, R. W. (2010). How sweet it is: Sugar-sweetened beverage consumption, obesity, and cardiovascular risk in childhhood. *Journal of the American Dietetic Association. 110(*10), 1456-1460.

Kilty, H. & Prentice, D. (2010) Adolescent cardiovascular risk factors: A follow-up study of nurse referrals to physicians. *Clinical Nursing Research Journal, 19* (1), 6-20.

King, A. J. C. & Coles, B. (1992). *The health of Canadian Youth.* Health and Welfare Canada, Ottawa, ON.

Krebs, N. F., Baker, R. D., Greer, F. R., Hayman, M. B., Jaksic, T., et al. (2003). Policy Statement: Prevention of Pediatric Overweight and Obesity Prevention Committee on Nutrition. *Pediatrics, 112*(2), 424-435.

Krishnan, S., Copeland, K. C., Bright, B. C., Gardner, A. W., Blackett, P. R., & Fields, D. A. (2011). Impact of type 1 diabetes and body weight status on cardiovascular risk factors in adolescent children. *The Journal of Clinical Hypertension, 13* (5), 351- 356.

Laing, S.P., Swerdlow, A. J., & Slater, S.D. et al. (1999). The British Diabetic Association and cohort study, II: Cause-specific mortality in patients with insulin-treated diabetes mellitus. *Diabetic Medicine, 16,* 466-471.

Libby, P., Nathan, D. M., & Abraham, K. et al. (2005). Report of the National Heart, Lung and blood Institute - National Institute of Digestive and Kidney Diseases Working Group on Cardiovascular Complications of Type 1 Diabetes Mellitus. *Circulation, 111,* 3489-3493. .

Laudenbach, L., & Ford-Gilboe, M. (2004). Psychometric testing of health options scale with adolescents. *Journal of Family Nursing, 10*(1), 121-138.

Lee, C.M., Huxley, R., Wildman, R.P., & Woodward, M. (2008). Indices of abdominal obesity are better discriminators of cardiovascular risk factor than BMI: a meta analysis. *Journal of Clinical Epidemiology 61,* 646-653.

Lobelo, F., Pate, R. R., Dowda, M., Liese. A. D., & Daniles, S. R. (2010). Cardiorespiratory fitness and clustered cardiovascular disease risk in U.S. adolescents. *Journal of Adolescent Health, 47,* 352-359.

Lule, E., Rosen, J. E., Singh, S., Knowles, J. C., & Behrman, J. R. (2006). *Adolescent health programs. In disease control priorities in developing countries.*New York: Oxford University.

Luma, G. B. & Spiotta, R. T. (2006). Hypertension in children and adolescents. *American Family Physician, 73* (9), 1558-1566.

Ma, G.S., Ji, C.Y., Ma, J., Mi, J., Sung, R.Y., Xiong, F., Yan, W.L., Hu, X.Q., Li, Y.P., Du, S.M., Fang, H., Y., & Jiang, J.,X. (2010). Waist circumference reference values for screening cardiovascular risk factors in Chinese children and adolescents. *Biomedical and Environmental Sciences 23,* 21-31.

Maggio, A. B. R., Aggoun, Y., Martin, X. E., Marchand, L. M., Beghetti, M., & Farpour-Lambert, N. J. (2010). Long-termfollow-up of cardiovascular risk factors after exercise training in obese children. *International Journal of Pediatric Obesity,* 6(2), 603-610.

Manios, Y., Magkos, F., Christakis, G. & Kafatos, A. G. (2005). Twenty-year dynamics in adiposity and blood lipids of Greek children: Regional differences in Crete persist. *Acta Paediatric, 94*(7), 859-865.

Mathers, C. D. (1998). *Health differentials among adult Australians aged 25-64.* Canberra: Australian Institute of Health and Welfare. Health Series WO-1.

McCrindle, B. W. (2000). Screening and management of hyperlipidemia in children. *Pediatric Annals, 29* (8), 500-508.

McCrindle, B., Manlhiot, C., Millar, K., Gibson, D., Stearne, K., Kilty, H., Prentice, D., Wong, H., Chatal, N & Stafford, D. (2010). Population trends towards increasing cardiovascular risk factors in Canadian adolescents. *The Journal of Pediatrics, 157* (5), 837-843.

McCusker, M. E., Yoon, P. W., Gwinn, M., Malarcher, A. M., Neff, L., & Khoury, M. J. (2004). Family history of heart disease and cardiovascular disease risk-reducing behaviors. *Genetic Medicine, 6*(3), 153-158.

McGill, H.C., McMahan, C. A., Zieskie, Malcolm, G. T. Oalmann, M. C. & Strong, J. P. (1997). Effects of serum lipoproteins and smoking on arthrosclerosis in young men and women. The PDAY Research Group. Pathobiological determinants of atherosclerosis in youth. *Arterioscler, Throm. Vasc Bio, 17*(1), 95-106.

Meininger, J. C. (2000). School-based interventions for primary prevention of cardiovascular disease: Evidence of effect for minority populations. *American Review of Nursing Research, 18,* 219-244.

Michos,E. D., Nasir, K., Rumberger, J. A., Vasamreddy, V., Braunstein, J. B., Budoff, M. J., & Blumenthal, R. S. (2004). Relation of family history of premature coronary heart disease and metabolic risk factors to risk of coronary arterial calcium in asymptomatic subjects. *The American Journal of Cardiology, 95*(5), 655-657.

Murabito, J. M., Nam, B. H., D'Agostino, S. B. Jr., Lloyd-Jones, D. M., O'Donnell, C. J., & Wilson, P. W. (2004). Accuracy of offspring reports of parental cardiovascular disease history: The Framingham Offspring Study. *Annuals of Internal Medicine, 140,* 434-440.

Nakumura, T., Tsubono,Y., Kameda-Takemura, K., Funahashi, T., Yamashita et al. (2001). Magnitude of sustained multiple risk factors for ischemic heart disease in Japanese employees: A case-control study. *Japanese Circ Journal, 65,* 11-17.

Nasir, K., Michos, E. D., Rumberger, J. B., Braunstein, W. S., Post, Budoff, M. J., & Blumenthal, R. S.(2004). Coronary artery calcification and family history of premature coronary heart disease: sibling history is more strongly associated than parental history. *Circulation, 110*, 2150-2156.

National High Blood Pressure Education Program Working Group on High Blood Pressure in Children and Adolescents (2004). The Fourth Report on the diagnosis, evaluation, and treatment of high blood pressure in children and adolescents. *Pediatrics, 114*, 555-576.

Newman, W.P., Freedman, D. S. Voors, A. W. et al., (1986) Relation of serum lipoprotein levels and systolic blood pressure to early atherosclerosis: The Bogalusa Heart Study. *New England Journal of Medicine, 314*(3), 138-144.

O'Donnell, C. J. (2004). Family history, subclinical atherosclerosis, and coronary heart disease risk: Barriers and opportunities for the use of family history information in risk prediction and prevention. *Circulation, Journal of the American Heart Association, 110*, 2074-2076.

Ogden, C. L., Carroll, M. D., Curtin, L. R., Lamb, M. M.& Flegal, K. M. (2010). Prevalence of high body mass index in US children and adolescents. *JAMA, 303*, 242-249.

Ogden, C. L., Flegal, K. M., Carroll, M. D., & Johnson, C. L. (2002). Prevalence trends in overweight among US children and adolescents 1999-2000. *Journal of the American Medical Association, 288*, 1728-1732.

Onkamo,P.,Vaananen, P., Karvonen, M., & Tuomilehto, J. (1999). Worldwide increase in incidence of Type 1 diabetes – the analysis of data on published incidence trends. *Diabetologia, 43*(10), 1334-1336.

Paradis, G., Lambert, M., O'Laughlin, J., et al. (2003). The Quebec child and adolescent health and social survey: Design and methods of a cardiovascular risk factor survey for youth. *Canadian Journal of Cardiology, 19*, 523-531.

Park, J. W., Yun, J. E., Park, T., Cho, E., Jee, S. H. Jang, Y., Beaty, T. H., Samet, & J. M. (2007). Family history of diabetes and risk of atherosclerosis cardiovascular disease in Korean men and women. *Atherosclerosis*, 197(1), 224-231.

Pollitt, R. A., Rose, K. M. & Kaufman, J. S. (2005). Evaluating the evidence for models of the life course socioeconomic factors and cardiovascular outcomes: A systematic review. *BMC Public Health, 5*, 7.

Prentice, D., Kilty, H. L., Stearne, K. & Dobbin, S. (2008). Prevalence of cardiovascular risk factors in grade nine students. *The Canadian Journal of Cardiovascular Nursing 18*(3), 12-16.

Prentice, D. Kilty, H., Stearne, K., & Dobbin, S. (2006). *An adolescent healthy heart program: A three year review.* Unpublished manuscript.

Rafraf, M., Gargari, B. P., & Safaiyan, A. (2010). Prevalence of prehypertension and hypertension among adolescent high school girls in Tabriz, Iran. *Food and Nutrition Bulletin, 31*(3), 461-465.

Raj, M., & Kumar, K. (2010). Obesity in children and adolescents. *India Journal of Medical Research*, 598-607.

Reed, K. E., Warburton, D. E. R., & McKay, H. A. (2007). Determining cardiovascular disease risk in elementary school children: Developing a healthy heart score. *Journal of Sports Science and Medicine, 6*, 142-148.

Reedy, J., & Krebs-Smith, S. M. (2010). Dietary sources of energy, solid fats, and added sugars among children and adolescents in the United States. *Journal of the American Dietetic Association, 110*(10), 1477-1484.

Resnico, K., Baranawski, T., Ahluwahlia, J. S., & Braithwaite, R. L. (1999). Cultural sensitivity in public health defined and demystified. *Ethnicity and Disease, 9,* 10-21. et al. (1996).

Robinson,T. N. (1999).Reducing children's television viewing to prevent obesity: A randomized controlled trail. *JAMA, 282,* 1561-1567.

Schreier, H. M. C., & Chen, E. (2010). Socioeconomic status in one's childhood predict offspring cardiovascular risk. *Brain, Behaviour, and Immunity, 24,* 1324-1331.

Shuener, M. T. (2004). Clinical application of genetic risk assessment strategies for coronary artery disease: genotypes. *Primary Care, 34,* 711-737.

Singh, A. S., Chin, M. J. M., Paw, A., Kremmers, S. P. J., Visscher, T. L. S., Brug, J., Mechelen, W. (2006). Design of the Dutch intervention in teenagers (NRG-DOiT): systematic development, implementation and evaluation of a school-based intervention aimed at the prevention of excessive weight gain in adolescents. *BMC Public Health, 6,* 304.

Sdringola, S., Patel, D., & Gould, K. L. (2001). High prevalence of myocardial perfusion abnormalities on positron emission tomography in asymptomatic persons with a parent or sibling with coronary artery disease. *Circulation, 103,* 496-501.

Shakley, D. C., & Clarke, N. W. (2005). Impact of socio-economic status on bladder cancer outcome. *Current Opinion Urology, 15,* 328-331.

Shatoor, A. S., Mahfouz, A. A., Khan, M. Y., Daffalla, A. A. Mostafa, O., & Hammad, R. K. (2010). Cardiovascular risk factors among adolescent secondary school boys in Ahad Rufeida, Southwestern Saudi Arabia. *Journal of Tropical Pediatrics, 57*(5), 382-384.

Shields, M. (2005). Youth smoking. Statistics Canada. Catalogue 82-003. *Health Reports, 16* (3).

Siega-Riz, A. M., Popkin, B. M., & Carson, T. (1998). Trends on breakfast concumption for children in the United States from 1965-1991. *American Journal of Clinical Nutrition, 67*(4), 7485-7565.

Smith, K. J., Gall, S. L., McNaughton, S. M., Blizzard, L. Dwyer, T., & Venn, A. J. (2010). *American Journal of Clinical Nutrition, 92,* 316-1325.

Spicuzza, L. Leonardi, E., & La Rosa, M. (2009). Pediatric sleep apnea: Early onset of the 'syndrome?" *Sleep Medicine Reviews, 13,* 111-112.

Stanton, W.R., Willis, M., & Balanda, K. P. (2000). Development of an instrument for monitoring adolescent health issues. *Health Education Research, 15*(2), 181-190.

Stary, H. C. (1989). Evolution and progression of atherosclerosis lesions in coronary arteries of children and young adults. *Atherosclerosis, 9,* 119-132.

Tanusputro, P., Manuel, D. G., Leung, M. et al.(2003). Risk factors for cardiovascular disease in Canada. *Canadian Journal of Cardiology, 19,* 1249-1269.

Toprak, A., Wand, H., Chen, W., Paul, T., Ruan, I., Srinivasan, S., & Berenseon, G. (2009). Prehypertension and black-white contrasts in cardiovascular risk in young adults: Bogalus Heart Study. *Journal of Hypertension, 27*(2), 243-250.

Walker, Z., Townsend, J., Oakey, L., Donovan, C., Smith, H., Hurst, J. et al. (2002). Health promotion for adolescents in primary care: A randomized clinical trial. *BMJ, 325,* 524-527.

Walker, Z. A., & Townsend, J. (1998). Promoting adolescent mental health in primary care: A review of the literature. *Journal of Adolescence, 21,* 621-634.

Wang, M. Q.,Fitzhugh, E. C., Eddy, J. M., Westerfield, R. C. & Fu, Q. (1998). Tobacco use among school adolescents: National socio-demographic risk profiles. *Journal of Health Education, 29*(3), 174-178.

Welsh, J., Sharma, A., Abramson, J. L., Vaccarino, V., Gillespie, M. S., & Vos, M. B. (2010). Caloric sweetener consumption and dyslipidemia among US adults. *JAMA, 303*(15), 1490-1497.

Williams, C. L., Hayman, L. L., Daniels, S. R., Robinson, T. M., Steinberger, J., Paridon, S., & Bizarre, T. (2002). *Circulation, 106*(9), 1178.

Winter, A., L., de Guia, N. A., Ferrence, R., & Cohen, J. E. (2002). The relationship between body weight perceptions, weight control behaviours and smoking status in adolescents. *Canadian Journal of Public Health, 93*(5), 362-365.

Wissler, R. W., Strong, J. P. (1998). Risk factors and progression of atheroscerlosis in youth. PDAY Research Group. Pathological Determinants of athrosclerosis in youth. *American Journal of Pathology, 153*(4), 1023-1033.

Wong, N. D., Black, H. R., & Gardin, J. M. (2000). *Preventive cardiology: A practical approach.* New York, NY: McGraw Hill.

World Health Organization (2011). *Waist Circumference and Waist-Hip Ratio: Report of a WHO Expert Consultation.* WHO, Geneva, 8-11.

World Health Organization (2009). Global health risks. WHO, Geneva, Switzerland.

World Health Organization. (2008). *Inequalities to young people's health: Key findings from the Health Behaviour in School-aged Children (HBSC) 2005/2006 survey*. WHO, Geneva, Switzerland,

World Health Organization. (2002).Adolescent friendly health services: An agenda for change. WHO, Geneva. WHO/FCH/CAH/02/14.

World Health Organization. (2005). *Preventing chronic diseases: A vital investment.* World Global Report. Geneva: World Health Organization.

World Health Organization (1995). *Physical status: The use and interpretation of anthropometry.* WHO Technical Report Series 854

Yoshinaga, M., Takahashi, H., Shinomiya, M., Miyazaki, A., Kuribayashi, N., & Ichida, F. (2010). Impact of having one cardiovascular risk factor on other cardiovascular risk factor levels in adolescents. *Journal of Atherosclerosis and Thrombosis, 17*(11), 1167-1175.

Yoshinaga, M., Sameshina, K., Tanaka, Y., Arata, M., Wada, A., & Takahashi, H. (2008). Association between the number of cardiovascular risk factors and each risk factor in elementary school children *Circulation, 72*, 1594-1597.

Yusuf, S., Reddy, S., Ounpuu, S., & Anand, S. (2001). Global burden of cardiovascular diseases Part I: General considerations, the epidemiologic transition, risk factors, and impact of urbanization. *Circulation, 104*, 2746-2753.

Yusuf, S., Hawken, S., Ounpuu, S., Dans, T., Avezum, A., Lanasa, F., McQueen, M., Budaj, A., Pais, P., Varigos, J., & Lisheng. (2004). Effect of potentially modifiable risk factors associated with myocardial infarction in 52 countries (the INTERHEART study): case-control study. *The Lancet, 364*, 937-952.

3

Novel and Traditional Cardiovascular Risk Factors in Adolescents

Alice P.S. Kong[1] and Kai Chow Choi[2]
[1]Department of Medicine and Therapeutics, Faculty of Medicine, The Chinese University of Hong Kong,
[2]The Nethersole School of Nursing, Faculty of Medicine, The Chinese University of Hong Kong, Hong Kong

1. Introduction

Cardiovascular diseases are prevalent conditions which impose significant negative impacts on the healthcare system. According to World Health Organization (WHO), non-communicable diseases (NCD) including cardiovascular diseases account for more than 60% of all deaths globally. Overweight/obesity, diabetes, hypertension and dyslipidemia are all traditional cardiovascular risk factors in adults. Of particular concern, adolescence obesity and its associated cardiovascular risk and co-morbidities have substantial tracking into adulthood (1-4).

Advances in technology of agriculture have helped to increase food production resulting in easily available, excessive provision of food in many developed countries. Urbanization also leads to changes in leisure activities from doing sports to television viewing and computer games. As a consequence to increasing demand from school and leisure activities, sleep deprivation is another novel risk factor contributing to the escalation of cardiovascular risk in the youth populations. In addition, exposure to heavy metals is increasingly recognized as a consequence of urbanization and may contribute to premature atherosclerosis.

2. Traditional cardiovascular risk factors in adolescents

2.1 Overweight and obesity

Overweight/obesity is an important and well-known cardiovascular risk factor in children, adolescents and adults. Obesity is closely associated with clustering of cardiovascular risk factors with insulin resistance being the possible link(5). Obesity is also associated with increased risk of a number of co-morbidities and premature mortality in both adult and the youth populations (2, 6-11). In a British cohort followed up for 57 years, overweight in childhood was associated with 1.5 times increased risk of all-cause mortality and two-fold increased risk of ischemic heart disease (6). Co-morbidities of adolescence obesity include type 2 diabetes mellitus, micro-inflammation, atherogenic dyslipidemia, hypertension, left ventricular hypertrophy, premature atherosclerosis leading to cardiovascular diseases, obstructive sleep apnoea, gastroesophageal reflux disease, depression and other psychosocial abnormalities (2, 12-16). Clustering of traditional cardiovascular risk factors, namely metabolic syndrome, is noted to have ethnic disparities (17)and the prevalence also varies according to the different definitions of metabolic syndrome adopted(11, 18). Despite the controversies regarding the exact definitions of metabolic syndrome in both adults and children(19, 20), International Diabetes Federation (IDF) recently suggests abdominal obesity as the core criteria in making a diagnosis of metabolic syndrome(21), highlighting the pivotal role of obesity in linking these cardiometabolic abnormalities and cardiovascular diseases.

Childhood obesity can predict the cardiovascular risk in adulthood (22). With increasing childhood obesity, there is increasingly early onset of atherosclerosis(23). In a study involving Hong Kong Chinese overweight children aged 9-12 years (mean BMI 25 ± 3 kg/m^2), BMI was independently associated with impaired arterial endothelial function and increased carotid intimal medial thickness, which are early markers of atherosclerosis (24). An important message from this study is that these obesity-related early vascular dysfunctions are partially reversible by lifestyle modifications (25).

Prevalence of childhood and adolescence overweight/obesity has marked variation among developed and developing countries. The prevalence of childhood and adolescence obesity has tripled between 1980 and 2000 in United States (US) and doubled between 1985 and 1995 in Australia(26). In a systemic review of published literatures examining data of prevalence of overweight/obesity among children living in developing countries, lowest prevalence was found in India and Sri Lanka whereas highest prevalence was found in Eastern Europe and the Middle East(27).When comparing epidemiological and clinical studies examining childhood and adolescence overweight/obesity, the diagnostic criterion used to define overweight/obesity should be interpreted with cautions. Despite the importance to identify overweight/obese individuals and screen for associated cardiovascular risk factors early, there is no consensus regarding the diagnostic criteria of childhood and adolescence obesity (28). Compared to adults, assessment of overweight and obesity in children and adolescents are different and not that straightforward. We need to take growth and puberty into consideration because BMI is anticipated to change with age and depends on gender. Gender difference is particularly important in the assessment of childhood and adolescence obesity as girls and boys enter puberty at different pace. In children and adolescents, there are ongoing debates regarding the optimal cutoff values of BMI and waist circumference (WC) to define childhood and adolescence overweight and obesity with various diagnostic criteria adopted by different countries and authorities (28-32).

From published pediatric literatures, at least four diagnostic criteria have been used for the definition of overweight and obesity in children and adolescents (11, 28):

1. An international BMI-for-age reference curve for defining overweight and obesity in children 2 to 18 years of age by the US National Center for Health Statistics, Centers for Disease Control and Prevention (CDC) and the International Obesity Task Force (IOTF) in 2000 (IOTF criteria) (31).

These criteria were based on median BMI by age and gender in six nationally representative datasets from Brazil, Hong Kong, Netherlands, Singapore, United Kingdom (UK) and the US from an international growth survey in 2000. These surveys had over 10,000 subjects each and altogether covered 97,876 boys and 94,841 girls. Overweight and obesity were defined as BMI-for-age ≥25 and ≥30 kg/m² respectively.

2. A national BMI reference curve for Chinese children and adolescents reported by the Group of China Obesity Task Force (COTF) in 2004 (COTF criteria) (33).

These criteria were based on the Chinese National Survey on Students Constitution and Health in 2000 involving 244,200 primary and secondary Chinese students aged 7–18 years. Overweight and obesity were defined as BMI-for-age ≥24 and ≥28 kg/m² respectively.

3. CDC 2000 Growth Charts for the US (CDC criteria) (34).

These criteria were based on the US National data collected in a series of 5 surveys between 1963 and 1994 for children and adolescents aged 2–20 years. Overweight and obesity were defined as BMI-for-age ≥85th and ≥95th percentiles respectively.

4. The Hong Kong Growth Survey (HKGS) conducted in 1993 with sex-specific reference charts of weight-for-height (HKGS criteria) (35).

This was a territory-wide cross-sectional growth survey which covered around 25,000 Hong Kong Chinese children from birth to 18 years of age. Childhood obesity in this survey was defined as weight > median weight for height × 120%. No definition for childhood overweight was set in this survey.

In recent years, increasing clinical attention has been drawn to central obesity because central body fat is a better predictor than overall body fat for cardiovascular risk factors in both adults (36, 37) and children (7, 38, 39). Central obesity reflects excess visceral adiposity which is a major culprit for insulin resistance and associated cardiovascular disease in both adults and children (7, 38, 40-43). WC and WC-derived indexes such as waist-to-hip ratio (WHR) and waist-to-height ratio (WHTR) are commonly employed anthropometric measurements as proxy measures of central obesity. In Caucasian adults, WC ≥102cm in men and ≥ 88cm in women are used to define central obesity (1,3). The corresponding cutoff values in Chinese and South Asian men and women are ≥ 90cm and ≥ 80cm respectively (5, 44). In adults, there are at least 14 different methods to quantify WC (19). In pediatric literatures, measurements of WC have been described at 5 different sites: 1) midway between the lowest rib and superior iliac crest (45-49); 2) at the umbilical level (50, 51); 3) at the narrowest point of the torso (52); 4) at the level of the right upper iliac crest (53); and 5) at the level of 2 cm above the umbilicus (54). Based on the 2005/2006 Hong Kong Growth Survey including 14,842 Hong Kong Chinese school children aged 6 to 18 years, reference values and percentile curves for WC and WHRT are established (49). These charts are based on WC measured midway between the lowest rib and superior iliac crest and provide reference values for estimation of central obesity in local Hong Kong Chinese youth populations.

In summary, adolescence obesity is a global concern because obesity associated cardiovascular risk factors and abnormalities are potentially reversible in early disease stage. Despite the epidemic of childhood and adolescence obesity worldwide, the most appropriate criterion to ascertain the diagnosis is still inconclusive. Given the high rates of adolescence obesity, adolescents are important population for monitoring and intervention.

2.2 Diabetes

Diabetes is a disorder of glucose metabolism with complex interplays between genetic, lifestyle and environmental factors. Historically, type 2 diabetes is much less common in children and adolescents compared to autoimmune type 1 diabetes and type 2 diabetes has once been thought to be non-existent in children (55). However, with increasing prevalence of obesity worldwide, type 2 diabetes in children and adolescents is increasing at an alarming pace (55). Atherosclerosis starts in young people with type 2 diabetes(56). The general awareness of type 2 diabetes in adolescents should be escalated, particularly in those with obesity and family history of type 2 diabetes. American Diabetes Association (ADA) (57)has recommended the testing for type 2 diabetes in asymptomatic children and adolescents who are: aged 10 years or at onset of puberty, overweight (BMI>85th percentile for age and sex, weight for height >85th percentile, or weight>120% of ideal for height), plus any two of the following risk factors:

1. family history of type 2 diabetes in first- or second-degree relative;
2. race/ethnicity (Native American, African American, Latino, Asian American, Pacific Islander);
3. clinical evidence and/or association of insulin resistance, e.g. polycystic ovarian syndrome, metabolic syndrome, acanthosis nigricans, etc;
4. maternal history of gestational diabetes during the child's gestation.

ADA recommends a three yearly screening in these at-risk young individuals (57). In making the diagnosis of diabetes in adolescents, the possibility of "hybrid" disease with obesity and concomitant diseases with compromised insulin secretion such as maturity-onset diabetes of the young (MODY) or latent autoimmune diabetes in adult (LADA) should always be considered(58).

For adolescents with type 1 diabetes who present with acute decompensation and diabetic ketoacidosis (DKA), insulin therapy is the standard therapy. Insulin use is also advised in youth with type 2 diabetes who present with severe hyperglycemia (≥11.1 mmol/L), HbA_{1c}>8.5% or severe manifestation of insulin deficiency such as DKA (59). Although oral antidiabetic agents are not recommended in treatment of type 1 diabetes traditionally, metformin use in conjunction with insulin in adolescents with poorly controlled diabetes has been reported to improve their glycemic control (60). Despite the escalating rate of type 2 diabetes in the youth, therapeutic modalities remain limited with metformin being the only U.S. Food and Drug Administration (FDA)-approved oral treatment for youth with type 2 diabetes (61). Similar recommendation has been adopted in other countries (62).

2.3 Hypertension

The global epidemic of obesity is leading to a shift in the diabetes, as well as hypertension distribution towards increasing levels in children and adolescent (63, 64). In addition, physical inactivity and high salt/sodium intake contribute to the rise in the prevalence of hypertension in the youth. Similar to childhood and adolescence obesity, there is also tracking of high blood pressure from childhood into adulthood(65, 66). Autopsy findings from Bogalusa Heart Study and the Pathobiologic Determinates of Atherosclerosis in Youth (PDAY) have shown that higher blood pressure in the youth populations is associated with increased atherosclerosis(67, 68).

Accurate measurement of blood pressure and correct diagnosis of hypertension or pre-hypertension in the youth populations are important to prevent end-organ damage in adults. The fourth report on the diagnosis, evaluation and treatment of high blood pressure in children and adolescents has suggested a diagnosis of hypertension as >95th percentile for gender, age and height on ≥ 3 occasions. Stage 1 hypertension is diagnosed if systolic or diastolic blood pressure reaches 95th to 99th percentile plus 5 mmHg on at least 3 separate occasions(69) whereas stage 2 hypertension is defined as >99th percentile plus 5mmHg. Various diagnostic cutoff values have been suggested for defining hypertension and pre-hypertension in the youth population (Table 1). Pre-hypertension is defined as >120/80 mmHg or ≥ 90th to <95th percentile (69). Blood pressure increases with age, yet there is limited information regarding the time course for children and adolescents with pre-hypertension to progress to hypertension. For early diagnosis of pre-hypertension and hypertension, reference blood pressure standards by sex-, age-, weight- and height are clinically important (70, 71).

The 4th report on the diagnosis, evaluation, and treatment of high BP in children and adolescents(69)	**Cool et al (76) , (77) and Kong et al (39, 78)**	**Cruz et al (79) and de Ferranti et al (75)**	**Weiss et al (80)**	**Zimmet et al (21)**
BP > 95th percentile for gender, age and height on ≥3 occasions	BP ≥ 90th percentile for gender, age and height	BP > 90th percentile for gender, age and height	BP > 95th percentile for gender, age and height	BP≥ 130/85 mmHg

Table 1. Diagnostic criteria used in pediatric literatures for definition of hypertension. Blood pressure: BP.

White coat hypertension is a well recognized phenomenon of transiently high blood pressure related to stress. Home-clinic blood pressure difference can vary substantially by age in children with the difference reduced with advancing age and substantially diminshed after 12 year-old(72). Therefore, ambulatory blood pressure (AMBP) is gaining popularity in both children and adults due to the stronger correlation between high AMBP with target organs damage observed in an emerging number of studies in both adults and paediatric populations (73).

For youth with pre-hypertension and hypertension, a search and thorough evaluation for secondary causes is recommended as secondary hypertension is more common in children than adults(69). If secondary hypertension is ruled out, children and adolescents with pre-hypertension should start lifestyle modifications(69). For stage 2 hypertension, drug therapy should be initiated but for those with stage 1 hypertension, pharmacological treatment is recommended if symptomatic, evidence of end-organ damage, concomitant diabetes or persistent high blood pressure despite non-pharmacological measures(69). A detailed elaboration of the dosage, dosing interval and precautions of different types of antihypertensive drugs for children with hypertension has been described in the fourth report on the diagnosis, evaluation and treatment of high blood pressure in children and adolescents(69).

2.4 Dyslipidemia

Dyslipidemia continue to track from childhood into adulthood(74). Similar to the controversies in diagnosis of obesity and hypertension, there is no consensus regarding the definition of dyslipidemia in children and adolescents. Typical dyslipidemia in children and adults with obesity and insulin resistance include increased triglyceride and decreased high-density lipoprotein (HDL) cholesterol levels. The definitions of high triglyceride level in the youth range from ≥ 1.1 mmol/l (ie ≥ 100 mg/dL) (75), ≥ 1.2 mmol/l (39, 76, 77) to ≥ 1.7 mmol/l (21, 39, 78). Some researchers adopt age-, sex- and/or race-specific percentile cutoff to diagnose hypertriglyceridemia with triglyceride ≥ 90th percentile (79)and >95th percentile (80) used. For defining low HDL cholesterol levels in the pediatric literatures, a cutoff value of ≤ 1.03 mmol/l (ie< 40mg/dL) for all ages/sexes (39, 76-78), < 1.03 mmol/l (21), <1.3 mmol/l (ie <50mg/dL)(75), or gender-specific cutoff ≤ 1.03 mmol/l for boys and ≤ 1.3 mmol/l for girls (81), or percentile specific cutoff <5th percentile (age-, sex- and race-specific)(80) and ≤ 10th percentile (age-, sex- and height-specific) (79, 82) have been reported.

Low density lipoprotein (LDL) cholesterol remains to be the primary target of lipid control to prevent cardiovascular events in adults (83). Hence, majority of randomized controlled trials carried out in pediatric populations have also focused on the use of statins in youth with elevated LDL cholesterol levels. There is general consensus that statin should be initiated, in combination with diet and lifestyle modification if LDL cholesterol level > 4.1 mmol/l (ie 160mg/dl) in at-risk youth (84, 85). Fibrates and niacin are lipid lowering drugs targeted to treat high triglyceride and low HDL cholesterol in adults, but neither drugs is approved for use by US FDA in the pediatric population.

3. Novel cardiovascular risk factors in adolescents

3.1 Sleep

Physiologically, average sleep duration decreases with progression from infancy, childhood to adolescence (86). With increasing demand from school and work, as well as changes in leisure activities such as television watching and computer games, the average sleep duration in the US adults has decreased from 9 hours per night a century ago to 6.9 hours per night in 2005 (87). In Sweden, the average sleep time has decreased from 9 hours per night in 1910 to 7.5 hours in 1990's in adults aged 20-64 years (88).

Sleep deprivation is now increasingly recognized as a lifestyle factor contributing to the global epidemic of childhood obesity and a novel, potentially reversible cardiovascular risk factor. Both laboratory and epidemiological studies suggested associations of obesity, insulin resistance, diabetes and cardiovascular disease with sleep debt in children, adolescents and adults (89-91). Increasing number of epidemiological studies show close association between sleep duration and obesity, which is evident as early as during early childhood (92-96). Short duration of sleep at age of 3 years predict future risk of obesity in childhood (92). In a Japanese study of 8274 children aged 6-7 years, an inverse relationship between hours of sleep and risk of childhood obesity was observed (93). Cross-sectional studies from US, Canada, UK, France, Germany and Japan suggest increased risk for overweight or obesity in Caucasian, Hispanic, African-American and Japanese children who sleep long hours than those with short sleep duration (93, 97-101). Prospective studies also suggest a predictive role of short sleep duration for overweight and obesity in Caucasians children (92, 102). Similar data from Chinese children and adolescents are comparatively sparse. A recent survey in Taiwan involving 656 boys and girls aged 13-18 years showed that sleep deprivation (defined as sleep <6 hours on schooldays) was associated with poor health status as measured by health-related behaviors in self-reported questionnaires (103).

Although the exact underlying mechanism linking sleep and obesity is not fully understood, preliminary results suggest a possible neurohormonal basis. There is evidence showing that sleep curtailment can activate the hypothalamo-pituitary-adrenal (HPA) axis (104). Van Cauter *et al* have demonstrated a significant rise in plasma cortisol levels in the following evening amongst subjects after partial (0400-0800 hours) and total sleep deprivation (37% and 45% increases, p=0.03 and 0.003 respectively) compared to those with normal sleep duration (2300-0700 hours) (104). In another study by Van Cauter *et al*, sleep debt was associated with adverse effects on carbohydrate metabolism and endocrine function (105). Glucose tolerance and thyrotropin concentrations were reduced while evening cortisol concentrations and activity of sympathetic nervous system were increased in the sleep debt group (4 hours per night) (105). Interestingly, these hormonal and metabolic changes are very similar to that accompanying normal ageing. Based on rodent studies, positive relation between sleep curtailment and hyperphagia has been noted. Van Cauter *et al* further demonstrated an inverse relationship between sleep debt and leptin, an important anorexigenic hormone secreted by adipocytes mediating the signals between adipose tissues and the hypothalamic regulatory centers (106, 107). In concert with this phenomenon, elevated ghrelin levels, the orexigenic hormone, were observed with reduced sleep duration accompanied by increased hunger and appetite (106). Similar results have also been reported by other workers showing associations between high BMI, short sleep duration, decreased leptin and elevated ghrelin levels (95). In addition, lipid and energy metabolism are regulated by circadian rhythm (108). Sleep problems may result in dysregulation of lipid metabolism and metabolic syndrome. In a national study in Japan, sleep duration in adults was closely related with serum lipid and lipoprotein levels (109). Recently, an association between atherogenic dyslipidemia and reduced sleep duration is reported in both U.S. and Hong Kong Chinese adolescents(110, 111).

3.2 Inflammation

Atherosclerosis can be regarded as a state of chronic, low-grade inflammation of the arterial wall, resulting from the interactions between plasma lipoproteins, peripheral blood mononuclear cells (PBMC) and the endothelium (112). It has been increasing recognized the clinical utility and prognostic role of serum inflammatory markers levels, in addition to traditional cardiovascular risk factors, in estimating cardiovascular risk in both adults and the youth populations. Both high circulating white cell counts and high serum high sensitivity C-reactive protein (hsCRP) are associated with increased risk of diabetes and associated complications in adults (113, 114). Increasing clinical evidence also suggest a link between inflammation, insulin resistance and cardiovascular risk factors in children and adolescents (13, 115-117). In a school children study including over 2,000 Hong Kong Chinese adolescents (median age: 16 years), overweight/obesity was associated with two to six-fold increased risk of having high hsCRP tertiles(13). In another cross-sectional study including 326 obese children aged 6-12 years (mean age 8.9 years), white blood cell counts were associated with plasma lipid profile (triglyceride, total and LDL cholesterol) and obesity indices (body mass index and WC)(117).

3.3 Heavy metals and environmental pollutants

Apart from changes in habits and lifestyle, exposure to heavy metals is increasingly recognized as a consequence of urbanization. Most heavy metals cannot be metabolized by our body, and excessive accumulation in the body will disturb the normal functions of cells. Kidney is the key organ to eliminate heavy metals from the body. Heavy metals might lead to albuminuria through inducing oxidative stress to renal tubular cells(118, 119). Certain heavy metals have additive effect in inducing nephrotoxicity. For example, synergistic effect of arsenic (As) and cadmium (Cd) in causing renal damage has been demonstrated in Chinese general population(120). In addition, chronic exposure to toxic heavy metals may promote atherosclerosis and contribute to the development of chronic kidney disease and cardiovascular diseases (119, 121). Furthermore, air pollutants can provoke systemic pro-inflammatory and pro-thrombotic response and lead to increase in platelet counts and platelet activation(122). The significance of platelet activation and whether anti-platelet therapies can help reducing cardiovascular risk profiles in the youth populations is still a debatable subject(123). Further studies are required to examine the impact of heavy metals and environmental pollutants, as novel cardiovascular risk factors, in accelerating the development of cardiovascular disease in both adults and the youth populations(124).

4. Controversies and the unmet needs to be addressed

Lifestyle modification including regular exercise and diet are cornerstones of management of traditional cardiovascular risk factors including obesity, diabetes, dyslipidemia and hypertension. With recent evidence demonstrating the importance of adequate sleep duration in adolescents, education for a healthy sleep habit becomes one of the essential targets of lifestyle modification to prevent cardiovascular risk factors in the youth. Childhood and adolescence are vulnerable periods for habit formation due to substantial tracking of lifestyle habits and cardiovascular risk from this period into adulthood (125, 126). Thus, promoting healthy eating habit, regular exercise and healthy sleep habit in the youth are important strategies to curb the public health problem of obesity.

The optimal dietary approach to combat obesity and reduce cardiovascular risk factors is still a matter of controversies. Indeed, modern food-processing technology produces many food products with high glycemic index (GI). There is now emerging evidence showing that both the quality and quantity of dietary components can impact upon various physiological processes underlying energy metabolism and control of satiety which can provide the basis for dietary intervention in diabetes and obesity (127, 128). Epidemiological studies from US and China indicate that the risks of chronic diseases such as type 2 diabetes and coronary heart disease are strongly related to dietary GI (129, 130). High GI food, especially rice, the main carbohydrate-contributing food in Chinese, may increase risk of diabetes (130). WHO and Food and Agriculture Organization (FAO) recommend low-GI diet to prevent common chronic diseases of affluence, including obesity and type 2 diabetes (131). Recently, it has been suggested that low GI diet may have a role in the management of childhood obesity(132).

Promotion of regular exercise is another important aspect of lifestyle modifications in reducing cardiovascular risk in adolescents. Physical inactivity has been reported to be associated with obesity and other cardiovascular risk factors in adolescents(133). The role of exercise in weight management and control of cardiovascular risk factors is usually associated with its direct impact on energy expenditure and its potential to alter various components of appetite control and eating behavior. Low physical activity level predicts weight gain in different ethnic groups (134, 135). Regular physical activity maintains good health and prevents myocardial infarction, cardiovascular events and premature mortality (136, 137). Since early 1990s, many studies have demonstrated the beneficial effects of physical activity on promoting weight reduction and fat loss as well as reducing risk of diabetes and hypertension (138-141). Beneficial effects of exercise and diet are possibly beyond weight reduction. In a small scale study of obese Hong Kong Chinese children, combined intervention with diet and exercise reduced adiposity as well as improved lipid profiles and endothelial function compared to diet alone (25). In another study, a 6-week intervention with diet and strength training improved lipid profile in obese Chinese children (142).

WHO recommends regular and accumulated physical activities to prevent premature death and other adverse health outcomes (143). However, there are ongoing debates on the optimal frequency, duration and intensity of physical activity. Most international guidelines recommend moderate activity in adults, especially those who are older and less active (136). In a systematic review of over 850 published literatures, the authors recommended ≥ 60 minutes physical activity of moderate to vigorous level in school-age youth (144). In 1988, the American College of Sports Medicine first recommended children and adolescents to have 20-30 minutes of vigorous exercise daily (145). In 2007, the Regional Office for Europe of the WHO made similar recommendations (146). Other guidelines suggested physical activity of moderate intensity at least twice or more weekly to enhance and maintain muscular strength, flexibility and bone health (20) while others suggested high levels and long duration of regular exercise (e.g. daily physical activity lasting at least 90 minutes) in the youth population (147).

As previously discussed, despite the escalating rate of diabetes and dyslipidemia in the youth population, therapeutic modalities remain limited with metformin and statin being the only US FDA approved oral treatment for youth with type 2 diabetes (61, 62) and dyslipidemia respectively (84, 85). More clinical researches are required to demonstrate the efficacy and safety for more therapeutic options in managing adolescents with type 2 diabetes and dyslipidemia.

5. Conclusion

In conclusion, cardiovascular disease is an increasing world health problem. In view of the substantial tracking of cardiovascular risk factors from adolescents to adulthood, there is an urgent need to intervene early with efficacious strategies to identify and treat the youth with cardiovascular risk factors. The traditional cardiovascular risk factors, namely overweight/obesity, diabetes, hypertension and dyslipidemia do not account for all cardiovascular deaths and novel factors, including lifestyle (e.g. sleep deprivation) and environmental (e.g. heavy metal poisoning), as well as the consequences and interactions related to these traditional and novel risk factors (e.g. inflammation and platelet activation) appear to be important, accounting for the dramatic recent changes in prevalence and would be of public health concern. Moreover, more intensive program for lifestyle modification and aggressive approach of pharmacological treatment should be considered in the youth at-risk of cardiovascular events.

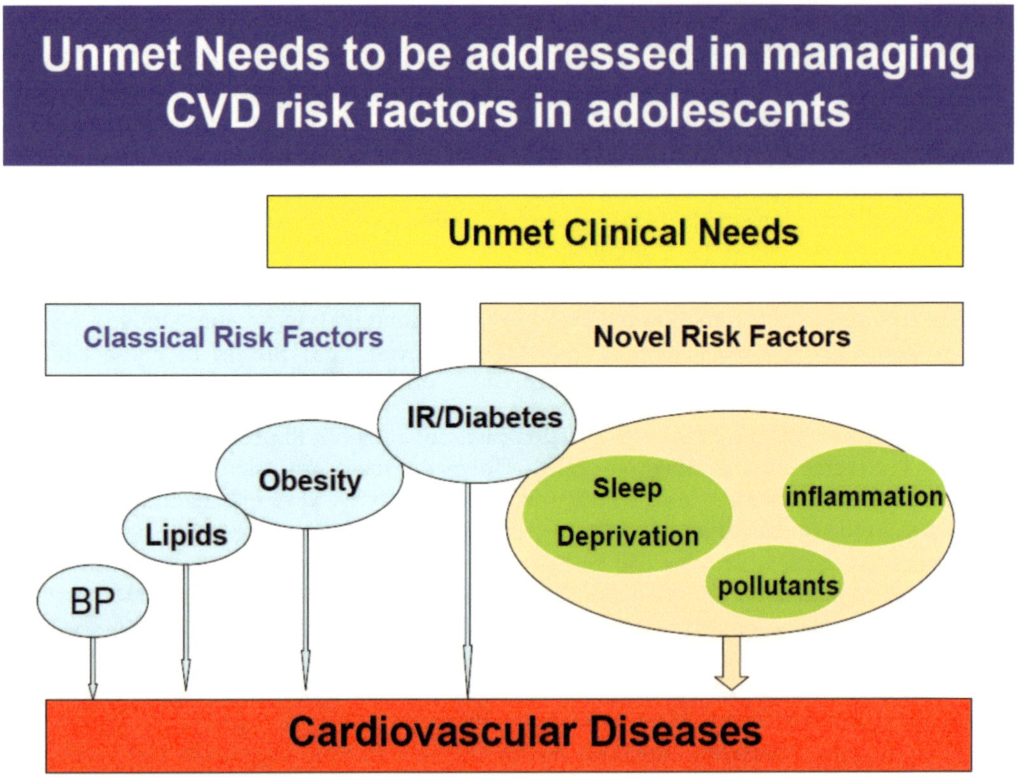

Fig. 1. Traditional and Novel Cardiovascular Risk Factors in Adolescents.

6. Acknowledgement

This book chapter and some of the cited studies were partially supported by funding from the Research Grants Council (RGC reference no.: CUHK 4055/01M, CUHK 4465/06M and CUHK 467410).

7. References

[1] Singh AS, Mulder C, Twisk JW, van Mechelen W, Chinapaw MJ. Tracking of childhood overweight into adulthood: a systematic review of the literature. Obes Rev 2008;9(5):474-88. Epub 2008 Mar 5.

[2] Daniels SR, Arnett DK, Eckel RH, Gidding SS, Hayman LL, Kumanyika S, et al. Overweight in children and adolescents: pathophysiology, consequences, prevention, and treatment. Circulation 2005;111(15):1999-2012.

[3] Srinivasan SR, Bao W, Wattigney WA, Berenson GS. Adolescent overweight is associated with adult overweight and related multiple cardiovascular risk factors: the Bogalusa Heart Study. Metabolism 1996;45(2):235-40.

[4] Guo SS, Huang C, Maynard LM, Demerath E, Towne B, Chumlea WC, et al. Body mass index during childhood, adolescence and young adulthood in relation to adult

overweight and adiposity: the Fels Longitudinal Study. Int J Obes Relat Metab Disord 2000;24(12):1628-35.

[5] Kong AP, Chan NN, Chan JC. The Role of Adipocytokines and Neurohormonal Dysregulation in Metabolic Syndrome. Current Diabetes Reviews 2006;2:397-407.

[6] Gunnell DJ, Frankel SJ, Nanchahal K, Peters TJ, Davey Smith G. Childhood obesity and adult cardiovascular mortality: a 57-y follow-up study based on the Boyd Orr cohort. Am J Clin Nutr 1998;67(6):1111-8.

[7] Freedman DS, Dietz WH, Srinivasan SR, Berenson GS. The relation of overweight to cardiovascular risk factors among children and adolescents: the Bogalusa Heart Study. Pediatrics 1999;103(6 Pt 1):1175-82.

[8] Ebbeling CB, Pawlak DB, Ludwig DS. Childhood obesity: public-health crisis, common sense cure. Lancet 2002;360(9331):473-82.

[9] Patel DA, Srinivasan SR, Xu JH, Chen W, Berenson GS. Persistent elevation of liver function enzymes within the reference range is associated with increased cardiovascular risk in young adults: the Bogalusa Heart Study. Metabolism 2007;56(6):792-8.

[10] Romero-Corral A, Montori VM, Somers VK, Korinek J, Thomas RJ, Allison TG, et al. Association of bodyweight with total mortality and with cardiovascular events in coronary artery disease: a systematic review of cohort studies. Lancet 2006;368(9536):666-78.

[11] Kong AP, Chow CC. Medical consequences of childhood obesity: a Hong Kong perspective. Res Sports Med 2010;18(1):16-25.

[12] Berenson GS, Srinivasan SR, Bao W, Newman WP, 3rd, Tracy RE, Wattigney WA. Association between multiple cardiovascular risk factors and atherosclerosis in children and young adults. The Bogalusa Heart Study. N Engl J Med 1998;338(23):1650-6.

[13] Kong AP, Choi KC, Ko GT, Wong GW, Ozaki R, So WY, et al. Associations of overweight with insulin resistance, beta-cell function and inflammatory markers in Chinese adolescents. Pediatr Diabetes 2008;9(5):488-95.

[14] Lauer RM, Lee J, Clarke WR. Factors affecting the relationship between childhood and adult cholesterol levels: the Muscatine Study. Pediatrics 1988;82(3):309-18.

[15] Lauer RM, Clarke WR. Childhood risk factors for high adult blood pressure: the Muscatine Study. Pediatrics 1989;84(4):633-41.

[16] Lumeng JC, Gannon K, Cabral HJ, Frank DA, Zuckerman B. Association between clinically meaningful behavior problems and overweight in children. Pediatrics 2003;112(5):1138-45.

[17] Schwandt P, Kelishadi R, Haas GM. Ethnic disparities of the metabolic syndrome in population-based samples of German and Iranian adolescents. Metab Syndr Relat Disord 2010;8(2):189-92.

[18] Kong AP, Ko GT, Ozaki R, Wong GW, Tong PC, Chan JC. Metabolic syndrome by the new IDF criteria in Hong Kong Chinese adolescents and its prediction by using body mass index. Acta Paediatr 2008;97(12):1738-42. Epub 2008 Oct 6.

[19] Reaven GM. The metabolic syndrome: requiescat in pace. Clin Chem 2005;51(6):931-8.

[20] Goodman E. Pediatric metabolic syndrome: smoke and mirrors or true magic? J Pediatr 2006;148(2):149-51.

[21] Zimmet P, Alberti KG, Kaufman F, Tajima N, Silink M, Arslanian S, et al. The Metabolic Syndrome in Children and Adolescents - an IDF consensus report. Pediatr Diabetes 2007;8(5):299-306.

[22] Sun SS, Liang R, Huang TT, Daniels SR, Arslanian S, Liu K, et al. Childhood obesity predicts adult metabolic syndrome: the Fels Longitudinal Study. J Pediatr 2008;152(2):191-200.

[23] McGill HC, Jr., McMahan CA, Herderick EE, Malcom GT, Tracy RE, Strong JP. Origin of atherosclerosis in childhood and adolescence. Am J Clin Nutr 2000;72(5 Suppl):1307S-1315S.

[24] Woo KS, Chook P, Yu CW, Sung RY, Qiao M, Leung SS, et al. Overweight in children is associated with arterial endothelial dysfunction and intima-media thickening. Int J Obes Relat Metab Disord 2004;28(7):852-7.

[25] Woo KS, Chook P, Yu CW, Sung RY, Qiao M, Leung SS, et al. Effects of diet and exercise on obesity-related vascular dysfunction in children. Circulation 2004;109(16):1981-6.

[26] Ogden CL, Flegal KM, Carroll MD, Johnson CL. Prevalence and trends in overweight among US children and adolescents, 1999-2000. JAMA 2002;288(14):1728-32.

[27] Kelishadi R. Childhood overweight, obesity, and the metabolic syndrome in developing countries. Epidemiol Rev 2007;29:62-76.

[28] Ko GT, Ozaki R, Wong GW, Kong AP, So WY, Tong PC, et al. The problem of obesity among adolescents in Hong Kong: a comparison using various diagnostic criteria. BMC Pediatr 2008;8:10.

[29] Power C, Lake JK, Cole TJ. Measurement and long-term health risks of child and adolescent fatness. Int J Obes Relat Metab Disord 1997;21(7):507-26.

[30] Dietz WH, Robinson TN. Use of the body mass index (BMI) as a measure of overweight in children and adolescents. J Pediatr 1998;132(2):191-3.

[31] Cole TJ, Bellizzi MC, Flegal KM, Dietz WH. Establishing a standard definition for child overweight and obesity worldwide: international survey. BMJ 2000;320(7244):1240-3.

[32] Reilly JJ. Assessment of childhood obesity: national reference data or international approach? Obes Res 2002;10(8):838-40.

[33] Group of China Obesity Task Force. [Body mass index reference norm for screening overweight and obesity in Chinese children and adolescents]. Zhonghua Liu Xing Bing Xue Za Zhi 2004;25(2):97-102.

[34] Ogden CL, Kuczmarski RJ, Flegal KM, Mei Z, Guo S, Wei R, et al. Centers for Disease Control and Prevention 2000 growth charts for the United States: improvements to the 1977 National Center for Health Statistics version. Pediatrics 2002;109(1):45-60.

[35] Leung SSF, Lau JTF, Tse LY, Oppenheimer SJ. Weight-for-age and weight-for height references for Hong Kong children from birth to 18 years. Journal of Paediatrics and Child Health 1996;32:103-9.

[36] Despres JP, Moorjani S, Lupien PJ, Tremblay A, Nadeau A, Bouchard C. Regional distribution of body fat, plasma lipoproteins, and cardiovascular disease. Arteriosclerosis 1990;10(4):497-511.

[37] Kahn HS, Valdez R. Metabolic risks identified by the combination of enlarged waist and elevated triacylglycerol concentration. Am J Clin Nutr 2003;78(5):928-34.

[38] Kelishadi R, Gheiratmand R, Ardalan G, Adeli K, Mehdi Gouya M, Mohammad Razaghi E, et al. Association of anthropometric indices with cardiovascular disease risk factors among children and adolescents: CASPIAN Study. Int J Cardiol 2007;117(3):340-8. Epub 2006 Jul 21.

[39] Ng VW, Kong AP, Choi KC, Ozaki R, Wong GW, So WY, et al. BMI and waist circumference in predicting cardiovascular risk factor clustering in Chinese adolescents. Obesity (Silver Spring) 2007;15(2):494-503.

[40] Kannel WB, Cupples LA, Ramaswami R, Stokes J, 3rd, Kreger BE, Higgins M. Regional obesity and risk of cardiovascular disease; the Framingham Study. J Clin Epidemiol 1991;44(2):183-90.

[41] Björntorp P. Metabolic implications of body fat distribution. Diabetes Care 1991;14:1132-1143.

[42] Maffeis C, Pietrobelli A, Grezzani A, Provera S, Tato L. Waist circumference and cardiovascular risk factors in prepubertal children. Obes Res 2001;9(3):179-87.

[43] Seidell JC, Perusse L, Despres JP, Bouchard C. Waist and hip circumferences have independent and opposite effects on cardiovascular disease risk factors: the Quebec Family Study. Am J Clin Nutr 2001;74(3):315-21.

[44] Alberti KG, Zimmet P, Shaw J. The metabolic syndrome--a new worldwide definition. Lancet 2005;366(9491):1059-62.

[45] Moreno LA, Fleta J, Mur L, Rodriquez G, Sarria A, Bueno M. Waist circumference values in Spanish children--gender related differences. Eur J Clin Nutr 1999;53(6):429-33.

[46] McCarthy HD, Jarrett KV, Crawley HF. The development of waist circumference percentiles in British children aged 5.0-16.9 y. Eur J Clin Nutr 2001;55(10):902-7.

[47] Fredriks AM, van Buuren S, Fekkes M, Verloove-Vanhorick SP, Wit JM. Are age references for waist circumference, hip circumference and waist-hip ratio in Dutch children useful in clinical practice? Eur J Pediatr 2005;164(4):216-22. Epub 2005 Jan 21.

[48] Kelishadi R, Gouya MM, Ardalan G, Hosseini M, Motaghian M, Delavari A, et al. First reference curves of waist and hip circumferences in an Asian population of youths: CASPIAN study. J Trop Pediatr 2007;53(3):158-64. Epub 2007 Feb 17.

[49] Sung RY, So HK, Choi KC, Nelson EA, Li AM, Yin JA, et al. Waist circumference and waist-to-height ratio of Hong Kong Chinese children. BMC Public Health 2008;8:324.

[50] Zannolli R, Morgese G. Waist percentiles: a simple test for atherogenic disease? Acta Paediatr 1996;85(11):1368-9.

[51] Savva SC, Kourides Y, Tornaritis M, Epiphaniou-Savva M, Tafouna P, Kafatos A. Reference growth curves for cypriot children 6 to 17 years of age. Obes Res 2001;9(12):754-62.

[52] Katzmarzyk PT. Waist circumference percentiles for Canadian youth 11-18y of age. Eur J Clin Nutr 2004;58(7):1011-5.

[53] Fernandez JR, Redden DT, Pietrobelli A, Allison DB. Waist circumference percentiles in nationally representative samples of African-American, European-American, and Mexican-American children and adolescents. J Pediatr 2004;145(4):439-44.

[54] Weili Y, He B, Yao H, Dai J, Cui J, Ge D, et al. Waist-to-height ratio is an accurate and easier index for evaluating obesity in children and adolescents. Obesity (Silver Spring) 2007;15(3):748-52.

[55] Jones KL. Role of obesity in complicating and confusing the diagnosis and treatment of diabetes in children. Pediatrics 2008;121(2):361-8.

[56] Kong AP, Chan JC. Atherosclerosis in young people with type 2 diabetes. International Diabetes Monitor 2010;22(5):223-224.

[57] American Diabetes Association. Standards of Medical Care in Diabetes-2010. Diabetes Care 2010;33 (Suppl):S11-61.

[58] Kong AP, Chan JC. Other Disorders with Type 1 Phenotype. Textbook of Diabetes 2010(4th Edition):9.14-9.21.

[59] Flint A, Arslanian S. Treatment of type 2 diabetes in youth. Diabetes 2011;34(Suppl 2):S177-83.

[60] Sarnblad S, Kroon M, Aman J. Metformin as additional therapy in adolescents with poorly controlled type 1 diabetes: randomised placebo-controlled trial with aspects on insulin sensitivity. Eur J Endocrinol 2003;149(4):323-9.

[61] Weigensberg MJ, Goran MI. Type 2 diabetes in children and adolescents. Lancet 2009;373(9677):1743-4.

[62] Rosenbloom AL, Silverstein JH, Amemiya S, Zeitler P, Klingensmith GJ. Type 2 diabetes in children and adolescents. Pediatr Diabetes 2009;10(Suppl 12):17-32.

[63] Muntner P, He J, Cutler JA, Wildman RP, Whelton PK. Trends in blood pressure among children and adolescents. JAMA 2004;291(17):2107-13.

[64] Leung LC, Sung RY, So HK, Wong SN, Lee KW, Lee KP, et al. Prevalence and risk factors for hypertension in Hong Kong Chinese adolescents: waist circumference predicts hypertension, exercise decreases risk. Arch Dis Child 2011;96(9):804-9.

[65] Raitakari OT, Porkka KV, Rasanen L, Ronnemaa T, Viikari JS. Clustering and six year cluster-tracking of serum total cholesterol, HDL-cholesterol and diastolic blood pressure in children and young adults. The Cardiovascular Risk in Young Finns Study. J Clin Epidemiol 1994;47(10):1085-93.

[66] Bao W, Threefoot SA, Srinivasan SR, Berenson GS. Essential hypertension predicted by tracking of elevated blood pressure from childhood to adulthood: the Bogalusa Heart Study. Am J Hypertens 1995;8(7):657-65.

[67] Tracy RE, Newman WP, 3rd, Wattigney WA, Srinivasan SR, Strong JP, Berenson GS. Histologic features of atherosclerosis and hypertension from autopsies of young individuals in a defined geographic population: the Bogalusa Heart Study. Atherosclerosis 1995;116(2):163-79.

[68] Homma S, Ishii T, Malcom GT, Zieske AW, Strong JP, Tsugane S, et al. Histopathological modifications of early atherosclerotic lesions by risk factors--findings in PDAY subjects. Atherosclerosis 2001;156(2):389-99.

[69] National High Blood Pressure Education Program Working Group on High Blood Pressure in Children and Adolescents. The fourth report on the diagnosis, evaluation, and treatment of high blood pressure in children and adolescents. Pediatrics 2004;114(2 Suppl 4th Report):555-76.

[70] Sung RY, Choi KC, So HK, Nelson EA, Li AM, Kwok CW, et al. Oscillometrically measured blood pressure in Hong Kong Chinese children and associations with anthropometric parameters. J Hypertens 2008;26(4):678-84.
[71] Falkner B, Gidding SS, Portman R, Rosner B. Blood pressure variability and classification of prehypertension and hypertension in adolescence. Pediatrics 2008;122(2):238-42.
[72] Stergiou GS, Rarra VC, Yiannes NG. Changing relationship between home and office blood pressure with increasing age in children: the Arsakeion School study. Am J Hypertens 2008;21(1):41-6.
[73] Urbina E, Alpert B, Flynn J, Hayman L, Harshfield GA, Jacobson M, et al. Ambulatory blood pressure monitoring in children and adolescents: recommendations for standard assessment: a scientific statement from the American Heart Association Atherosclerosis, Hypertension, and Obesity in Youth Committee of the council on cardiovascular disease in the young and the council for high blood pressure research. Hypertension 2008;52(3):433-51.
[74] Nicklas TA, von Duvillard SP, Berenson GS. Tracking of serum lipids and lipoproteins from childhood to dyslipidemia in adults: the Bogalusa Heart Study. Int J Sports Med 2002;23(Suppl 1):S39-43.
[75] de Ferranti SD, Gauvreau K, Ludwig DS, Neufeld EJ, Newburger JW, Rifai N. Prevalence of the metabolic syndrome in American adolescents: findings from the Third National Health and Nutrition Examination Survey. Circulation 2004;110(16):2494-7.
[76] Cook S, Weitzman M, Auinger P, Nguyen M, Dietz W. Prevalence of a metabolic syndrome phenotype in adolescents. Findings from the Third National Health and Nutrition Examination Survey, 1988-1994. Arch Pediatr Adolesc Med 2003;157:821-827.
[77] Ford ES, Ajani UA, Mokdad AH. The metabolic syndrome and concentrations of C-reactive protein among U.S. youth. Diabetes Care 2005;28(4):878-81.
[78] Kong AP, Choi KC, Cockram CS, Ho CS, Chan MH, Ozaki R, et al. Independent associations of alanine aminotransferase (ALT) levels with cardiovascular risk factor clustering in Chinese adolescents. J Hepatol 2008;49(1):115-122.
[79] Cruz ML, Weigensberg MJ, Huang TT, Ball G, Shaibi GQ, Goran MI. The metabolic syndrome in overweight Hispanic youth and the role of insulin sensitivity. J Clin Endocrinol Metab 2004;89(1):108-13.
[80] Weiss R, Dziura J, Burgert TS, Tamborlane WV, Taksali SE, Yeckel CW, et al. Obesity and the metabolic syndrome in children and adolescents. N Engl J Med 2004;350(23):2362-74.
[81] Grundy SM. Metabolic syndrome scientific statement by the American Heart Association and the National Heart, Lung, and Blood Institute. Arterioscler Thromb Vasc Biol 2005;25(11):2243-4.
[82] Goodman E, Daniels SR, Meigs JB, Dolan LM. Instability in the diagnosis of metabolic syndrome in adolescents. Circulation 2007;115(17):2316-22.
[83] Expert Panel on Detection Evaluation and Treatment of high blood cholesterol in adults. Executive summary of the Third Report of the National Cholesterol Education Program Expert Panel on Detection, Evaluation and Treatment of

high blood cholesterol in adults (Adult Treatment Panel III). JAMA 2001;285:2486-97.
[84] McCrindle BW, Urbina EM, Dennison BA, Jacobson MS, Steinberger J, Rocchini AP, et al. Drug therapy of high-risk lipid abnormalities in children and adolescents: a scientific statement from the American Heart Association Atherosclerosis, Hypertension, and Obesity in Youth Committee, Council of Cardiovascular Disease in the Young, with the Council on Cardiovascular Nursing. Circulation 2007;115(14):1948-67.
[85] McNeal C, Wilson DP. Metabolic syndrome and dyslipidemia in youth. J Clin Lipidol 2008;2(3):147-55.
[86] Iglowstein I, Jenni OG, Molinari L, Largo RH. Sleep duration from infancy to adolescence: reference values and generational trends. Pediatrics 2003;111(2):302-7.
[87] National Sleep Foundation. National Sleep Foundation 2005 Omnibus "Sleep in America" Poll. 2005:Available at: http://www/sleepfoundation.org.
[88] Broman JE, Lundh LG, Hetta J. Insufficient sleep in the general population. Neurophysiol Clin 1996;26(1):30-9.
[89] Van Cauter E, Knutson K. Sleep and the epidemic of obesity in children and adults. Eur J Endocrinol 2008:[Epub ahead of print].
[90] Van Cauter E, Knutson K. Sleep and the epidemic of obesity in children and adults. Eur J Endocrinol 2008;159(Suppl):S59-66.
[91] Van Cauter E, Holmback U, Knutson K, Leproult R, Miller A, Nedeltcheva A, et al. Impact of sleep and sleep loss on neuroendocrine and metabolic function. Horm Res 2007;67(Suppl 1):2-9.
[92] Taheri S. The link between short sleep duration and obesity: we should recommend more sleep to prevent obesity. Arch Dis Child 2006;91(11):881-4.
[93] Reilly JJ, Armstrong J, Dorosty AR, Emmett PM, Ness A, Rogers I, et al. Early life risk factors for obesity in childhood: cohort study. BMJ 2005;330(7504):1357.
[94] Sekine M, Yamagami T, Hamanishi S, Handa K, Saito T, Nanri S, et al. Parental obesity, lifestyle factors and obesity in preschool children: results of the Toyama Birth Cohort study. J Epidemiol 2002;12(1):33-9.
[95] Shigeta H, Shigeta M, Nakazawa A, Nakamura N, Yoshikawa T. Lifestyle, obesity, and insulin resistance. Diabetes Care 2001;24(3):608.
[96] Taheri S, Lin L, Austin D, Young T, Mignot E. Short sleep duration is associated with reduced leptin, elevated ghrelin, and increased body mass index. PLoS Med 2004;1(3):e62.
[97] Vorona RD, Winn MP, Babineau TW, Eng BP, Feldman HR, Ware JC. Overweight and obese patients in a primary care population report less sleep than patients with a normal body mass index. Arch Intern Med 2005;165(1):25-30.
[98] Chaput JP, Brunet M, Tremblay A. Relationship between short sleeping hours and childhood overweight/obesity: results from the 'Quebec en Forme' Project. Int J Obes (Lond) 2006;30(7):1080-5.
[99] Gupta NK, Mueller WH, Chan W, Meininger JC. Is obesity associated with poor sleep quality in adolescents? Am J Hum Biol 2002;14(6):762-8.

[100] Locard E, Mamelle N, Billette A, Miginiac M, Munoz F, Rey S. Risk factors of obesity in a five year old population. Parental versus environmental factors. Int J Obes Relat Metab Disord 1992;16(10):721-9.

[101] von Kries R, Toschke AM, Wurmser H, Sauerwald T, Koletzko B. Reduced risk for overweight and obesity in 5- and 6-y-old children by duration of sleep--a cross-sectional study. Int J Obes Relat Metab Disord 2002;26(5):710-6.

[102] Knutson KL. Sex differences in the association between sleep and body mass index in adolescents. J Pediatr 2005;147(6):830-4.

[103] Agras WS, Hammer LD, McNicholas F, Kraemer HC. Risk factors for childhood overweight: a prospective study from birth to 9.5 years. J Pediatr 2004;145(1):20-5.

[104] Chen MY, Wang EK, Jeng YJ. Adequate sleep among adolescents is positively associated with health status and health-related behaviors. BMC Public Health 2006;6:59.

[105] Leproult R, Copinschi G, Buxton O, Van Cauter E. Sleep loss results in an elevation of cortisol levels the next evening. Sleep 1997;20(10):865-70.

[106] Spiegel K, Leproult R, Van Cauter E. Impact of sleep debt on metabolic and endocrine function. Lancet 1999;354(9188):1435-9.

[107] Spiegel K, Tasali E, Penev P, Van Cauter E. Brief communication: Sleep curtailment in healthy young men is associated with decreased leptin levels, elevated ghrelin levels, and increased hunger and appetite. Ann Intern Med 2004;141(11):846-50.

[108] Spiegel K, Leproult R, L'Hermite-Baleriaux M, Copinschi G, Penev PD, Van Cauter E. Leptin levels are dependent on sleep duration: relationships with sympathovagal balance, carbohydrate regulation, cortisol, and thyrotropin. J Clin Endocrinol Metab 2004;89(11):5762-71.

[109] Kudo T, Horikawa K, Shibata S. Circadian rhythms in the CNS and peripheral clock disorders: the circadian clock and hyperlipidemia. J Pharmacol Sci 2007;103(2):139-43.

[110] Kaneita Y, Uchiyama M, Yoshiike N, Ohida T. Associations of usual sleep duration with serum lipid and lipoprotein levels. Sleep 2008;31(5):645-52.

[111] Gangwisch JE, Malaspina D, Babiss LA, Opler MG, Posner K, Shen S, et al. Short sleep duration as a risk factor for hypercholesterolemia: analyses of the National Longitudinal Study of Adolescent Health. Sleep 2010;33(7):956-61.

[112] Kong AP, Wing YK, Choi KC, Li AM, Ko GT, Ma RC, et al. Associations of sleep duration with obesity and serum lipid profile in children and adolescents. Sleep Medicine 2011;12(7):659-65.

[113] Kelishadi R. Inflammation-induced atherosclerosis as a target for prevention of cardiovascular diseases from early life. Open Cardiovasc Med J 2010;4:24-9.

[114] Schmidt MI, Duncan BB, Sharrett AR, Lindberg G, Savage PJ, Offenbacher S, et al. Markers of inflammation and prediction of diabetes mellitus in adults (Atherosclerosis risks in communities study): a cohort study. Lancet 1999;353:1649-52.

[115] Tong PCY, Lee KF, So WY, Ng MCY, Chan WB, Lo MKW, et al. Association of white blood cell counts with macrovascular and microvascular complications in Chinese patients with type 2 diabetes. Diabetes Care 2004;27:216-222.
[116] Misra A. C-reactive protein in young individuals: problems and implications for Asian Indians. Nutrition 2004;20(5):478-81.
[117] Eckel RH, Grundy SM, Zimmet PZ. The metabolic syndrome. Lancet 2005;365(9468):1415-28.
[118] Kelishadi R, Hashemipour M, Ashtijou P, Mirmoghtadaee P, Poursafa P, Khavarian N, et al. Association of cell blood counts and cardiometabolic risk factors among young obese children. Saudi Med J 2010;31(4):406-12.
[119] Huang M, Choi SJ, Kim DW, Kim NY, Park CH, Yu SD, et al. Risk assessment of low-level cadmium and arsenic on the kidney. J Toxicol Environ Health A 2009;72(21-22):1493-8.
[120] Houston MC. The role of mercury and cadmium heavy metals in vascular disease, hypertension, coronary heart disease, and myocardial infarction. Altern Ther Health Med 2007;13(2):S128-33.
[121] Hong F, Jin T, Zhang A. Risk assessment on renal dysfunction caused by co-exposure to arsenic and cadmium using benchmark dose calculation in a Chinese population. Biometals 2004;17(5):573-80.
[122] Navas-Acien A, Silbergeld EK, Sharrett R, Calderon-Aranda E, Selvin E, Guallar E. Metals in urine and peripheral arterial disease. Environ Health Perspect 2005;113(2):164-9.
[123] Poursafa P, Kelishadi R, Amini A, Amini A, Amin MM, Lahijanzadeh M, et al. Association of air pollution and hematologic parameters in children and adolescents. J Pediatr (Rio J) 2011;87(4):350-6.
[124] Poursafa P, Kelishadi R. Air pollution, platelet activation and atherosclerosis. Inflamm Allergy Drug Targets 2010;9(5):387-92.
[125] Alissa EM, Ferns GA. Heavy metal poisoning and cardiovascular disease. J Toxicol 2011;2011:870125.
[126] Kristensen PL, Moller NC, Korsholm L, Wedderkopp N, Andersen LB, Froberg K. Tracking of objectively measured physical activity from childhood to adolescence: the European youth heart study. Scand J Med Sci Sports 2008;18(2):171-8.
[127] Baker JL, Olsen LW, Sorensen TI. Childhood body-mass index and the risk of coronary heart disease in adulthood. N Engl J Med 2007;357(23):2329-37.
[128] Ludwig DS. The glycemic index: physiological mechanisms relating to obesity, diabetes, and cardiovascular disease. JAMA 2002;287(18):2414-23.
[129] Brand-Miller J, McMillan-Price J, Steinbeck K, Caterson I. Carbohydrates--the good, the bad and the whole grain. Asia Pac J Clin Nutr 2008;17(Suppl 1):16-9.
[130] Krishnan S, Rosenberg L, Singer M, Hu FB, Djousse L, Cupples LA, et al. Glycemic index, glycemic load, and cereal fiber intake and risk of type 2 diabetes in US black women. Arch Intern Med 2007;167(21):2304-9.
[131] Villegas R, Liu S, Gao YT, Yang G, Li H, Zheng W, et al. Prospective study of dietary carbohydrates, glycemic index, glycemic load, and incidence of type 2 diabetes mellitus in middle-aged Chinese women. Arch Intern Med 2007;167(21):2310-6.

[132] Obesity: preventing and managing the global epidemic. Report of a WHO consultation. World Health Organ Tech Rep Ser;2000;894:i-xii.
[133] Kong AP, Chan RS, Nelson EA, Chan JC. Role of low-glycemic index diet in management of childhood obesity. Obes Rev 2011;12(7):492-8.
[134] Kong AP, Choi KC, Li AM, Hui SS, Chan MH, Wing YK, et al. Association between physical activity and cardiovascular risk in Chinese youth independent of age and pubertal stage. BMC Public Health 2010;10:303.
[135] Esparza J, Fox C, Harper IT, Bennett PH, Schulz LO, Valencia ME, et al. Daily energy expenditure in Mexican and USA Pima indians: low physical activity as a possible cause of obesity. Int J Obes Relat Metab Disord 2000;24(1):55-9.
[136] Bell AC, Ge K, Popkin BM. Weight gain and its predictors in Chinese adults. Int J Obes Relat Metab Disord 2001;25(7):1079-86.
[137] Erlichman J, Kerbey AL, James WP. Physical activity and its impact on health outcomes. Paper 1: The impact of physical activity on cardiovascular disease and all-cause mortality: an historical perspective. Obes Rev 2002;3(4):257-71.
[138] Inoue M, Iso H, Yamamoto S, Kurahashi N, Iwasaki M, Sasazuki S, et al. Daily total physical activity level and premature death in men and women: results from a large-scale population-based cohort study in Japan (JPHC study). Ann Epidemiol 2008;18(7):522-30.
[139] Ballor DL, Keesey RE. A meta-analysis of the factors affecting exercise-induced changes in body mass, fat mass and fat-free mass in males and females. Int J Obes 1991;15(11):717-26.
[140] Baba R, Koketsu M, Nagashima M, Inasaka H. Role of exercise in the prevention of obesity and hemodynamic abnormalities in adolescents. Pediatr Int 2009;51(3):359-63.
[141] Knowler WC, Barrett-Connor E, Fowler SE, Hamman RF, Lachin JM, Walker EA, et al. Reduction in the incidence of type 2 diabetes with lifestyle intervention or metformin. N Engl J Med 2002;346:393-403.
[142] Khan NA, Hemmelgarn B, Herman RJ, Bell CM, Mahon JL, Leiter LA, et al. The 2009 Canadian Hypertension Education Program recommendations for the management of hypertension: Part 2--therapy. Can J Cardiol 2009;25(5):287-98.
[143] Sung RY, Yu CW, Chang SK, Mo SW, Woo KS, Lam CW. Effects of dietary intervention and strength training on blood lipid level in obese children. Arch Dis Child 2002;86(6):407-10.
[144] World Health Organization. Global strategy on diet, physical activity and health. Geneva 2004;World Health Organization:2004.
[145] Strong WB, Malina RM, Blimkie CJ, Daniels SR, Dishman RK, Gutin B, et al. Evidence based physical activity for school-age youth. J Pediatr 2005;146(6):732-7.
[146] American College of Sports Medicine. Physical fitness in children and youth. Med Sci Sports Exerc 1998;20:422-23.
[147] World Health Organization 2007. Steps to Health: A European Framework to Promote Physical Activity for Health. http://www.euro.who.int/Document/E90191.pdf.

[148] Andersen LB, Harro M, Sardinha LB, Froberg K, Ekelund U, Brage S, et al. Physical activity and clustered cardiovascular risk in children: a cross-sectional study (The European Youth Heart Study). Lancet 2006;368(9532):299-304.

4

Cardiovascular Risk Factors in the Elderly

Melek Z. Ulucam
Baskent University Cardiology Dept., Ankara, Turkey

1. Introduction

The twenty-first century is often called the age of aging. Old age, though one of the most difficult concept to define, is frequently used to describe those older than 60 years of age. Ages can also be divided according to decade: sexagenarian (60 to 69 years), septuagenarian (70 to 79 years), octogenarian (80 to 89 years), nonagenarian 90 to 99 years and centenarian (>100 years) etc. Today, with improved quality of life resulting in longer life spans, the percentage of elderly in the total population is increasing. Because they live longer than men, women constitute the majority of older persons. Since 1950, the proportion of the world's population aged 60 and over has changed from one in thirteen to one in ten, with some developing countries aging faster than developed countries. Marked differences exist between regions. In Europe, one in five people are aged 60 and over as compared to one in 20 in Africa. According to the United Nations Population Division, one in every ten persons is now aged 60 and over. It is projected that by the year 2050 this figure will increase to one in five and by 2150 it will be one in three (**Figure 1**, United Nations Department of Economic and Social Affairs Population Division Report, 2009). The older population is also aging in itself. Currently, octogenarians constitute 11 percent of the world's older population. By 2050, 27 percent of the older population will be 80 years and over (Troisi, 2005).

2. Information on aging, atherogenesis and risk factors

Markers of cardiovascular aging in humans are the progressive **rise** of systolic blood pressure, pulse pressure, pressure pulse rate, left ventricular mass, coronary artery disease and atrial fibrillation prevalence. In parallel with aging a **decrease** can be seen in early diastolic filling rate, maximal heart rate, maximal cardiac output, maximum aerobic capacity, left ventricular contractility index, maximal O2 consumption, ejection fraction and reflex heart rate augmentation during exercise, heart rate variability, vasodilator response to beta-adrenergic stimulation, endothelium-mediated vasodilatation.

With aging, cardiovascular (CV) diseases become more frequent and complicated. They are usually not isolated, but are associated with other medical problems (Ulucam & Muderrisoglu, 2008) and they continue to be the most important cause of morbidity and mortality in the elderly. More than 15% of deaths in the world are due to CV diseases (Ozturk & Kutlu, 2010) for both women and men >65 years of age (Ulucam & Muderrisoglu, 2008). Among CV diseases, more than 75-80% of the population aged 65 and over die from vascular diseases, in particular coronary heart disease. The most important pathologic cause is atherosclerosis, which results in coronary and cerebrovascular events and other major health problems (Ozturk & Kutlu, 2010). Thus, the prevention of CV disease and atherosclerosis plays a key role in the formation of a healthy elderly population (Packard et al., 2005). Maintaining an optimized cardiovascular risk profile seems likely to improve the chance of becoming a centenarian, especially for males (Benatti et al., 2010).

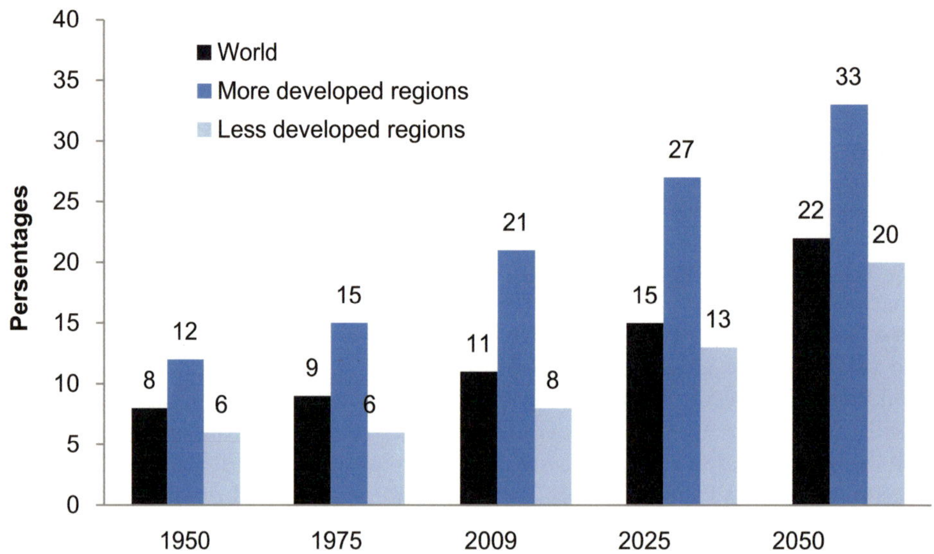

Fig. 1. Population aged 60 or over: world and development regions, 1950-2050 (United Nations Department of Economic and Social Affairs Population Division Report, 2009)

3. Cardiovascular risk factors in the elderly

The most well known **CV risk factors in the elderly** are high blood pressure (BP), wide pulse pressure, age (male > 55, women > 65), smoking, dyslipidemia (total cholesterol >190 mg/dL, or LDL cholesterol >115 mg/dL, or HDL cholesterol in men <40 mg/dL, female <46 mg/dL, triglyceride >150 mg/dL), fasting glucose 102-125 mg/dL, abnormal glucose tolerance test, diabetes mellitus, abdominal obesity (abdominal circumference: M > 102 cm, F > 88 cm), and a family history of premature CV disease (Mancia et al., 2007).

There are of course some major difficulties associated with identifying subjects with a higher CV risk in the elderly populations; every old person may have different nutritional, coagulative, renal, psychogenic, cognitive, and immunity disorders, which all affect CV risk factors and make every old person unique (Redgrave, 2004).

4. Hypertension in the elderly

The European Society of Cardiology describes hypertension (HT) as systolic and diastolic BP values that are over 140 and 90 mm Hg respectively and isolated systolic hypertension (ISH) as systolic BP at ≥ 140 mm Hg and diastolic BP <90 mm Hg respectively. Both types of HT can be divided into 3 phases according to severity (Mancia et al., 2007, 2009). Based on this definition, >50% of elderly people are hypertensive and 30% of the population over age 80 suffers from ISH (Staessen et al., 2000). Given the increasing life span of the older population, this poses a higher risk for the elderly, as indicated by the Framingham study which suggested that the lifetime probability of an elderly person developing HT is as high as 90% (Splansky et al., 2007).

4.1 Blood pressure in the elderly

The **pathophysiological reasons for HT in the elderly** are stiffness and compliance reduction of the aorta and great vessels, the increase in systemic vascular resistance, weakness of baroreceptor reflexes, reduction of CV beta-receptor activity, and low plasma renin activity despite a fall in volume reduction and environmental factors (diet, stress, inactivity, and obesity). As a result, systolic BP increases, diastolic BP decreases and pulse pressure rises. All of these combine to create ISH, a natural result of aging (Izzo, 2005; Hajjar et al. 2001). Although ISH is the most frequent type of HT in the elderly, systolic and diastolic HT can also be seen, albeit to a lesser extent (**Figure 2**, Chobanian, 2007).

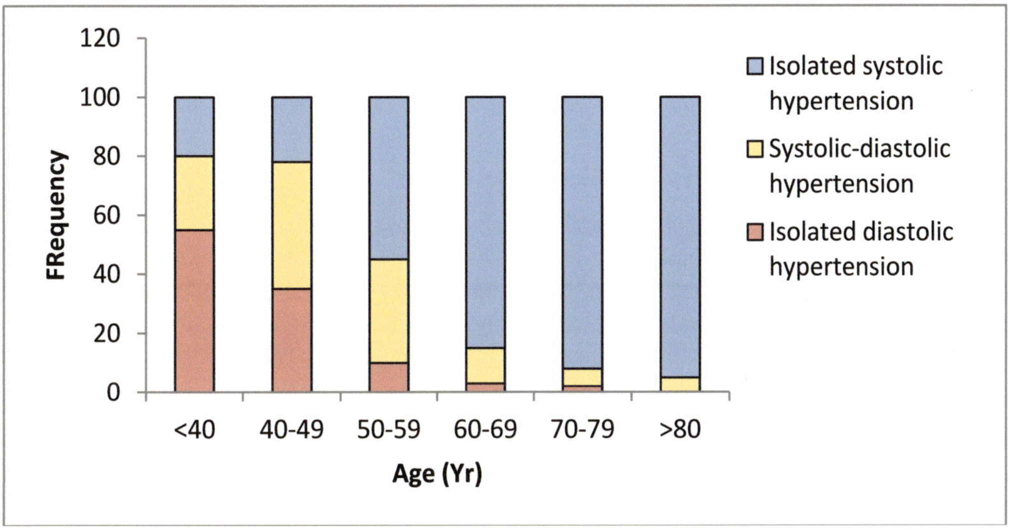

Fig. 2. Frequency of hypertension according to subtype and age (Chobanian, 2007).

ISH creates different clinical manifestations in the elderly and young people. In **young people**, aortic regurgitation, high output states, hyperkinetic circulation, tachycardia, high left ventricular ejection rate, high cardiac index, normal systemic vascular resistance accompanied by high plasma volume are components of **ISH** whereas the main characteristics of the **ISH in the elderly** are loss of aortic compliance, normokinetic circulation, normal heart rate, decreased left ventricular ejection rate and cardiac index, increased systemic vascular resistance and low plasma volume (Adamopoulos et al., 1975).

The specifics of HT in the elderly have been described abundantly in the literature. Baroreflex sensitivity decreases with age, leading to an impaired baroreflex-mediated increase in the heart rate and total systemic vascular resistance in response to decreased BP

(Gribbin et al., 1971). Therefore, elderly people are more likely than younger people to develop **orthostatic and postprandial hypotension** when treated with antihypertensive medications. Another specific condition called **pseudohypertension** is a frequent finding in the elderly, and refers to a falsely high systolic BP resulting from markedly sclerotic arteries that do not collapse during inflation of the BP cuff. Pseudohypertension can be confirmed by measuring intra-arterial pressure.

The importance of hypertension lies in its being an independent and strong risk factor for atherosclerotic cardiovascular disease (CVD), heart failure, stroke, kidney failure, and death in all age groups. The relationship between HT and risk of CVD is linear, progressive and continuous, in that the higher the BP, the greater the risk of CVD (Mancia et al., 2009). However, compared with diastolic BP, systolic BP is a much more accurate predictor of cardiovascular morbidity and mortality (Mancia et al., 2007).

In the elderly, combined HT and ISH increase the risk of congestive heart failure, coronary artery disease, transient ischemic attacks, and incidences of strokes and death (Joint National Committee, 1993). Even with the same BP values, elderly people with HT are 3-4 times more likely than younger hypertensives to suffer from CVD. (Chobanian et al., 2003). Although BP control rates are lower in elderly hypertensives (Hyman & Pavlik, 2001), the results of treatment are better in the elderly (Staessen, 2000). Another striking finding shows that in same age normotensives both type of HT increase the risks of congestive heart failure 6 times and CV mortality 8 times in women and 2 times in men (Sowers, 1987).

4.2 Clinical studies about hypertension in the elderly

Many studies have examined the **benefits of pharmacological treatment of systolic and/or diastolic HT** in the elderly, and have demonstrated a positive effect of medication on the prevention of strokes, coronary artery disease, heart failure, and all CVD (Amery et al., 1982; Ekbom et al., 1992; Hypertension Detection and Follow-up Program Cooperative Group, 1988; Medical Research Council Working Party, 1985; Thijs et al., 1992).

Studies have also compared the **effectiveness of different antihypertensive drugs in elderly hypertensive** patients, and have shown that diuretics, beta-blockers, angiotensin converting enzyme inhibitors, angiotensin receptor blockers, and calcium channel blockers all have similar effects (Brown et al., 2000; Hansson et al., 1999). Subgroup analysis of another study showed that alpha-blocker increases heart failure in older hypertensives and klortalidon is shown to be superior to other pharmacological agents (Antihypertensive and Lipid-Lowering Treatment to Prevent Heart Attack Trial Collaborative Research Group, 2003). In studies dealing with the **ISH in the elderly**, thiazide diuretics and dihydropyridine calcium channel blockers were shown to have similar effects (SHEP Cooperative Research Group, 1991; Staessen et al., 1997; Wang et al., 2000). Both decreased the incidence of strokes by 30%, the risk of CV events by 23%, and the total number of mortality cases by 13%. Those who were shown to benefit most from this treatment were males of an age > 70 years, and who suffered from wide pulse pressure and CV complications.

All of these studies are compatible with the conclusion that treatment of elderly hypertensives reduces cardiac and cerebral mortality and morbidity. Treatment compliance was good and drugs were well tolerated. These studies also show us that diuretics, calcium channel blockers, as well as beta-blockers, angiotensin receptor blockers and angiotensin converting enzyme inhibitors may be started as an initial drug, but alpha-blockers should not be used as the first drug and/or as monotherapy.

In studies on **very old** (80-99 years) hypertensives, treatment was shown to severely reduced stroke, fatal and nonfatal CV disease, but total mortality did not change (Staessen et al., 2000). In a pilot study, the risk of strokes decreased by 53% and the risk of fatal strokes decreased by 43% in the combined treatment groups, as compared with the placebo group; however, there was an unexpected increase in total mortality (Bulpitt et al., 2003). However, the study Hypertension in the Very Elderly (HYVET) has shown that antihypertensive treatment caused a reduction in heart failure, strokes and also total mortality **(Figure 3,** Beckett et al., 2008). The prevalence of CV disease was only 12% at baseline in HYVET patients. Therefore, the absolute reduction in CV events resulting from antihypertensive drug therapy in an elderly population with a high prevalence of CV disease could be much greater than observed in HYVET. In conclusion, for hypertensive patients older than 80 years, if there is adequate quality of life and a life expectancy of more than 2 years, it makes sense to apply the same guidelines for younger hypertensives.

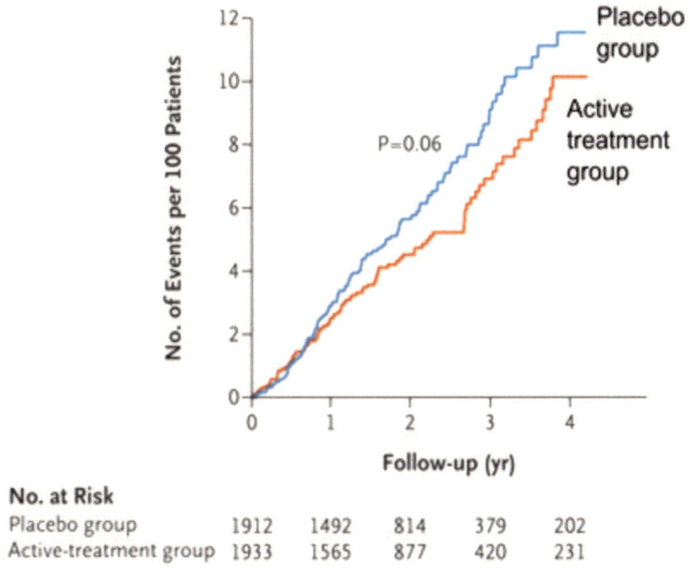

Fig. 3. Kaplan–Meier estimates of the rate of death from cardiovascular causes in HYVET study (Beckett et al., 2008).

In the first observational studies of **hormone replacement therapy (HRT)** in postmenopausal women, it was shown that HRT prevents the development of CVD. However, in the Heart and Estrogen/Progestin Replacement Study (HERS) (Hulley et al., 1998) and Heart and Estrogen/Progestin Study II (HERS II) (Grady et al., 2002) studies, performed some years later, no long- or short-term benefits of HRT were observed. In the Women's Health Initiative WHI (Wassertheil-Smoller et al., 2004) study of patients being treated with HRT, deaths resulting from coronary heart disease, strokes, pulmonary embolisms, venous thromboembolisms, and risk of ischemic strokes increased and BP rose slightly. For these reasons, HRT should not be given to prevent CV endpoints, without knowing the baseline BP, if any, and patients should be monitored closely.

4.3 Treatment rules of hypertension in the elderly

Factors to be taken into account in deciding when to start treatment in elderly and young hypertensives are not fundamentally different. The decision is based on both BP level and the patient's CV risk factors (Mancia et al., 2007, 2009). For a hypertensive patient in stage 1, who does not display any risk factors, it is possible to monitor him or her for several months with non-drug therapies, whereas non drug therapies must be started immediately in patients with established CV or renal disease (Mancia et al., 2007., 2009).

Non-drug treatments, such as sodium restriction, maintaining ideal weight, regular exercise, smoking cessation, reducing dietary fat content, etc., have proven efficacy and should be administered before pharmacological treatment, or with it. Lifestyle changes are the first, primary, and permanent treatment recommendations in The Seventh Report of the Joint National Committee on Prevention, Detection, Evaluation, and Treatment of High Blood Pressure (JNC 7) (Chobanian et al., 2003), as well as the European Society of Cardiology (ESC) hypertension guidelines (Mancia et al., 2007). In the Tone study (Trial of Non Pharmacologic Interventions in the Elderly) (Kostis et al., 2002) salt restriction, weight loss, or both were attempted in 985 patients between the ages of 60-80. Each method alone reduced BP, but the combination of the two methods had the most successful results.

In elderly hypertensives, there is no evidence that any drug dramatically affects combined HT or ISH. Most elderly hypertensives suffer from other health problems (target organ damage and associated CV cases), and so the choice of drug should be based on each patients personal requirements. Although there is no clear difference in the results, tolerability, cost, compatibility with other drugs and patient preference affects the choice of the initial antihypertensive drug. A recently published meta-analysis (Staessen et al., 2000), showed that drug selection is less important than the reduction BP for the prevention of CV outcomes (Mancia et al., 2007). It is difficult to lower BP below 140 mm Hg in many old patients, so often two or more drugs are required (Fagard et al., 2002; Mancia et al., 2002). In such cases, the general rules about which drugs may be combined with each other will guide the selection of agents (Mancia et al., 2007).

Compared with younger patients, however, older patients are at an increased risk for serious adverse effects, including effects of drug interactions related to the use of multiple medications. Drug dosage is half that prescribed to young people, and it is important that BP be lowered at a slow pace. Syncope in elderly persons may be caused by orthostatic or postprandial hypotension, and frail elderly persons are at an increased risk for these adverse consequences of antihypertensive therapy. Blood pressure should be measured regularly, especially after eating, with the patient sitting in an upright position. Marked orthostatic or postprandial hypotension should prompt a reduction in drug dosage or substitution to another antihypertensive agent.

According to hypertension guidelines, the goal of treatment of hypertension in elderly persons is to reduce the blood pressure to less than 140/90 mm Hg and to less than 130/80 mm Hg in those with diabetes mellitus or chronic renal insufficiency (Chobanian et al., 2003; Mancia et al., 2007). There is sufficient evidence to recommend that SBP be lowered below 140 mm Hg (and DBP below 90 mm Hg) in all hypertensive patients, both those at low moderate risk and those at high risk. Evidence is less available for elderly hypertensive patients, in whom the benefit of lowering SBP below 140 and 130 mmHg has never been tested in randomized trials. The optimum diastolic blood pressure goal in elderly persons is unclear (Aronow, 2010). Based on current data, it may be prudent to recommend lowering systolic and diastolic BP values within the range 130–139/80–85 mmHg, and possibly close to the lower values in this range, in all hypertensive patients. More critical evidence from specific-randomized trials is needed for more specific conclusions (Mancia et al., 2009).

5. Dyslipidemia in the elderly

Atherosclerosis is a continuous degenerative process, and its burden increases progressively with aging. The pathology consists of chronic remodeling of the vascular wall and participation of the calcification process. Hyperlipidaemia is one of the most important risk factors in the development of atherosclerosis. Older studies indicated that serum cholesterol was related to CV disease, but the relationship between serum cholesterol and CV mortality was not clear. A few decades later, a study gave us the first scientific clue showing that lowering serum cholesterol decreases the CV morbidity by decreasing atherosclerosis (The Lipid Research Clinics, 1984). Significant reduction in cholesterol levels and CV disease morbidity can be achieved through lifestyle changes and drug therapy. Our information and knowledge on the importance of cholesterol plaque stability and its relationship with lipid lowering drugs developed subsequently. The current accepted theory is that the main mechanism of action of lipid lowering drugs is to ensure a more stable formation of atherosclerotic plaques (Streja, D. & Streja, E., 2011).

5.1 Atherogenic particles and aging

Atherogenic particles are defined as total cholesterol, low-density lipoprotein (LDL) cholesterol, non-high density lipoprotein (HDL) cholesterol (Total cholesterol-HDL cholesterol) or Apolipoprotein B (Apo B). Their role in CV diseases is shared by other risk factors, such as high BP, obesity, smoking and alcohol.

Elderly individuals have different properties of lipid metabolism compared with younger individuals, as **physiological changes can be seen in the lipid profile** of the elderly. In general, **atherogenic particles increase with age**. Age-related changes in the total serum cholesterol concentration primarily result from an increase in LDL cholesterol levels. Apolipoprotein B and LDL cholesterol show a progressive increase with age (Aslam et al., 2009). The mechanisms responsible for the progressive age-related elevation in LDL cholesterol have not been fully explained; however, various data suggest a decrease in the fractional catabolic rate of LDL cholesterol as playing a primary role. This reduction in LDL cholesterol catabolism is believed to result from diminished activity of hepatic LDL cholesterol receptors (Ericsson et al., 1991). Triglycerides (TG) increase with age, and reaches maximum values in men at age 50-59 and in women at 60-69. In contrast, HDL cholesterol levels do not vary much with age, being approximately 10 mg/dL higher in women than men throughout their lifetime (Aslam et al., 2009).

5.2 Clinical studies about atherogenic particles and cardiovascular risk

Numerous studies, including those with elderly subjects, reported a high risk of coronary artery disease in subjects with only high, but also low, **total cholesterol** concentrations (Abbott et al., 2002, Higgins & Keller, 1992; Manolio et al., 1992; Tyroler & Ford, 1992). However, there are some confusing data, in that a meta-analysis about the relationship between total cholesterol and coronary events shows a significant association for men aged 65-80 years, but none for women over 65 years or men over 80 years (Anum & Adera, 2004). This suggests that total cholesterol may not be a good parameter to predict coronary events in the elderly (Krumholz et al., 1994). This lack of association is especially valid for elderly women (Barrett-Connor, 1992).

One meta-analysis showed that high **triglyceride** levels are strongly associated with a significantly higher CV risk in middle age cohorts (Sarwar et al., 2007). Another study reported that in the highest TG quintile an 80% increase in the risk of coronary events, a 70% increased risk of coronary death and a 50% increased risk of stroke was observed in all age groups and genders (Patel et al., 2004). A specific study for participants aged 65 years and older showed a gender specific risk of triglycerides, which were shown to be powerful independent predictors of CVD in women only (Mazza et al., 2005). Therefore, it seems that high TG levels increase CVD in the elderly, but women are more affected.

HDL cholesterol is the parameter of strongest association with CV risk in lipid particles, especially for middle-aged men and women. Subjects with high HDL cholesterol are more likely to have long life expectancy (Arai & Hirose, 2004; Barter, 2004). In The Prospective Study of Pravastatin in the Elderly at Risk (PROSPER) Study, it is reported that low HDL cholesterol in elderly people determines both the risk of fatal and nonfatal coronary and cerebrovascular events and the efficiency of statin therapy (Packard et al., 2005).

Non-HDL cholesterol does not appear to be a reliable predictor of CV risk in older subjects. Some studies have reported that **Apo B and Apo A1** might be superior to the measurement of standard lipid parameters (Bruno et al., 2006).

Randomized controlled trials of the last 30 years used groups of older individuals, which was often not the case in earlier studies. Most of these recent studies have shown that lipid-lowering **statine therapy for both primary and secondary prevention reduced CV events in elderly individuals.**

Two randomized **primary prevention clinical trials** (CARDS, Neil et al., 2006 and ASCOT, Sever et al., 2003) reported separately that elderly and young individuals showed similar results after lipid-lowering drug therapy. Cardiovascular event rates in treated individuals in both groups were significantly less frequently observed. In other words, the treatment of hyperlipidemia, are useful in both younger and elderly individuals. However, data on primary prevention in the elderly are less clear. There is a significant reduction in coronary events, coronary deaths and all cause mortality but numbers needed to treat are higher than in secondary prevention (Berthold et al., 2011).

Cholesterol And Recurrent Events (CARE) (Sacks et al., 1996), Scandinavian Simvastatin Survival Study (4S) (The Scandinavian Simvastatin Survival Study Group, 1994), and Long-term Intervention with Pravastatin in Ischemic Disease (LIPID) (LIPID Study Group, 1998) are three large **secondary prevention clinical trials**. They include large numbers of elderly patient subgroups and analyses of these studies have demonstrated similar results. In not only the middle aged, but also in the elderly, CV events were seen less in treated cases, (Lewis et al., 1998).

Some current studies are designed specifically for elderly patients. The PROSPER trial (Packard et al., 2005), was designed to determine whether pravastatin 40 mg/d reduces coronary and cerebral events in older patients aged 70-82 years who have preexisting vascular disease or who are at high risk for vascular disease and stroke. This double-blind randomized trial included 5804 patients on either placebo or 40 mg of pravastatin. The primary composite endpoint was definite or suspected death from coronary heart disease, nonfatal myocardial infarction, or fatal or nonfatal stroke. After 3 years, coronary events were significantly reduced by 19%, and coronary mortality was reduced by 24%in patients on pravastatin; however, this therapy had no effect on stroke or cognitive function. The PROSPER study clearly showed that the benefits of statin therapy observed among middle-aged adults can also be extended to older patients (>70 years). Study Assessing Goals in the Elderly (SAGE) trial (Deedwania et al., 2007), enrolled 893 people aged 65-85 who had coronary heart disease and one or more past episodes of myocardial ischemia. They were randomized according to intensive (atorvastatin 80 mg/day) vs. moderate (pravastatin 40 mg/day) lipid-lowering therapy. After one year, intensive therapy was shown to reduce cardiac events by 28%, indicating the benefit of intensive statin therapy in older men and women.

It is widely accepted that age is not a factor affecting the benefits of lipid-lowering drugs. Therefore, today's guidelines for the prevention and treatment of CV diseases, recommend lipid-lowering drugs without specifying an age limit. Despite the satisfactory results obtained from the statin trials that included elderly patients, there are still knowledge gaps regarding the benefits of therapy with other hypolipidemic agents, such as fibrates and niacin, in the elderly.

5.3 Treatment rules of dyslipidemia in the elderly

The National Cholesterol Education Program Adult Treatment Panel 3 **(Table 1,** The National Cholesterol Education Program expert panel, 2001**)** and the American Heart Association (AHA) and American College of Cardiology (ACC) (Smith et al, 2006) suggest LDL cholesterol goals for lipid lowering therapy. For all patients with coronary artery disease, ACC/AHA recommends LDL set the goal at <70 mg/dL.

Not all guidelines accept old age as a parameter affecting treatment methods of dyslipidemia, but they suggest evaluating and treating every old person individually. This is because guidelines are based on risk scoring, but most of the risk assessment tools are not adaptable to the elderly. So, when deciding which drug (especially statin) therapy to use in the elderly, instead of applying the algorithms routinely prescribed for persons with multiple risk factors, the physician's decision must be based on the HDL cholesterol level, other vascular diseases, accompanying chronic diseases, frailty, benefit/cost assessment, safety, tolerability, and patient preference. The AHA Evidence-based Guidelines for Cardiovascular Disease Prevention in Women **(**Mosca et al., 2007**)** also declares that treatment rules are not clear for the treatment of very elderly women, because of the exclusion criteria of many studies. Uncertainty about the benefits of hipolipidemic treatment in these patient groups and the resulting question marks indicate the need for more clinical trials that included men and women patients at a very advanced age.

Risk Level	LDL Goal
Coronary heart disease and coronary heart disease risk equivalent*	<100 mg/dl
Multiple (2+) risk factors	<130 mg/dl**
0-1 risk factor	<160 mg/dl

*Diabetes, chronic kidney disease
**LDL cholesterol goal for multiple risk factors and 10 year risk >20 percent is 100 mg/dL.

Table 1. Low-density lipoprotein goals for three risk levels (The National Cholesterol Education Program expert panel, 2001).

Most guidelines for CV prevention recommend **lifestyle change** as an important measure for therapy of dyslipidemia in all age groups. Their suggestions are based on several randomized clinical trials. There is no specific advice for the elderly in these trials. Beyond the randomized clinical trials, there are many positive observations about the use of grains, nuts (Hu et al., 1999), the Mediterranean diet (particularly walnuts), monounsaturated fat (olive oil), smoking cessation, and strong negativities about foods with high glycemic index or containing trans fatty acids (Lemaitre et al., 2006).

Statins decrease cholesterol synthesis by inhibiting HMG CoA Reductase, the most important enzyme in the synthesis of cholesterol. All statins also perform anti-inflammatory and anti-proliferative functions in other metabolic ways. These properties, referred to as "pleiotropic effects," (Arnaud & Mach, 2005; Athyros et al., 2009; Gotto& Farmer, 2001; Liao & Laufs, 2005) are improvement in endothelial function, decreased smooth muscle cell proliferation and prevention of vascular remodeling. Statins also reduce the level of anti-inflammatory markers such as C-reactive protein (CRP) (Jialal et al., 2001). **Fibrates** increase fatty acid oxidation and reduce very light density lipoprotein (VLDL) and Apo C3 concentration (Chinetti-Gbaguidi et al., 2005; Robillard et al., 2005). A process of activation of lipoprotein lipase increases VLDL catabolism. Fibrates have pleiotropic effects too. Other lipid lowering drugs are **bile acid binding resins**, **niacin**, **cholesterol absorption inhibitors**, and **omega-3 fatty acids**. **Serum antioxidants** have been associated with a reduced CV mortality in the elderly, however, the benefit of antioxidant therapy on CV mortality is yet to be proven (Buijsse et al., 2005; Fletcher et al., 2003).

5.4 Safety and toxic effects of lipid-lowering drugs in elderly individuals

The safety of using lipid-lowering drugs is diminished in the older age group. With age, the glomerular filtration rate, hepatic blood flow, and elimination of drugs can decrease (Redgrave, 2004). All of these may result in the drugs, including statins, causing **augmented toxic effect**. In addition, aging increases the number of co-morbidities requiring pharmacologic intervention and this in turn results in polypharmacy. All these factors contribute to a modification of the risk/benefit ratio of preventative interventions. This further decreases the safety of lipid lowering drugs.

The most important side effects of statins are **rhabdomyolysis**. Although it has been suggested, it has not yet been definitively proven that statins cause decreased cognitive function. Meta analyses of statins have not confirmed the hypothesis that they may increase cancer prevalence. Some studies recorded decreased colorectal cancer frequency (Poynter et al., 2005), but other studies were not able to confirm this (Bailey et al., 2007; Bouchard et al., 2007; Gibson et al., 2006; Goodpaster et al., 2006; Ho et al., 2006; Fonarow GC, 2005; Naughton et al., 2007). Another study (Setoguchi et al., 2007) concluded that it is unlikely that statins have any relationship with cancer incidence. Larger studies are needed to be performed in order to use statins for the prevention of cancer in medical practice. An old study that compared fibrates (Committee of Principal Investigators, 1978) showed a decrease in the risk of myocardial infarction, but an increase in the risk gastro-intestinal cancer. There is no such indication in currently used fibrates.

6. Smoking in the elderly

Smoking in old age has been a subject of much attention in past years. In studies across the board, smoking was seen to jeopardize the health of individuals in every age group. The risks were caused not only by smoking in elderly individuals, but also by exposure to passive smoke.

Many health problems are likely to occur in old age. Hypertension, heart and vascular diseases, cancer, chronic diseases are associated with, and more frequently experienced during this period. Smoking tobacco products increases the risk of each of these conditions, and if they occur at the same time, the risk greatly increases. Smoking cessation decreases the associated risks for each organ, and increases physical capacity, which results in a decrease in the threats to the health of the heart and blood vessels.

The relationship between smoking and adverse cardiovascular events and death is well established. Numerous studies have demonstrated that cigarette smoking increases CV morbidity and mortality in elderly patients with CAD. Smoking also aggravates angina pectoris and precipitates silent myocardial ischemia in older patients who have CAD. At 40 month follow-up of 644 older men, mean age 80 years, and at 48-month follow up of 1488 older women, mean age 82 years, current cigarette smoking increased the relative risk of new coronary events (nonfatal or fatal myocardial infarction [MI], or sudden cardiac death) by a factor of 2.2 in older men and 2.0 in older women (Aronow & Ahn, 1996).

There are three main approaches for smoking cessation: to never begin smoking, to quit smoking, and to prevent passive smoking. From a prevention standpoint, goals should be the same for each age group, but abstinence by never beginning to smoke remains the best method of preventing the adverse CV effects of smoking. However, if it is not possible, based on the available data, older men and women who smoke cigarettes should be strongly encouraged to stop smoking because cessation of smoking will reduce CV and all-cause mortality after MI. However, changes in an individual's perception of health in old age may create difficulty in an attempt at smoking cessation. The elderly are often more resistant to changing their behavior patterns than younger patients. There is a widely accepted perception in old age that, "there is little point to quitting smoking at this age." This perception is not based on reality, as stopping smoking is beneficial at all ages. In order to change such false perceptions, a smoking cessation program should be instituted (Smith et al., 2006). They are frequently applied toward young people, adults and the elderly quite successfully. Intervention programs that use behavioral approaches, physician counseling, close clinical follow-up, and pharmacologic therapy are recommended to help older adults who are tobacco dependent (Williams et al., 2002).

Quitting smoking has an early impact on mortality risk, reducing mortality by as much as 50% in those with prior MI, with most of this mortality benefit occurring in the first year (Sparrow & Dawber, 1978). In patients over the age of 70 years with CAD, participating in the Coronary Artery Surgery Study (CASS) registry, morbidity and mortality rates were reduced among those who stopped smoking, with risk reductions similar to those seen among younger patients (Hermanson et al., 1988). The risk of new coronary events falls immediately after cessation of smoking, returning to that of non-smoking elderly persons within 5 years.

7. Inflammation and heart in the elderly

Inflammation markers related to CV risk have been known for a long time. Some **meta-analyses** clearly show that high sensitivity C-reactive protein (hs-CRP) is useful in predicting CV risk. It is believed that hsCRP gives information about intravascular inflammation and unstable atherosclerotic plaque (Kubo et al., 2009). hs-CRP represents the atherosclerotic burden like ankle brachial index, increased carotid intima-media thickness or vascular calcifications (Cao et al., 2003) not only in young but also old patients.

A prospective big **study** has shown that hs-CRP accurately predicts CV mortality (Clarke et al., 2008). However, it is suggested that high CRP is also a good independent marker for nonvascular mortality. In another study, mortality risk was much greater if there was more than one inflammatory marker (Wang et al., 2006). Results of these **studies** suggest to measure hs-CRP levels in order to measure the benefit of statin therapy. The AHA suggests to measure hs-CRP in order to determine higher risk of CV events and to limit the use of hipolipidemic therapy in specific groups of patients. Some **cardiovascular risk estimation models** have added hs-CRP to their parameters (Cook et al., 2006; Ridker et al., 2008). These models are suggested to be used in patients up to 79 years of age.

Most data detailing the importance of hs-CRP in the **elderly** uses The Cardiovascular Health Study as its main source. This study implicated that CRP is a strong and independent predictor of 10-year coronary artery disease risk in patients over age 65 (Cushman et al., 2005).

hs-CRP indicates the risk of CV events and other causes of mortality for all ages (Kaptoge et al., 2010). But its specificity decreases with increasing age. hs-CRP increase is a part of the aging process and high hs-CRP values are frequent in healthy older people (Streja, 2011). It not only increases progressively with healthy aging, it may also be due to of the higher number of disease in the elderly, so the specificity of CRP for CV risk is lower than younger patients. Furthermore, according to some studies, well-known traditional risk factors predict CV risk but hs-CRP adds only a few, or it does not change the risk status. Because of the abovementioned reasons, there are still hesitations about adding hs-CRP to the process of CV risk determination in the elderly.

Other inflammatory parameters are also found to be related with mortality but we do not have too much information about them compared with CRP. Some studies compare interleukin 6 (IL-6) and hs-CRP and conclude that the ability of IL-6 to estimate risk is modest, while the ability of hs-CRP is only borderline (Rodondi et al., 2010). Furthermore, there are some close associations between inflammatory markers, Factor VIII, and D-dimer, which are the risk factors for increased risk of death in the elderly (Zakai et al., 2007).

8. References

Abbott, RD., Curb, JD., Rodriguez, BL., Masaki, KH., Yano, K., Schatz, IJ., Ross, GW., & Petrovitch, H. (2002). Age-related changes in risk factor effects on the incidence of coronary heart disease. *Ann Epidemiol*, Vol. 12, No. 3, pp. 173-181. ISSN: 1047-2797

Adamopoulos, P.N., Chrysanthakopoulis, S.G., & Frohlich, E.D. (1975). Systolic hypertension: nonhomogeneous diseases. *Am J Cardiol*, Vol. 36, No. 5, pp. 697-701. ISSN: 0002-9149

Amery, A., Birkenhäger, W., Bogaert, M., Brixko, P., Bulpitt, C., Clement, D., De Leeuw, P., De Plaen, JF., Deruyttere, M., De Schaepdryver, A., Fagard, R., Forette, F., Forte, J., Hamdy, R., Hellemans, J., Henry, JF., Koistinen, A., Laaser, U., Laher, M., Leonetti, G., Lewis, P, Lund-Johansen, P., MacFarlane, J., Meurer, K., Miguel, P., Morris J., Mutsers, A., Nissinen, A., O'Brien E., Ohm, OJ., O'Malley, K., Pelemans, W., Perera N., Tuomilehto, J., Verschueren, LJ., Willemse, P., Williams, B., & Zanchetti, A. (1982). Antihypertensive therapy in patients above age 60 with systolic hypertension. A progress report of the European Working Party on High Blood Pressure in the Elderly (EWPHE). *Clin Exp Hypertens A*, Vol. 4, No. 7, pp. 1151-1176. ISSN: 1064-1963

Antihypertensive and Lipid-Lowering Treatment to Prevent Heart Attack Trial Collaborative Research Group. (2003). Diuretic versus alpha-blocker as first-step antihypertensive therapy: final results from the Antihypertensive and Lipid-Lowering Treatment to Prevent Heart Attack Trial (ALLHAT). *Hypertension*. Vol. 42, No. 3, pp. 239-46. ISSN: 0194-911X

Anum, EA., & Adera, T. (2004) Hypercholesterolemia and coronary heart disease in the elderly: a meta-analysis. *Ann Epidemiol*, Vol. 14, No. 9, pp 705-721. ISSN: 1047-2797

Arai, Y., & Hirose, N. (2004). Aging and HDL metabolism in elderly people more than 100 years old. *J Atheroscler Thromb*, Vol. 11, No: 5, pp. 246-252. ISSN: 1340-3478

Arnaud, C., & Mach, F. (2005). Pleiotropic effects of statins in atherosclerosis: role on endothelial function, inflammation and immunomodulation. *Arch Mal Coeur Vaiss*, Vol 98, No 6, pp. 661-666. ISSN: 0003-9683

Aronow, WS., & Ahn, C. (1996). Risk factors for new coronary events in a large cohort of very elderly patients with and without coronary artery disease. *Am J Cardiol*, Vol. 77, No. 10, pp. 864-866. ISSN: 0002-9149

Aronow, WS. (2010). Why and how we should treat elderly patients with hypertension? *Curr Vasc Pharmacol*, Vol. 8, No.6, pp. 780-787. ISSN: 1570-1611

Aslam, F., Haque, A., Lee, V.L., & Foody, J. A. (2009). Hyperlipidemia in older adults. *Clin Geriatr Med*, Vol. 25, pp. 591-606. ISSN: 0749-0690

Athyros, VG., Kakafika, AI., Tziomalos, K., Karagiannis, A., & Mikhailidis, DP. (2009). Pleiotropic effects of statins--clinical evidence. *Curr Pharm Des*, Vol. 15, No. 5, pp 479-489. ISSN: 1381-6128

Bailey, TC., Noirot, LA., Blickensderfer, A., Rachmiel, E., Schaiff, R., Kessels, A., Braverman, A., Goldberg, A., Waterman B., & Dunagan, W.C. (2007). An intervention to improve secondary prevention of coronary heart disease. *Arch Intern Med,* Vol 167, No. 6, pp. 586-90. ISSN: 0003-9926

Barrett-Connor, E. (1992). Hypercholesterolemia predicts early death from coronary heart disease in elderly men but not women. The Rancho Bernardo Study. *Ann Epidemiol,* Vol 2, No. 1-2, pp. 77-83. ISSN: 1047-2797

Barter, P. (2004). HDL: a recipe for longevity. *Atheroscler* Suppl. Vol. 5, No. 2, pp. 25-31. ISSN: 0021-9150

Beckett, NS., Peters, R., Fletcher, AE., Staessen, JA., Liu, L., Dumitrascu, D., Stoyanovsky, V., Antikainen, RL., Nikitin, Y., Anderson, C., Belhani, A., Forette, F., Rajkumar, C., Thijs, L., Banya, W., & Bulpitt, CJ; HYVET Study Group. (2008). Treatment of hypertension in patients 80 years of age or older. *N Engl J Med,* Vol. 358, No. 18, pp. 1887-1898. ISSN: 0028-4793

Bennati, E., Murphy, A., Cambien, F., Whitehead, AS., Archbold, GP., Young, IS., Rea, IM. (2010). BELFAST centenarians: a case of optimised cardiovascular risk? *Curr Pharm Des.* Vol. 16,No. 7, pp. 789-795. ISSN: 1381-6128

Berthold, HK., Gouni-Berthold, I. (2011). Lipid-lowering drug therapy in elderly patients. *Curr Pharm Des.* Vol. 17, No. 9, pp. 877-893. ISSN: 1381-6128

Bouchard, MH., Dragomir, A., Blais, L., Bérard, A., Pilon, D., & Perreault S. (2007). Impact of adherence to statins on coronary artery disease in primary prevention. *Br J Clin Pharmacol,* Vol. 63, No. 6, pp 698-708. ISSN: 0306-5251

Brown, MJ., Palmer, CR., Castaigne, A., de Leeuw, PW., Mancia, G., Rosenthal, T., & Ruilope, LM. (2000). Morbidity and mortality in patients randomised to double-blind treatment with a long-acting calcium-channel blocker or diuretic in the International Nifedipine GITS study: Intervention as a Goal in Hypertension Treatment (INSIGHT). *Lancet.* Vol. 356, No. 9227, pp. 366-72. ISSN: 0140-6736

Bruno, G, Merletti, F., Biggeri, A., Bargero, G., Prina-Cerai, S., Pagano, G., & Cavallo-Perin, P. (2006). Effect of age on the association of non-high-density-lipoprotein cholesterol and apolipoprotein B with CV mortality in a Mediterranean population with type 2 diabetes: the Casale Monferrato study. *Diabetologia,* Vol. 49, No. 5, pp. 937-944. ISSN: 0012-186X

Buijsse, B., Feskens, EJ., Schlettwein-Gsell, D., Ferry, M., Kok, FJ., Kromhout, D., & de Groot, LC. (2005). Plasma carotene and alpha-tocopherol in relation to 10-y all-cause and cause-specific mortality in European elderly: the Survey in Europe on Nutrition and the Elderly, a Concerted Action (SENECA). *Am J Clin Nutr,* Vol 82, No. 4, pp 879-886. ISSN: 0002-9165

Bulpitt, CJ., Beckett, NS., Cooke, J., Dumitrascu, DL., Gil-Extremera, B., Nachev, C., Nunes, M., Peters, R., Staessen, JA., & Thijs, L.; Hypertension in the Very Elderly Trial Working Group. (2003). Results of the pilot study for the Hypertension in the Very Elderly Trial. *J Hypertens.* Vol 21, No 12, pp: 2409-17. ISSN: 0263-6352

Cao, JJ., Thach, C., Manolio, TA., Psaty, BM., Kuller, LH., Chaves, PH., Polak, JF., Sutton-Tyrrell., K, Herrington, DM., Price, TR., & Cushman, M. (2003). C-reactive protein, carotid intima-media thickness, and incidence of ischemic stroke in the elderly: the Cardiovascular Health Study. *Circulation.* Vol 15, No 108, pp. 166-70. ISSN: 0009-7322

Chinetti-Gbaguidi, G., Fruchart, JC., & Staels, B. (2005). Pleiotropic effects of fibrates. *Curr Atheroscler Rep.* Vol. 7, No. 5, pp. 396-401. ISSN: 1523-3804

Chobanian, AV., Bakris, GL., Black, HR., Cushman, WC., Green LA., Izzo, JL. Jr., Jones, DW., Materson, BJ., Oparil, S., Wright, JT. Jr., & Roccella, EJ.; Joint National Committee on Prevention, Detection, Evaluation, and Treatment of High Blood Pressure. National Heart, Lung, and Blood Institute; National High Blood Pressure Education Program Coordinating Committee. (2003). Seventh report of the Joint National Committee on Prevention, Detection, Evaluation, and Treatment of High Blood Pressure. *Hypertension*, Vol, 42, No. 6, pp. 1206-1252. ISSN: 0194-911X

Chobanian, AV. (2007) Clinical Practice. Isolated systolic hypertension in the elderly. *N Engl J Med.* Vol. 357, No. 8. pp 789-96. ISSN: 0028-4793

Clarke R., Emberson, JR., Breeze, E., Casas, JP., Parish, S., Hingorani, AD., Fletcher, A., Collins, R., & Smeeth, L. (2008). Biomarkers of inflammation predict both vascular and non-vascular mortality in older men. *Eur Heart J.* Vol. 29, No. 6. pp:800-9. ISSN: 0195-668X

Committee of Principal Investigators. (1978). A co-operative trial in the primary prevention of ischaemic heart disease using clofibrate. Report from the Committee of Principal Investigators. *Br Heart J.* Vol. 40, No. 10, pp. 1069-118. ISSN: 0007-0769

Cook, NR., Buring, JE., & Ridker, PM. (2006). The effect of including C-reactive protein in cardiovascular risk prediction models for women. *Ann Intern Med,* Vol. 145, No. 1, pp 21-29. ISSN: 0003-4819

Cushman, M., Arnold, AM., Psaty, BM., Manolio, TA., Kuller, LH., Burke, GL., Polak, JF., & Tracy RP. (2005). C-reactive protein and the 10-year incidence of coronary heart disease in older men and women: the cardiovascular health study. *Circulation.* Vol. 112, No. 1, pp.25-31. ISSN: 0009-7322

Deedwania, P., Stone, PH., Bairey Merz., CN, Cosin-Aguilar, J., Koylan, N., Luo, D., Ouyang, P., Piotrowicz, R., Schenck-Gustafsson, K., Sellier, P., Stein, JH., Thompson, PL., & Tzivoni, D. (2007). Effects of intensive versus moderate lipid-lowering therapy on myocardial ischemia in older patients with coronary heart disease: results of the Study Assessing Goals in the Elderly (SAGE). *Circulation.* Vol 115, No. 6, pp 700-707. ISSN: 0009-7322

Ekbom, T., Dahlöf, B., Hansson, L., Lindholm, L.H., Scherstén, B., & Wester, P.O. (1992). Antihypertensive efficacy and side effects of three beta-blockers and a diuretic in elderly hypertensives: a report from the STOP-Hypertension study. *J Hypertens.* Vol. (10), No. 12, pp.1525-1530. ISSN: 0263-6352

Ericsson, S., Eriksson, M., Vitols, S.,Einarsson, K., Berglund, L., Angelin, B.(1991). Influence of age on the metabolism of plasma low density lipoproteins in healthy males. *J Clin Invest;* Vol. 87, No. 2, pp. 591-596. ISSN: 0021-9738

Expert Panel on Detection, Evaluation, and Treatment of High Blood Cholesterol in Adults. (2001). Executive Summary of The Third Report of The National Cholesterol Education Program (NCEP) Expert Panel on Detection, Evaluation, And Treatment of High Blood Cholesterol In Adults (Adult Treatment Panel III). *JAMA.*Vol. 285, No. 19, pp. 2486-97. ISSN: 0098-7484

Fagard, R.H., Van Den Enden, M., Leeman, M., & Warling, X. (2002). Survey on treatment of hypertension and implementation of World Health Organization/International Society of Hypertension risk stratification in primary care in Belgium. *J Hypertens.* Vol. 20, No. 7, pp. 1297-302. ISSN: 0263-6352

Fletcher, A.E., Breeze, E., & Shetty, P.S. (2003). Antioxidant vitamins and mortality in older persons: findings from the nutrition add-on study to the Medical Research CouncilTrial of Assessment and Management of Older People in the Community. *Am J Clin Nutr.* Vol 78, No. 5, pp. 999-1010. ISSN: 0002-9165

Fonarow, GC. (2005). In-hospital initiation of statin therapy in acute coronary syndromes: maximizing the early and long-term benefits. *Chest.* Vol. 128, No. 5, pp. 3641-3651. ISSN: 0012-3692

Gibson, T.B., Mark, T.L., Axelsen, K., Baser, O., Rublee, DA., & McGuigan, KA. (2006). Impact of statin copayments on adherence and medical care utilization and expenditures. *Am J Manag Care.* Vol 12, No 11-19. ISSN: 1088-0224

Goodpaster, B.H., Park, S.W., Harris, T.B., Kritchevsky, S.B., Nevitt, M., Schwartz, A.V., Simonsick, E.M., Tylavsky, F.A., Visser, M., & Newman A.B. (2006). The loss of skeletal muscle strength, mass, and quality in older adults: the health, aging and body composition study. *J Gerontol A Biol Sci Med Sci.* Vol. 61, No. 10. Pp. 1059-1064. ISSN: 1079-5006

Gotto Jr, A.M. Jr, & Farmer, J.A. (2001). Pleiotropic effects of statins: do they matter? *Curr Opin Lipidol.* Vol 12, No. 4, pp: 391-394. ISSN: 0957-9672

Grady, D., Herrington, D., Bittner, V., Blumenthal, R., Davidson, M., Hlatky, M., Hsia, J., Hulley, S., Herd, A., Khan, S., Newby, LK., Waters, D., Vittinghoff, E., & Wenger, N.; HERS Research Group. (2002). Cardiovascular disease outcomes during 6.8 years of hormonetherapy: Heart and Estrogen/progestin Replacement Study follow-up (HERS II). *JAMA.* Vol 288, No 1, pp:49-57. ISSN: 0098-7484

Gribbin B., Pickering, TG., Sleight P., & Peto R.(1971). Effect of age and high blood pressure on baroreflex sensitivity in man. *Circ Res.* Vol 29, No. 4, pp 424-431. ISSN: 0009-7330

Hajjar, I.M. , Grim C.E., George, V., & Kotchen, T.A. (2001), Impact of diet on blood pressure and age-related changes in blood pressure in the US population: analysis of NHANES III. *Arch Intern Med.* Vol. 161, No 4, pp:589-593. ISSN: 0003-9926

Hansson, L., Lindholm, L.H., Ekbom, T., Dahlöf, B., Lanke, J., Scherstén., B., Wester, P.O., Hedner, T., & de Faire, U. (1999). Randomised trial of old and new antihypertensive drugs in elderly patients: cardiovascular mortality and morbidity the Swedish Trial in Old Patients with Hypertension-2 study. *Lancet.* Vol. 354, No. 9192, pp:1751-6. ISSN: 0140-6736

Hermanson, B, Omenn, GS, Kronmal, RA, & Gersh, BJ. (1988). Beneficial six-year outcome of smoking cessation in older men and women with coronary artery disease. Results from the CASS registry. *N Engl J Med.* Vol. 319, No. 21, pp:1365-69. ISSN: 0028-4793

Higgins, M. & Keller, JB. (1992). Cholesterol, coronary heart disease, and total mortality in middle-aged and elderly men and women in Tecumseh. *Ann Epidemiol.* Vol.2 No.1-2, pp:69-76. ISSN: 1047-2797

Hajjar, I.M., Grim, C.E., George, V., Kotchen, T.A. (2001). Impact of diet on blood pressure and age-related changes in blood pressure in the US population: analysis of NHANES III. *Arch Intern Med.* Vol. 26, No. 161, pp. 589-593. ISSN: 0003-9926

Ho, P.M., Magid, D.J., Masoudi, F.A., McClure, D.L., & Rumsfeld, J.S. (2006). Adherence to cardioprotective medications and mortality among patients with diabetes and ischemic heart disease. *BMC Cardiovasc Disord.* Vol 6, pp. 48. ISSN: 1471-2261

Hu, F.B., & Stampfer, M.J. (1999). Nut consumption and risk of coronary heart disease: a review of epidemiologic evidence. *Curr Atheroscler Rep.* Vol. 1, No. 3, pp 204-209. ISSN: 1523-3804

Hulley, S., Grady, D., Bush, T., Furberg, C., Herrington, D., Riggs, B., & Vittinghoff, E. (1998). Randomized trial of estrogen plus progestin for secondary prevention of coronary heart disease in postmenopausal women. Heart and Estrogen/progestin Replacement Study (HERS) Research Group. *JAMA.* Vol. 280, No. 7. pp:605-613. ISSN: 0098-7484

Hyman, D.J. & Pavlik, V.N. (2001). Characteristics of patients with uncontrolled hypertension in the United States. *N Engl J Med.* Vol. 345, No 7, pp 479-86. ISSN: 0028-4793

Hypertension Detection and Follow-up Program Cooperative Group. (1988). Persistence of reduction in blood pressure and mortality of participants in the Hypertension Detection and Follow-up Program. *JAMA.* Vol. 259, No. 14, pp. 2113-2122. ISSN: 0098-7484

Izzo, JL. (2005). Aging, arterial stiffness, and systolic hypertension. In: Hypertension in the elderly, Prisant M, pp 23-34, Humana Press, ISBN: 1-58829-197-9, NJ.

Jialal, I., Stein, D., Balis, D., Grundy, S.M., Adams-Huet, B., & Devaraj, S. (2001). Effect of hydroxymethyl glutaryl coenzyme a reductase inhibitor therapy on high sensitive C-reactive protein levels. *Circulation.* Vol 103, No 15, pp.1933-1935. ISSN: 0009-7322

Joint National Committee (1993). The fifth report of the Joint National Committee on Detection, Evaluation, and Treatment of High Blood Pressure (JNC V). *Arch Intern Med.* Vol. 153, No. 2, pp. 154-183. ISSN: 0003-9926

Kaptoge, S., Di Angelantonio, E., Lowe, G., Pepys, M.B., Thompson, S.G., Collins, R., & Danesh, J. (2010). Emerging Risk Factors Collaboration, C-reactive protein concentration and risk of coronary heart disease, stroke, and mortality: an individual participant meta-analysis. *Lancet.* Vol. 375, No. 9709, pp. 132-40. ISSN: 0140-6736

Kostis, J.B., Wilson, A.C., Shindler, D.M., Cosgrove, N.M., & Lacy, C.R. (2002) Persistence of normotension after discontinuation of lifestyle intervention in the trial of TONE. Trial of Nonpharmacologic Interventions in the Elderly. *Am J Hypertens.* Vol. 15, No. 8, pp. 732-4. ISSN: 0895-7061

Krumholz, HM, Seeman, T.E., Merrill, S.S., Mendes de Leon, CF, Vaccarino, V, Silverman, DI, Tsukahara, R, Ostfeld, AM, & Berkman, LF. (1994). Lack of association between cholesterol and coronary heart disease mortality and morbidity and all-cause mortality in persons older than 70 years. *JAMA.* Vol. 272, No. 17, pp:1335-1340. ISSN: 0098-7484

Kubo, T., Matsuo, Y., Hayashi, Y., Yamano, T., Tanimoto, T., Ino, Y., Kitabata, H., Takarada, S, Hirata, K., Tanaka, A., Nakamura, N., Mizukoshi, M., Imanishi, T., & Akasaka, T. (2009). High-sensitivity C-reactive protein and plaque composition in patients with stable angina pectoris: a virtual histology intravascular ultrasound study. *Coron Artery Dis.* Vol 20, No. 8, pp:531-535. ISSN: 0954-6928

Lemaitre, R.N., King, I.B., Mozaffarian, D., Sotoodehnia, N., Rea, T.D., Kuller, L.H., Tracy, R.P., & Siscovick, D.S. (2006). Plasma phospholipid trans fatty acids, fatal ischemic heartdisease, and sudden cardiac death in older adults: the cardiovascular health study. *Circulation.* Vol 114, No 3, pp. 209-215. ISSN: 0009-7322

Lewis, S.J., Moye, L.A., Sacks, F.M., Johnstone, D.E., Timmis, G., Mitchell, J., Limacher, M., Kell, S., Glasser, S.P., Grant, J., Davis, B.R., Pfeffer, M.A., & Braunwald, E. (1998). Effect of pravastatin on cardiovascular events in older patients with myocardial infarction and cholesterol levels in the average range. Results of the Cholesterol and Recurrent Events (CARE) trial. *Ann Intern Med.* Vol. 129, No. 9, pp. 681-689. ISSN: 0003-4819

Liao, J.K., & Laufs, U. (2005). Pleiotropic effects of statins. *Annu Rev Pharmacol Toxicol.* Vol 45, pp. 89-118. ISSN: 0362-1642

Mancia, G., De Backer, G., Dominiczak, A., Cifkova, R., Fagard, R., Germano, G., Grassi, G.,Heagerty, A.M., Kjeldsen, S.E., Laurent, S., Narkiewicz, K., Ruilope, L., Rynkiewicz, A., Schmieder, R.E., Struijker Boudier, H.A., Zanchetti, A., Vahanian, A., Camm, J., De Caterina, R., Dean, V., Dickstein, K., Filippatos, G., Funck-Brentano, C., Hellemans, I., Kristensen, S.D., McGregor, K., Sechtem, U., Silber, S., Tendera, M., Widimsky, P., Zamorano, J.L., Kjeldsen, S.E., Erdine, S., Narkiewicz, K., Kiowski, W., Agabiti-Rosei, E., Ambrosioni, E., Cifkova R., Dominiczak, A., Fagard, R., Heagerty, A.M., Laurent, S., Lindholm, L.H., Mancia, G., Manolis, A., Nilsson, P.M., Redon, J., Schmieder, R.E., Struijker-Boudier, H.A., Viigimaa, M., Filippatos, G., Adamopoulos, S., Agabiti-Rosei, E., Ambrosioni, E., Bertomeu, V., Clement, D., Erdine, S., Farsang, C., Gaita, D., Kiowski, W., Lip, G., Mallion, J.M., Manolis, A.J., Nilsson, P.M., O'Brien, E., Ponikowski, P., Redon, J., Ruschitzka, F., Tamargo, J., van Zwieten, P., Viigimaa, M., Waeber, B., Williams, B., & Zamorano J.L., The task force for the management of arterialhypertension of the European Society of Hypertension, The task force for the management of arterial hypertension of the European Society of Cardiology. (2007). 2007 Guidelines for the management of arterial hypertension: The Task Force for the Management of Arterial Hypertension of the European Society of Hypertension (ESH)and of the European Society of Cardiology (ESC). *Eur Heart J.* Vol. 28, No. 12, pp. 1462-1536. ISSN: 0195-668X

Mancia, G., & Grassi, G. (2002). Systolic and diastolic blood pressure control in antihypertensive drug trials. *J Hypertens.* Vol. 20, No. 8, pp. 1461-1464. ISSN: 0263-6352

Mancia, G., Laurent, S., Agabiti-Rosei, E., Ambrosioni, E., Burnier, M., Caulfield, M.J., Cifkova, R., Clément, D., Coca, A., Dominiczak, A., Erdine, S., Fagard, R., Farsang, C., Grassi, G., Haller, H., Heagerty, A., Kjeldsen, S.E., Kiowski, W., Mallion, J.M., Manolis, A., Narkiewicz, K., Nilsson, P., Olsen, M.H., Rahn, K.H., Redon, J., Rodicio, J., Ruilope L., Schmieder, R.E., Struijker-Boudier, H.A., van Zwieten, P.A., Viigimaa, M., & Zanchetti, A.; European Society of Hypertension. (2009). Reappraisal of European guidelines on hypertension management: a European Society of Hypertension Task Force document. *J Hypertens.* Vol. 27, No. 11, pp 2121-2158. ISSN: 0263-6352

Manolio, T.A., Pearson, T.A., Wenger, N.K., Barrett-Connor, E., Payne, GH., & Harlan WR. (1992). Cholesterol and heart disease in older persons and women. Review of an NHLBI workshop. *Ann Epidemiol.* Vol. 2, No. 1-2, : pp. 161-176. ISSN: 1047-2797

Mazza A., Tikhonoff, V., Schiavon, L., & Casiglia, E. (2005). Triglycerides + high-density-lipoprotein-cholesterol dyslipidaemia, a coronary risk factor in elderly women: the

CArdiovascular Study in the ELderly. *Intern Med J.* Vol. 35, No. 10, pp. 604-610. ISSN: 1444-0903

Medical Research Council Working Party. (1985) MRC trial of treatment of mild hypertension: principal results. *Br Med J (Clin Res Ed).* Vol. 291, No. 6488, pp. 97-104. ISSN: 0959-535X

Mosca, L., Banka, C.L., Benjamin, E.J., Berra, K., Bushnell, C., Dolor, R.J., Ganiats, T.G., Gomes, A.S., Gornik, H.L., Gracia, C., Gulati, M., Haan, C.K., Judelson, D.R., Keenan, N., Kelepouris, E., Michos, E.D., Newby, L.K., Oparil, S., Ouyang, P., Oz, M.C., Petitti, D., Pinn, V.W., Redberg, R.F., Scott, R., Sherif, K., Smith, SC. Jr., Sopko, G., Steinhorn, R.H., Stone, N.J., Taubert, K.A., Todd, B.A., Urbina, E., & Wenger, N.K. (2007) Evidence-based guidelines for cardiovascular disease prevention in women: 2007 update. *J Am Coll Cardiol.* Vol. 49, No. 11, pp. 1230-50. ISSN: 0735-1097

Naughton, C, Feely, J, & Bennett, K. (2007). A clustered randomized trial of the effects of feedback using academic detailing compared to postal bulletin on prescribing ofpreventative cardiovascular therapy. *Fam Pract.* Vol 24, No. 5, pp. 475-480. ISSN: 0263-2136

Neil, H.A., DeMicco, D.A., Luo, D., Betteridge, D.J., Colhoun, H.M., Durrington, P.N., Livingstone, S.J., Fuller, J.H., & Hitman, G.A. (2006) Analysis of efficacy and safety in patients aged 65-75 years at randomization: Collaborative Atorvastatin Diabetes Study (CARDS). *Diabetes Care.* Vol. 29, No. 11, pp. 2378-2384. ISSN: 0149-5992

Ozturk, S., & Kutlu M. (2010). Hyperlipidemia in older patients and methods of treatment. *Turkish Journal of Geriatrics* Supp 2, pp. 41 -46. ISSN: 1304-2947

Packard, C.J., Ford I., Robertson, M., Shepherd, J., Blauw, G.J., Murphy, M.B., Bollen, E.L., Buckley, B.M., Cobbe, S.M., Gaw A., Hyland, M., Jukema, J.W., Kamper, A.M., Macfarlane, P.W., Perry, I.J., Stott, D.J., Sweeney, B.J., Twomey, C., & Westendorp, R.G.; PROSPER Study Group. (2005). Plasma lipoproteins and apolipoproteins as predictors of cardiovascular risk and treatment benefit in the PROspective Study of Pravastatin in the Elderly at Risk (PROSPER). *Circulation.* Vol. 112, No. 20, pp. 3058-3065. ISSN: 0009-7322

Patel, A., Barzi F., Jamrozik K., Lam TH., Ueshima H., Whitlock G., & Woodward M.; Asia Pacific Cohort Studies Collaboration. (2004) Serum triglycerides as a risk factor for cardiovascular diseases in the Asia-Pacific region. *Circulation.* Vol. 110, No. 17, pp. 2678-86. ISSN: 0009-7322

Pedersen, T.R., Kjekshus, J., Berg, K., Haghfelt, T., Faergeman, O., Faergeman, G., Pyörälä, K., Miettinen, T., Wilhelmsen, L., Olsson, A.G., & Wedel, H.; Scandinavian Simvastatin Survival Study Group. (2004). Randomised trial of cholesterol lowering in 4444 patients with coronary heart disease: the Scandinavian Simvastatin Survival Study (4S). 1994. *Atheroscler Suppl.* Vol. 5, No. 3, pp. 81-87.

Poynter, J.N., Gruber, S.B., Higgins, P.D., Almog, R., Bonner, J.D., Rennert, H.S., Low, M., Greenson, J.K., & Rennert, G. (2005). Statins and the risk of colorectal cancer. *N Engl J Med.* Vol. 352, No. 21, pp. 2184-2192. ISSN: 0098-7484

Redgrave, T.G. (2004). Chylomicron metabolism. Biochem Soc Trans. Vol. 32, No. 1, pp. 79-82. ISSN: 0300-5127

Ridker, PM., Paynter, N.P., Rifai, N., Gaziano, J.M., & Cook, N.R. (2008). C-reactive protein and parental history improve global cardiovascular risk prediction: the Reynolds Risk Score for men. *Circulation*. Vol. 118, No. 22, pp. 2243-2251. ISSN: 0009-7322

Robillard, R, Fontaine, C., Chinetti, G., Fruchart, J.C., & Staels, B. (2005). Fibrates. *Handb Exp Pharmacol*. Vol. 170, pp.389-406. ISSN: 0171-2004

Rodondi, N., Marques-Vidal, P., Butler, J., Sutton-Tyrrell, K., Cornuz, J., Satterfield, S., Harris, T., Bauer, D.C., Ferrucci L., Vittinghoff, E., & Newman, A.B.; Health, Aging, and Body Composition Study. (2010). Markers of atherosclerosis and inflammation for prediction of coronary heart disease in older adults. *Am J Epidemiol*. Vol. 171 No. 5, pp. 540-9. ISSN: 0002-9262

Sacks, FM, Pfeffer, MA, Moye, LA, Rouleau, JL, Rutherford, JD, Cole, TG, Brown, L,Warnica, JW, Arnold, JM, Wun, CC, Davis, BR, & Braunwald, E (1996). The effect of pravastatin on coronary events after myocardial infarction in patients with average cholesterol levels. Cholesterol and Recurrent Events Trial investigators. *N Engl J Med*. Vol. 335, No. 14, pp. 1001-1009. ISSN: 0028-4793

Sarwar, N., Danesh, J., Eiriksdottir, G., Sigurdsson, G., Wareham, N., Bingham S., Boekholdt, SM., Khaw, K.T., & Gudnason, V. (2007). Triglycerides and the risk of coronary heart disease: 10,158 incident cases among 262,525 participants in 29 Western prospective studies. *Circulation*. Vol. 115, No. 4, pp. 450-458. ISSN: 0009-7322

Setoguchi, S., Glynn, R.J., Avorn, J., Mogun, H., & Schneeweiss, S. (2007). Statins and the risk of lung, breast, and colorectal cancer in the elderly. *Circulation*. Vol. 115, No. 1, pp. 27-33. ISSN: 0009-7322

Sever, P.S., Dahlöf, B., Poulter, N.R., Wedel, H., Beevers, G., Caulfield, M., Collins, R., Kjeldsen, S.E., Kristinsson, A., McInnes, GT, Mehlsen, J., Nieminen, M., O'Brien, E., & Ostergren, J.; ASCOT investigators. (2003). Prevention of coronary and stroke events with atorvastatin in hypertensive patients who have average or lower-than-average cholesterol concentrations, in the Anglo-Scandinavian Cardiac Outcomes Trial--Lipid Lowering Arm (ASCOT-LLA): a multicentre randomised controlled trial. *Lancet*. Vol. 361, No. 9364, pp. 1149-1158. ISSN: 0140-6736

SHEP Cooperative Research Group. (1991). Prevention of stroke by antihypertensive drug treatment in older persons with isolated systolic hypertension. Final results of the Systolic Hypertension in the Elderly Program (SHEP). *JAMA*. Vol. 265, No. 24, pp. 3255-64. ISSN: 0098-7484

Smith, S.C. Jr., Allen, J., Blair, S.N., Bonow, R.O., Brass, L.M., Fonarow, G.C., Grundy, S.M., Hiratzka, L., Jones, D., Krumholz, H.M., Mosca, L., Pasternak, R.C., Pearson, T., Pfeffer, M.A., & Taubert, K.A.; AHA/ACC; National Heart, Lung, and Blood Institute. (2006). AHA/ACC guidelines for secondary prevention for patients with coronary and other atherosclerotic vascular disease: 2006 update: endorsed by the National Heart,Lung, and Blood Institute. *Circulation*. Vol. 113, No. 19, pp. 2363-2372. ISSN: 0009-7322

Sowers, JR. (1987). Hypertension in the elderly. *Am J Med*. Vol. 82, No. 1B, pp. 1-8. ISSN: 0002-9343

Sparrow, D. & Dawber, T.R. (1978). The influence of cigarette smoking on prognosis after a first myocardial infarction. A report from the Framingham study. *J Chronic Dis*. Vol. 31, No. 6-7, pp. 425-432. ISSN: 0021-9681

Splansky, GL, Corey, D, Yang, Q, Atwood, LD, Cupples, LA, Benjamin, EJ, D'Agostino, RB Sr, Fox, CS, Larson, MG, Murabito, JM, O'Donnell, CJ, Vasan, RS, Wolf, PA, & Levy, D. (2007). The Third Generation Cohort of the National Heart, Lung and Blood Instiyute's Framingham Heart Study: Design, recruitment and initial examination. *Am J Epidemiol.* Vol. 165, No. 11, pp. 1328-1335. ISSN: 0002-9262

Staessen, J.A., Fagard, R., Thijs, L., Celis H., Arabidze, G.G., Birkenhäger, W.H., Bulpitt, C.J., de Leeuw, P.W., Dollery, C.T., Fletcher, A.E., Forette, F., Leonetti, G., Nachev, C., O'Brien, E.T., Rosenfeld, J., Rodicio, J.L., Tuomilehto J., & Zanchetti, A. (1997) Randomised double-blind comparison of placebo and active treatment for older patients with isolated systolic hypertension. The Systolic Hypertension in Europe (Syst-Eur) Trial Investigators. *Lancet.* Vol. 350, No. 9080, pp. 757-764. ISSN: 0140-6736

Staessen, JA, Gasowski, J, Wang, JG, Thijs, L, Den Hond, E, Boissel, JP, Coope, J, Ekbom, T, Gueyffier, F, Liu, L, Kerlikowske, K, Pocock, S, & Fagard, RH. (2000). Risks of untreated and treated isolated systolic hypertension in the elderly: meta-analysis of outcome trials. Lancet. Vol. 355, No. 9207, pp. 865-72. ISSN: 0140-6736

Streja, D., Streja, E. (2011). Management of Dyslipidemia in the Elderly, In: *Endocrinology of aging,* Hershman J, published by mdtext.com, inc, S.Dartmouth, MA., retrieved from www.endotext.org website, version of January/5/2011.

The Lipid Research Clinics. (1984). The Lipid Research Clinics Coronary Primary Prevention Trial results. I. Reduction in incidence of coronary heart disease. *JAMA.* Vol. 251, No. 3, pp. 351-364. ISSN: 0098-7484

The Long-Term Intervention with Pravastatin in Ischaemic Disease (LIPID) Study Group. (1998) Prevention of cardiovascular events and death with pravastatin in patients with coronary heart disease and a broad range of initial cholesterol levels. *N Engl J Med.* Vol. 5, No. 339, pp. 1349-1357. ISSN: 0098-7484

The National Cholesterol Education Program Expert Panel. (2001). 2001 Executive Summary of The Third Report of The National Cholesterol Education Program (NCEP) Expert Panel on Detection, Evaluation, And Treatment of High Blood Cholesterol In Adults (Adult Treatment Panel III). *JAMA.* Vol. 285, No. Pp. 2486-2497. ISSN: 0098-7484

The Scandinavian Simvastatin Survival Study Group. (1994). Randomised trial of cholesterol lowering in 4444 patients with coronary heart disease: (4S). *Lancet.* Vol. 344, No. 8934, pp. 1383-1389. ISSN: 0140-6736

Thijs, L., Fagard, R., Lijnen, P, Staessen, J., Van Hoof, R., & Amery, A. (1992). A meta-analysis of outcome trials in elderly hypertensives. *J Hypertens.* Vol. 10, No. 10, pp. 1103-1109. ISSN: 0263-6352

Troisi, J. (2005). Ethical issues in the elderly. *Journal of The Indian Academy of Geriatrics,* Vol. 1, No. 2, pp. 70-76.

Tyroler, H.A., & Ford, C.E. (1992). Serum cholesterol and coronary heart disease risk in female and older hypertensives. The experience under usual community care in the Hypertension Detection and Follow-up Program. *Ann Epidemiol.* Vol. 2, No. 1-2, pp. 155-160. ISSN: 1047-2797

Ulucam, M., & Muderrisoglu, H. (2008). Current therapeutic methods for the hypertension in the elderly. *Turkish Journal of Geriatrics,* Vol. 11, No. 4, pp. 208-216 ISSN: 1304-2947

United Nations Department of Economic and Social Affairs Population Division Report. (2009). *World Population Ageing 2009*. Available from: http ://www.un.org/ esa/ population/ publications/ WPA2009/ WPA2009-report.pdf

Wang, J.G., Staessen, J.A, Gong, L., & Liu, L. Systolic Hypertension in China (Syst-China) Collaborative Group. (2000). Chinese trial on isolated systolic hypertension in the elderly. *Arch Intern Med*. Vol. 160, no. 2, pp. 211-220. ISSN: 0003-9926

Wang, T.J., Gona, P, Larson, M.G., Tofler, G.H., Levy, D., Newton-Cheh, C., Jacques, P.F., Rifai., N., Selhub, J., Robins, S.J., Benjamin, E.J, D'Agostino, R.B., & Vasan, R.S.. (2006). Multiple biomarkers for the prediction of first major cardiovascular events and death. *N Engl J Med*. Vol. 355, No. 25, pp. 2631-2639. ISSN: 0098-7484

Wassertheil-Smoller, S., Psaty, B., Greenland, P., Oberman, A., Kotchen, T., Mouton, C., Black, H., Aragaki, A., & Trevisan, M. (2004). Association between cardiovascular outcomes and antihypertensive drug treatment in older women. *JAMA*. Vol. 292, No. 23, pp. 2849-59 ISSN: 0098-7484

Williams, M.A., Fleg, J.L., Ades, P.A., Chaitman, B.R., Miller, N.H., Mohiuddin, S.M., Ockenel, S., Taylor, C.B., & Wenger, N.K.; American Heart Association Council on Clinical Cardiology Subcommittee on Exercise, Cardiac Rehabilitation, and Prevention. (2002). Secondary prevention of coronary heart disease in the elderly (with emphasis on patients > or =75 years of age): an American Heart Association scientific statement from the Council on Clinical Cardiology Subcommittee on Exercise,Cardiac Rehabilitation, and Prevention. *Circulation*. Vol. 105, No. 14, pp. 1735-1743. ISSN: 0009-7322

Zakai, N.A., Katz, R., Jenny, N.S., Psaty, B.M., Reiner, A.P., Schwartz, S.M., & Cushman, M. (2007), Inflammation and hemostasis biomarkers and cardiovascular risk in the elderly: the Cardiovascular Health Study. *J Thromb Haemost*. Vol. 5, No. 6, pp. 1128-1135. ISSN: 0340-6245

5

Vascular Inflammation: A New Horizon in Cardiovascular Risk Assessment

Vinayak Hegde and Ishmael Ching
Akron General Medical Center, Ohio, USA

1. Introduction

Coronary artery disease (CAD) remains the leading cause of death across the globe (Rosamond et al., 2008). Although it was thought in the past that coronary artery disease was a disease of the Western world, it is now well known that the developing countries are not spared of the risk (see Figure 1). In fact, recent studies have indicated that in the next decade or so, 80% of the deaths from cardiovascular diseases are projected to occur in developing countries (Yusuf et al., 2001). It is also quite interesting that despite tremendous advances in cardiovascular medicine, myocardial infraction and sudden death are still the initial presentation in half of the patients with coronary artery disease. In the last few decades, cardiac developments have improved the care, and prolonged longevity of patients who suffer an acute coronary syndrome. Unfortunately, the efforts in primary prevention of cardiovascular disease have not quite paralleled the advances in secondary prevention (Rosamond, 2008).

Given the silent nature of the disease and the significant repercussions, it is imperative for physicians to identify at risk individuals early, and implement effective primary prevention of coronary artery disease. Even when selecting pharmacotherapy for cholesterol and blood pressure management, guidelines rely on the patients risk to dictate the intensity of treatment. Thus, cardiovascular risk assessment is the first and most crucial step in the management of the cardiovascular patient. Such risk assessment has traditionally been guided by clinical tools such as the Framingham Risk Score (FRS) from the Framingham Heart Study in the United States, or the Systemic Coronary Risk Evaluation, "SCORE" from European studies on cardiovascular risk assessment (Conroy et al., 2003). Additionally, clinicians use laboratory markers, chiefly total and LDL cholesterol to assess an individual's risk.

Developing a stellar risk determinant requires thorough understanding of the process of atherosclerosis. Atherosclerosis is an ongoing process that occurs through out the life of an individual. We now know that plaque ruptures rather than gradually developing coronary stenoses are the culprits in acute coronary syndromes. A variety of chemokines are involved in the process, and an individual's genetic susceptibility to these enzymes plays a vital role in determining who is at risk for plaque ruptures and cardiac events (KJ Williams et al., 2008). A truly preventative and comprehensive risk assessment algorithm should detect asymptomatic atherosclerosis by making room for inflammatory markers capable of predicting downstream coronary events. Although lipid panels and Framingham scores provide an assessment of an individual's overall risk, neither of them specifically indicates arterial inflammation or an individual's susceptibility for plaque rupture, the two fundamental culprits in acute coronary syndromes. The goal of medical research is to combine clinical criteria along with pertinent laboratory values and atherosclerosis imaging to generate an inclusive risk assessment tool for patients. Another desirable attribute of this tool is that it should go above and beyond the barriers of gender and ethnicity, and be applicable to a global population. This chapter discusses the role of novel risk factors, focusing mainly on coronary calcium scoring (CCS), while touching upon high sensitivity C reactive protein (CRP), and apolipoproteins in cardiovascular disease. It is important to understand where the traditional risk factors fall short of risk prediction, and where these novel markers could improve our assessment.

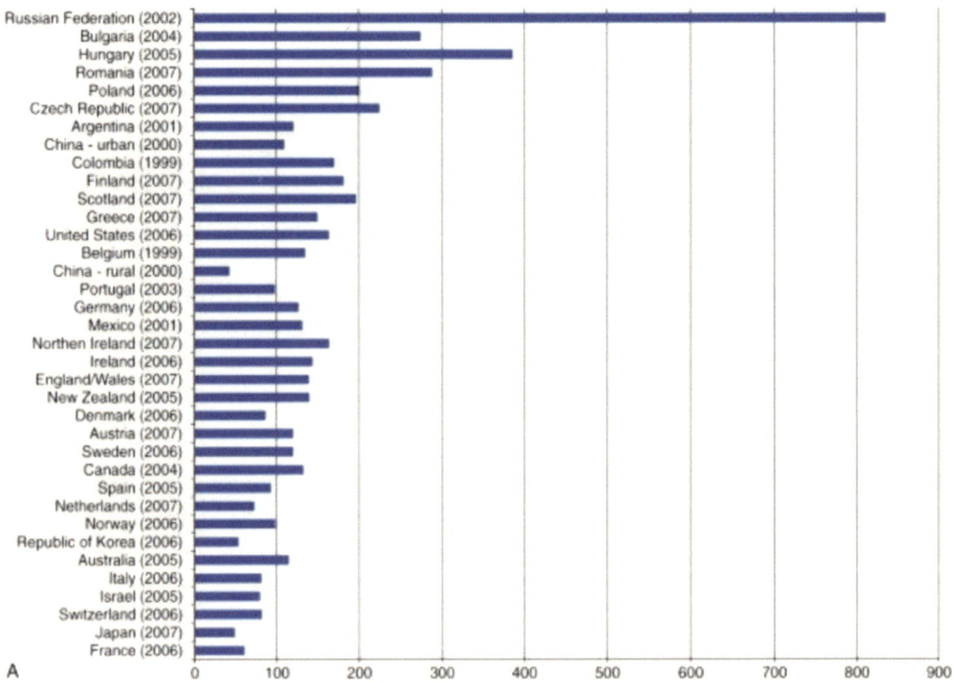

Adapted with permission from American Heart Association: Heart disease & stroke statistics—2010 update. A report from the American Heart Association, Dallas, Tex, 2010, American Heart Association.

Fig. 1. Age-adjusted rates of death from coronary heart disease (per 100,000 population) among men aged 35 to 74 in selected countries.

1.1 Atherosclerosis an inflammatory process

Atherogenesis in blood vessels has been described to occur in four major steps. The first step is initiation of endothelial activation. Lipoproteins play a key role in this step. During this stage, the intima of susceptible arteries areas (those subjected to hemodynamic stresses) gets infiltrated by atherogenic lipoproteins including low-density lipoproteins (LDL), very low density lipoproteins (VLDL) and other triglyceride rich lipoproteins (TGRL). Under appropriate genetic and environmental triggers, the modified lipoproteins release inflammatory signals to activate endothelial cells. Recently, the role of platelets has been explored in endothelial activation. Platelets release inflammatory mediators such as interleukin 1 beta(IL-1β), CD40L, which lead to endothelial activation. This is particularly pronounced in patients with diabetes, hypertension, obesity, dyslipidemia, and in smokers (Vasina et al 2010, Gasparyan et al 2011). The activated endothelial cells express intracellular cell adhesion molecules such as (ICAM)-1 and glycoprotein I-B (GpIB), which promote platelet adhesion and activation. The activated endothelial cells also release chemoattractant and adhesion molecules such as monocyte chemoattractant protein (MCP-1) and vascular cell adhesion molecule1 (VCAM-1). These molecules attract phagocytic cells such as monocytes in to the intima of the vessel wall. These monocytes ingest the modified lipoproteins and turn in to foam cells. In the mean while platelets release platelet derived growth factor (PDGF), which attracts smooth muscle cells (Hopkins & RR Williams, 1981).

During the promotion phase, lipoprotein infiltration continues in proportion to their plasma levels. The growth or necrosis of the plaque is controlled by a balance between lipoprotein entry, foam cell formation and reverse cholesterol transport out of the plaque (Tabas, 2002). During the progression phase, macrophages secrete matrix metalloproteinases (MMPs) that weaken the fibrous cap of the plaque. Additionally, Interferon-γ secreted by activated T cells strongly inhibits collagen synthesis (Libby, 2009). The weakened cap allows cholesterol crystals to erode through the endothelium, causing encroachment of the plaque in to the vessel lumen. Thus, inflammation appears to be the key to plaque destabilization and rupture (Crisby et al., 2001) (see Fig 2).

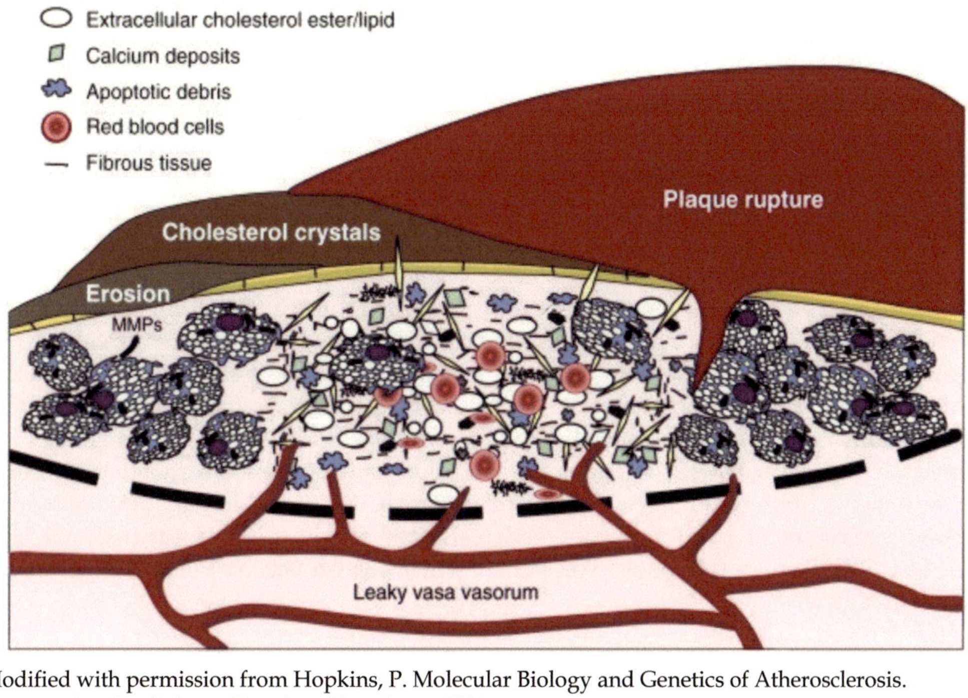

Modified with permission from Hopkins, P. Molecular Biology and Genetics of Atherosclerosis. Preventative Cardiology. Elseviers/Saunders, c2011.

Fig. 2. Atherosclerotic plaque destabilization, rupture and calcification.

Shearing stress on the vessel wall from uncontrolled hypertension, contributes to endothelial activation. This stress, in conjunction with other risk factors determines plaque composition with regards to percentage of fibrous versus lipid components (Cheng et al., 2006). Calcium starts to appear inside plaques during the healing and remodeling phase of ruptured plaques. Higher the intimal calcium in a blood vessel, more are the number of prior silent or manifest plaque rupture events inside it (Sangiorgi et al., 1998).

2. Assessment of atherosclerosis and cardiovascular risk

Risk identification and stratification for a clinician begins with an office based assessment of the patient. The presence of CAD/CAD equivalents such as diabetes, peripheral vascular disease automatically places the patient in the high-risk category, needing no further stratification. In the absence of CAD equivalents, risk factors such as hypertension, cigarette smoking, low HDL, family history of premature CAD are considered. When two or more risk factors are present, clinicians currently use risk assessment algorithms such as Framingham Heart Study from the United States or from the Prospective Cardiovascular Münster (PROCAM) study in Germany, or the European risk prediction system called SCORE (Systemic Coronary Risk Evaluation). These algorithms project an individual' s 10 year, absolute risk for cardiovascular events such as myocardial infarction (MI), cardiac death (see Table 1). It should be noted that the derived risk is short to intermediate term, and not a lifetime assessment. The cumulative effects of risk factors depend on the duration of an individual's exposure to them. 10-year risk may not be sufficient enough to manifest such effects. It is a known fact that the incidence of coronary artery disease increases exponentially with age (McDermott, 2007; Petersen et al., 2005). Thus, if one decides to go by 10-year prediction algorithms alone, a significant number of patients with coronary artery disease would be classified as low risk. Their lifetime risk would be missed because of the myopic nature of the algorithm.

Long-term risk assessment is particularly relevant for younger patients, in whom initiation of healthy lifestyle modifications and treatment may be delayed or even avoided due to lack of risk awareness. To evade such neglect, the author recommends that physicians should get in to the habit of estimating the lifetime risk. This paradigm has not yet been enforced by clinical guidelines. Lifetime risk assessment is generally performed using the modified technique of survival, and Kaplan Meyer analysis (Lloyd-Jones et al., 2006). These analyses although useful for statistical purposes, are fairly complicated and may not be feasible for day-to-day use in a clinical setting. The alternative is to assess long-term cardiac risk using markers for subclinical atherosclerosis. The traditional risk assessment algorithms suffer from a complete lack of such markers (both biochemical and imaging). Among chemical markers, high sensitivity CRP and apolipoprotein analysis may herald early atherosclerosis. On the imaging front, carotid intimal medial thickness (CIMT) and coronary calcium scoring are two indicators of subclinical atherosclerosis that can be easily measured. CIMT is reviewed elsewhere in this book. The author will focus on coronary calcification in the sections to follow.

2.1 Assessment of coronary artery calcium

As discussed before, the presence of calcium speaks for plaque rupture and healing events within the vessel wall. Calcification of plaques is an active process involving deposition of hydroxyapatite crystals, as opposed to simple mineral precipitation. The concept of visualizing coronary calcium was first proposed in the early 1980's by a team of physicists at University of California, San Francisco. They invented the Electron Beam Tomography (EBT) scanner, formerly known as the Ultrafast Computed Tomography (CT) (UIC, 2011). It was only in the early 1990's, after years of rigorous testing at major medical centers around the world, that medical institutions began offering Coronary Artery Calcification Scans to the general public.

10-Year Absolute Risk Category	Definition of Category
High risk	CHD*, CHD risk equivalents† including 2+ major risk factors‡ plus a 10-year risk for hard CHD greater than 20%§
Moderately high risk	2+ major risk factors‡ plus a 10-year risk for hard CHD 10% to 20%
Moderate risk	2+ major risk factors plus a 10-year risk for hard CHD less than 10%
Lower risk	0 to 1 major risk factor (10-year risk for hard CHD usually less than 10%)§

*CHD includes history of myocardial infarction, unstable angina, stable angina, coronary artery procedures (angioplasty or by-pass surgery), or evidence of clinically significant myocardial ischemia. †CHD risk equivalents include clinical manifestations of non-coronary forms of atherosclerotic disease (peripheral arterial disease, abdominal aortic aneurysm, and carotid artery disease [transient ischemic attacks or stroke of carotid origin or greater than 50% obstruction of a carotid artery]), diabetes, and 2 risk factors with 10-year risk for hard CHD less than 20%. ‡Major risk factors include cigarette smoking, hypertension (BP greater than or equal to 140/90 mm Hg or on antihypertensive medication), low HDL cholesterol (less than 40 mg/dL), family history of premature CHD (CHD in male first-degree relative less than 55 years; CHD in female first-degree relative less than 65 years), and age (men greater than or equal to 45 years; women greater than or equal to 55 years). §Almost all people with 0 to 1 risk factor have a 10-year risk less than 10%, and 10-year risk assessment in people with 0 to 1 risk factor is thus not necessary.
Modified with permission from Grundy SM, Cleeman JI, Merz CN, et al. Implications of recent clinical trials for the National Cholesterol Education Program Adult Treatment Panel III guidelines. Circulation 2004; 110: 227–39 (16).
BP blood pressure; CHD coronary heart disease; HDL high-density lipoprotein.

Table 1. Absolute Risk Categories as per the National Cholesterol Education Program (NCEP) Update, 2004

In the present day, there are two modalities for detection of coronary artery calcification. Traditionally, EBT scans were used for this purpose. However, with the development of Multidetector Computed Tomography (MDCT) scanners within the last decade, MDCT has become increasingly popular for the same purpose. Imaging continuously moving structures such as the heart can be fairly challenging. The scan has to be gated off the patient's electrocardiogram (ECG). Coronary arteries are best imaged during diastole, when there is little cardiac motion. Thus, the ECG triggering is done during end systole or early diastole. In clinical practice, 75% of the patient's R-R interval is most favorable for cardiac imaging. Factors such as heart rate irregularities, and tachycardia may necessitate the use of values anywhere between 40-80% of R-R interval for cardiac triggering.

EBT is an ultrafast single slice, high resolution CT scan. Like any form of CT scans, the X-ray source-point moves along a circle in space around an object to be imaged. In EBT, however, the X-ray tube itself is large and stationary, and partially surrounds the imaging circle. Rather than moving the tube itself, the electron-beam focal point (and hence the X-ray source point) is swept electronically along a tungsten anode in the tube, tracing a large circular arc on its inner surface. This motion can be very fast. The resultant scan provides 3 mm thick continuous nonoverlapping slices with an acquisition time of 100 msec/tomogram in a prospective manner (Agatston et al., 1990; Callister et al., 1998a).

As opposed to EBT, MDCT is capable of acquiring clinical images of the heart with multislice imaging technology that captures up to 64 simultaneous anatomical slices of 0.5 mm through an advanced 64-row data acquisition system in a single gantry rotation. In addition, the system's sensitivity and accuracy are enhanced with a process called isotropic scanning. This fast scanning capability allows important diagnostic information concerning the heart to be obtained within a single breath-hold, less than ten seconds, and a CT angiogram can be imaged within 15 seconds. The latest generation of MDCT scanners can acquire up to 320 sections of the heart simultaneously with ECG triggering in either a retrospective or prospective fashion. The patient lies on the CT couch, and the couch is advanced gradually either continuously (helical or spiral scanning) at a fixed speed or in a stepwise fashion (axial/conventional scanning). Figure 3 demonstrates the two scanning modes of MDCT. The gantry speed is up to 330 msec (Agatston, 1990).

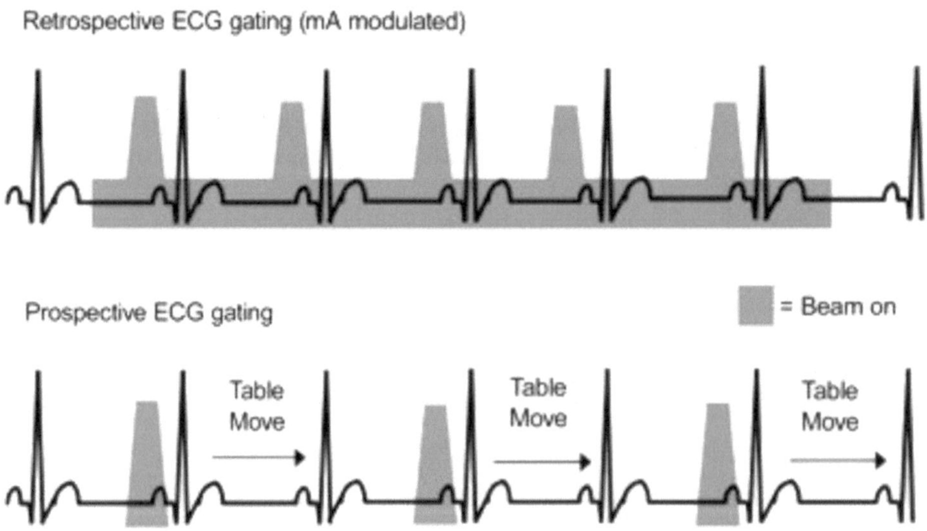

Adapted with permission from Shuman W.P. et al. Prospective versus Retrospective ECG Gating for 64-Detector CT of the Coronary Arteries: Comparison of Image Quality and Patient Radiation Dose. August 2008 Radiology, 248, 431-437.

Fig. 3. Retrospective and Prospective Gating Techniques for Coronary Computed Tomography Angiography.

2.2 Calcium scoring

Coronary calcium scans are performed using the axial mode and with prospective ECG gating. Either EBT or MDCT scanners can be used for this purpose. No intravenous contrast is necessary. Coronary calcium is diagnosed when as two or three hyperattenuated adjacent pixels with tomographic density of >130 Hounsefeld (HU) units for EBT and 90-130 HU for MDCT, are visualized within the coronary tree. The computer software then computes a calcium score for the patient using either the Agatston or Callister methods. The Agatston method involves multiplying the calculated area of the calcification (measured every 3 mm slice thickness) by the CT density of the same area. Partial volume averaging artifacts could theoretically pose a threat to the validity of this calculation. This artifact results when the computer yields a CT number representative of the average attenuation of the materials within a voxel. Also scanning at 3 mm slice thickness overestimates the area of smaller lesions that are 1mm or less (Barrett & Keat, 2004). As a result, some smaller lesions receive higher peak values for intensity and area. Despite this theoretical concern, there is evidence to suggest that the Agatston score correlates well with that calculated using the Callister method (Callister et al., 1998a). The latter involves computing volume rather than area for lesions with HU density above specified threshold. This partially corrects for slice thickness induced artifacts. Figure 4 summarizes coronary artery calcification (CAC) score calculation.

In comparing EBT and MDCT head to head, studies have revealed an excellent correlation between the two for the presence of calcium (Mao et al., 2009; Daniell et al, 2005; Budoff et al., 2006). This being said, there were some minor differences. Compared to EBT, MDCT had more motion artifacts, and also had higher mean HU for calcific lesions ($p<0.001$). The Agatston and volumetric scores were not significantly different between EBT and MDCT. However, the study by Mao et al used heart rate control for calcium scoring scans (Mao et al., 2009). Majority of centers do not routinely use heart rate control for this purpose alone, unless a coronary CT Angiogram is also requested. Even in the absence of heart rate control, Daniell et al did not report any significant difference between the two scanners. At our center, MDCT is routinely employed for this purpose, without heart rate control.

Using either of the two methods described above, the computer generates a Calcium Artery Calcification (CAC) Score report. The report compares the patient's calcium score to age and gender matched controls, and generates a percentile value for the patient in question.

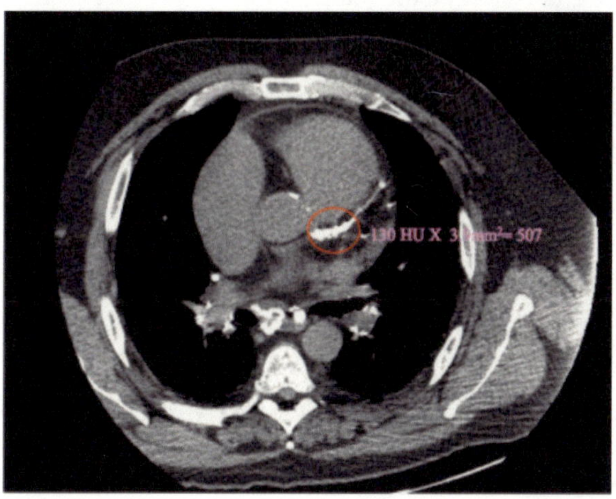

Fig. 4. Coronary Calcium Score (CCS) calculation in a patient with extensive coronary calcification

The figure depicts extensive coronary artery calcification involving the left main and the left anterior descending arteries. Agatston score is calculated by multiplying the area of the calcification (mm^2) by its density in Hounsefeld units (HU). The total calcium score is much higher than that for the lesion depicted.

2.3 Radiation dose

Recently, significant concerns have been raised about the radiation exposure to patients from CT scans. Typical radiation dose from a retrospectively gated coronary CT angiograms (CTA) ranges from 10-18 mSv (Gopal & Budoff, 2009). With the introduction of radiation dose reducing techniques such as dose modulation, reduction of kilovoltage for thinner patients, limitation of vertical scan field and prospective gating, the exposure to radiation can be decreased by 80-90%. In fact, studies have reported that the use of prospective gating alone, without any other dose sparing techniques, cuts down radiation exposure by 70-80%. The typical radiation dose for a prospectively gated CTA is about 4.2 mSv (about the same or slightly lower than a diagnostic cardiac catheterization) (Hirai et al., 2008; De Backer et al., 2003).

Although these concerns are valid for coronary CT angiograms (both prospectively and retrospectively gated), radiation exposure is certainly not an issue for calcium scoring. Radiation exposure from CCS scans alone is approximately 1 mSv from either EBT or MDCT scanners. This exposure is negligible, and is nearly equivalent to that from a single X ray. Thus, the benefit of assessing coronary calcium in at risk individuals justifies the minor risk of radiation exposure in most patients.

2.4 Coronary artery calcium scoring in asymptomatic patients

It has been proven that plaque rupture and acute coronary syndromes are generally a function of the total atherosclerotic burden (Kullo & Ballantyne, 2005). Since calcium is known to appear at an advanced stage of atherosclerosis, it has been proposed that patients with calcific plaques also likely have "soft" plaques that could be vulnerable to rupture. The co occurrence of calcific and noncalcific plaques forms the basis of using CCS as a predictor of acute coronary syndromes. Although CAC may not identify a vulnerable plaque per se, it defines a patient's risk for coronary events by virtue of its association with total plaque burden (Rumberger et al., 1995; O'Rourke et al., 2000; Agatston et al., 1990). This is the very basis of testing asymptomatic patients for coronary calcification. Detection of coronary artery calcifications in this group of individuals can help direct decisions on intensity of lipid lowering, aspirin therapy etc. Whether this strategy is useful across all risk groups is questionable, and is discussed later. In the sections to follow, we review data from metaanalyses, observational and prospective cohort studies on prognostic value of CCS.

2.5 Observational studies

Several observational studies have suggested the utility of CCS in cardiac risk stratification. Earlier studies often focused on endpoints such as coronary revascularization. These studies were criticized for a lack of hard endpoints such as cardiac death, myocardial infarctions (MI) etc, and were thought to overestimate the prognostic value of calcium scoring (Pletcher et al., 2004). However, we now have more than a few studies looking at hard endpoints described above. Table 2 summarizes the salient findings of these studies (Arad et al., 2000, 2005; Wong et al., 2000; Raggi et al., 2001; Kondos et al, 2003; Shaw et al., 2003; Greenland et al., et al, 2004; Vliegenthart et al., 2005; Taylor et al., 2005; LaMonte et al., 2005; Budoff et al., 2007; Becker et al., 2008; Anand et al., 2006; Polonsky et al., 2010). Briefly, the study by Arad et al (2000) showed that among 1172 asymptomatic patients observed for 3.6 years after an initial EBT screening, no events occurred in patients without coronary calcification, and in patients with a CAC score <100. The negative predictive value of a normal CCS scan was 99.8% for hard cardiac endpoints. Also the authors described increasing cardiac event rates in individuals with a CAC score ≥80, ≥160, and ≥600. Raggi and coworkers (2001) studied more than 600 asymptomatic patients who underwent EBT and were then followed for 32 ± 7 months. They showed that both the absolute CAC score and the relative score percentiles predicted subsequent death and nonfatal MI. Additionally, hard cardiac events occurred in only 0.3% of subjects with a normal CAC score, but increased to 13% in those with a CAC score >400. The largest observational study with the longest duration of follow up was reported by Budoff and colleagues (2007). They followed 25,253 patients out to 6.8 years, and reported relative risk ratios of 4.5 for CAC scores between 101 and 299, and 12.5 for scores more than 1000. Shaw and colleagues (2003) demonstrated that mortality significantly increased with increasing CAC score, within men and women separately as well as within each Framingham risk group (low, intermediate, and high-risk). This finding contradicts a report from Kondos et al. (2003) describing the futility of CCS in patients with low Framingham risk. With the exception of minor differences, most studies indicate that CAC is an independent predictor of CAD adverse outcome as well as of all-cause mortality after adjusting for traditional risk factors. It should be noted that these studies consistently quote impressive relative risk ratios, but when one looks at the absolute risk, the difference is not as impressive in majority of the studies. Also most data has been reported in Caucasian population. Thus, the author does advise caution in extrapolating these vivid results to one's practice, and ethnically diverse patient population.

2.6 Prospective studies and meta-analysis

Prospective studies have confirmed these results, and have additionally indicated an independent role for CCS above traditional risk factors. The South Bay Heart Watch study included 1196 asymptomatic patients who were observed for a median of 7.0 years, and it was demonstrated that the CAC score added predictive power beyond that of standard coronary risk factors and C-reactive protein (Greenland et al., 2004). Registry data from the St. Francis Heart Study, a prospective population based study of over 5000 asymptomatic individuals confirmed the higher event rates associated with increasing CAC scores (Arad et al., 2005). CAC scores >100 were associated with relative risks of 12 to 32, thus achieving secondary prevention equivalent event rates >2%/year (superior to FRS). The Rotterdam Heart Study studied CCS in a slightly older cohort, i.e. 1795 asymptomatic patients with mean age of 71 years (Vliegenthart et al., 2005). During a mean follow-up of 3.3 years, the multivariate-adjusted relative risk of coronary events was 3.1 for calcium scores of 101 to 400, 4.6 for calcium scores of 401 to 1000, and 8.3 for calcium scores >1000. In a younger cohort of asymptomatic persons, the 3-year mean follow-up in 2000 participants (mean age, 43 years) showed that coronary calcium was associated with an 11.8 fold increased risk for incident CAD (P <0.002) while controlling for the FRS (Taylor et al., 2005).

Budoff and colleagues (2007) showed risk-adjusted hazard ratios of 2.2 for total mortality for CAC score categories of 11-100, and 12.5 for category >1000. CAC scores provided significant incremental information over traditional risk factors. In Europe, Becker and coworkers (2008) reported their data in 924 patients aged 59.4 ± 18.7 years During the 3-year follow-up period, the event rates for coronary revascularization, MI, and cardiac death in patients with volume scores above the 75th percentile were significantly higher compared with the total study group, and no cardiovascular events occurred in patients with scores of zero. In fact, their statistical analysis demonstrated that it outperformed both PROCAM and Framingham models (P <0.0001), in which 36% and 34% of MIs occurred in the high-risk cohorts, respectively.

The studies discussed this far did not include particularly high-risk subgroups. Anand et al (2006) evaluated CCS in asymptomatic diabetic patients. CAC scores were prospectively measured in 510 asymptomatic type 2 diabetic subjects (mean age, 53 ± 8 years; 61% men) without prior CVD, with a median follow-up of 2.2 years. In the multivariable model, the CAC score and extent of myocardial ischemia by nuclear stress testing were the only independent predictors of outcome. Performance analysis using receiver operative curve (ROC) analysis (described in detail later) demonstrated that CCS predicted cardiovascular events with the best accuracy, area under the curve (0.92), significantly better than the United Kingdom Prospective Diabetes Study risk score (0.74) and Framingham score (0.60). The relative risk to predict a cardiovascular event for a CAC score of 101 to 400 was 10.13, and it increased to 58.05 for scores >1000 (P <0.0001). Even in this diabetic population, no cardiac events or perfusion abnormalities occurred in subjects with CAC ≤10 Agatston units up until 2 years of follow-up. These results emphasize the value of screening for subclinical disease in diabetics who often do not feel regular symptoms of coronary artery disease and thereby labeled as "asymptomatic".

Combining results of several studies, a meta-analysis of six trials was published in the ACC/AHA consensus document on CCS (Greenland et al., 2007). The meta-analysis reported a relative risk ratio of 4.3 for any measurable calcium, as compared with zero CAC score, thus implying a four-fold increase in the 3-5 year risk. Also, the annual incidence of coronary events increased with increasing tertiles of CAC scores (see fig 5). Although critics tend to point to limitations such as study generalizability of self-referral cohorts, validity of the risk factor measures and risk of test-induced bias, the meta-analysis still remains a stellar piece of evidence supporting the prognostic value of coronary artery calcium scoring.

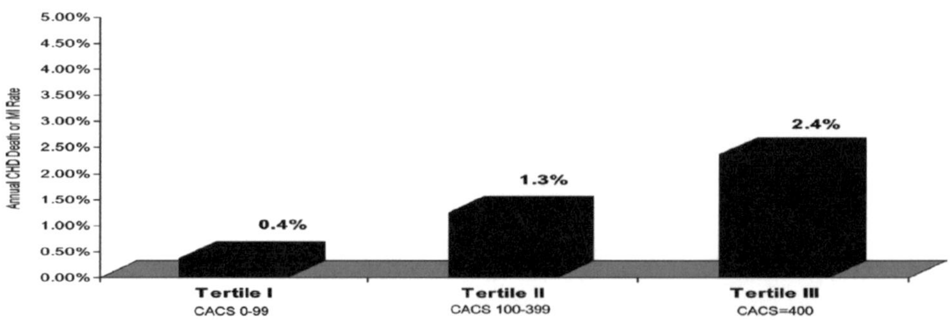

Adapted with permission from Greenland et al. JACC Vol. 49, No. 3, 2007. ACCF/AHA Expert Consensus Document on Coronary Artery Calcium Scoring January 23, 2007:378 – 402

Fig. 5. Annual incidence of Coronary Artery Disease related events in different tertiles of Coronary Calcium Scores.

Author (Year)	Study and Population	Follow Up (Years)	Number of Events	Results
Arad et al (2000)	Observational N = 1172	3.6	15 nonfatal MI, 21 revascularizations, 3 deaths	OR of 20 for CAC scores ≥160
Wong et al (2000)	Observational N = 926	3.3	6 nonfatal MI, 20 revascularizations, 2 CVA	Overall, patients with CAC score ≥271 had a risk ratio of 9 for a CAD event.
Raggi et al (2001)	Observational N = 676	2.7	21 nonfatal MI, 9 deaths	OR of 22 for cardiac events for CAC score > 90 percentile
Kondos et al (2003)	Observational N = 5635	3.1	37 nonfatal MI, 166 revascularizations, 21 deaths	RR of 124 for cardiac events in men; incremental prognostic value of CCS
Shaw et al (2003)	Observational N = 10,377	5	249 all-cause mortality	CAC score an independent predictor of mortality with RR 4.0 for score of 401-1000
Greenland et al (2004)	Prospective N = 1312	7	68 nonfatal MI, 16 deaths	RR of 3.9 for CAC score >301 CAC score incremental to FRS
Arad et al (2005)	Prospective N = 4613	4.3	40 nonfatal MI, 59 revascularizations, 7 CVA	RR for CAD events with CAC >100 11. CCS superior to FRS in prediction of cardiac events
Vliegenthart et al (2005)	Prospective N = 1795	3.3	40 nonfatal MI, 38 CVA	RR >8, for CAC scores >1000 regardless of FRS
Taylor et al (2005)	Prospective N=1983	3	9 ACS events	CAC had an independent12-fold increase in RR.
LaMonte et al (2005)	Retrospective N=10746	3.5	81 MI/CAD death, 206 revascularizations	Increasing cardiac event rates with higher CAC scores
Anand et al (2006)	Prospective N= 510 (diabetics)	2.2	Total 22 events (cardiac and cerebral)	Rate of death or MI increased by CAC categories

Budoff et al (2007)	Observation referral-based N = 25,253	6.8	510 all-cause deaths	Rate of death or MI increased by CAC categories
Detrano et al (2008)	Prospective N=6,814	3.4	162 CAD events	FRS-adjusted risk 28% higher with CAC scores doubling. CAC predictive in all ethnic groups
Becker et al (2008)	Prospective	3.3	179 (65 cardiac death, 114 MI)	CAC score ≥75th percentile associated with higher annualized event rate for MI. No cardiac events in patients with CAC = 0.

(CAC: Coronary Artery Calcium, CAD: Coronary Artery Disease, CVA: Cerebrovascular Accident, FRS: Framingham Risk Score, MI: Myocardial infraction, OR: odds Ratio, RR: relative risk)

Table 2. Clinical Trials summarizing data on Coronary Calcium Scoring.

2.7 Independent prognostic value of CAC scores over cardiac risk factors

Several authors in the preceding section have described an incremental role for CCS. Wong and colleagues (2000) showed that the CAC score severity predicted subsequent cardiovascular events independent of age, gender, and patient risk factor profile. Recent reports have included univariable and multivariable models that have evaluated the independent contribution of CAC in models evaluating risk factors or the FRS. The CAC score strongly predicted mortality, with 43% additional predictive value beyond risk factors alone (Greenland et al., 2004). In the St. Francis Heart Study, both univariable and multivariable models supported CAC scores as independent predictors of CAD outcome above and beyond traditional risk factors (Arad et al., 2000). Of note, CAC scores were also predictive of outcome in a multivariable model containing high-sensitivity C-reactive protein, a relatively newer marker for CAD (Taylor et al., 2005), similar to a previous report by Park et al. (Park et al., 2002). Other authors have evaluated the prognostic contribution of CCS in multivariable models that controlled for risk factors such as a family history of premature CHD or body mass index, that are not in the FRS, and proved CCS to be independently predictive in these settings too (LaMonte et al., 2005; O'Malley et al., 2003.

2.8 Coronary calcium scoring: Complementary to Framingham scores and global risk assessment?

Since CCS has shown to have incremental value over risk factors, the next step is to assess whether it can be integrated in to risk assessment algorithms. The concept of Bayesian theory provides a framework to evaluate the expected relationship between the predictive values of CAC score in individuals with low- to high-risk FRS. As dictated by Bayesian theory, a test's post-test likelihood of events is partially dependent upon a patient's pretest risk estimate. Thus, for patients with a low risk FRS very few events would be expected during follow-up and the resulting post-test risk estimate for patients with an abnormal CAC score would be expected to remain low. Not surprisingly, several reports have documented the futility of CAC score in risk prediction for low-risk populations (Kondos et al., 2003; Greenland et al., 2004). Such studies demonstrate the importance of selecting optimal cohorts for whom CAC testing will be of greater value. In addition, the recent data provide support for the concept that use of CAC testing is most useful in terms of incremental prognostic value for populations with an intermediate FRS (Redberg et al., 2003). In a secondary analysis of patients with an intermediate FRS from 4 reports (Greenland et al., 2004; Arad et al., 2005; Vliegenthart et al., 2005; LaMonte et al., 2005), annual CAD death or MI rates were 0.4%, 1.3%, and 2.4% for each tertile of CAC score where scores ranged from less than 100, 100 to 399, and greater than or equal to 400, respectively. From this analysis, intermediate-risk FRS patients with a CAC score greater than or equal to 400 would be expected to have coronary event rates that place them in the CAD risk equivalent status i.e >20% event rate in the next ten years.

One way to determine additive utility of a new test is through the use of Receiver Operative Curve (ROC) analyses. The ROC curve is a plot of true-positive rate versus false-positive rate over the entire range of possible cutoff values. The area under the ROC curve (AUC) ranges between 1.0 for the perfect test and 0.5 for a useless test. Studies comparing predictive capacity of conventional and newer biomarkers for prediction of cardiovascular events consistently demonstrate that adding a number of newer biomarkers (such as C-reactive protein, interleukins, and other proposed risk stratifiers) change the C-statistic by only 0.009 ($P = 0.08$). Such small changes such as these in the C-statistic suggest rather limited improvement in risk discrimination with additional risk markers. The costs involved in implementing the use of such biomarkers may not be justified by the magnitude of the observed benefit. However, CAC scanning has been shown to markedly improve the C-statistic in the studies described above, suggesting robust improvement in risk discrimination (Anand et al 2006; Budoff et al 2007).

2.9 Calcium scoring in symptomatic patients

This far, we have discussed the utility of CCS in asymptomatic patients. Researchers have investigated the role of CCS in symptomatic patients also. If a patient does not have coronary artery calcification, it would be very unlikely that they have high grade obstructive CAD. However, once calcium is discovered, theoretically, one cannot definitively opine if the plaque is obstructive or not. Nevertheless, this topic has been a target of active research. Trials investigating this subject have studied symptomatic patients referred for coronary angiography.

A meta-analysis including 3683 patients from 16 studies was performed to evaluate the diagnostic accuracy of coronary calcium scoring (O'Rourke et al., 2000). The entry criteria included diagnostic catheterization for patients without prior history of coronary disease or prior cardiac transplantation. Patients were symptomatic and referred to the cardiac catheterization laboratory for exclusion of obstructive CAD. On average, significant coronary disease (defined as greater than 50% by some or 70% luminal stenosis by others on coronary angiography) was reported in 57.2% of the patients. Presence of CAC was reported on average in 65.8% of patients. The odds of obstructive CAD were found to be elevated 20-

fold with a positive CAC. Additionally, higher coronary calcium scores were associated with higher degrees of obstructive coronary artery disease.

Similar to data in asymptomatic patients, some other authors have described the independent predictability of CAC in symptomatic patients. A large case series by Guerci et al (1998) found that coronary calcium score of greater than 80 (Agatston score) was associated with increased likelihood of obstructive coronary artery disease regardless of the number of risk factors. Also, the series by Kennedy et al (1998) clearly reported that in their multivariate analyses, only male sex and coronary calcium score were significantly related to the extent of angiographic disease. The ROC analysis for CAC showed a much larger area under the curve, as compared to conventional risk factors, thus establishing its role as a disease discriminator.

2.10 CAC in comparison to other tests for diagnosis of coronary artery disease

As a new test for CAD, it is important to assess and compare CCS to the currently accepted modalities for CAD diagnosis. Schermund et al (1999) compared EBT derived CAC measurement to nuclear stress tests using technetium in a cohort of 308 symptomatic patients referred for cardiac catheterization. They found a strong association of CAC score with perfusion defects on Single Photon Emission Computed Tomography (SPECT) scans and angiographically obstructive CAD. This association remained significant after excluding the influence of interrelated risk factors and SPECT variables.

Other authors have reported similar results using thallium exercise stress testing (Kajinami et al., 1995; Yao et al., 1997). In fact, a study by Shavelle et al (2000) indicated that CAC might be more accurate for diagnosis for CAD. The relative risk for obstructive CAD in this study was 4.43, and was significantly higher than that for treadmill ECG (1.72) or technetium stress (1.96). The overall accuracy of CAC was 80%, as opposed to 71 and 74% for exercise treadmill ECG and technetium stress respectively. When combined with an abnormal treadmill ECG response, CAC was found to be 83% specific for obstructive CAD. He et al (2000) suggest a complementary role for CCS based on their finding of a threshold phenomenon. In their study, no myocardial hypoperfusion was noted in patients with CAC less than 100, and a marked increase in perfusion abnormalities with increasing CAC scores. If indeed, the absence of coronary calcium in symptomatic patients can exclude obstructive disease, it can possibly be used in the triage of patients with chest pain in the emergency rooms in the future. Some groups have looked at this possibility, and although their results favor CAC as a triage tool (Georgiou et al., 2001; McLaughlin et al., 1999), the author personally has some concerns about adopting this paradigm as a standard of care, at least for now. This is mainly because of small sample sizes of these studies, and the fact that it may not be safe to discharge every patient with absent coronary calcifications. Some of these patients could have noncalcified soft plaques that may be prone to rupture. Absence of coronary calcification may lead to a false sense of security in such patients, and they may be discharged. A small proportion of these patients could develop a full-blown acute coronary syndrome outside of hospital settings. The medico-legal implications of such mishaps are far from few. In our opinion, until further data become available, CAC scoring should not be recommended as a triage tool in the emergency room setting. This issue is further elaborated in the section on absent coronary artery calcifications in CAD.

2.11 Using CCS in patients with established CAD

While there is limited utility to CCS in patients with documented CAD, a recognized use of CAC screening is to track atherosclerotic changes over time by serial measurements. A large prospective study was designed to evaluate the impact of aggressive lipid-lowering and antioxidant therapy on the progression of CAC. The study included 4613 asymptomatic persons between 50 to 70 years of age, with coronary arteries EBT scanning at baseline and again at 2 years and 4.3 years (Arad et al, 2005). Whereas the intervention did not seem to significantly affect progression of CAC, it was noted that patients who sustained a coronary event demonstrated a median increase in CAC score of 247 as compared to a CAC score increase of 4 in those who did not sustain a coronary event. Multiple logistic regressions demonstrated that 2-year change in calcium score ($P = 0.0001$) was significantly associated with subsequent CAD events. Increasing calcium scores were seen to most strongly correlate with coronary events in this study, as in another observational study by Raggi et al. (2004).

Since statins are known to stabilize coronary artery plaques, one would expect that coronary calcification would not progress, and if anything, regress with aggressive statin therapy. However, the results of clinical trials have been controversial in this regard. In a retrospective study, Callister and associates (1998b) demonstrated a 45% slowing in the rate of CAC progression in patients receiving statins. Budoff and coworkers (2000), in a prospectively designed study, demonstrated a 61% decrease in the rate of CAC score progression in dyslipidemic patients on statin therapy. Similarly, Achenbach and colleagues (2002) showed that with a standard dose of 0.3 mg/day of open-label cerivastatin in dyslipidemic patients, the median annual relative increase in CAC scores was 25% during the untreated period before study entry versus 9% during the treatment period ($P <0.0001$). Reduction of CAC score was most pronounced in those patients who achieved an LDL level <100 mg/dL.

On the other hand, at least three randomized controlled trials have failed to replicate these results. The SALTIRE trial (Scottish Aortic Stenosis and Lipid Lowering Trial, Impact on Regression) randomized 102 patients to atorvastatin or placebo and assessed CAC progression during an average follow-up of 2 years. Despite a significant reduction in LDL and C-reactive protein levels, there was a insignificant increase in percentage CAC progression (Houslay et al., 2006). Schermund and coworkers (2006) also failed to show reduced progression of CAC in asymptomatic patients randomized to 80 mg of atorvastatin, despite a 20% reduction in LDL level as compared to the group receiving 10-mg atorvastatin during one year of follow up. Similarly, the BELLES (Beyond Endorsed Lipid Lowering with EBCT Scanning) study, which randomized hyperlipidemic postmenopausal women to atorvastatin 80 mg or pravastatin 40 mg, found no effect on CAC progression in either arms. Although atorvastatin reduced LDL concentration by 47% ± 20% and pravastatin reduced LDL by 25% ± 19%, there was no significant decrease in CAC progression after 12 months, and rather, a statistically insignificant increase of 15% and 14% in CAC scores in the atorvastatin and pravastatin arms, respectively (Raggi et al., 2005). The authors were unable to justify this increase in CAC scores despite LDL reduction.

Based on the conflicting data, the ACC/AHA guidelines do not recommend following CAC scores longitudinally to track coronary atherosclerosis over time (Greenland et al., 2007).

2.12 Absence of coronary artery calcium and its implications

So far, we have reviewed data on the presence and absence of coronary calcium in symptomatic and asymptomatic cohorts. It appears that absence of CAC reliably excludes obstructive coronary disease in asymptomatic and selected symptomatic individuals. Also the absence of coronary calcium appears to be associated with a low cardiovascular event rate, suggesting that less aggressive pharmacotherapy may be acceptable in this population. However, published event rates for individuals with zero CAC vary, probably because of differences in baseline risk, follow-up period, and very different endpoints in studies.

Overall, absence of coronary calcium appears to be favorable in terms of prognosis for coronary events. However, we do need to elaborate on the few patients with coronary artery disease, who are missed by CCS. In a cohort of asymptomatic middle-aged individuals, Blaha et al. (2009) observed that relatively more coronary events occurred among diabetics and smokers, even in the absence of CAC. The likely mechanisms include non-calcified soft plaques, rapid development of atherosclerosis, and plaque destabilization. Even so, whereas the relative risk of events is higher in the presence of low CAC, the absolute event rate remains low. Thus, in an appropriately selected non–high-risk patient, the absence of CAC can likely be used as a rationale to emphasize lifestyle therapy, while refraining from expensive preventive pharmacotherapy, and frequent cardiac imaging or testing.

Given the low 10-year risk in this population, a drug such as a statin that produces a 30% relative risk reduction would have to be given to more than 300 patients for 10 years to prevent one death i.e. number needed to treat (NNT) is approximately 333 for 10 years (Blaha et al., 2009). Although current guidelines do not recommend that preventive therapies such as lipid-lowering medications be stopped or dosed lower in the absence of CAC, data from the aforementioned studies suggest that aggressive management in this cohort is probably not warranted if one does not qualify according to NCEP guidelines. This strategy will allow those with absent CAC to follow healthy lifestyle modifications with little or no medical therapy, whereas intense therapy is focused on a population of patients with an actual higher risk of events demonstrated by atherosclerotic burden on CCS. Again, in implementing this standard of care, one needs to remember the caveat about smokers and diabetic patients described above.

The ACC/AHA guidelines echo these results, recommending against invasive diagnostic procedures or hospital admission in patients with absent CAC (Greenland et al., 2007). The ACC/ASNC appropriateness criteria also mention that the absence of CAC generally precludes the need for assessment by myocardial perfusion imaging (Brindis et al., 2005). This strategy can significantly cut down radiation exposure and coronary angiography related complications.

2.13 Applying coronary calcium screening in every day life: The practicalities and challenges

2.13.1 Is calcium scoring valid across various ethnicities and races?

Demographic data suggest that African American patients have lower incidence of coronary artery calcifications despite a higher overall prevalence of coronary artery disease (Greenland et al., 2007). Most literature on CCS has been described in white populations. Two studies have addressed the value of CAC in other ethnic groups. First, Nasir and coworkers (2007) in nearly 15,000 ethnically diverse self-referred patients assessed the role of CAC for the prediction of all-cause mortality. In comparison of prognosis by CAC scores in ethnic minorities, relative risk ratios were highest for African Americans, with scores ≥400 exceeding 16.1 ($P < 0.0001$). Hispanics with CAC scores ≥400 had relative risk ratios from 7.9 to 9.0; Asians with CAC scores ≥1000 had relative risk ratios 6.6-fold higher than those of non-Hispanic whites ($P < 0.0001$). The second study to address this question is the prospective Multi-Ethnic Study of Atherosclerosis (MESA) study by Detrano et al., (2008). MESA was designed to investigate the prevalence and progression of subclinical CAD in a population-based sample of 6814 men and women between 45 to 84 years of age. The cohort was selected from six United States field centers and included approximately 38% white, 28% African American, 23% Hispanic, and 11% Asian (primarily of Chinese descent) patients. Their results indicated that when compared with whites, the relative risks for having coronary calcification were 0.78 (95% CI, 0.74 to 0.82) in blacks, 0.85 (95% CI, 0.79 to 0.91) in Hispanics, and 0.92 (95% CI, 0.85 to 0.99) in Chinese. Despite this difference in prevalence of CAC, the predictive value of coronary calcium in various ethnic groups remains valid. These results strongly support the role of CCS as a global coronary event risk stratifier.

2.13.2 Is CCS equally predictive in both men and women?

Women develop atherosclerosis about 10 years later than men. The appearance of coronary calcium tracks with this later onset of CAD. Thus cut off values for CAC scores are different in men and women. However, these differences start to diminish after the age of sixty years. Premenopausal women generally have a low likelihood of obstructive coronary artery disease and vulnerable plaques compared to age matched men. Premenopausal women who have any degree of CAC before sixty years of age are at much higher risk of coronary events and deserve particular attention to aggressive lipid therapy and risk factor modification. These gender differences highlight the importance of age and gender specific reference points for CAC scoring (Hoff et al., 2001). In this regard, one also needs to remember that we presently do not have any guidelines about applying these scores to younger women who have been rendered menopausal iatrogenically via surgical hysterectomy or oophorectomy. Due to small numbers, this cohort has not been systematically studied yet. It is unclear whether these women should be treated as though they have the same level of risk as their age matched male controls.

2.13.3 Is CAC scoring valid in end stage renal disease patients?

It is well known that the subset of patients with end stage renal disease, especially those on hemodialysis have a higher prevalence of coronary artery calcification. Although this cohort as a whole is at higher risk for coronary events, one cannot use coronary artery calcifications to prognosticate this group in the same way as patients without renal disease. Some studies suggest that such patients develop calcification of the tunica media as opposed to the typical intimal calcification associated with atherosclerotic plaques (Moe et al., 2002). The role of medial calcification remains to be explored in CAD. Studies have reported conflicting data about correlation between coronary calcium detected on CT scanning and luminal narrowing on coronary angiography (Haydar et al., 2004; Sharples et al., 2004). In the absence of firm recommendations in this cohort, it is best to individualize care to each patient as much as possible.

2.13.4 Who is an appropriate patient for CCS?

The ACC/AHA consensus document on CCS mentions "it may be reasonable to consider use of CAC measurement in asymptomatic individuals who are at intermediate risk by the FRS" (Greenland et al., 2007pp 378-402). Such individuals are most likely to be reclassified to a higher risk status on the basis of high CAC score, thus modifying subsequent patient management. However, the committee did not find enough evidence for the utility of CAC testing in risk stratification of those considered at low risk as well as of those considered at high risk for CAD in the next 10 years.

Patients with a 10-year risk >20% already qualify for aggressive lipid-lowering management with optional LDL-C goals of <70 mg/dL, and further CAC testing may not change treatment goals. The current guidelines do not recommended CAC testing for those with a 10-year estimated risk of <10% (low risk). However, by current criteria, most non-diabetic women who are younger than 60 years would not be candidates for further risk stratification with CAC testing. This approach will exclude a large number of women at higher risk for CAD from CAC testing. One should remember that those at <10% 10-year risk of CAD are frequently at significant longer term risk of CHD, particularly those women with a family history of premature CAD. Since family history of premature CAD does not factor into most global risk algorithms, it may be advisable to screen a subset of women with low 10-year risk with CAC if they have family history of premature CAD. At least 25% of individuals with family history of premature CAD have significant CAC. Clinical studies have strongly supported family history of premature CAD to be an independent risk factor associated strongly with higher burden of subclinical atherosclerosis. Nasir and coworkers (2007) demonstrated that among those with premature family history of CAD (especially with sibling history), nearly one-third to one-quarter of self-referred patients with no or one CAD risk factor had CAC ≥100.

Another way to work around this problem may be to look for alternative definitions of the "intermediate risk" category. The 2003 American College of Cardiology Bethesda Conference on atherosclerosis imaging defines "intermediate-risk groups" as those at 6% to 20% 10-year risk, as opposed to FRS, which defines intermediate risk as 10-20% 10-year risk (Wilson et al., 2003). By this definition, more higher risk women would be placed in the intermediate-risk group, and thus qualify for risk factor modification, especially regarding LDL-C control, aggressive preventive strategies, such as statin, aspirin, and possibly blood pressure-lowering therapies if they additionally have increased levels of CAC. The recommendations involving low FRS risk category and women with family history of premature CAD were not incorporated in the 2007 consensus document on CCS. The author himself uses these pearls in clinical practice and looks forward to them being integrated in a future consensus document from the ACC/AHA.

2.14 Does CAC scoring improve healthy life style adherence and medication compliance?

Some working groups have demonstrated that the discovery of any calcium on a CAC scan independently lead to initiation of aspirin and/or statin therapy by physicians (Wong et al., 1996). The same group also demonstrated that initiation of healthful lifestyle changes, including losing weight and decreasing dietary fat often accompanied an abnormal CAC scan. Although the initiation of appropriate lifestyle and pharmacotherapy by physicians correlated with abnormal CAC scores, it is still unclear whether routine atherosclerotic imaging improves medication adherence. Kalia et al (2006) reported that in a study of 505 asymptomatic individuals that continuation of lipid-lowering medication was lowest (44%) among those with a CAC score in the first quartile (0-30), whereas 91% of individuals with a CAC score in the fourth quartile (>526) adhered to lipid-lowering medication. In multivariable analysis, after adjustment for other cardiovascular risk factors, higher baseline CAC scores were strongly associated with adherence to statin therapy. Most data in this regard seem to be coming from only one group of investigators. Moreover, a randomized clinical trial assessing the effects of CAC scanning on estimated risk of CAD after 1 year, determined by changes in FRS, found no difference in mean absolute risk change in 10-year FRS comparing the groups who received CAC score results with those who did not. In this study, the prevalence of CAC was fairly low (15%), with generally low CAC scores even in those with CAC. It is possible that the study was not powered enough to detect the difference between the study groups (O'Malley et al., 2003).

2.15 Is this technology cost effective?

Establishing cost effectiveness of diagnostic tests is quite challenging. To establish effectiveness, CAC measurement has to be shown to enhance quality of life, prolong life or both. While this is feasible for therapies having randomized control trials, no such studies exist for CAC measurement (Douglas & Ginsburg, 1996).

In the absence of clinical trial data, cost effectiveness is approached with simulations in which decisions, test results and outcomes are estimated with as much information from medical literature. Despite significant challenges, three studies have attempted to study cost effectiveness of CAC scoring (O'Malley & Greenberg, 2004; Taylor et al., 2005; Shaw et al., 2003). Most studies assessing cost effectiveness of diagnostic modalities use the Incremental Cost Effectiveness Ratio (ICER) as a measure of cost effectiveness. ICER is defined as the ratio of the change in costs secondary to an intervention/test (compared to the alternative, such as doing nothing or using the best available alternative treatment) to the change in effects of the same (O'Malley & Greenberg, 2004). O'Malley and colleagues (2004) were able to demonstrate an ICER of $86752. The Prospective Army Coronary Calcium project found an ICER of $31,500 (Taylor et al., 2005) and Shaw et al (2003) demonstrated an ICER of $500,000 with estimated coronary risk of <0.6% per year, $42,339 for an incidence of 1%, and $30742 for an incidence of 2% per year. The consensus committee felt that neither of these models were strong or grounded enough to justify establishing a policy at this time.

In our opinion, although the proposed cost effectiveness models are weak, their respective authors do offer a valid argument. The basis of their assertion is that both noninvasive testing and invasive angiography rates are low in individuals with low CAC scores. In the absence of CCS data, this patient population will be subjected to functional testing such as myocardial perfusion assessment, and possibly even invasive coronary angiography, both of which drive medical costs up significantly. With its valuable attributes of very little radiation exposure, strong risk stratification evidence, and relative inexpensiveness, CCS appears to be a cost effective alternative in cardiovascular care. Figure 6 summarizes the merits of CAC scoring as an ideal risk stratifier and an economically feasible alternative.

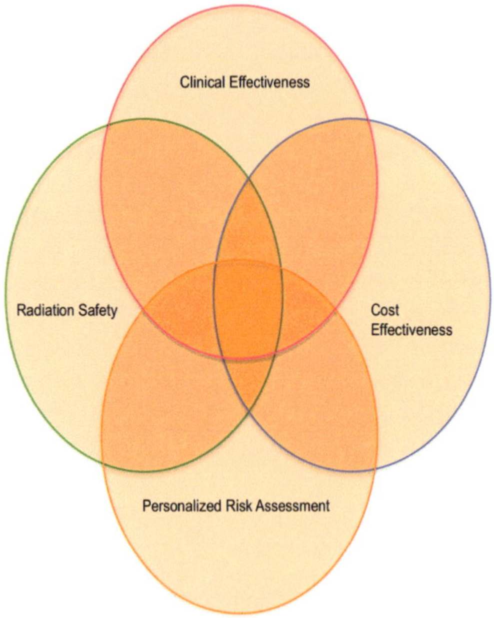

(A)

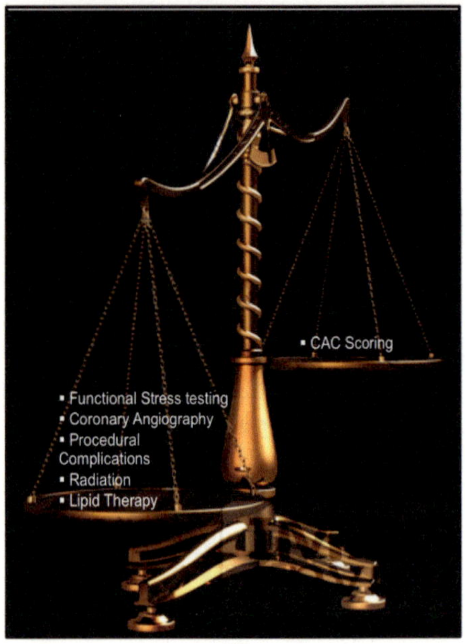

(B)

Fig. 6. Clinical (A) and Economic (B) Attributes of Coronary Calcium Scoring (CCS)

3. Other markers for CAD

After the extensive discussion on calcium scoring and its role in assessment of CAD, we will now briefly discuss other novel risk markers for CAD.

3.1 C-reactive protein

3.1.1 Historical background and function

C-reactive protein (CRP) is a nonspecific marker of inflammation. C-reactive protein (CRP) was first described by the laboratory of Oswald Avery at the Rockefeller Institute in New York (Ghose, 2004). It was tested for an association with cardiovascular disease when inflammation was implicated as the culprit in the pathogenesis of atherosclerosis (Ross, 1999). CRP occurs in two forms, a pentameric (pCRP) form and a monomeric (mCRP) form (Eisenhardt et al, 2009a). The pentameric form is produced by hepatocytes as an acute phase reactant, elevating up to a 1,000-fold within 24-72 hours in response to infection, inflammation and tissue injury (Pepys & Baltz, 1983). Monomeric CRP is believed to be derived from dissociation of pCRP (Eisenhardt et al., 2009b) and possibly produced in extrahepatic cells such as smooth muscle in arterial walls, adipose tissue and macrophages (Yasojima et al., 2001).

Interestingly, pCRP is believed to promote both inflammatory and anti-inflammatory effects. There is even considerable data suggesting that pCRP may have vasculoprotective potential. mCRP however, has been documented to directly induce expression of VCAM-1 and to play a key role in the promotion of platelet aggregation (Eisenhardt et al., 2009) . Fig 7 summarizes the vascular inflammatory process.

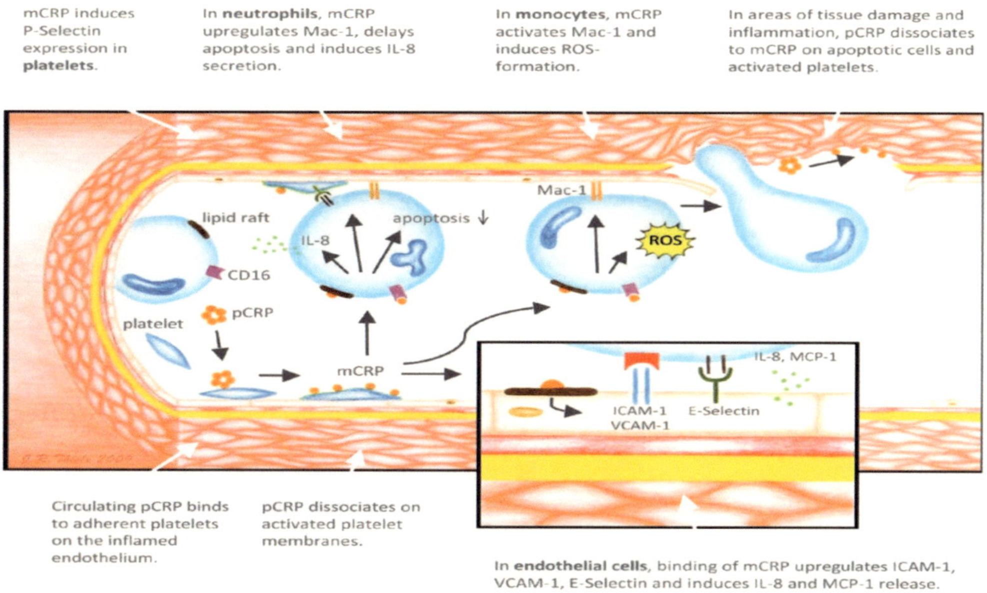

Adapted with permission from: Eisenhardt SU, Thiele JR, Bannasch H et al. C-reactive protein: how conformational changes influence inflammatory properties. Cell Cycle 2009; 8:23, 3885-3892.

Fig. 7. Role of CRP in vascular inflammation Dissociation and pro-inflammatory effects of mCRP in the peripheral circulation. CRP circulates as a disc shaped pentamer and is dissociated by its exposure to bioactive lipids on cell membranes of activated platelets and apoptotic/necrotic cells. The resulting mCRP then exerts its pro-inflammatory effects that are depicted in the figure.

3.1.2 Nonspecific CRP

The controversy with CRP stems from its nonspecific nature. A great degree of variability was noted in a study in which serial measurements of serum CRP were obtained in 159 patients with stable ischemic heart disease. In this trial, risk stratification was performed using 3 risk categories (CRP <1, 1-3 and >3mg/L). In this process, 40% of patients changed risk categories between the first and second measurements (Ockene et al., 2001). Even a minor inflammatory ailment such as an upper respiratory tract infection can produce significant fluctuations in CRP levels, thus making it difficult to rely on it as a cardiovascular disease marker.

Further, it is extremely difficult to assess CRP in the milieu of other chronic inflammatory disease such as rheumatoid arthritis or systemic lupus erythematosus, which independently raise CRP levels. A study by Breland and associates (2010) evaluated plasma levels of CRP in patients with CAD without inflammatory rheumatologic disease (IRD), CAD with IRD, IRD without CAD, and healthy subjects. They found that plasma levels of CRP in patients with CAD without IRD, CAD with IRD and IRD without CAD were significantly elevated relative to healthy individuals (p=0.002) . No significant difference was detected in levels of CRP in patients with CAD with or without IRD, and in patients with IRD without CAD.

Gasparyan et al (2010), in their review of the literature, noted that CRP plays a universal role in the enhanced atherogenesis in all rheumatologic diseases. Elevations in CRP levels have been linked to antiphospholipid antibodies in SLE (Feinboom & Bauer, 2005 as cited in Gasparyan et al., 2010) and anti-CCP in RA (del Val Del Amo et al., 2006). CRP as a prognostic marker for CAD in patients with IRD needs further studies with larger sample sizes, however preliminary data is suggestive that an elevated CRP does incur increased risk for CAD. A multiethnic lupus cohort study conducted in the USA determined that CRP independently predicted arterial events (hazard ratio [HR] 3.9, 95%CI 1.5-10.1) (Toloza et al., 2004 as cited in Gasparyan et al., 2010). While in the UK, a cohort of RA patients with CRP levels >5 mg/L were found to be at risk of cardiovascular death (HR 3.9, 95%CI 1.2-13.4 for men and 4.22, 95% CI 1.4-12.6 for women) (Goodson et al., 2005 as cited in Gasparyan et al., 2010).

Cirrhosis complicates the interpretation of CRP, as it is a cause of decreased production of CRP from the liver. Also medications such as oral contraceptives have also been documented to increase CRP levels (Mackenzie & Woodhouse, 2006). In the recent years, high sensitivity CRP (hs-CRP) has generated significant interest among researchers. hs-CRP detects concentrations down to 0.3 mg/L and below, as compared to more traditional assays which detect in the range of 3 to 5 mg/L. hsCRP assays are used to assess cardiovascular risk because these tests are able to quantify CRP levels normally observed in asymptomatic patients (Marrow, 2011).

3.1.3 CRP and CAD link

The added value of high hsCRP to risk stratification was initially evaluated by Ridker and colleagues (Cook et al., 2006). In their model they added hsCRP to variables utilized in the Framingham risk score (i.e., age, total cholesterol level, high-density lipoprotein cholesterol level, smoking and blood pressure) in the Women's Health Study (Cook et al., 2006). Their results showed only a marginal improvement in the area under the receiver operating characteristic curve (AUC-ROC) (Cook et al., 2006). The same group then explored whether risk prediction of hsCRP could be improved when used together with several other novel biomarkers such as hemoglobin A1c (HbA1c), homocysteine, soluble intercellular adhesion molcule-1, and apolipoproteins (Ridker et al., 2007). The Women's Health Study was divided into a model derivation cohort (n = 16,400) and a model validation cohort (n = 8158) (Ridker et al., 2007). The amalgamation that produced the best fitting model consisted of age, systolic blood pressure, current smoking, hsCRP, parental history of MI < age 60, HbA1c in diabetics, apolipoprotein B-100 level, apolipoprotein A-I level and lipoprotein (a) levels. This algorithm was simplified for more efficient clinical utility into the Reynolds Risk Score (RRS) (Ridker et al., 2007) (see Table 3). The RRS reclassified 40-50% of intermediate-risk, as predetermined by the FRS, to higher risk or lower risk. The FRS and RRS differ in the addition of hsCRP and parental history of MI < age 60 to the latter. However, it is important to point out that none of the subjects were reclassified from a low risk to a high risk category and vice versa, emphasizing the importance of determining prior probability of disease in those recommended to have further testing. The RRS was later validated in men. When compared to a traditional risk stratification model, the RRS reclassified 18% of subjects in the Physicians Health Study II, and was associated with better model fit and discrimination (Ridker et al., 2008a).

Best-Fitting Model	Clinically Simplified Model
Age	Age
Systolic blood pressure	Systolic blood pressure
Current smoking	Current smoking
hsCRP	hsCRP
Parental history of MI <age 60	Parental history of MI <age 60
Hemoglobin A1c (if diabetic)	Hemoglobin A1c (if diabetic)
Apo B-100	Total Cholesterol
Apo A-I	HDL-C
Lp(a) [if apo B-100 ≥ 100]	

Adapted with permission from Ridker PM, Buring JE, Rifai N, et al. Development and validation of improved algorithms for the assessment of global cardiovascular risk in women: the Reynolds Risk Score. JAMA 2007; 297:611-619.

Table 3. Reynolds Risk Score

Most recently, evaluation of the therapeutic benefit of statin therapy in patients with LDL-C levels lower than 130 mg/dL, with elevated hsCRP levels greater than 2mg/L was examined in the Justification for the Use of Statins in Primary Prevention: an Interventional Trial Evaluating Rosuvastatin (JUPITER). Patients who met these criteria were treated with Rosuvastatin. Treatment with this therapy was associated with a 44% relative risk reduction in major cardiovascular events. The trial was discontinued early due to the early observation of clear benefit from such therapy (Ridker et al., 2008b). The Atherosclerosis Risk in Communities (ARIC) study was then conducted analyzing data on participants with the entry criteria of the JUPITER trial (Yang et al., 2009). The results of the ARIC trial suggested that elevated hsCRP conferred high risk regardless of LDL-C levels (<130mg/dL or ≥ 130mg/dL) (Yang et al., 2009).

3.2 Lipoprotein associated phospholipase A_2

3.2.1 Form and function

Lipoprotein Associated Phospholipase A_2 (Lp-PLA_2) was first cloned in 1995. It is a modified LDL particle in which a large glycoprotein, apolipoprotein (a), is covalently bound to apo B by a disulfide bridge (Streyer et al., 1994). The apo(a) chain has five cysteine rich domains known as "kringles". The fourth kringle is homologous is structure to the fibrin-binding domain of plasminogen, the plasma protein responsible for dissolving clots. This structural similarity unfortunately sets up a competition between Lp-PLA2 and plasminogen for binding sites, thus causing interference with fibrinolysis. Lp-PLA_2 induces foam cell formation and encourages cholesterol deposition in atherosclerotic plaques (McLean et al., 1987). Lp-PLA_2 is also thought to propogate inflammation via its action on oxidized phospholipids and nonesterified fatty acids, both of which are capable of inducing expression of adhesion molecules and attracting monocytes (Caslake & Packard, 2005).

3.2.2 Cardiovascular risk and Lp-PLA$_2$

Studies have contended Lp-PLA$_2$ as another biomarker associated with both cardiovascular disease and stroke (Ballantyne et al., 2004; Blake et al., 2001). The ARIC study that evaluated the increase in predictive risk provided by 19 markers including hsCRP showed that only Lp-PLA$_2$ significantly increased the AUC-ROC when added to traditional risk factors for cardiovascular disease (Folsom et al., 2006). The largest prospective analysis, that assessed the association between increased Lp-PLA$_2$ and coronary artery disease revealed an odds ratio of 1.60 (95% CI 1.09-1.18) for those patients with Lp-PLA2 values in the upper third tertile as compared to the lowest third tertile after adjusting for traditional risk factors (Bennet et al., 2008). The best data summarizing the relationship between Lp-PLA$_2$ and cardiovascular disease comes from a meta-analysis of individual patient records from 120,000 subjects in 36 prospective studies (Erqou et al., 2009). This study was able to show that Lp-PLA$_2$ was associated with a continuous risk for cardiovascular events (Erqou et al., 2009).

3.2.3 Who should be screened?

Although Lp-PLA$_2$ is a valid cardiovascular disease marker, it may not be feasible to screen everybody for the same. Stein and Rosenson (1997) put forth some recommendations for screening and treatment of Lp-PLA$_2$. Based on their recommendations, screening should only be performed in the following circumstances:

1. Patients with coronary heart disease and no other identifiable dyslipidemia.
2. Patients with strong family history of coronary heart disease and no other dyslipidemia.
3. Patients with hypercholesterolemia refractory to therapy with LDL cholesterol lowering therapies.

The last recommendation stemmed from the observation that Lp-PLA$_2$ does not respond to usual the therapy for LDL-C. The Friedewald formula, which is commonly used to calculate LDL cholesterol, does not distinguish between Lp-PLA$_2$, and LDL-cholesterol. Often, patients who present with elevated LDL may not have true LDL excess, but may instead have significant Lp-PLA$_2$ accumulation (Berresen et al., 1981). Such patients may be "refractory"to traditional LDL lowering therapy with statins, bile acid sequestrants, fibric acid derivatives etc.

3.2.4 Treatment

The most effective treatment to reduce Lp-PLA$_2$ levels is nicotinic acid (Carlson et al., 1989). Estrogen replacement therapy has also been reported to reduce Lp-PLA$_2$ by 50% (Sacks et al., 1994). Apheresis is a newer therapy that has been investigated for treatment of elevated Lp-PLA$_2$ (Keller, 2007).

3.3 Apolipoprotein B

Forty years ago Fredrickson and associates recognized that atherosclerosis is more closely related to the total number of apolipoprotein B (apo B)-containing particles rather than to LDL-C (Ridker et al., 2007). Apo B is an integral part of LDL, oxidized LDL, VLDL, and triglycerides (TG). It thus provides a direct measure of all circulating atherogenic lipoproteins (Ridker et al., 2008b). Also, measurement of LDL may sometimes be inaccurate in the setting of hypertriglyceridemia, particularly in diabetic patients. The utility of Apo-B in cardiovascular risk stratification is discussed in the paragraphs to follow. The author and his working group of clinicians use this marker frequently in day-to-day practice.

3.3.1 Combining apolipoproteins with CCS

Having discussed the above biomarkers in detail, it is now time to deliberate on how they can be incorporated in to an algorithm for clinical use. At the present time, there are no randomized trials or guidelines describing such combinations. The thoughts and possibilities presented in this section of the chapter are entirely based on the author's personal clinical experience. We present the risk stratification algorithm followed at our institution. We wish to emphasize that this approach should be considered experimental in the absence of evidence-based data supporting this paradigm.

Like most clinicians, we start our patient risk assessment by calculating Framingham risk scores. When patients are identified to have a 10-year risk of 10-20%, particular attention is paid to their HDL status. When these patients have low HDL, cardiologists consider the possibility of premature atherosclerosis in certain subtypes of patients within this class. Two main categories of dyslipidemias with risk of premature atherosclerosis include Familial hypertriglyceridemia (High TG, Low HDL, near normal LDL; otherwise known as Type IV Hyperlipidemia) and Familial Combined Hyperlipidemia (high TG, high LDL, low HDL; otherwise known as Type IIb Hyperlipidemia). These disorders are not very uncommon, and such patients have high levels of small dense LDL in their circulation (Genest et al, 1992). Particularly, the subgroup with Type IV hyperlipidemias is often clinically undertreated because of normal to near normal LDL levels. While lipoprotein analysis is not the routine standard of care for every patient at our institution, we do recommend checking Apo B 100 levels for further risk stratification in the class patients described above, particularly if they have family history of premature CAD. The apo B levels reflect their potential for early subclinical atherosclerosis.

If the Apo B levels are reported to be within normal limits, further testing is not encouraged and annual follow up of lipid panels, along with statin therapy is advised per the NCEP guidelines. However, in the presence of elevated Apo B 100 levels, these patients are aggressively treated with statins, with or without niacin to achieve LDL goals of <70 mg/dl. We also follow their Apo B levels with therapy with a goal to maintain Apo B levels less than 80 mg/dl. In such patients, a one-time screening with coronary calcium scoring is offered. The rationale for this protocol is that these patients, by virtue of their small dense LDL particles are at much higher risk for plaque inflammation and rupture. In the absence of coronary artery calcifications, no further workup for CAD is recommended, and patients are encouraged to keep up with lifestyle modifications, while maintaining their cholesterol levels at those dictated by the NCEP guidelines. The detection of coronary calcium alerts the physician that the patient in question has already developed vulnerable plaques with silent plaque ruptures. This finding reinforces life style modifications and compliance with/modification of lipid therapy. Further, we quantify the CAC scores. The presence of calcium scores >100, suggests high risk for cardiovascular events, and suggests the need for further assessment of atherosclerotic coronary disease with either functional stress testing or coronary CT Angiography. In the absence of coronary calcification, the life style behaviors and lipid pharmacotherapy are still recommended, and the option of repeating calcium scoring every 2-3 years with/ without coronary CTA is offered.

Thus, we clinically use Apo B 100 as a surrogate for soft plaque and coronary calcification as a surrogate for ruptured plaques. In our experience, we do find it cost effective to avoid routine stress testing in the presence of normal Apo B levels and absent coronary calcification in asymptomatic patients even with family history of premature CAD. Although our data are not enough to present our thoughts in the form of a study yet, we have had very good success rate with detection of subclinical disease and prevention of acute coronary syndromes in patients with intermediate Framingham risk scores. Our group is working on designing an observational study to test this clinical algorithm. Figure 8 summarizes our algorithm.

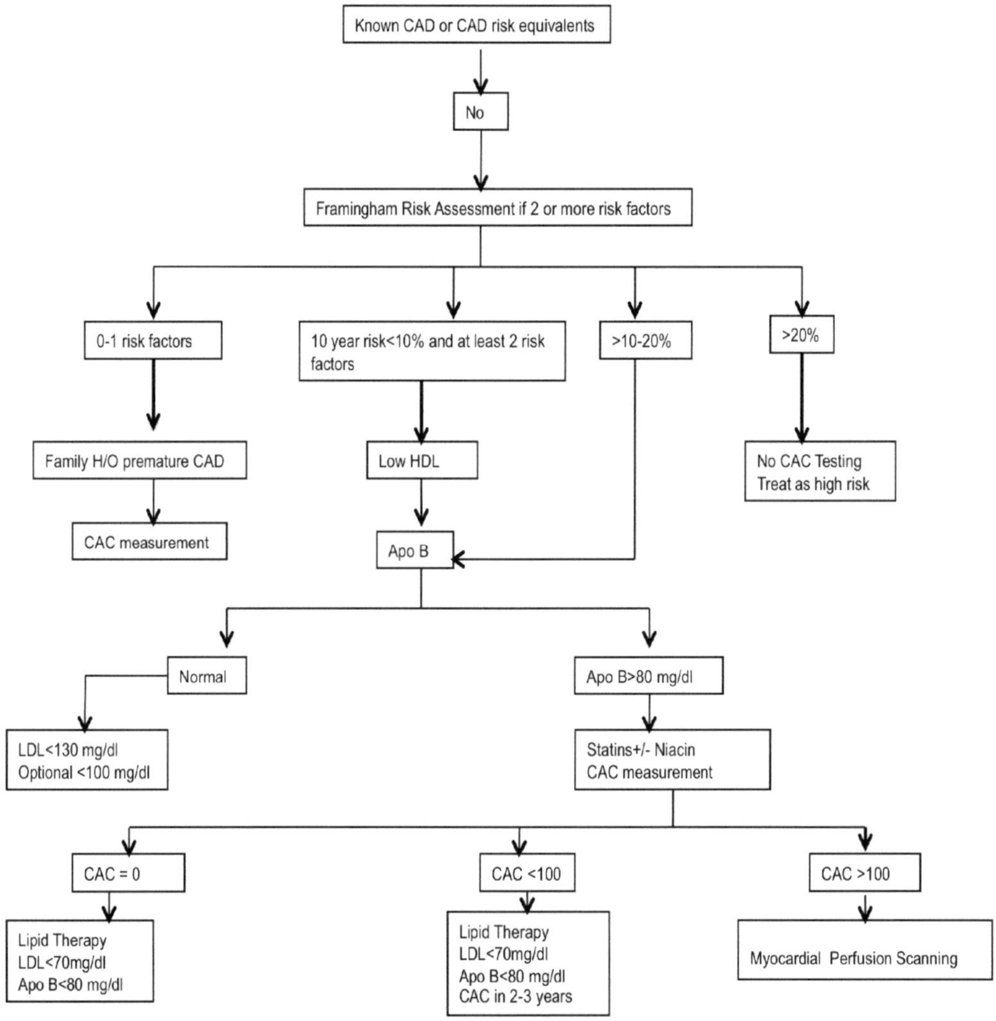

Fig. 8. Cardiovascular Risk stratification Algorithm proposed by Hegde et al

3.3.2 Platelet volume as a marker of cardiovascular risk

Although the author has focused mainly on the role of CCS and lipoproteins in this chapter, there are emerging data on the role of other novel markers such as platelet morphology and volumes as markers of cardiovascular disease. Mean platelet volume (MPV) has been studied as a marker of both vascular inflammation and thromboses (Gasparyan et al 2011). Diabetic patients have hyperactive platelets that are hyposensitive to anti aggregatory effects of prostacyclins and nitric oxide (Watala C. 2005). They also have higher MPV values as compared to normal controls. In fact, Zuberi et al have described that MPV reaches its highest level with increasing insulin resistance, and transition from prediabetes to diabetes, indicating a major increase in the level of risk. Vander Loo and colleagues have indicated that high MPV may herald the occurrence of an acute coronary syndrome in the near future. Inflammatory cytokines such as IL-6 and CRP alter the morphology of platelets released from the bone marrow weeks before an acute coronary syndrome. This finding could potentially be utilized to risk stratify asymptomatic individuals in to low, intermediate versus high risk groups for cardiovascular events. This idea has also been explored in the setting of an actual acute cornary syndrome. Pizzulli et al observed that in subgroups of patients with acute coronary syndromes, patients requiring percutaneous interventions had higher MPV as compared to those with normal MPVs. Although the concept is interesting, the data are not coherent cross studies. Case control studies by other authors such as Glud et al (1986) and Erne et al (1988) have failed to demonstrate such correlation between acute coronary syndromes and MPV. The role of MPV needs to be confirmed in larger clinical trials before we recommend its use as a cardiovascular risk stratifier.

4. Summary and key points

1. Subclinical atherosclerosis is the new target of early detection and treatment strategies to prevent acute coronary syndromes and decrease cardiac mortality.
2. Plaque inflammation and ruptures are the culprits in acute coronary syndromes. Future cardiac event risk stratifiers should include biomarkers that reflect inflammation within vascular tree.
3. Coronary Calcium Scoring (CCS) is a strong indicator of overall atherosclerotic burden in an individual. The total CCS, by virtue of its association with soft plaques, is an indicator of patient's overall risk for future cardiac events. It has established validity across several ethnicities and age groups.
4. CCS appears to be a strong and viable risk stratifier for patients within the intermediate risk category of CAD (10 year FRS 10-20%). CCS may help to redefine goals for life style modifications, lipid therapy and overall management for this patient population.
5. CCS is a valid prognosticator of coronary events across multiple ethnicities including Caucasian, African American, Hispanic and Asian origin.
6. CCS has limited utility and is best avoided in patients with Framingham risk scores of <10%, unless they have strong family history of premature CAD. CCS should also be avoided in patients with FRS of > 20%, since the results are unlikely to change therapeutic decisions anyways.
7. CCS may be useful in symptomatic patients in the setting of equivocal stress testing results.
8. There are insufficient data to support the routine use of CCS as a filter in the triage of symptomatic patients presenting to acute care facilities with chest pain.

9. Apolipoprotein and high sensitivity CRP may be combined with CCS to improve risk stratification in patients with intermediate Framingham scores, although the data are limited in this regard.

5. Future research

Future studies should focus on incorporating simple, yet effective novel imaging and/or biochemical markers in to cardiovascular risk stratification algorithms, with a goal to improve detection of subclinical atherosclerosis. Markers with substantial clinical evidence (Lp-PLA2 and Apo B) should be incorporated in to risk stratification algorithms, along with platelet volume indices. Clinical trials should be designed to assess the performance of such newer algorithms. Genetic and enzymatic markers including matrix metalloproteinases, interferon gamma are on the horizon, and may indeed provide incremental information that could improve cardiovascular care in the future. However, these markers lack sufficient clinical human data. Further evaluation of their efficacy and cost effectiveness is warranted.

6. Acknowledgements

My parents, wife Shwetha Kamath, son to be born Vihaan Hegde, and family for their support

My coauthor Ishmael David Christian Ching, MD for his hard work and assistance with the manuscript

My librarians Judy Knight MLS, Suzanne Cable, Melissa Trace for their help with referencing

Akron General Medical Center for its ongoing support

In Tech publications for this wonderful opportunity

7. References

Achenbach, S., Ropers, D., & Pohle, K., et al. (2002). Influence of lipid-lowering therapy on the progression of coronary artery calcification - A prospective evaluation. Circulation, Vol.106, No.9, (August 2002), pp. 1077-1082, ISSN 0009-7322

Agatston, A., Janowitz, W., & Hildner, F., et al. (1990). Quantification of coronary-artery calcium using ultrafast computed-tomography. Journal of the American College of Cardiology, Vol.15, No.4, (March 1990), pp. 827-832, ISSN 0735-1097

Anand, D., Lim, E., & Hopkins, D., et al. (2006). Risk stratification in uncomplicated type 2 diabetes: prospective evaluation of the combined use of coronary artery calcium imaging and selective myocardial perfusion scintigraphy. European Heart Journal, Vol.27, No.6, (March 2006), pp. 713-721, ISSN 0195-668X

Arad, Y., Goodman, K., & Roth, M., et al. (2005). Coronary calcification, coronary disease risk factors, C-reactive protein, and atherosclerotic cardiovascular disease events - The St. Francis Heart Study. Journal of the American College of Cardiology, Vol.46, No.1, (July 2005), pp. 158-165, ISSN 0735-1097

Arad, Y., Spadaro, L., & Goodman, K., et al. (2000). Prediction of coronary events with electron beam computed tomography. Journal of the American College of Cardiology, Vol.36, No. 4, (October 2000), pp. 1253-1260, ISSN 0735-1097

Ballantyne, C., Hoogeveen, R., & Bang, H., et al. (2004). Lipoprotein-associated phospholipase A2, high-sensitivity C-reactive protein, and risk for incident coronary heart disease in middle-aged men and women in the Atherosclerosis Risk in Communities (ARIC) study. Circulation, Vol.109, No.7, (February 2004), pp. 837-842, ISSN 0009-7322

Barrett, J., Keat, N. (2004). Artifacts in CT: Recognition and avoidance. Radiographics, Vol.24, No.6, (November-December 2004), pp. 1679-1691, ISSN 0271-5333

Barter, P., Ballantyne, C., & Carmena, R., et al. (2006). Apo B versus cholesterol in estimating cardiovascular risk and in guiding therapy: report of the thirty-person/ten-country panel. Journal of Internal Medicine, Vol.259, No.3, (March 2006), pp. 247-258, ISSN 0954-6820

Becker, A., Leber, A., & Becker, C., et al. (2008). Predictive value of coronary calcifications for future cardiac events in asymptomatic individuals. American Heart Journal, Vol.155, No.1, (January 2008), pp. 154-160, ISSN 0002-8703

Bennet, A., Di Angelantonio, E., & Erqou, S., et al. (2008). Lipoprotein(a) levels and risk of future coronary heart disease. Archives of Internal Medicine, Vol.168, No.6, (March 2008), pp. 598-608, ISSN 0003-9926

Blaha, M., Budoff, M., & Shaw, L., et al. (2009). Absence of coronary artery calcification and all-cause mortality. Jacc-Cardiovascular Imaging, Vol.2, No.6, (June 2009), pp. 692-700, ISSN 1936-878X

Blake, G., Dada, N., & Fox, J., et al. (2001). A prospective evaluation of lipoprotein-associated phospholipase A(2) levels and the risk of future cardiovascular events in women. Journal of the American College of Cardiology, Vol.38, No.5, (November 2001), pp. 1302-1306, ISSN 0735-1097

Borresen, A., Berg, K., & Dahlen, G., et al. (1981). The effect of gemfibrozil on human-serum apolipoproteins and on serum reserve cholesterol binding-capacity (SRCBC). Artery, Vol.9, No.1, pp. 77-86, ISSN 0098-6127

Brindis, R. (2005). ACCF/ASNC appropriateness criteria for single-photon emission computed tomography myocardial perfusion imaging (SPECT MPI) - A report of the American College of Cardiology Foundation Quality Strategic Directions Committee Appropriateness Criteria Working Group and the American Society of Nuclear Cardiology. Journal of the American College of Cardiology, Vol.46, No.8, (October 2005), pp. 1587-1605, ISSN 0735-1097

Budoff, M., Achenbach, S., & Blumenthal, R., et al. (2006). Assessment of coronary artery disease by cardiac computed tomography - A scientific statement from the American Heart Association committee on cardiovascular imaging and intervention, council on cardiovascular radiology and intervention, and Committee on Cardiac Imaging, Council on Clinical Cardiology. Circulation, Vol.114, No.16, (October 2006), pp. 1761-1791, ISSN 0009-7322

Budoff, M., Lane, K., & Bakhsheshi, H., et al. (2000). Rates of progression of coronary calcium by electron beam tomography. American Journal of Cardiology, Vol.86, No.1, (July 2000), pp. 8-11, ISSN 0002-9149

Budoff, M., McClelland, R., & Nasir, K., et al. (2009). Cardiovascular events with absent or minimal coronary calcification: The Multi-Ethnic Study of Atherosclerosis (MESA). American Heart Journal, Vol.158, No. 4, (October 2009), pp. 554-561, ISSN 0002-8703

Budoff, M., Shaw, L., & Liu, S., et al. (2007). Long-term prognosis associated with coronary calcification - Observations from a registry of 25,253 patients. Journal of the American College of Cardiology, Vol.49, No.18, (May 2007), pp. 1860-1870, ISSN 0735-1097

Callister, T., Cooil, B., & Raya, S., et al. (1998). Coronary artery disease: Improved reproducibility of calcium scoring with an electron-beam CT volumetric method. Radiology, Vol.208, No.3, (September 1998), pp. 807-814, ISSN 0033-8419

Callister, T., Raggi, P., & Cooil, B., et al. (1998). Effect of HMG-Coa reductase inhibitors on coronary artery disease as assessed by electron-beam computed tomography. New England Journal of Medicine, Vol.339, No.27, (December 1998), pp. 1972-1978, ISSN 0028-4793

Carlson, L., Hamsten, A., & Asplund, A. (1989). Pronounced lowering of serum levels of lipoprotein LP(A) in hyperlipemic subjects treated with nicotinic-acid. Journal of Internal Medicine, Vol.226, No. 4, pp. 271-276, ISSN 0954-6820.

Caslake, M., & Packard, C. (2005). Lipoprotein-associated phospholipase A(2) as a biomarker for coronary disease and stroke. Nature Clinical Practice Cardiovascular Medicine, Vol.2, No.10, (October 2005), pp. 529-535, ISSN 1743-4297

Cheng, C., Tempel, D., & van Haperen, R., et al. (2006). Atherosclerotic lesion size and vulnerability are determined by patterns of fluid shear stress. Circulation, Vol.113, No.23, (June 2006), pp. 2744-2753, ISSN 0009-7322

Conroy, R., Pyorala, K., & Fitzgerald, A., et al. (2003). Estimation of ten-year risk of fatal cardiovascular disease in Europe: the SCORE project. European Heart Journal, Vol.24, No.11, (June 2003), pp. 987-1003, ISSN 0195-668X

Cook, N., Buring, J., & Ridker, P. (2006). The effect of including C-reactive protein in cardiovascular risk prediction models for women. Annals of Internal Medicine, Vol.145, No.1, (July 2006), pp. 21-29, ISSN 0003-4819

Crisby, M., Nordin-Fredriksson, G., & Shah, P., et al. (2001). Pravastatin treatment increases collagen content and decreases lipid content, inflammation, metalloproteinases, and cell death in human carotid plaques - Implications for plaque stabilization. Circulation, Vol.103, No.7, (February 2001), pp. 926-933, ISSN 0009-7322

Cui, Y., Blumenthal, R., & Flaws, J., et al. (2001). Non-high-density lipoprotein cholesterol level as a predictor of cardiovascular disease mortality. Archives of Internal Medicine, Vol.161, No.11, (June 2001), pp. 1413-1419, ISSN 0003-9926

Daniell, A., Wong, N., & Friedman, J., et al. (2005). Concordance of coronary artery calcium estimates between MDCT and electron beam tomography. American Journal of Roentgenology, Vol.185. No.6, (December 2005), pp. 1542-1545, ISSN 0361-803X

De Backer, G., Ambrosioni, E., & Borch-Johnsen, K., et al. (2003). European guidelines on cardiovascular disease prevention in clinical practice - Third Joint Task Force of European and other Societies on Cardiovascular Disease Prevention in Clinical Practice. European Heart Journal, Vol.24, No.17, (September 2003), pp. 1601-1610, ISSN 0195-668X

Detrano, R., Guerci, A., & Carr, J., et al. (2008). Coronary calcium as a predictor of coronary events in four racial or ethnic groups. New England Journal of Medicine, Vol.358, No.13, (March 2008), pp. 1336-1345, ISSN 0028-4793

Douglas, P., & Ginsburg, G. (1996). The evaluation of chest pain in women. New England Journal of Medicine, Vol.334, No.20, (May 1996), pp. 1311-1315, ISSN 0028-4793

Eisenhardt, S., Habersberger, J., & Murphy, A., et al. (2009). Dissociation of pentameric to monomeric C-reactive protein on activated platelets localizes inflammation to atherosclerotic plaques. Circulation Research, Vol.105, No.2, (July 2009), pp. 128-37, ISSN 0009-7330

Eisenhardt, S., Thiele, J., & Bannasch, H., et al. (2009). C-reactive protein: How conformational changes influence inflammatory properties. Cell Cycle, Vol.8, No.23, (December 2009), pp. 3885-3892, ISSN 1538-4101

Electron Beam Tomography (EBT). (n.d.) Accessed August 18, 2011, Available from http://www.uic.edu/orgs/heart/EBT.htm

Erne, P., Wardle, J., Sanders, K., et al. Mean Platelet Volume and size distribution and their sensitivity to agonists in patients with coronary artery disease and congestive heart failure. Thromb Haemost, Vol 59, No2, (April 1988), pp. 259-263, ISSN 0340-6245

Erqou, S., Kaptoge, S., & Perry, P., et al. (2009). Lipoprotein(a) Concentration and the risk of coronary heart disease, stroke, and nonvascular mortality. Jama-Journal of the American Medical Association, Vol.302, No.4, (July 2009), pp. 412-423, ISSN 0098-7484

Folsom, A., Chambless, L., & Ballantyne, C., et al. (2006). An assessment of incremental coronary risk prediction using C-reactive protein and other novel risk markers - The atherosclerosis risk in communities study. Archives of Internal Medicine, Vol.166, No.13, (July 2006), pp. 1368-1373, ISSN 0003-9926

Gasparyan, AY., Ayvazyan, L., Dimitri, P. et al. Mean Platelet Volume: A Link Between Thrombosis and Inflammation? Current Pharmaceutical Design, Vol 17, No 1, (2011), pp. 47-58. ISSN 1381-6128

Genest Jr, J., Martin-Munley, S, & McNamara JR, et al. (1992). Familial lipoprotein disorders in patients with premature coronary artery disease. Circulation, Vol. 85, No. 6, (June 1992); pp. 2025-2033, ISSN: 1524-4539

Georgiou, D., Budoff, M., & Kaufer, E., et al. (2001). Screening patients with chest pain in the emergency department using electron beam tomography: A follow-up study. Journal of the American College of Cardiology, Vol.38, No.1, (July 2001), pp. 105-110, ISSN 0735-1097

Ghose, T. (2004). Oswald Avery: the professor, DNA, and the Nobel Prize that eluded him. Canadian Bulletin of Medical History, Vol.21, No.1, pp. 135-144, ISSN 0823-2105

Glud, T., Schmidt, EB., Kristensen, SD., et al. Platelet number and volume during myocardial infarction in relation to infarct size. Acta Med Scand; Vol 220, No 5, (1986), pp. 401-405 ISSN 0001-6101

Gopal, A., & Budoff, M. (2009). A new method to reduce radiation exposure during multi-row detector cardiac computed tomographic angiography. International Journal of Cardiology, Vol.132, No.3, (March 2009), pp. 435-436, ISSN 0167-5273

Greenland, P., Bonow, R., & Brundage, B., et al. (2007). ACCF/AHA 2007 Clinical Expert Consensus document on coronary artery calcium scoring by computed tomography in global cardiovascular risk assessment and in evaluation of patients with chest pain. Journal of the American College of Cardiology, Vol.49, No.3, (January 2007), pp. 378-402, ISSN 0735-1097

Greenland, P., LaBree, L., & Azen, S., et al. (2004). Coronary artery calcium score combined with Framingham score for risk prediction in asymptomatic individuals. Jama-Journal of the American Medical Association, Vol.291, No.2, (January 2004), pp. 210-215, ISSN 0098-7484

Guerci, A., Spadaro, L., & Goodman, K., et al. (1998). Comparison of electron beam computed tomography scanning and conventional risk factor assessment for the prediction of angiographic coronary artery disease. Journal of the American College of Cardiology, Vol.32, No.3, (September 1998), pp. 673-679, ISSN 0735-1097

Haydar, A., Hujairi, N., & Covic, A., et al. (2004). Coronary artery calcification is related to coronary atherosclerosis in chronic renal disease patients: a study comparing EBCT-generated coronary artery calcium scores and coronary angiography. Nephrology Dialysis Transplantation, Vol.19, No.9, (September 2004), pp. 2307-2312, ISSN 0931-0509

He, Z., Hedrick, T., & Pratt, C., et al. (2000). Severity of coronary artery calcification by electron beam computed tomography predicts silent myocardial ischemia. Circulation, Vol.101, No.3, (January 2000), pp. 244-251, ISSN 0009-7322

Hirai, N., Horiguchi, J., & Fujioka, C., et al. (2008). Prospective versus retrospective ECG-gated 64-detector coronary CT angiography: assessment of image quality, stenosis, and radiation dose. Radiology, Vol.248, No.2, (August 2008), pp. 424-430, ISSN 0033-8419

Hoff, J., Chomka, E., & Krainik, A., et al. (2001). Age and gender distributions of coronary artery calcium detected by electron beam tomography in 35,246 adults. American Journal of Cardiology, Vol.87, No.12, (June 2001), pp. 1335-1339, ISSN 0002-9149

Hopkins, P., & Williams, R. (1981). A survey of 246 suggested coronary risk factors. Atherosclerosis, Vol.40, No.1, (August-September 1981), pp. 1-52, ISSN 0021-9150

Houslay, E., Cowell, S., & Prescott, R., et al. (2006). Progressive coronary calcification despite intensive lipid-lowering treatment: a randomised controlled trial. Heart, Vol.92, No.9, (September 2006), pp. 1207-1212, ISSN 1355-6037

Kajinami, K., Seki, H., Takekoshi, N., & Mabuchi, H. (1995). Noninvasive prediction of coronary atherosclerosis by quantification of coronary-artery calcification using electron-beam computed-tomography – comparison with electrocardiographic and thallium exercise stress test-results. Journal of the American College of Cardiology, Vol.26, No.5, (November 1995), pp. 1209-1221, ISSN 0735-1097

Kalia, N., Miller, L., & Nasir, K., et al. (2006). Visualizing coronary calcium is associated with improvements in adherence to statin therapy. Atherosclerosis, Vol.185, No.2, (April 2006), pp. 394-399, ISSN 0021-9150

Keller, C. (2007). Apheresis in coronary heart disease with elevated Lp (a): a review of Lp (a) as a risk factor and its management. Therapeutic Apheresis and Dialysis, Vol.11, No.1, (February 2007), pp. 2-8, ISSN 1744-9979

Khaleeli, E., Peters, S., & Bobrowsky, K., et al. (2001). Diabetes and the associated incidence of subclinical atherosclerosis and coronary artery disease: Implications for management. American Heart Journal, Vol.141, No.4, (April 2001), pp. 637-644, ISSN 0002-8703

Kondos, G., Hoff, J., & Sevrukov, A., et al. (2003). Electron-beam tomography coronary artery calcium and cardiac events - A 37-month follow-up of 5635 initially asymptomatic low- to intermediate-risk adults. Circulation, Vol.107, No.20, (May 2003), pp. 2571-2576, ISSN 0009-7322

Kullo, I., & Ballantyne, C. (2005). Conditional risk factors for atherosclerosis. Mayo Clinic Proceedings, Vol.80, No.2, (February 2005), pp. 219-230, ISSN 0025-6196

LaMonte, M., FitzGerald, S., & Church, T., et al. (2005). Coronary artery calcium score and coronary heart disease events in a large cohort of asymptomatic men and women. American Journal of Epidemiology, Vol.162, No.5, (September 2005), pp.421-429, ISSN 0002-9262

Libby, P. (2009). Molecular and cellular mechanisms of the thrombotic complications of atherosclerosis. Journal of Lipid Research, Vol.50, Suppl., (April 2009), pp. S352-S357, ISSN 0022-2275

Lloyd-Jones, D., Leip, E., & Larson, M., et al. (2006). Prediction of lifetime risk for cardiovascular disease by risk factor burden at 50 years of age. Circulation, Vol.113, No.6, (February 2006), pp. 791-798, ISSN 0009-7322

Mackenzie, I., & Woodhouse, J. (2006). C-reactive protein concentrations during bacteraemia: a comparison between patients with and without liver dysfunction. Intensive Care Medicine, Vol.32, No.9, (September 2006), pp. 1344-1351, ISSN 0342-4642

Mao, S., Pal, R., & Mckay, C., et al. (2009). Comparison of coronary artery calcium scores between electron beam computed tomography and 64-multidetector computed tomographic scanner. Journal of Computer Assisted Tomography, Vol.33, No.2, (March-April 2009), pp. 175-178, ISSN 0363-8715

Marrow, D. (2011) Screening for cardiovascular risk with C-reactive protein, In: UpToDate, Kaski, J & Downey B (Eds.), Waltham, MA.

McDermott, M. (2007). The international pandemic of chronic cardiovascular disease. Jama-Journal of the American Medical Association, Vol.297, No.11, (March 2007), pp. 1253-1255, ISSN 0098-7484

McLaughlin, V., Balogh, T., & Rich, S. (1999). Utility of electron beam computed tomography to stratify patients presenting to the emergency room with chest pain. American Journal of Cardiology, Vol.84, No.3, pp. 327-8, A8, ISSN 1879-1913

McLean, J., Tomlinson, J., & Kuang, W., et al. (1987). CDNA sequence of human apolipoprotein(A) is homologous to plasminogen. Nature, Vol.330, No.6144, (November 1987), pp. 132-137, ISSN 0028-0836

Michos, E., Nasir, K., & Braunstein, J., et al. (2006). Framingham risk equation underestimates subclinical atherosclerosis risk in asymptomatic women. Atherosclerosis, Vol.184, No.1, (January 2006), pp. 201-206, ISSN 0021-9150

Moe, S., O'Neill, K., & Duan, D., et al. (2002). Medial artery calcification in ESRD patients is associated with deposition of bone matrix proteins. Kidney International, Vol.61, No.2, (February 2002), pp. 638-647, ISSN 0085-2538

Nambi, V., Brautbar, A., Ballantyne C. (2011). Novel Biomarkers and the Assessment of Cardiovascular Risk, In: *Preventive Cardiology: A Companion to Braunwald's Heart Disease,* Blumenthal, R.S., Foody, J.M., Wong, N.D., pp. 56-63, Published by Saunders, ISBN 978-1-4377-1366-4, Philidelphia, PA

Nasir, K., Budoff, M., & Wong, N., et al. (2007). Family history of premature coronary heart disease and coronary artery calcification - Multi-ethnic study of atherosclerosis (MESA). Circulation, Vol.116, No.6, (August 2007), pp. 619-626, ISSN 0009-7322

Nasir, K., Michos, E., & Rumberger, J., et al. (2004). Coronary artery calcification and family history of premature coronary heart disease - Sibling history is more strongly associated than parental history. Circulation, Vol.110, No.15, (October 2004), pp. 2150-2156, ISSN 0009-7322

Nasir, K., Shaw, L., & Liu, S., et al. (2007). Ethnic differences in the prognostic value of coronary artery calcification for all-cause mortality. Journal of the American College of Cardiology, Vol.50, No.10, (September 2007), pp. 953-960, ISSN 0735-1097

O'Malley, P., Feuerstein, I., & Taylor, A. (2003). Impact of electron beam tomography, with or without case management, on motivation, behavioral change, and cardiovascular risk profile - A randomized controlled trial. Jama-Journal of the American Medical Association, Vol.289, No.17, (May 2003), pp. 2215-2223, ISSN 0098-7484

O'Malley, P., Greenberg, B., & Taylor, A. (2004). Cost-effectiveness of using electron beam computed tomography to identify patients at risk for clinical coronary artery disease. American Heart Journal, Vol.148, No.1, (July 2004), pp. 106-113, ISSN 0002-8703

O'Rourke, R., Brundage, B., & Froelicher, V., et al. (2000). American College of Cardiology/American Heart Association expert consensus document on electron-beam computed tomography for the diagnosis and prognosis of coronary artery disease. Journal of the American College of Cardiology, Vol.36, No.1, (July 2000), pp. 326-340, ISSN 0735-1097

Ockene, I., Matthews, C., & Rifai, N., et al. (2001). Variability and classification accuracy of serial high-sensitivity C-reactive protein measurements in healthy adults. Clinical Chemistry, Vol.47, No.3, (March 2001), pp. 444-450, ISSN 0009-9147

Park, R., Detrano, R., & Xiang, M., et al. (2002). Combined use of computed tomography coronary calcium scores and C-reactive protein levels in predicting cardiovascular events in nondiabetic individuals. Circulation, Vol.106, No.16, (October 2002), pp. 2073-2077, ISSN 0009-7322

Pepys, M., & Baltz, M. (1983). Acute phase proteins with special reference to C-reactive protein and related proteins (pentaxins) and serum amyloid A-protein. Advances in Immunology, Vol.34, pp. 141-212, ISSN 0065-2776

Pletcher, M., Tice, J., & Pignone, M., et al. (2004). Using the coronary artery calcium score to predict coronary heart disease events - A systematic review and meta-analysis. Archives of Internal Medicine, Vol.164, No.12, (June 2004), pp. 1285-1292, ISSN 0003-9926

Polonsky, T., McClelland, R., & Jorgensen, N., et al. (2010). Coronary artery calcium score and risk classification for coronary heart disease prediction. Jama-Journal of the American Medical Association, Vol.303, No.16, (April 2010), pp. 1610-1616, ISSN 0098-7484

Raggi, P., Callister, T., & Shaw, L. (2004). Progression of coronary artery calcium and risk of first myocardial infarction in patients receiving cholesterol-lowering therapy. Arteriosclerosis, Thrombosis, and Vascular Biology, Vol.24, No.7, (July 2004), pp. 1272-1277, ISSN 1079-5642

Raggi, P., Cooil, B., & Callister, T. (2001). Use of electron beam tomography data to develop models for prediction of hard coronary events. American Heart Journal, Vol.141, No.3, (March 2001), pp. 375-382, ISSN 0002-8703

Raggi, P., Davidson, M., & Callister, T., et al. (2005). Aggressive versus moderate lipid-lowering therapy in hypercholesterolemic postmenopausal women - beyond endorsed lipid lowering with EBT scanning (BELLES). Circulation, Vol.112, No.4, (July 2005), pp. 563-571, ISSN 0009-7322

Raggi, P., Shaw, L., & Berman, D., et al. (2004). Prognostic value of coronary artery calcium screening in subjects with and without diabetes. Journal of the American College of Cardiology, Vol.43, No.9, (May 2004), pp. 1663-1669, ISSN 0735-1097

Redberg, R. F., Vogel, R. A., & Criqui, M. H., et al. (2003). 34th Bethesda Conference: Task force #3--What is the spectrum of current and emerging techniques for the noninvasive measurement of atherosclerosis? Journal of the American College of Cardiology, Vol.41, No.11, (June 2003), pp. 1886-1898, ISSN 0735-1097

Ridker, P., Buring, J., & Rifai, N., et al. (2007). Development and validation of improved algorithms for the assessment of global cardiovascular risk in women - The Reynolds Risk Score. Jama-Journal of the American Medical Association, Vol.297, No.6, (February 2007), pp. 611-619, ISSN 0098-7484

Ridker, P., Danielson, E., & Fonseca, F., et al. (2008). Rosuvastatin to prevent vascular events in men and women with elevated C-reactive protein. New England Journal of Medicine, Vol.359, No.21, (November 2008), pp. 2195-2207, ISSN 0028-4793

Ridker, P., Paynter, N., & Rifai, N., et al. (2008). C-reactive protein and parental history improve global cardiovascular risk prediction: The Reynolds Risk Score for Men. Circulation, Vol.118, No.22, (November 2008), pp. 2243-2244, ISSN 0009-7322

Rosamond, W., Flegal, K., & Furie, K., et al. (2008). Heart disease and stroke statistics - 2008 update - A report from the American Heart Association Statistics Committee and

Stroke Statistics Subcommittee. Circulation, Vol.117, No.4, (January 2008), pp. E25-E146, ISSN 0009-7322

Rumberger, J., Sheedy, P., & Breen, J., et al. (1995). Coronary calcium, as determined by electron-beam computed-tomography, and coronary-disease on arteriogram - effect of patients sex on diagnosis. Circulation, Vol.91, No.5, (March 1995), pp. 1363-1367, ISSN 0009-7322

Rumberger, J., Simons, D., & Fitzpatrick, L., et al. (1995). Coronary-artery calcium area by electron-beam computed-tomography and coronary atherosclerotic plaque area - a histopathologic correlative study. Circulation, Vol.92, No.8, (October 1995), pp. 2157-2162, ISSN 0009-7322

Sacks, F., McPherson, R., & Walsh, B. (1994). Effect of postmenopausal estrogen replacement on plasma LP(A) lipoprotein concentrations. Archives of Internal Medicine, Vol.154, No.10, (May 1994), pp. 1106-1110, ISSN 0003-9926

Sangiorgi, G., Rumberger, J., & Severson, A., et al. (1998). Arterial calcification and not lumen stenosis is highly correlated with atherosclerotic plaque burden in humans: A histologic study of 723 coronary artery segments using nondecalcifying methodology. Journal of the American College of Cardiology, Vol.31, No.1, (January 1998), pp. 126-133, ISSN 0735-1097

Sarwar, A., Shaw, L., & Shapiro, M., et al. (2009). Diagnostic and prognostic value of absence of coronary artery calcification. Jacc-Cardiovascular Imaging, Vol.2, No.6, (June 2009), pp. 675-688, ISSN 1876-7591

Schmermund, A., Achenbach, S., & Budde, T., et al. (2006). Effect of intensive versus standard lipid-lowering treatment with atorvastatin on the progression of calcified coronary atherosclerosis over 12 months - A multicenter, randomized, double-blind trial. Circulation, Vol.113, No.3, (January 2006), pp. 427-437, ISSN 0009-7322

Schmermund, A., Denktas, A., & Rumberger, J., et al. (1999). Independent and incremental value of coronary artery calcium for predicting the extent of angiographic coronary artery disease - Comparison with cardiac risk factors and radionuclide perfusion imaging. Journal of the American College of Cardiology, Vol.34, No.3, (September 1999), pp. 777-786, ISSN 0735-1097

Sharples, E., Pereira, D., & Summers, S., et al. (2004). Coronary artery calcification measured with electron-beam computerized tomography correlates poorly with coronary artery angiography in dialysis patients. American Journal of Kidney Diseases, Vol.43, No.2, (February 2004), pp. 313-319, ISSN 1523-6838

Shavelle, D., Budoff, M., & LaMont, D., et al. (2000). Exercise testing and electron beam computed tomography in the evaluation of coronary artery disease. Journal of the American College of Cardiology, Vol.36, No.1, (July 2000), pp. 32-38, ISSN 0735-1097

Shaw, L., Raggi, P., & Berman, D., et al. (2003). Cost effectiveness of screening for cardiovascular disease with measures of coronary calcium. Progress in Cardiovascular Diseases, Vol.46, No.2, (September-October 2003), pp. 171-184, ISSN 0033-0620

Shaw, L., Raggi, P., & Schisterman, E., et al. (2003). Prognostic value of cardiac risk factors and coronary artery calcium screening for all-cause mortality. Radiology, Vol.228, No.3, (September 2003), pp. 826-833, ISSN 0033-8419

Stein, J., & Rosenson, R. (1997). Lipoprotein Lp(a) excess and coronary heart disease. Archives of Internal Medicine, Vol.157, No.11, (June 1997), pp. 1170-1176, ISSN 0003-9926

Steyrer, E., Durovic, S., & Frank, S., et al. (1994). The role of lecithin - cholesterol acyltransferase for lipoprotein (A) assembly - structural integrity of low-density lipoproteins is a prerequisite for LP(A) formation in human plasma. Journal of Clinical Investigation, Vol.94, No.6, (December 1994), pp. 2330-2340, ISSN 0021-9738

Tabas, I. (2002). Consequences of cellular cholesterol accumulation: basic concepts and physiological implications. Journal of Clinical Investigation, Vol.110, No.7, (October 2002), pp. 905-911, ISSN 0021-9738

Taylor, A., Bindeman, J., & Feuerstein, I., et al. (2005). Coronary calcium independently predicts incident premature coronary heart disease over measured cardiovascular risk factors - Mean three-year outcomes in the Prospective Army Coronary Calcium (PACC) project. Journal of the American College of Cardiology, Vol.46, No.5, (September 2005), pp. 807-814, ISSN 0735-1097

Van der LooB, Martin JF. A role for changes in platelet production in the cause of acute coronary syndromes. Arteriosc Thromb Vasc Biol, Vol 19, (March 1999), pp. 672-679 ISSN 1524-4636

Vasina, E., Heemskerk, J., Weber, C., et al. (2010). Platelets and Platelet Derived Microparticles in vascular Inflammatory Disease. Inflammation & Allergy- Drug targets, Vol. 9, No.5, (December 2010), pp. 346-354, ISSN 1871-5281

Vliegenthart, R., Oudkerk, M., & Hofman, A., et al. (2005). Coronary calcification improves cardiovascular risk prediction in the elderly. Circulation, Vol.112, No.4, (July 2005), pp. 572-577, ISSN 0009-7322

Watala C. Blood Platelet Reactivity and its pharmacological modulation in (people with) diabetes mellitus. Curr Pharm Des, Vol.11, No. 18, (2005), pp. 2331-2365, ISSN: 1381-6128

Williams, K., Feig, J., & Fisher, E. (2008). Rapid regression of atherosclerosis: insights from the clinical and experimental literature. Nature Clinical Practice Cardiovascular Medicine, Vol.5, No.2, (February 2008), pp. 91-102, ISSN 1743-4300

Wilson, P. W., Smith, S. C., & Blumenthal, R. S., et al. (2003). 34th Bethesda Conference: Task force #4--How do we select patients for atherosclerosis imaging? Journal of the American College of Cardiology, Vol.41, No.11, (June 2003), pp. 1898-1906, ISSN 0735-1097

Wong, N., Detrano, R., & Diamond, G., et al. (1996). Does coronary artery screening by electron beam computed tomography motivate potentially beneficial lifestyle behaviors? American Journal of Cardiology, Vol.78, No.11, (December 1996), pp. 1220-1223, ISSN 0002-9149

Wong, N., Hsu, J., & Detrano, R., et al. (2000). Coronary artery calcium evaluation by electron beam computed tomography and its relation to new cardiovascular events.

American Journal of Cardiology, Vol.86, No.5, (September 2000), pp. 495-498, ISSN 0002-9149

Yang, E., Nambi, V., & Tang, Z., et al. (2009). Clinical Implications of JUPITER (Justification for the Use of statins in Prevention: an Intervention Trial Evaluating Rosuvastatin) in a US Population Insights From the ARIC (Atherosclerosis Risk in Communities) Study. Journal of the American College of Cardiology, Vol.54, No.25, (December 2009), pp. 2388-2395, ISSN 0735-1097

Yao, Z., Liu, X., & Shi, R., et al. (1997). A comparison of Tc-99m-MIBI myocardial SPET with electron beam computed tomography in the assessment of coronary artery disease. European Journal of Nuclear Medicine, Vol.24, No.9, (September 1997), pp. 1115-1120, ISSN 0340-6997

Yasojima, K., Schwab, C., & McGeer, E., et al. (2001). Generation of C-reactive protein and complement components in atherosclerotic plaques. American Journal of Pathology, Vol.158, No.3, (March 2001), pp. 1039-1051, ISSN 0002-9440

Yusuf, S., Reddy, S., & Ounpuu, S., et al. (2001). Global burden of cardiovascular diseases - Part I: General considerations, the epidemiologic transition, risk factors, and impact of urbanization. Circulation, Vol.104, No.22, (November 2001), pp. 2746-2753, ISSN 0009-7322

6

Alterations in the Brainstem Preautonomic Circuitry May Contribute to Hypertension Associated with Metabolic Syndrome

Bradley J. Buck[1], Lauren K. Nolen[2], Lauren G. Koch[3], Steven L. Britton[4] and Ilan A. Kerman[5]
[1]*College of Medicine, The University of Toledo, OH,*
[2] *Genetics and Genomic Sciences Theme, Graduate Biomedical Sciences Program, University of Alabama at Birmingham, AL,*
[3]*Department of Anesthesiology, University of Michigan,*
[4]*Department of Physical Medicine and Rehabilitation, University of Michigan,*
[5]*Department of Psychiatry and Behavioral Neurobiology, University of Alabama at Birmingham, AL, USA*

1. Introduction

Metabolic syndrome (MetS) is defined as a co-occurrence of insulin resistance, obesity (specifically visceral adipose tissue accumulation), hypertriglyceridemia, and hypertension (HTN) (Grundy et al., 2004; Fig. 1). MetS has been implicated in the development of atherosclerosis, heart disease, type-2 diabetes, and has significantly contributed to morbidity and mortality around the world (Rizzo et al., 2006; Lorenzo et al., 2006). The number of people living with MetS in the United States has steadily increased in recent years. It was estimated that in the year 2000 over 47 million Americans had MetS (Ford et al., 2002), while in 2005 that number increased to 50 million (Alberti et al., 2005). Due to the serious consequences of the above conditions, timely research is needed to discover and understand the underlying pathophysiology of this illness.

1.1 Genetic basis of metabolic syndrome

Recent evidence indicates a complex genetic background for MetS. Rather than being defined by specific mutations in a small number of genes, it is best described as a cluster of genetic traits that differs from patient to patient. Many studies have reported associations between various single nucleotide polymorphisms (SNPs) and individual defining traits of MetS; however, none of these studies has been able to extend that association to the disease as a whole. For instance, a genome wide association study (GWAS) of Indian Asian men by Zabaneh and Balding (2010) found numerous SNPs that were significantly associated with metabolic traits such as high HDL-cholesterol, type-2 diabetes, and increased diastolic blood pressure, but none were also associated with the overall MetS phenotype. In a similar study, Wong et al. (2007) described a polymorphism in the gene for human melanocortin receptor

3, which was significantly associated with insulin resistance in the Maori kindred but did not predict the syndrome as a whole.

Diagnostic criteria for Metabolic Syndrome

Central obesity

- BMI >30 kg/m^2

Plus any two of the following:

Raised triglycerides

- >150 mg/dL
- Treatment for this lipid abnormality

Reduced HDL-cholesterol

- <40 mg/dL in men
- <50 mg/dL in women
- Treatment for this lipid abnormality

Raised blood pressure

- Systolic ≥130 mm Hg
- Diastolic ≥85 mm Hg
- Medicinal treatment for hypertension

Raised fasting plasma glucose

- Fasting plasma glucose ≥100 mg/dL
- Type 2 diabetes

*Adapted from Alberti et al., 2005.

Fig. 1. Diagnostic criteria for metabolic syndrome as proposed by the International Diabetes Federation. Abbreviations: BMI, body mass index – weight (kg) divided by the square of the height (m).

One possible reason for past struggles, as reported by Mei et al. (2010), is the phenomenon of gene pleiotropy, or the instance of one gene affecting multiple phenotypes. In the case of single-trait association studies, gene pleiotropy may cause a loss of statistical power and thus the ability to find significant effects. Using a computational model that accounts for such effects, Mei et al. (2010) were able to identify eleven gene variants that were significantly associated with MetS. Several of these genes had even been previously associated with individual metabolic traits, but had failed to be significantly correlated with the syndrome itself. Even without advanced computational methods, some investigators have reported certain genotypes that predict the development of MetS.

For example, Leu et al. (2011) reported an adiponectin gene variant that was significantly correlated with MetS as well as the development of hypertension, and Devaney et al. (2011), found that the H1 haplotype of the *akt1* gene was strongly associated with metabolic syndrome in a population of African-American and European-American subjects. Taken together, recent data indicate a strong, yet evolving, genetic component to MetS. This evidence yields support for using selectively-bred animal strains as appropriate models for the disease.

1.2 Animal models of metabolic syndrome

In the past several decades, multiple animal models of MetS have been proposed, most of them in rats (see review by Artinano and Castro, 2009). Currently, obese Zucker rats are the most commonly used model. These rats exhibit many of the features of MetS, including obesity, dyslipidaemia, insulin resistance, and hypertension (Zucker and Zucker, 1961). While these phenotypes represent the key components of MetS in humans, one major drawback of the obese Zucker model is its reliance on disruption of the leptin receptor gene, which does not reflect the genetic background of the disease in humans (Chua et al., 1996). Several strains of spontaneously hypertensive rats (SHRs) have also been used to model MetS, but suffer the drawback of the same genetic basis as the obese Zucker rats (Ishizuka et al., 1998).

A more realistic model was developed in 2007 by Kovacs et al. The Wistar Ottawa Karlsburg W (WOKW) rats, like other models, exhibit the key features of MetS but have a polygenic background that makes the model more applicable to human disease (Kovacs et al., 2000). Recently, the WOKW rats have been used to identify quantitative trait loci for several of the major traits of MetS, as well as to establish an association between MetS and impaired coronary function (Grisk et al., 2007).

Recently a new animal model of MetS was developed. Selective breeding of a population of rats based on their intrinsic running capacity produced rats exhibiting physiological characteristics similar to those seen in metabolic syndrome. Low capacity runners (LCRs), those rats unable to run extensive distances, exhibited, compared to their high capacity runner counterparts (HCRs), elevated fasting glucose levels, triglyceride levels, free fatty acid levels, visceral adipose tissue accumulation, and blood pressure (Wisloff et al., 2005). Additionally, elevated levels of insulin were also discovered in LCRs, while the difference in c-peptide levels, the peptide sequence released when proinsulin is cleaved to insulin and c-peptide, between HCRs and LCRs was not significant. These data implicate insulin resistance in the LCRs, as exhibited by the decrease in insulin clearance (the ratio between measured insulin and c-peptide). Taken together, these data by Wisloff et al. (2005) suggest that the LCR rat may be used as a model of MetS.

The goal of the current study is to investigate possible brainstem neural mechanisms of hypertension associated with MetS in the LCR model. Previous work has documented a 13.2% increase in the 24-hour mean arterial pressure (MAP) in the LCR rats as compared to their HCR counterparts (Wisloff et al. 2005).

1.3 Brainstem cardiovascular circuitry

Brainstem regulation of vascular tone is a delicate balance between excitatory and inhibitory influences. To understand and appreciate this pathway we provide the reader with: (1) the major transmitters within the circuit; (2) the discrete brainstem nuclei involved in the circuit; and (3) the interplay between the nuclei resulting in altered vascular tone. We begin here with a discussion of the main neurotransmitters, followed by a review of the involved nuclei and their circuitry.

1.3.1 Neurotransmitters

Brainstem cardiovascular circuitry overwhelmingly involves but two transmitters: γ-aminobutyric acid (GABA) and glutamate (Talman et al, 1980; Andersen et al., 2001; Suzuki et al., 1996; Gordon & Sved, 2002; Minson et al., 1997).

GABA is synthesized intra-cellularly from glutamate in a decarboxylation reaction guided by the enzyme glutamic acid decarboxylase, or GAD. Interestingly, GAD has two isoforms, or variants, coded for on separate chromosomes. These are referred to GAD65 and GAD67, with the numbers representing their atomic mass in kilodaltons. While the significance of having two isoforms is yet to be determined, some believe GAD65 is responsible for local control of GABA synthesis while GAD67 is responsible for long-term maintenance of baseline GABA levels within neural tissue (Esclapez et al., 1994; Esclapez & Houser, 1999). Additionally, it is generally believed the two isoforms are localized within different cellular compartments. GAD67 is associated predominantly with cytoplasmic pools of GABA, while GAD65 is associated with vesicular pools of GABA (Soghomonian & Martin, 1998). Thus, it is likely that GAD67 regulates GABA synthesis for metabolic functions of the cell, while GAD65 regulates GABA synthesis for synaptic release (Soghomonian & Martin, 1998).

Glutamate, conversely, is predominantly derived from extra-cellular stores and concentrated in neural tissue via cytoplasmic transporters (Danbolt, 2001; Kang et al., 2001). For this reason, quantification is much more difficult and includes, at the very least, expression analysis of glutamate transporters, and more accurately, direct sampling of synaptic cleft concentrations.

1.3.2 Neural control of cardiovascular function

Within the last 20 years a number of investigators have used expression of the immediate early gene, c-fos, as a marker of baro-sensitive neurons following alterations in blood pressure. In such studies hyper- or hypo- tension was experimentally induced by administration of specific vasoactive drugs (e.g. phenylephrine to increase blood pressure). These studies have pointed to three main brain regions being involved in cardiovascular regulation: the nucleus tractus solitarius (NTS), the caudal ventrolateral medulla (CVLM), and the rostral ventrolateral medulla (RVLM) (Chan and Sawchenko, 1994; Graham et al., 1995; Miura, 1994). Phenotyping of these barosensitive neurons demonstrates an intricate relay of information between these nuclei resulting in end organ modulation.

The brainstem cardiovascular network begins in the stretch sensitive baroreceptors of the carotid sinus and aortic arch. It is here that afferent signals are produced. Traveling via the glossopharyngeal and vagus nerves, the signal is relayed to caudal NTS neurons of the medulla (Spyer, 1994). These afferent projections are likely glutamatergic (Talman et al,

1980; Andersen et al., 2001). And while the NTS contains heterogeneous neuronal populations, including those that are glycinergic, glutamatergic, and nitric oxide positive (Chan and Sawchenko, 1998), barosensitive NTS neurons have been shown to be primarily glutamatergic (Sapru, 2002; Suzuki et al., 1996).

Interestingly, the NTS also contains a population of non-barosensitive GABAergic neurons which project onto the barosensitive, excitatory NTS cells. The inputs to such inhibitory NTS interneurons to date are not well characterized, yet some believe they may receive inputs from rostral nuclei including the mesencephalic locomotor region and the hypothalamus (Degtyarenko and Kaufman, 2005). Chen et al. (2009) have also indicated that this population of GABAergic neurons receives inputs from muscle afferents and that following exercise they contribute to the phenomenon of post-exercise hypotension. In addition, Tsukamoto and Sved (1993) have reported that microinjection of a $GABA_B$ receptor antagonist into the NTS leads to a significant drop in blood pressure. This suggests that although the main phenotype of the barosensitive neuron within the NTS is glutamatergic, GABA secretion from NTS interneurons appears to play an important role in the regulation of blood pressure through inhibition of glutamatergic NTS efferents.

From the NTS the signal is relayed to the CVLM (Gordon & Sved, 2002; Kawai & Emiko, 2000). Because of its robust collection of GABAergic cell bodies, the CVLM has been termed the 'depressor region.' For instance, Agrawal et al. (1989) demonstrated that excitation of the CVLM with L-glutamate microinjections leads to marked decreases in mean arterial pressure, MAP. Conversely, inhibition of the CVLM cells via administration of the $GABA_A$ receptor agonist muscimol leads to significant increases in MAP (Willette et al., 1984), and as expected, destruction of the CVLM leads to drastic increases in MAP (Imaizumi, 1985).

The inhibitory, GABAergic efferents of the CVLM project to the RVLM (Chan & Sawchenko, 1998; Minson et al., 1997), and their functional importance has been documented by microinjections of the $GABA_A$ agonist muscimol into the RVLM, which cause large decreases in MAP (Schreihofer et al., 2000). The RVLM contains glutamatergic cells that project down the spinal cord, modulating end organ function. For example, electrical and pharmacological activation of the RVLM cell bodies results in large increases in MAP, while its bilateral destruction leads to a drop in MAP equivalent to that observed in spinalized animals (Ross et al., 1984). These studies, along with evidence of glutamatergic RVLM projections to the intermediolateral cell column (Matsumoto et al., 1994), bolster the current notion of the RVLM as a source of excitatory drive to sympathetic vasomotor efferents.

While activity of RVLM neurons is under tonic suppression from the CVLM, the source of its excitatory inputs remains to be elucidated. To answer this question, Guyenet and colleagues (1987) blocked excitatory amino acid (EAA) receptors within the RVLM with EAA receptor antagonists. This resulted in no overall change in MAP. More recently, Kiely and Gordon (1994) and Horiuchi et al. (2004) report the same phenomenon. At the current time no excitatory inputs to the RVLM have been reported except for sparse projections from the NTS (Ross et al., 1985). Such claims have been dismissed by electrophysiological (Agarwal & Calaresu, 1991) and pharmacological (Blessing, 1988) evidence of an NTS-CVLM-RVLM pathway (Chan & Sawchenko, 1998). As a result of this, some have attributed the RVLM's firing to intrinsic, pulse-mediated auto-activity (Horiuchi et al., 2004).

In summary, excitatory afferent signals originating at baroreceptors within the carotid sinus and aortic arch synapse onto NTS neurons. The NTS also receives input from more rostral nuclei. These rostral projections appear to synapse on GABAergic, inhibitory NTS interneurons. Once integration within the NTS has taken place, its excitatory, glutamatergic cell population projects to the CVLM. The CVLM relays the signal via its inhibitory GABAergic projections to the RVLM. From the RVLM the signal is sent down the spinal cord toward the target vasculature (Fig. 2).

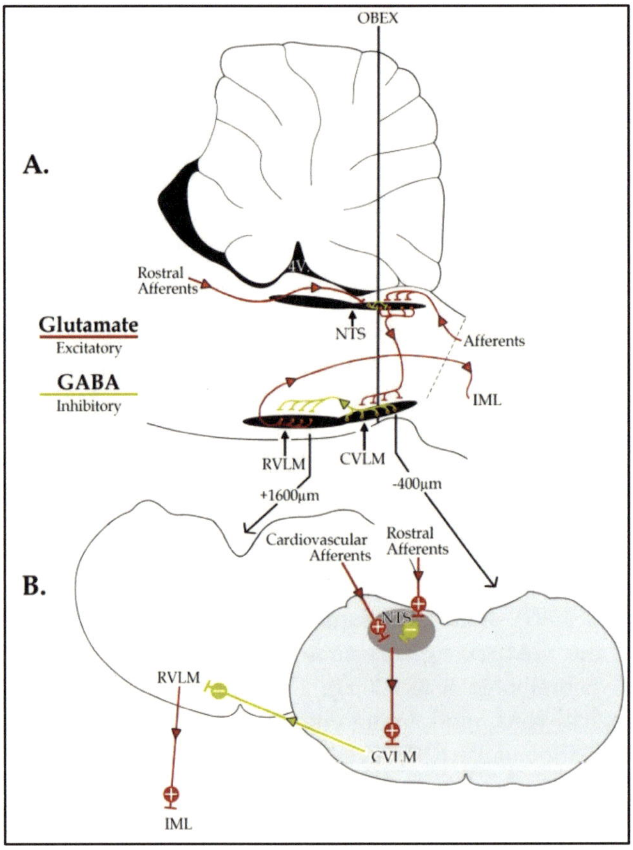

Fig. 2. Central cardiovascular circuitry. (A) Sagittal brainstem section showing the main regions involved in cardiovascular regulation. Baroreceptor afferents terminate within the NTS, which sends projections to CVLM, which in turn sends GABAergic projections to RVLM. (B) Coronal brainstem sections at +1,600 μm and -400 μm relative to the obex. Abbreviations: CVLM, caudal ventrolateral medulla; NTS, nucleus of the solitary tract; RVLM rostral ventrolateral medulla; VMM, ventromedial medulla; MLR, mesencephalic locomotor region; 4V, fourth ventricle; IML, intermediolateral cell column.

1.4 Concluding introductory remarks

Central cardiovascular control regions within the high and low aerobic capacity strains of rat used in this study are yet to be characterized. The objectives of the present study are: (1) to characterize the expression of both *Gad65* and *Gad67* within the NTS and VLM nuclei of high and low aerobic capacity rats; and (2) to propose a neural mechanism underlying hypertension within the LCR phenotype.

2. Materials and methods

All procedures conducted were approved by the University Committee on the Use and Care of Animals at the University of Michigan and adhered to the outlines described in the Guide for the Care and Use of Laboratory Animals (National Academy of Sciences, 1996).

2.1 Rat strain

The HCR and LCR phenotypes were developed as described by Koch and Britton (2001). Briefly, 96 male and 96 genetically heterogeneous female rats were obtained from the N:NIH stock at the National Institutes of Health (Bethesda, MD). At 10 weeks of age all rats were given treadmill education for a period of 1 week. Education consisted of familiarizing the rats to the treadmill and the mild shock stimulus (1.2 mA at 3 Hz for ~1.5 s) given when they traveled off the back of the treadmill. Once the rats learned to run in avoidance of the stimulus they were tested. In the event a rat did not become acclimated to the treadmill after the prescribed education period, it was not further tested and was excluded from the study.

The following week, at the age of 12 weeks, those rats which reached threshold were tested on 5 consecutive days. Using their single best day the rats were sorted, and the 13 highest and 13 lowest capacity rats for each sex were randomly paired within their newly acquired phenotype for breeding. The offspring from these pairs were weaned 28 days after birth and began treadmill education at the age of 10 weeks, at which time the process, as stated above, was repeated. In following generations (F1 onward), the only deviation from the above protocol was that no minimum threshold was required for inclusion in the study. Additionally, it should be noted that after initiation of the F1 generation from the founder population, all subsequent generations were bred using within-family rotational breeding methods between the original 13 families for each phenotype in order to minimize inbreeding.

2.2 Tissue collection and sectioning

8 adult HCR and 8 adult LCR male rats were obtained from the 18th generation. Animals were housed in pairs, with each cage containing a pair of either HCR or LCR male rats. Food and water were readily available to all animals, and cages were kept in a 12 hour light, 12 hour dark environment.

Rats were sacrificed via rapid decapitation using a guillotine. The brains were extracted, flash frozen in 2-methylbutane at -30˚C, and stored at -80˚C until further processing took place. At the time of sectioning each brain was removed from -80˚C and allowed to equilibrate at -20˚C within the cryostat for 5 minutes. At this time each brain was dissected in two at the level of the anterior thalamus to allow for mounting of the tissue on a block. The caudal half of the dissected tissue was mounted and subsequently embedded with M-1 embedding matrix (Thermo Shandon, Pittsburgh, PA). The tissue was then sectioned on a cryostat (Leica CM1850) at -20˚C at a thickness of 10μm in the coronal plane throughout the entire rostro-caudal extent of the medulla. Sections were mounted 4 per slide on Superfrost slides (Fischer Scientific) by apposing the slides kept at room temperature onto the cryostat stage. A total of 100 slides were taken per animal, resulting in a total sectioned distance of 4.0 mm. Following sectioning, slides were stored at -80°C until further processing.

2.3 Tissue mapping

To standardize tissue levels between animals, every tenth slide was pulled from storage and allowed to equilibrate at room temperature for ~2 minutes. Slides were then stained for 5 minutes in a 1% cresyl violet solution containing 1% glacial acetic acid. Following the 5 minute incubation, sections were placed in water for 30 seconds and then dehydrated as follows: 30 seconds each in 50% ethanol, 70% ethanol, 85% ethanol, 95% ethanol (twice), and 100% ethanol (twice). Following the final 100% ethanol wash, slides were placed in xylene for at least 5 minutes and pulled to be coverslipped with Permount (Fischer Scientific) and standard laboratory coverglass.

Following a 2 day drying period slides were examined under a microscope. The obex, which we classify as the opening of the 4th ventricle, was located and recorded for all brains. By using these reference slides we were able to align all brains relatiave to each other and in relation to the obex (Fig. 3).

2.4 *In situ* hybridization

Gene expression of *Gad65* and *Gad67* was quantified using radioactive *in situ* hybridization. Total rat brain RNA was obtained, reverse-transcribed, and then subjected to the polymerase chain reaction (PCR) to amplify *Gad65* and *Gad67* mRNA. *Gad* PCR products were then purified via agarose gel electrophoresis. Representative bands were excised, and the resulting RNA was purified. Purified RNA was then subcloned into Bluescript SK vectors containing both T3 and T7 promoter sequences (Stratagene, San Diego, CA). Vectors were introduced into *E. Coli* bacteria and stored at -80°C in a 50% glycerol stock until further processing.

Prior to the execution of the below experiments, plasmid DNA containing the *Gad* insert was extracted from bacteria clones and sequenced. Sequencing results obtained by automated deoxynucleotide sequencing at the University of Michigan DNA sequencing core matched those provided by NCBI's local alignment search tool (BLAST) available at www.ncbi.nlm.nih.gov/BLAST/.

Radioactive probe manufacturing: E. Coli containing Bluescript vectors with the *Gad65* or *Gad67* insert were removed from -80°C storage and grown at 37°C for 16 hours in a shaker set to 250 rpms. Following the 16 hour incubation the bacterial clones were removed from the shaker and centrifuged at 7000 rpms in a Beckman centrifuge (SM-24 rotor) for 10 minutes. The less dense supernatant was poured off, and the plasmids were extracted and purified using a Qiagen QIAprep Spin Miniprep Kit (Qiagen, Hilden, Germany). "The bench protocol: QIAprep Spin Minipred Kit using a microcentrifuge" protocol was follow precisely except for the last step, where 40µl of Buffer EB was used to elute DNA rather than 50µl.

At this time a reaction to "pop-out" the insert was conducted to ensure the insert was of the expected size – 640 nt for *Gad65* (NCBI accession number: M72422) and 900 nt for *Gad67* (NCBI accession number: M34445). 2µl of the eluted DNA was added to 14µl of distilled water, 2µl of 10x React3 buffer (Invitrogen, Carlsbad, CA), 1µl of EcoR1 enzyme (Invitrogen, 10U/µl), and 1µl of BamH1 enzyme (Invitrogen, 10units/µl). The mix was incubated at 37°C for 1 hour. Simultaneously, 20µl of the eluted DNA was linearized by adding 10µl of 10x React2 buffer (for anti-sense; Invitrogen) or 10x React3 buffer (Sense), 50µl of distilled water, and 5µl of Hind3 (Anti-Sense; Invitrogen, 10units/µl) or BamH1 (Sense; Invitrogen, 10uU/µl). This mixture was incubated at 37°C for 2 hours. Following the incubations the products were run out on a 2% agarose gel and visualized using ethidium bromide.

Sense and anti-sense cRNA probes were synthesized as follows: 4µl ^{35}S-UTP (10µCi/µl; Amersham Biosciences, Piscataway, NJ) and 3µl ^{35}S-CTP (10µCi/µl; Amersham Biosciences) were added to 5µl of 5x T3/T7 buffer (Invitrogen), 5µl of filtered water, 1µl ATP (10mM), 1µl GTP (10mM), 1µl RNAse inhibitor (40U/µl; GeneChoice, Frederick, MD), 2µl 0.1M DTT (Invitrogen), 2µl of linearized DNA, and 1µl of T3 polymerase (40units/µl; Invitrogen). The contents were allowed to incubate in a water bath set to 37°C for 2 hours. Following the 2 hour incubation, 1µl of RNAse-free DNAse (10U/µl; Roche Scientific, Basel, Switzerland) was added, and the mixture was allowed to sit at room temperature for 15 minutes, after which the contents were transferred to a drained BioRad Micro Bio-Spin Chromatography column (BioRad, Hercules, CA). The manufacturer's protocol was followed except for the last step. Briefly, the column was allowed to drain for 5 minutes followed by a 2 minute 1000g spin before the probe was added. The probe was diluted with 25µl of filtered, distilled water before being added to the prepared column. The column was then placed into a clean 1.5mL eppendorf tube and spun for 4 minutes at 1000g. The column was then discarded, and 1µl of 1M DTT was added to the purified probe. At this time 1µl of the purified probe was taken, and its radioactivity was quantified using a Packard 2200CA liquid scintillation analyzer (Packard, Wellesley, MA). The remaining probe was placed at -80°C for storage (< 3 days).

Preparation of the tissue: Slides were removed from storage at -80°C and placed in 4% paraformaldehyde at room temperature for 1 hour. They were then transferred to 2X sodium chloride/sodium citrate solution (SSC) for 5 minutes – this step was repeated 3 times for a total of three 5 minute washes. Slides were then placed in a 0.1M triethanolamine (TEA) wash (pH = 8.0, obtained through the addition of acetic anhydride) for 10 minutes. Lastly, the slides were dehydrated by running them through a series of ethanol washes for 30 seconds each (50%, 75%, 90%, 95% twice, and 100% twice). The slides were then allowed to air dry.

Hybridization: 70µl of hybridization buffer containing 10^6 cpm of the cRNA probe and 10mM DTT was pipetted onto each slide. The slides were cover-slipped with standard cover glass and put in incubation trays containing blotting paper dampened with 50% formamide. Each tray was covered with a lid, sealed in plastic wrap, and kept at 55°C for 18 hours.

Post-Hybridization: Following removal of coverslips, the slides were washed three times for 5 minutes in 2X SSC and were then transferred to a 37°C RNAse A solution for 1 hour. The slides were then taken through the following washes, each of which lasted 5 minutes: 2X SSC, 1X SSC, and 0.5X SSC. A 1 hour incubation in 65-70°C 0.1X SSC followed. Slides were then dipped in distilled water and dehydrated in ethanol (30 seconds each in 50%, 75%, 90%, 95% twice, and 100% twice).

Film/Exposure: Following dehydration, slides were allowed to dry for 15 minutes and then apposed to Kodak Biomax MR radiosensitive film. Each cassette contained alternating rows of slides with HCR or LCR tissue. Following a 72 hour exposure, cassettes were opened in the dark, and the film was developed using a Kodak X-OMAT 2000A processor (Eastman Kodak).

Emulsion dipping: In order to visualize individual hybridized probes, slides were emulsion dipped in K.5D emulsion gel containing silver bromide (Ilford Scientific, Cheshire, GB). Following an 11 day exposure at 10ºC the slides were developed by placing them in Kodak D19 developer (Eastman Kodak, Rochester, NY) for 2 minutes, followed by 30 seconds in water, 3 minutes in Kodak Liquid Rapid Fixer Solution (Eastman Kodak, Rochester, NY), 30 seconds in water to wash off the fixer, and 15 minutes under cool tap water. Slides were then stained using a 1% cresyl violet solution containing 1% glacial acetic acid for 2 minutes. Slides were then briefly rinsed in water and dehydrated by taking them through a series of graded alcohols as described above (2.3 - Tissue mapping). Following the 100% ethanol washes, slides were placed in xylene for at least 5 minutes and were then pulled to be coverslipped with Permount (Fischer Scientific) and standard laboratory coverglass.

2.5 Film and image analysis

The autoradiographs were illuminated using a Northern Light Illuminator (Imaging Research, St. Catharines, ON) and then digitized with a Sony XC-ST70 video camera connected to a computer running MCID Basic software (Imaging Research, St. Catherines, ON). Images were analyzed with Scion Image Beta 4.02 software (Scion Corp., Frederick, MA) using an in-house macro designed to count only those pixels which were 3.5 standard deviations above the average background value. Background was calculated for each image using an area of tissue containing no *Gad* expression such as white matter tracts. Signal and integrated optical density (IOD) values for each nucleus of interest within each section were calculated. IOD is defined as the area of highlighted pixels multiplied by the average density (i.e. signal) of each pixel, expressed in arbitrary units. Signal and IOD measurements were averaged between left and right sides. Each region of interest was analyzed across multiple rostro-caudal levels that were matched between HCR and LCR samples.

For illustration purposes, emulsion dipped slides were digitized using a Sony DXC 970MD color video camera (Sony Corp.) connected to a Leica DMRD microscope (Leica, Wetzlar, Germany). All equipment was connected to a computer running MCID Basic (Imaging Research).

2.6 Data analysis

Statistical analyses were performed using SPSS version 13 software (SPSS Inc., Chicago, IL). To assess for differences between the HCR and LCR phenotypes at various caudal-to-rostral levels, linear mixed effects model statistics were conducted. Within the model, repeated covariance types were selected based on Akaike's information criterion (AIC). In all cases, heterogeneous first-order autoregressive (ARH1) produced the smallest AIC value and was thus used for all analyses. In the event the model reached significance, post-hoc testing was conducted. P-values for multiple t-tests were corrected for using Bonferroni correction. Significance was set to $p<0.05$ in all cases. Data are presented as mean ± SEM.

3. Results

Our initial analysis focused on the distribution of *Gad65* and *Gad67* mRNA in the medulla of HCR and LCR rats. Labeling for *Gad65* and *Gad67* was present throughout the brainstem and included VLM, ventromedial medulla, NTS, area postrema, raphe nuclei, vestibular nuclei, and spinal trigeminal nucleus (Fig. 3). Labeling was absent in motor nuclei, such as the facial nerve nucleus and the hypoglossal nerve nucleus. Examination of emulsion dipped material revealed dense clustering of grains over cresyl violet stained nuclei within the same locations as revealed by the radiographs, including NTS (Fig. 4). The general patterns of *Gad65* and *Gad67* mRNA distributions were very similar.

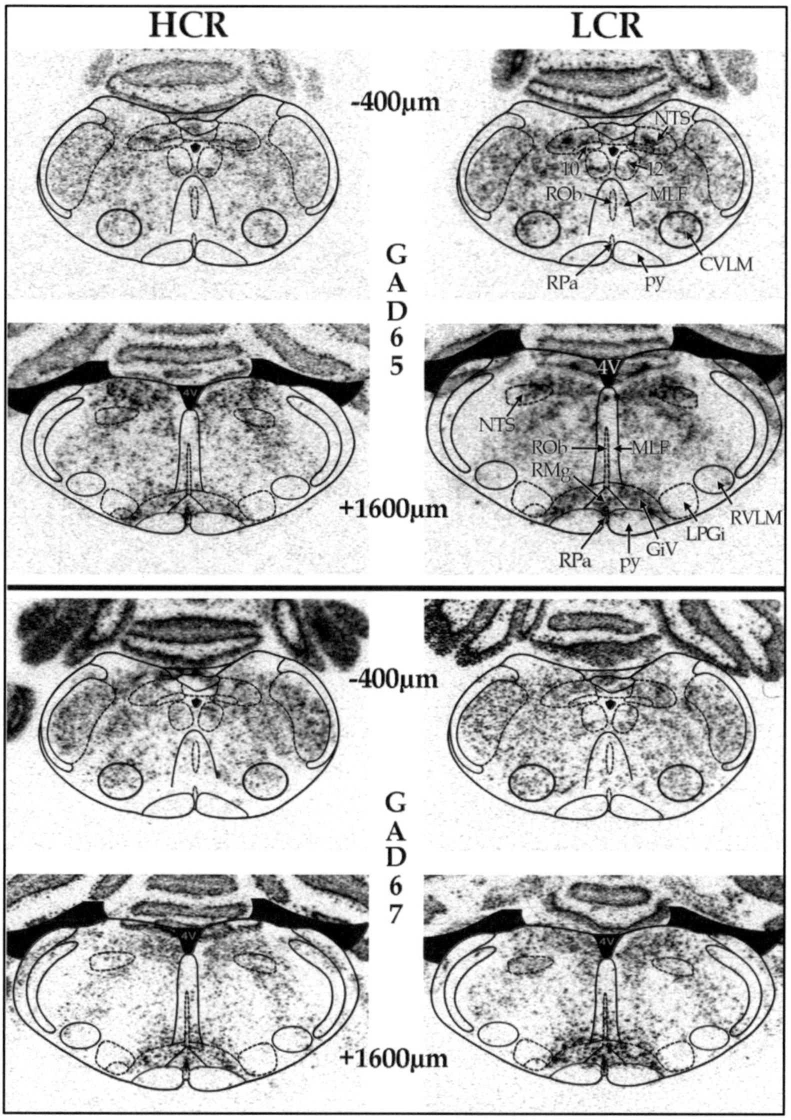

Fig. 3. Autoradiographs illustrating *Gad65* (top) and *Gad67* (bottom) expression at -400 μm and +1,600 μm relative to obex. Abbreviations: 10 - dorsal motor nucleus of the vagus; 12 - hypoglossal nerve nucleus; CVLM, caudal ventrolateral medulla; GiV, ventral gigantocellular nucleus; MLF - medial longitudinal fasciculus; LPGi, lateral paragigantocellular nucleus; py, pyramidal tract; RMg, raphe magnus; ROb, raphe obscurus, RPa, raphe pallidus; RVLM, rostral ventrolateral medulla.

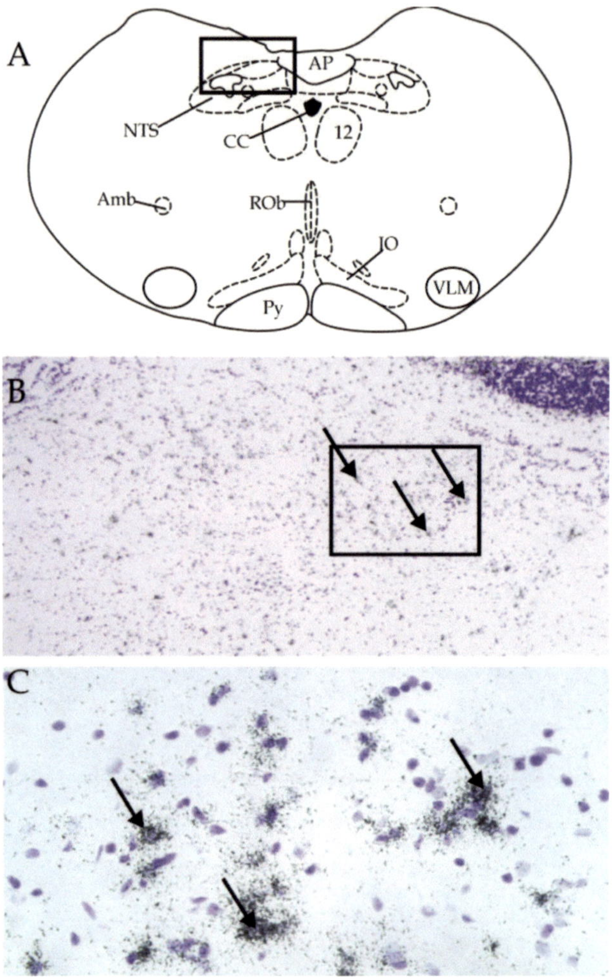

Fig. 4. Emulsion dipped material revealed dense clusters of dark grains corresponding to *Gad65* mRNA. (A) Drawing of the brainstem at -400 µm relative to obex, adapted from the atlas of Paxinos and Watson. (B) 5x image of NTS (see boxed area in 5A). Arrows indicate examples of dense GAD65 expression. (C) 63x image of boxed area in figure 5B. Slides were counter-stained with cresyl violet (purple) to highlight cell nuclei. Again arrows indicate dense grain clusters, corresponding to GABAergic neurons. Abbreviations: Amb, nucleus ambiguus; AP, area postrema; CC, central canal; IO, inferior olive; NTS, nucleus of the solitary tract; Py, pyramidal tract; ROb, raphe obscurus; VLM, ventrolateral medulla.

The expression of *Gad65* mRNA in LCR and HCR rats was quantified within NTS and VLM. Significant main effects of level and phenotype were observed within both regions ($p < 0.05$), indicating that LCR rats had higher levels of *Gad65* mRNA compared to HCR rats.

Analysis of the signal data revealed an upregulation in *Gad65* expression in LCR animals within the caudal NTS at -400 µm relative to the obex (Fig. 5A). We observed a similar upregulation in *Gad65* expression in the VLM of LCR rats both caudally (at -400 µm) and rostrally (at +400 µm and +1200 µm; Fig. 5B).

Analysis of the IOD data confirmed these observations and revealed increased *Gad65* expression in LCR animals at -800 µm and -400 µm in the NTS (Fig. 5C), as well as at +400 µm within the VLM (Fig. 5D).

In the case of *Gad67* mRNA, no significant differences in its expression were detected between HCR and LCR rats in either NTS or VLM.

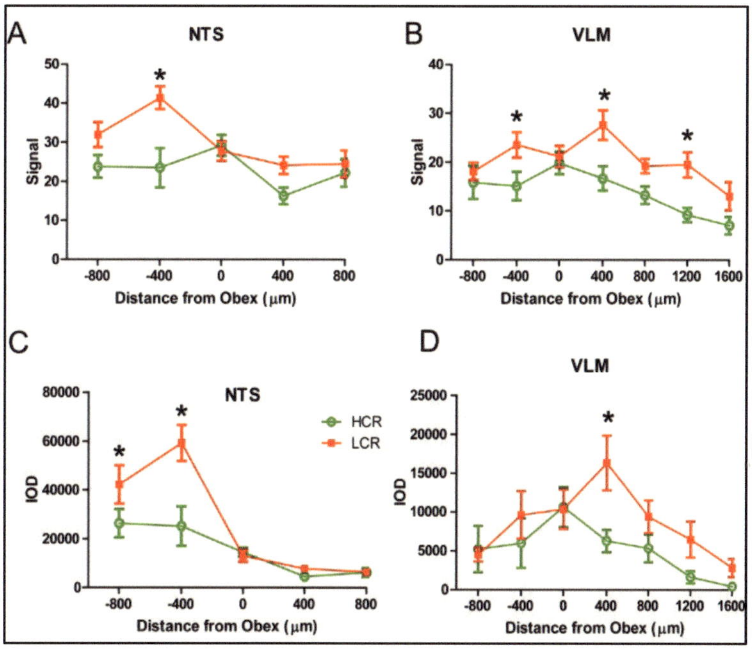

Fig. 5. Upregulation of *Gad65* expression within NTS and VLM in LCR rats. Note increase in expression at specific rostro-caudal levels. * - $p < 0.05$ compared to HCR. Adapted from Buck et al., 2007.

4. Discussion

The current study quantified expression of the GABA synthesizing enzymes *Gad65* and *Gad67* in the brainstem of a rat model of MetS (i.e. LCR) as compared to its high aerobic capacity counterpart (i.e. HCR rat). As described previously, the low capacity running rats, LCRs, exhibited dramatically poorer exercise capacity compared to their high capacity, HCR, counterparts. LCR rats became exhausted more quickly, ran for a shorter distance, and ran at a slower pace compared to HCR rats. The LCR animals also weighed significantly more than their HCR counterparts (Buck et al., 2007), and previous characterization demonstrates elevated mean blood pressures in the LCR strain equating to a roughly 13 mmHg difference (Wisloff et al., 2005). These findings together with prior observations of increased visceral adiposity and increased insulin resistance suggest that LCR animals may represent an animal model of metabolic syndrome (Wisloff et al., 2005).

Specifically, this study examined the distribution of *Gad65* and *Gad67* in baro-responsive nuclei in the brainstems of both the HCR and LCR phenotypes. Our hypothesis was that alterations in brainstem circuitry, specifically involving the inhibitory neurotransmitter

GABA, contribute to the observed variations in mean arterial pressure between the two groups.

4.1 Nucleus of the solitary tract, NTS

GABA containing neurons within the NTS were first described by Chan and Sawchenko (1998), who identified a small population of baro-sensitive GABAergic neurons within the NTS. More recently, however, Degtyarenko and Kaufman (2005) demonstrated a larger collection of non-barosensitive GAD- containing interneurons within the NTS. Significantly outnumbering the small population of baro-sensitive neurons, this newly characterized population likely exerts far more influence on the cardiovascular circuitry (Degtyarenko and Kaufman, 2005). It should be noted, however, that inputs to these NTS interneurons are still mostly undocumented, although some believe they receive their input from the mesencephalic locomotor region and are integral in resetting the circuitry during exercise (Degtyarenko and Kaufman, 2005). Other reports have indicated that this population receives inputs from muscle afferents (Chen et al., 2009), and that following exercise they contribute to the phenomenon of post-exercise hypotension. Full characterization of inputs to GAD containing NTS cells, however, is yet to be determined.

The present study set out to determine differences in expression of both *Gad65* and *Gad67* in the NTS of HCR and LCR rats. Our data suggest that increased levels of *Gad65* may lead to increased levels of GAD65 protein, which would result in increased synthesis of GABA within the caudal NTS. It seems likely that these changes predominantly impact inhibitory interneurons within the NTS. Such interneurons play a critical role in regulating excitatory output from the NTS and may contribute to elevated arterial pressure in the LCR rats through inhibition of excitatory influence on the CVLM.

No differences were seen in *Gad67* expression between the HCRs and LCRs. However, GAD67 is likely responsible for long-term maintenance of cytoplasmic pools of GABA and is used to set baseline levels (Esclapez et al., 1994; Soghomonian & Martin, 1998; Esclapez & Houser, 1999). GAD65, on the other hand, regulates local control of GABA synthesis and represents vesicular synthesis (Soghomonian & Martin, 1998), thus playing a prominent role in GABAergic neurotransmission.

4.2 Ventrolateral medulla, VLM

Past research involving microinjections of excitatory and inhibitory transmitters into the VLM led to the identification of physiologically defined pressor and depressor regions, respectively (Schreihofer & Guyenet, 2002). Schreihofer and Guyenet went on to map these two regions relative to the obex in the adult rat. Their experimentation resulted in a CLVM depressor region extending from -500μm to +1000μm relative to the obex and a RVLM pressor region extending from +700μm to +2000μm, ending at the caudal pole of the facial nerve nucleus.

In the present study we observed an upregulation in the expression of *Gad65* mRNA in both the rostral and caudal VLM in LCR rats. While upregulation of *Gad65* within the CVLM may be a compensatory response to chronic elevation in blood pressure, the findings in the RVLM do not fit the currently accepted model of central control of vascular tone. According to the classical model, increased GABAergic neurotransmission within the rostral VLM would lead to lower, not higher, blood pressure, as we observed in the LCR rats (Guyenet,

2006). Though the latter finding is difficult to resolve with existing literature, there may be other possibilities that may explain this observation. One option is that this alteration in *Gad65* mRNA expression occurs in non-cardiovascular neurons. Rostral VLM is a heterogeneous region that also contains neurons with respiratory functions (Richter & Spyer, 2001). Thus, up-regulation in expression of *Gad65* mRNA in the rostral VLM of LCR rats may represent potential alterations in respiratory function.

Another possibility is that the presumed increase in GABAergic neurotransmission activates an "accessory" vasomotor pathway originating from the rostral VLM (McAllen et al., 2005). This pathway is thought to activate "accessory" sympathetic preganglionic neurons, which are characterized by their unmyelinated axons and which drive hexamethonium-resistant transmission in sympathetic ganglia (McAllen et al., 2005). Unlike "regular" sympathetic preganglionic neurons, which are inhibited by administration of GABA in the rostral VLM, the "accessory" sympathetic preganglionic neurons are activated by this manipulation (McAllen et al., 2005). Thus, it may be that activation of this "accessory" pathway contributes to resting blood pressure differences between LCR and HCR rats.

Yet another possibility is that increased *Gad65* mRNA expression in the rostral VLM of LCR rats leads to increased GABA production and secretion within projection neurons, rather than local interneurons. Data from anatomical and pharmacological experiments suggest that neurons within the rostral VLM project to the NTS, where they inhibit the baroreceptor reflex (Len & Chan, 2001; Livingston & Berger, 1989; Loewy et al., 1981). This notion is supported by the observation that administration of glutamate into the rostral VLM, but not into surrounding regions, leads to the release of GABA in the caudal NTS (Len & Chan, 2001). This glutamate-induced increase in GABA secretion in the NTS is associated with the suppression of the baroreceptor reflex, an effect that is blocked by administration of $GABA_A$ and $GABA_B$ receptor antagonists in the NTS (Len & Chan, 2001). Such an increase in baroreflex inhibition would lead to higher resting blood pressure levels, which may contribute to increased blood pressure levels in LCR rats. Future studies will be required to test these hypotheses.

5. Conclusions and future directions

The present study examined potential differences in the expression of *Gad65* and *Gad67* mRNA within brainstem cardiovascular control nuclei in a rat model of metabolic syndrome. Our goal was to assess for differences in GABAergic tone as an explanation for hypertension in the LCR phenotype. We found increased levels of *Gad65*, but not *Gad67*, expression within the caudal NTS, caudal VLM, and rostral VLM of LCR rats compared to their HCR counterparts. These findings suggest a neural component in the development of hypertension in MetS.

To better understand brainstem contributions in the development of hypertension in MetS, further studies are needed to more fully characterize inputs to GABAergic NTS neurons. Additionally, past studies have highlighted an up-regulation of $GABA_B$ receptor mRNA in the NTS of hypertensive rats (Durgam et al., 1999). $GABA_B$ receptor expression appears to be important in mediating increases in MAP during rest (Tolstykh et al., 2003). Thus, examination of potential $GABA_B$ receptor expression and function differences between HCR and LCR rats may add additional insight into the pathophysiology of hypertension associated with MetS.

6. Acknowledgements

The authors would like to thank Dr. Stanley Watson who allowed us to conduct much of this work in his laboratory at the University of Michigan. We are grateful to Sharon Burke and Jennifer Fitzpatrick for their technical assistance. Without them this chapter would not have been possible. Additionally we acknowledge Huda Akil, Ph.D. for her support of the project, as well as Dr. Paul Burghardt and Dr. Sarah Clinton for sharing their knowledge of *in situ* hybridization and radiographic quantification. Supported by: 4R00MH081927-03 (IAK).

7. References

Agarwal SK, Calaresu FR (1991) Monosynaptic connection from caudal to rostral ventrolateral medulla in the baroreceptor reflex pathway. Brain Res 555:70-74.

Agarwal SK, Gelsema AJ, Calaresu FR (1989) Neurons in rostral VLM are inhibited by chemical stimulation of caudal VLM in rats. Am J Physiol 257:R265-270.

Alberti KG, Zimmet P, Shaw J (2005) The metabolic syndrome--a new worldwide definition. Lancet 366:1059-1062.

Altschuler SM, Bao XM, Bieger D, Hopkins DA, Miselis RR (1989) Viscerotopic representation of the upper alimentary tract in the rat: sensory ganglia and nuclei of the solitary and spinal trigeminal tracts. J Comp Neurol 283:248-268.

Andresen MC, Doyle MW, Jin YH, Bailey TW (2001) Cellular mechanisms of baroreceptor integration at the nucleus tractus solitarius. Ann N Y Acad Sci 940:132-141.

Blessing WW (1988) Depressor neurons in rabbit caudal medulla act via GABA receptors in rostral medulla. Am J Physiol 254:H686-692.

Blessing WW, Nalivaiko E (2001) Raphe magnus/pallidus neurons regulate tail but not mesenteric arterial blood flow in rats. Neuroscience 105:923-929.

Buck BJ, Kerman IA, Burghardt PR, Koch LG, Britton SL, Akil H, Watson SJ (2007) Upregulation of GAD65 mRNA in the medulla of the rat model of metabolic syndrome. Neurosci Lett 419:178-183.

Chan RK, Sawchenko PE (1994) Spatially and temporally differentiated patterns of c-fos expression in brainstem catecholaminergic cell groups induced by cardiovascular challenges in the rat. J Comp Neurol 348:433-460.

Chan RK, Sawchenko PE (1998) Organization and transmitter specificity of medullary neurons activated by sustained hypertension: implications for understanding baroreceptor reflex circuitry. J Neurosci 18:371-387.

Chen CY, Bechtold AG, Tabor J, Bonham AC (2009) Exercise reduces GABA synaptic input onto NTS baroreceptor second-order neurons via NK1 receptor internalization in spontaneously hypertensive rats. J Neurosci 29(9):2754-2761.

Chua SC, Chung WK, Wu-Peng XS, Zhang Y, Liu SM, Tartaglia L, Leibel RL (1996) Phenotypes of mouse *diabetes* and rat *fatty* due to mutations in the OB (leptin) receptor. Science 271(5251):994-996.

d'Ascanio P, Centini C, Pompeiano M, Pompeiano O, Balaban E (2002) Fos and FRA protein expression in rat nucleus paragigantocellularis lateralis during different space flight conditions. Brain Res Bull 59:65-74.

Dampney RA (1994) The subretrofacial vasomotor nucleus: anatomical, chemical and pharmacological properties and role in cardiovascular regulation. Prog Neurobiol 42:197-227.

Danbolt NC (2001) Glutamate uptake. Prog Neurobiol 65:1-105.

de Artinano AA, Castro MM (2009) Experimental rat models to study the metabolic syndrome. British Journal of Nutrition 102:1246-1253.

Degtyarenko AM, Kaufman MP (2005) MLR-induced inhibition of barosensory cells in the NTS. Am J Physiol Heart Circ Physiol 289:H2575-2584.

Devaney JM, Gordish-Dressman H, Harmon BT, Bradbury MK, Devaney SA, Harris TB, Thompson PD, Clarkson PM, Price TB, Angelopoulos TJ, Gordon PM, Moyna NM, et al. (2011) *AKT1* polymorphisms are associated with risk for metabolic syndrome. Hum Genet 129:129-139.

Durgam VR, Vitela M, Mifflin SW (1999) Enhanced gamma-aminobutyric acid-B receptor agonist responses and mRNA within the nucleus of the solitary tract in hypertension. Hypertension 33:530-536.

Erickson JT, Millhorn DE (1991) Fos-like protein is induced in neurons of the medulla oblongata after stimulation of the carotid sinus nerve in awake and anesthetized rats. Brain Res 567:11-24.

Esclapez M, Tillakaratne NJ, Kaufman DL, Tobin AJ, Houser CR (1994) Comparative localization of two forms of glutamic acid decarboxylase and their mRNAs in rat brain supports the concept of functional differences between the forms. J Neurosci 14:1834-1855.

Esclapez M, Houser CR (1999) Up-regulation of GAD65 and GAD67 in remaining hippocampal GABA neurons in a model of temporal lobe epilepsy. J Comp Neurol 412:488-505.

Fong AY, Stornetta RL, Foley CM, Potts JT (2005) Immunohistochemical localization of GAD67-expressing neurons and processes in the rat brainstem: subregional distribution in the nucleus tractus solitarius. J Comp Neurol 493:274-290.

Ford ES, Giles WH, Dietz WH (2002) Prevalence of the metabolic syndrome among US adults: findings from the third National Health and Nutrition Examination Survey. Jama 287:356-359.

Gordon FJ, Sved AF (2002) Neurotransmitters in central cardiovascular regulation: glutamate and GABA. Clin Exp Pharmacol Physiol 29:522-524.

Graham JC, Hoffman GE, Sved AF (1995) c-Fos expression in brain in response to hypotension and hypertension in conscious rats. J Auton Nerv Syst 55:92-104.

Grisk O, Frauendorf T, Schluter T, Kloting I, Kuttler B, Krebs A, Ludemann J, Rettig R (2007) Impaired coronary function in Wistar Ottawa Karlsburg W rats--a new model of the metabolic syndrome. Eur J Physiol 454:1011-1021.

Grundy SM, Brewer HB, Jr., Cleeman JI, Smith SC, Jr., Lenfant C (2004) Definition of metabolic syndrome: Report of the National Heart, Lung, and Blood Institute/American Heart Association conference on scientific issues related to definition. Circulation 109:433-438.

Guyenet PG, Filtz TM, Donaldson SR (1987) Role of excitatory amino acids in rat vagal and sympathetic baroreflexes. Brain Res 407:272-284.

Guyenet PG (2006) The sympathetic control of blood pressure. Nat. Rev. Neurosci. 7: 335–346.

Hermann GE, Bresnahan JC, Holmes GM, Rogers RC, Beattie MS (1998) Descending projections from the nucleus raphe obscurus to pudendal motoneurons in the male rat. J Comp Neurol 397:458-474.

Hisano S (2003) Vesicular glutamate transporters in the brain. Anat Sci Int 78:191-204.

Horiuchi J, Killinger S, Dampney RA (2004) Contribution to sympathetic vasomotor tone of tonic glutamatergic inputs to neurons in the RVLM. Am J Physiol Regul Integr Comp Physiol 287:R1335-1343.

Imaizumi T, Granata AR, Benarroch EE, Sved AF, Reis DJ (1985) Contributions of arginine vasopressin and the sympathetic nervous system to fulminating hypertension after destruction of neurons of caudal ventrolateral medulla in the rat. J Hypertens 3:491-501.

Ishizuka T, Ernsberger P, Liu S, Bedol D, Lehman TM, Koletsky RJ, Friedman JE (1998) Phenotypic consequences of a nonsense mutation in the leptin receptor gene (fak) in obese spontaneously hypertensive Koletsky rats (SHROB). J Nutr 128(12):2299-306.

Len WB, Chan JY (2001) Rostralventrolateralmedullasuppressesreflexbradycardia by the release of gamma-aminobutyric acid in nucleus tractus solitarii of the rat. Synapse 39: 23–31.

Kandler K, Herbert H (1991) Auditory projections from the cochlear nucleus to pontine and mesencephalic reticular nuclei in the rat. Brain Res 562:230-242.

Kang TC, Kim HS, Seo MO, Choi SY, Kwon OS, Baek NI, Lee HY, Won MH (2001) The temporal alteration of GAD67/GAD65 ratio in the gerbil hippocampal complex following seizure. Brain Res 920:159-169.

Kawai Y, Senba E (1996) Organization of excitatory and inhibitory local networks in the caudal nucleus of tractus solitarius of rats revealed in in vitro slice preparation. J Comp Neurol 373:309-321.

Kawai Y, Senba E (2000) Electrophysiological and morphological characteristics of nucleus tractus solitarii neurons projecting to the ventrolateral medulla. Brain Res 877:374-378.

Kiely JM, Gordon FJ (1994) Role of rostral ventrolateral medulla in centrally mediated pressor responses. Am J Physiol 267:H1549-1556.

Koch LG, Britton SL (2001) Artificial selection for intrinsic aerobic endurance running capacity in rats. Physiol Genomics 5:45-52.

Korsak A, Gilbey MP (2004) Rostral ventromedial medulla and the control of cutaneous vasoconstrictor activity following i.c.v. prostaglandin E(1). Neuroscience 124:709-717.

Kovacs P, van den Brandt J, Kloting K (2000) Genetic dissection of the syndrome X in the rat. Biochemical and Biophysical Research Communications 269:660-665.

Kuo JS, Hwa Y, Chai CY (1979) Cardio-inhibitory mechanism in the gigantocellular reticular nucleus of the medulla oblongata. Brain Res 178:221-232.

Lernmark A (1996) Glutamic acid decarboxylase--gene to antigen to disease. J Intern Med 240:259-277.

Leu HB, Chung CM, Lin SJ, Jong YS, Pan WH, Chen JW (2011) Adiponectin gene polymorphism is selectively associated with the concomitant presence of metabolic syndrome and essential hypertension. PLoS ONE 6(5):E19999.

Livingston CA, Berger AJ (1989) Immunocytochemical localization of GABA in neurons projecting to the ventrolateral nucleus of the solitary tract. Brain Res. 494: 143–150.

Loewy AD, Wallach JH, McKellar S (1981) Efferentconnectionsoftheventral medulla oblongata in the rat. Brain Res. 228: 63–80.

Lorenzo C, Williams K, Hunt KJ, Haffner SM (2006) Trend in the prevalence of the metabolic syndrome and its impact on cardiovascular disease incidence: the San Antonio Heart Study. Diabetes Care 29:625-630.

Matsumoto M, Takayama K, Miura M (1994) Distribution of glutamate- and GABA-immunoreactive neurons projecting to the vasomotor center of the intermediolateral nucleus of the lower thoracic cord of Wistar rats: a double-labeling study. Neurosci Lett 174:165-168.

McAllen RM, Allen AM, Bratton BO (2005) A neglected 'accessory' vasomotor pathway: implications for blood pressure control. Clin. Exp. Pharmacol. Physiol. 32: 473–477.

Mei H, Chen W, Dellinger A, He J, Wang M, Yau C, Srinivasan SR, Berenson GS (2010) Principal-component-based multivariate regression for genetic association studies of metabolic syndrome components. BMC Genetics 11:100.

Minson JB, Llewellyn-Smith IJ, Chalmers JP, Pilowsky PM, Arnolda LF (1997) c-fos identifies GABA-synthesizing barosensitive neurons in caudal ventrolateral medulla. Neuroreport 8:3015-3021.

Miura M, Takayama K, Okada J (1994) Neuronal expression of Fos protein in the rat brain after baroreceptor stimulation. J Auton Nerv Syst 50:31-43.

Nakamura K, Matsumura K, Kobayashi S, Kaneko T (2005) Sympathetic premotor neurons mediating thermoregulatory functions. Neurosci Res 51:1-8.

Potts J (2006) Inhibitory neurotransmission in the nucleus tractus solitarii: implications for baroreflex resetting during exercise. Exp Physiol 91(1):59-72

Richter DW, Spyer KM (2001) Studying rhythmogenesis of breathing: comparison of in vivo and in vitro models. Trends Neurosci. 24: 464– 472.

Rizzo M, Berneis K, Corrado E, Novo S (2006) The significance of low-density-lipoproteins size in vascular diseases. Int Angiol 25:4-9.

Ross CA, Ruggiero DA, Reis DJ (1985) Projections from the nucleus tractus solitarii to the rostral ventrolateral medulla. J Comp Neurol 242:511-534.

Ross CA, Ruggiero DA, Park DH, Joh TH, Sved AF, Fernandez-Pardal J, Saavedra JM, Reis DJ (1984) Tonic vasomotor control by the rostral ventrolateral medulla: effect of electrical or chemical stimulation of the area containing C1 adrenaline neurons on arterial pressure, heart rate, and plasma catecholamines and vasopressin. J Neurosci 4:474-494.

Ruggiero DA, Cravo SL, Golanov E, Gomez R, Anwar M, Reis DJ (1994) Adrenergic and non-adrenergic spinal projections of a cardiovascular-active pressor area of medulla oblongata: quantitative topographic analysis. Brain Res 663:107-120.

Sapru HN (2002) Glutamate circuits in selected medullo-spinal areas regulating cardiovascular function. Clin Exp Pharmacol Physiol 29:491-496.

Schreihofer AM, Guyenet PG (2002) The baroreflex and beyond: control of sympathetic vasomotor tone by GABAergic neurons in the ventrolateral medulla. Clin Exp Pharmacol Physiol 29:514-521.

Schreihofer AM, Stornetta RL, Guyenet PG (2000) Regulation of sympathetic tone and arterial pressure by rostral ventrolateral medulla after depletion of C1 cells in rat. J Physiol 529 Pt 1:221-236.

Seiders EP, Stuesse SL (1984) A horseradish peroxidase investigation of carotid sinus nerve components in the rat. Neurosci Lett 46:13-18.

Silva NF, Pires JG, Dantas MA, Futuro Neto HA (2002) Excitatory amino acid receptor blockade within the caudal pressor area and rostral ventrolateral medulla alters cardiovascular responses to nucleus raphe obscurus stimulation in rats. Braz J Med Biol Res 35:1237-1245.

Soghomonian JJ, Martin DL (1998) Two isoforms of glutamate decarboxylase: why? Trends Pharmacol Sci 19:500-505.

Spyer KM (1994) Annual review prize lecture. Central nervous mechanisms contributing to cardiovascular control. J Physiol 474:1-19.

Stornetta RL, McQuiston TJ, Guyenet PG (2004) GABAergic and glycinergic presympathetic neurons of rat medulla oblongata identified by retrograde transport of pseudorabies virus and in situ hybridization. J Comp Neurol 479:257-270.

Suzuki T, Takayama K, Miura M (1997) Distribution and projection of the medullary cardiovascular control neurons containing glutamate, glutamic acid decarboxylase, tyrosine hydroxylase and phenylethanolamine N-methyltransferase in rats. Neurosci Res 27:9-19.

Sved AF, Tsukamoto K (1992) Tonic stimulation of GABAB receptors in the nucleus tractus solitarius modulates the baroreceptor reflex. Brain Res 592:37-43.

Talman WT, Perrone MH, Reis DJ (1980) Evidence for L-glutamate as the neurotransmitter of baroreceptor afferent nerve fibers. Science 209:813-815.

Tolstykh G, Belugin S, Tolstykh O, Mifflin S (2003) Responses to GABA(A) receptor activation are altered in NTS neurons isolated from renal-wrap hypertensive rats. Hypertension 42:732-736.

Tsukamoto K, Sved AF (1993) Enhanced gamma-aminobutyric acid-mediated responses in nucleus tractus solitarius of hypertensive rats. Hypertension 22:819-825.

Vitela M, Mifflin SW (2001) gamma-Aminobutyric acid(B) receptor-mediated responses in the nucleus tractus solitarius are altered in acute and chronic hypertension. Hypertension 37:619-622.

Willette RN, Barcas PP, Krieger AJ, Sapru HN (1983) Vasopressor and depressor areas in the rat medulla. Identification by microinjection of L-glutamate. Neuropharmacology 22:1071-1079.

Willette RN, Punnen S, Krieger AJ, Sapru HN (1984) Interdependence of rostral and caudal ventrolateral medullary areas in the control of blood pressure. Brain Res 321:169-174.

Wisloff U, Najjar SM, Ellingsen O, Haram PM, Swoap S, Al-Share Q, Fernstrom M, Rezaei K, Lee SJ, Koch LG, Britton SL (2005) Cardiovascular risk factors emerge after artificial selection for low aerobic capacity. Science 307:418-420.

Wong J, Nock NL, Xu Z, Kyle C, Daniels A, White M, Yue DK, Elston RC, Mountjoy KG (2008) J Dia Res 10:1016.

Zabenah D, Balding DJ (2010) A genome-wide association study of the metabolic sydrome in Indian Asian Men. PLoS ONE 5(8):e11961.

Zaretsky DV, Zaretskaia MV, DiMicco JA (2003) Stimulation and blockade of GABA(A) receptors in the raphe pallidus: effects on body temperature, heart rate, and blood pressure in conscious rats. Am J Physiol Regul Integr Comp Physiol 285:R110-116.

Zhou SY, Gilbey MP (1995) Sympathoexcitatory influence of a fast conducting raphe-spinal pathway in the rat. Am J Physiol 268:R1230-1235.

Zucker LM, Zucker TF (1961) Fatty, a new mutation in the rat. J Hered 52(6):275-278.

7

Cardiometabolic Syndrome

Alkerwi Ala'a[1,2], Albert Adelin[2] and Guillaume Michèle[2]
[1]*Centre de Recherche Public-Santé, Centre for Health Studies,*
[2]*University of Liège, School of Public Health,*
[1]*Grand-Duchy of Luxembourg*
[2]*Belgium*

1. Introduction

The term "Metabolic Syndrome" is generally used to indicate a clinical entity of substantial heterogeneity, represented by the co-occurrence of hypertension, impaired glucose tolerance, atherogenic dyslipidemia, central fat accumulation, insulin resistance, as well as prothrombotic and inflammatory states[1]. This multiple metabolic and cardiovascular disorders clusters together in the same individual more often than might be expected by chance, leading to an increased probability of suffering from cardiovascular disease and type 2 diabetes mellitus[2], [3].

Notwithstanding the controversial concept[4], data from large prospective population-based studies, such as the Framingham offspring study[5], the Botnia study[2], the Kuopio Ischemic heart Disease study[3], the Italian study [6], and the Atherosclerosis Risk in Communities (ARIC) study[7], [8], confirmed that the presence of the metabolic syndrome was significantly associated with an increased risk of cardiovascular disease morbidity and mortality, thus providing substantial support for the metabolic syndrome hypothesis[1]. One important justification cited for the utility of the syndrome is that it changed medical perspective from a single-risk factor to the multiple-risk factors paradigm [9], [10].

During the last decade, this multiplex cardiometabolic disorder has progressively become a major worldwide public health problems, because of its association with increased risk of type 2 diabetes mellitus, atherosclerotic cardiovascular disease and all-cause mortality[2], [3], [1]. More than 100 million individuals suffer from this syndrome in the world. this number is set to increase rapidly, fuelled by the increase in obesity and diabetes epidemics[11]. The pathogenesis of the metabolic syndrome is complex and so far incompletely understood but the interaction of obesity, sedentary lifestyle, dietary, environmental and genetic factors are known to contribute to its development[12], [13], [14].

This chapter constitutes a review of the state-of-the-art of the metabolic syndrome, as regards the historical evolution of the concept, the debated key points and the evolution towards a new concept of global cardiometabolic risk. The last section provides an overview of the worldwide epidemiology of the metabolic syndrome, in terms of prevalence variation and determinants.

2. Historical evolution of the metabolic syndrome concept

Regardless of the disagreement about who first described the metabolic syndrome in the medical literature, its basic concept existed for at least 80 years[15]. According to a group of researchers[11], the constellation of metabolic disturbances was initially described in 1920s by Kylin, and later by Vague in 1947. The latter drew the attention to upper body adiposity (android or male-type obesity), as a metabolic abnormality commonly associated with type 2 diabetes and cardiovascular disease [16,17]. However, the frequent simultaneous presence of obesity, hypertension, diabetes and hyperlipidemia was described in 1965 by Avogaro et al, and then by Haller et al in 1977, who described their association with atherosclerosis[11].

Ten years later, the clinical importance of the syndrome was highlighted by Reaven who introduced the concept of Syndrome X, as a clustering of disturbances in glucose and insulin metabolism, dyslipidemia and hypertension. Reaven suggested that insulin resistance was a fundamental "disorder" associated with a set of metabolic abnormalities which not only increased the risk of type 2 diabetes but also contributed to the development of cardiovascular disease before the appearance of hyperglycemia. He emphasized that insulin resistance was at the centre of a cluster of metabolic abnormalities, which include hypertriglyceridemia, low high-density lipoprotein (LDL) cholesterol level, increased glycemia, and elevated blood pressure[13].

Following this early conceptual contribution, numerous studies have confirmed that insulin resistance was indeed associated with metabolic abnormalities that increase the risk of both diabetes and cardiovascular disease [18,19]. Syndrome X was also called Reaven's Syndrome, Insulin Resistance Syndrome, deadly quartet, and is now widely known as metabolic syndrome. A later key conceptual advance was the recognition of the central role of abdominal obesity [20] in the diagnosis of the metabolic syndrome, and its introduction as a clinically easy-measurable entity. This second hallmark put the abdominal obesity on the front line to diagnose the metabolic syndrome.

3. Debated key points

After a plethora of international publications, the metabolic syndrome concept is still ill-defined with many unanswered questions[11], [21]. So far, evidence-based outcomes concerning the components and cut-off values are limited and based principally on expert consensus[22].

3.1 Diversity of definitions

During the last decade, several definitions of the metabolic syndrome were suggested by a number of expert groups. Although these definitions were similar in their focus on basic criteria as obesity, dyslipidemia, hyperglycemia, and hypertension, substantial differences remained concerning the insulin resistance.

3.1.1 WHO definition

In an attempt to provide a tool for clinicians and researchers, the "WHO Working Group on Diabetes" proposed a set of criteria to define the metabolic syndrome [23]. The consensus was published on the WHO website in 1999, but reported clearly that the definition would be modified as new information became available about the components and their predictive power. The WHO definition, stated that diabetes type 2 or impaired glucose tolerance (IGT), together with at least 2 of 4 other factors (hypertension, hyperlipidemia, obesity and microalbuminuria) define the metabolic syndrome. In case of normal glucose tolerance, the evidence of insulin resistance is needed; this is defined as the lowest quartile of measures of insulin sensitivity. The definition of obesity is based either on overall obesity assessed by body mass index (BMI), or on central obesity assessed by waist-to-hip ratio (WHR)[23] (Table 1).

WHO definition of the metabolic syndrome 1999[23]
Glucose intolerance, Impaired Glucose Tolerance (IGT) or Diabetes mellitus and/or insulin resistance together with two or more of the following criteria listed below:
1. Obesity: BMI > 30 kg/m^2 and / or Waist-to-hip ratio > 90 cm in men or > 85 cm in women
2. Dyslipidaemia: serum triglycerides ≥ 150 mg/dl and/or HDL-C < 35 mg/dl in men and < 39 mg/dl in women
3. Urinary albumin excretion rate ≥ 20 µg/min or albumin: creatinine ratio ≥ 30 mg/g
4. Hypertension: Blood pressure ≥ 140/90 mmHg

Table 1. WHO definition of the metabolic syndrome 1999

The potential disadvantage of the WHO criteria is that special testing of glucose status, beyond routine clinical assessment, is necessary to diagnose the metabolic syndrome, for example: oral glucose tolerance test (OGTT) and insulin resistance measurement by hyperinsulinemic euglycemic clamp. Since insulin clamp evaluation was impractical, most epidemiological studies used hyperinsulinemia as a surrogate for insulin resistance[24], [3]. Another weak point was related to the non-reliable measurement of obesity by the BMI, especially in the elderly, due to the changes in height with advancing age compared to younger adults[25]. In addition, for any given BMI tertile, subjects in the top waist tertile had a worse risk factor profile than individuals with the same BMI but with lower waist circumference measures, meaning that the BMI and waist circumference did not predict the risk of metabolic disturbances equally[11]. The greater truncal adipose tissue was distinguished as the real risk factor for the metabolic syndrome [25]. Moreover, the frequency of microalbuminuria in non-diabetic individuals is very low and, therefore, this criterion was relevant only in the presence of diabetes[11].

3.1.2 EGIR definition

In 1999, the European Group for the Study of Insulin Resistance (EGIR) proposed an alternative definition[26], which was called the insulin resistance syndrome. While the WHO definition required an evaluation of insulin resistance under euglycemic hyperinsulinemic conditions and was applied alike to diabetic and non-diabetic subjects, the EGIR definition excluded the diabetic population and relied on fasting insulin as a surrogate marker of insulin resistance. The EGIR definition retained insulin resistance, as an essential component and major etiological determinant of the metabolic syndrome. However, waist circumference was used as surrogate for obesity measured by the BMI; this represented a major deviation in the conceptual development of the metabolic syndrome. In addition, the impaired glucose tolerance was not necessary for the recognition of the metabolic syndrome (Table 2).

EGIR definition of the metabolic syndrome1999[27]
Hyperinsulinaemia defined as fasting insulin concentration above the upper quartile for the non-diabetic subjects* (age and sexes combined) in addition to two or more of the following components:
1. Central obesity: waist circumference ≥ 94 cm in men or ≥ 80 cm in women
2. Dyslipidemia: serum triglycerides (TG) >180 mg/dl and/or HDL-C < 40 mg/dl and/or drug treatment for dyslipidemia
3. Hypertension: systolic blood pressure (SBP) ≥ 140 mmHg or diastolic blood pressure (DBP) ≥ 90 mmHg and/or drug treatment for hypertension
4. Fasting plasma glucose ≥ 110 mg/dL,
* The EGIR insulin resistance syndrome was defined only for non-diabetic subjects.

Table 2. EGIR definition of the metabolic syndrome1999

3.1.3 NCEP-ATPIII definitions

Two years later, the National Education Program's Adult Treatment Panel III (NCEP-ATPIII) formulated another definition, designed to have clinical utility. The ATPIII did not find enough evidence to recommend routine measurement of insulin sensitivity or the 2-hour post-challenge glucose intolerance, but included simply a fasting glucose testing[28]. Additionally, the cut-off points for each component of the cluster and the way of combining them to define the metabolic syndrome differed from the two previous definitions[28]. The ATPIII definition is based on a simple set of common clinical measures and diagnostic criteria, including waist circumference to identify central obesity, raised triglycerides (TG), reduced HDL-C, elevated blood pressure (BP) and raised fasting plasma glucose level. The metabolic syndrome diagnosis was established, when 3 out of 5 listed characteristics were present (Table 3). The ATPIII criteria were widely used in both clinical practice and epidemiological studies. This definition had the advantage of excluding the specific measure of insulin sensitivity, and treated all components with equal importance by avoiding the emphasis on a single cause [29].

NCEP-ATIII definition of the metabolic syndrome 2001[30]
Any 3 of 5 following criteria constituted the diagnosis of metabolic syndrome
1. Central obesity: waist circumference ≥ 102 cm in men or ≥ 88 cm in women
2. Hypertriglyceridamia: serum TG ≥ 150 mg/dl
3. Low HDL-C < 40 mg/dl in men and < 50mg/dl in women
4. Hypertension: SBP ≥ 130 mmHg or DBP ≥ 85 mmHg
5. Fasting plasma glucose ≥ 110 mg/dL

Table 3. NCEP-ATIII definition of the metabolic syndrome 2001

Subsequently, various modifications of the ATPIII definition were developed later by the American Heart Association/National Heart, Lung, Blood Institute (AHA/NHLBI) including adjustment of waist circumference to lower thresholds particularly in ethnic groups, for instance, the Asian American, who are more susceptible to insulin resistance. In addition, TG, HDL-C levels, and BP were counted as abnormal when a person was taking drug treatment for these factors. The threshold for elevated fasting plasma glucose was reduced from ≥ 110 mg/dL to ≥ 100 mg/dL, in accordance with the American Diabetes Association's guidelines [29] (Table 4).

Revised ATPIII definition of the metabolic syndrome 2005[29]
Any 3 of 5 criteria listed below constitute the diagnosis of metabolic syndrome
1. Elevated waist circumference ≥102 cm in men or ≥ 88 cm in women
2. Elevated TG ≥ 150 mg/dl and/or drug treatment for elevated TG*
3. Reduced HDL-C < 40 mg/dl in men and < 50 mg/dl in women and/or drug treatment for reduced HDL-C
4. Elevated BP ≥ 130 mmHg systolic BP or ≥ 85 mmHg diastolic BP or drug treatment for hypertension
5. Elevated fasting plasma glucose ≥ 100 mg/dL and/or drug treatment for elevated glucose
*Fibrates and nicotinic acid are the most commonly used drugs for elevated TG and reduced HDL-C. Patients taking 1 of these drugs were presumed to have high TG and low HDL

Table 4. Revised ATPIII definition of the metabolic syndrome 2005

3.1.4 IDF definition

In parallel, a consensus group, comprising members of the International Diabetes Federation (IDF) and representatives from organizations which contributed to the previous definitions, was formed in 2005 to establish a unified definition for the metabolic syndrome that would be suitable for use in both epidemiological and clinical practice. A major issue for the IDF consensus was that central (abdominal) obesity was a prerequisite risk factor for the diagnosis of the syndrome. The IDF provided, for the first time, different obesity cut-off points for different ethnic groups (Table 5 & 6). Waist circumference was a well accepted proxy measurement for abdominal obesity and served as the first screening test for the metabolic syndrome. The added advantage is that insulin resistance which is difficult to measure in routine clinical practice was not an essential requirement[31].

The IDF definition of the metabolic syndrome 2005[31]
Central obesity (defined as waist circumference with ethnicity specific values) plus any 2 of the following 4 factors:
1. Raised serum TG ≥ 150 mg/dl or specific treatment for this lipid abnormality
2. Reduced HDL-C < 40 mg/dl in men and < 50 mg/dl in women and/or specific treatment for this lipid abnormality
3. Elevated BP ≥ 130 mmHg systolic BP or ≥ 85 mmHg diastolic BP and/or treatment of previously diagnosed hypertension
4. Elevated fasting plasma glucose ≥ 100 mg/dL or previously diagnosed type 2 diabetes.
If Fasting plasma glucose was above 100 mg/dL, oral glucose tolerance test (OGTT) was strongly recommended but was not necessary to define the presence of the metabolic syndrome.

Table 5. The IDF definition of the metabolic syndrome 2005

The underlying principle behind the ethnic-specific thresholds was that for a given waist circumference, Asians, Blacks, Caucasians showed different levels of intra-abdominal adiposity, putting the subjects at different risk levels of cardiovascular disease and diabetes[32].

Country/Ethnic group		Waist circumference
Europids	Male	≥ 94 cm
In the USA, the ATP III values (102 cm male; 88 cm female) are likely to continue to be used for clinical purposes	Female	≥ 80 cm
South Asians	Male	≥ 90 cm
Based on a Chinese, Malay and Asian-Indian population	Female	≥ 80 cm
Chinese	Male	≥ 90 cm
	Female	≥ 80 cm
Japanese	Male	≥ 90 cm
	Female	≥ 80 cm
Ethnic South and Central Americans	Use South Asian recommendations until more specific data are available	
Sub-Saharan Africans	Use European data until more specific data are available	
Eastern Mediterranean and Middle East (Arab) populations	Use European data until more specific data are available	

Table 6. Ethnic specific values for waist circumference

3.1.5 Last Joint Interim Statement

In 2009, a Joint Interim Statement (JIS) of the IDF Task force on Epidemiology and prevention (National Heart, Lung, and Blood Institute; American Heart Association; World Heart Federation; International Atherosclerosis Society; and International Association for the Study of obesity) was published, in an attempt to harmonize the definition. The new definition is also known as Revised IDF 2005. Unlike the first IDF definition, the abdominal obesity should not be an obligatory criterion, though the waist circumference was agreed to be a useful preliminary screening tool. The remaining 4 diagnostic criteria were essentially identical to those provided by the R-ATPIII and IDF. The presence of 3 components out of 5 establishes the diagnosis of metabolic syndrome (Table 7).

This new definition recognizes that the risk associated with a particular waist measurement varies in different populations and ethnic groups. The WHO identified 2 levels of abdominal obesity in European population depending on risk for metabolic complications[34]. An increased risk occurs at waist circumferences of ≥ 94 cm in men or ≥ 80 cm in women, but risk is substantially higher at ≥ 102 cm in men or ≥ 88 cm in women. Until more data from research work become available, it was suggested to use national or regional cut-off points for waist circumference.

To sum up, the abundance of widely varying data, comparing the prevalence of metabolic syndrome by using different criteria across different populations reinforced the need for a standardized definition internationally. Now after the release of the JIS, the current question is whether this new definition is the last word or whether the scientific community needs further reconciliation.

Joint Interim Statement definition of the metabolic syndrome 2009 [33]
Any 3 of 5 criteria listed below constitute the diagnosis of metabolic syndrome
1. Elevated waist circumference according to population- and country-specific definitions (either the IDF or AHA/NHLBI cut points for people of European origin)
2. Elevated TG ≥ 150 mg/dl or drug treatment for elevated TG
3. Reduced HDL-C < 40 mg/dl in men and < 50 mg/dl in women or drug treatment for reduced HDL-C
4. Elevated BP ≥ 130 mmHg systolic BP or ≥ 85 mmHg diastolic BP and/or drug treatment for hypertension
5. Elevated fasting plasma glucose ≥ 100 mg/dL or drug treatment for elevated glucose

Table 7. Last Joint Interim Statement definition of the metabolic syndrome 2009

3.2 Ambiguous pathophysiologic mechanism

The pathogenesis of the metabolic syndrome is currently a subject of crucial discussion. The criteria of metabolic syndrome are interrelated, but the pathophysiology of their relation is not yet fully understood. The long-standing debate about how to define this syndrome led to the appearance of two distinct schools of thought: the insulin resistance-based and the ectopic fat deposition-based hypothesis. So far, both suggested mechanisms remain equivocal and debated.

The basic scientists and endocrinologists support the point of view that the insulin resistance and compensatory hyperinsulinemia are squarely responsible for the metabolic syndrome [13], [21], [35]. According to this group, obesity is thought to exacerbate insulin resistance and thus increase the likelihood of an associated adverse clinical condition. However, the obesity is not considered as a fundamental component of the syndrome, as the clustering of risk factors can occur in insulin resistant individuals of normal weight[36], [37]. The primary goal of this pathophysiological approach is to alert physicians to the idea that patients with insulin resistance are not only at risk for cardiovascular disease, but also to other multiple adverse clinical conditions such as polycystic ovarian syndrome, nonalcoholic fatty liver disease, breast cancer, sleep apnoea. Cardiovascular disease is just one of these important conditions. This group of researchers do not seek strict clinical definition for the metabolic syndrome[38].

In opposition, the other group consists of cardiologists and clinical epidemiologists. This group support the term "metabolic syndrome" and seek to assemble a set of related metabolic risk factors for cardiovascular prevention perspectives. In line with this viewpoint, obesity is considered as a core component of the metabolic syndrome rather than a modulator of the effects of insulin resistance[39]. The primary clinical goal of this school of thought is to suggest an operational tool to be used for long-term risk stratification of atherosclerosis patients [40], [29]. This group supports the idea that the abdominal obesity is the predominant driving force behind the metabolic syndrome and is a particularly detrimental factor in persons who have concomitant metabolic susceptibility from other causes.

Chronologically, the pathophysiological "Insulin Resistance Syndrome" transmuted into clinical "Metabolic Syndrome" in the 1990s[41]. This shift happened to help the scientists to translate science into practice in an area of major medical and public health concern. As insulin resistance was difficult to be measured by the glucose clamp technique, at the population level, fasting plasma insulin levels was used as a proxy to prompt the research for cheap, easy surrogates of insulin resistance[41]. However, this introduced a confusion because of the partial difference in the physiology of hyperinsulinemia and insulin resistance[42], as well as a lack of measurement standardization across studies[41].

Thereafter, anthropometric measures were suggested to replace insulin resistance in new definitions of the metabolic syndrome. The NCEP-ATPIII and particularly the IDF, took the position that obesity (especially abdominal obesity) is a dominant factor behind the multiplication of risk factors. According to the NCEP, the onset of obesity elicits a clustering of risk factors in persons who are metabolically susceptible[40].

In sum, the metabolic susceptibility has many contributing factors, including genetic forms of insulin resistance, increased abdominal fat, ethnic and racial influences, physical inactivity, advancing age, endocrine dysfunction, and genetic diversity[43]. However, the relevance of this application has not yet exclusively been established by the research[41].

3.3 Uncertain clinical utility

Although the suggested definitions provided some uniformity to researchers, a considerable confusion about the precise clinical utility of the "metabolic syndrome" exists and remains controversial.

The major polemic emerged in 2005 when a joint committee of the American Diabetes Association (ADA) and from the European Association for the Study of Diabetes (EASD) published a critical appraisal of the metabolic syndrome concept, and of its diagnostic utility in clinical practice[22]. This group of researchers opposed extending the concept of the metabolic syndrome to clinical practice and objected to characterize the metabolic syndrome as a risk factor for heart disease or diabetes[22], [44]. The claim was that the primary clinical emphasis should remain on treating the individual risk factors and that aggregating them into a syndrome has little clinical utility. Moreover, creating a diagnostic category of the metabolic syndrome was criticized by Reaven himself who was a pioneer in systemizing the concept of a risk factor syndrome. Reaven believed that this effort had little clinical or pedagogic utility and if necessary the WHO approach was the most rational one[44]. In this line, the WHO Expert Consultation, who edited the first definition 10 years earlier, released in 2009 a Position Statement, pertaining to evaluate the relevance and the clinical utility of the metabolic syndrome concept[38]. The statement critically concluded that though the metabolic syndrome may be considered useful as an educational concept, it has limited practical utility as a diagnostic or management tool.

The counter arguments, represented principally by the IDF and AHA, advocated that the diagnosis of the metabolic syndrome helps physicians to discover persons at increased lifetime risk for cardiovascular disease [45], [46]. They believe that the metabolic syndrome is a simple useful tool to call attention to patients who are at high lifetime risk for both atherosclerotic cardiovascular disease and diabetes; such persons deserve increased attention in clinical management and monitoring[23], [26], [29], [22],[44]. Grundy was the scientist who most thoroughly advocated the clinical utility of the metabolic syndrome, by linking the importance of clinical metabolic syndrome recognition to an "iceberg phenomenon"[43]. He explained that identifying the metabolic syndrome provides a simple means of recognising the risk, submerged in a tangle of metabolic derangement[43]. According to Grundy, seeing the tip of the iceberg can be lifesaving because most of the danger lies below. The same is true in case of finding aggregated metabolic signs such as high TG, low HDL-C, impaired fasting plasma glucose, and mildly elevated BP in a patient with an increased waist circumference [43].

Although the metabolic syndrome seemed to provide little advantage over the available risks scores (Framingham or European SCORE)[47], [22], several clinicians believe that the clinical diagnosis is useful because it determines the therapeutic strategy in patients at higher risk[43]. Moreover, the application of the available cardiovascular disease risk scores is still cumbersome and not routinely used in clinical practice. The metabolic syndrome may thus represent a simple convenient alternative tool to identify individuals at increased risk of atherosclerotic cardiovascular disease or type 2 diabetes mellitus[48], [46]. Beyond risk assessment, the presence of the metabolic syndrome can alert clinicians to the likelihood of related pathological conditions, e.g. obstructive sleep apnoea, fatty liver, cholesterol gallstones, and polycystic ovarian disease[45]. In addition, it helps to recognize that patients with a clustering of measured risk factors usually have several hidden metabolic risk factors, e.g, a prothrombotic state, a proinflammatory state, and multiple lipoprotein abnormalities[29], [46].

3.4 Debated therapeutic strategies

Globally, there are two viewpoints about the best therapeutic strategy for patients with the metabolic syndrome. One conventional approach holds that each of the metabolic risk factors should be singled out and treated separately. However, the concern about this prescription is that it may lead to an aggressive use of medications at the expense of lifestyle therapies, particularly, weight reduction and increased exercise[43]. Alternatively, the other view emphasizes the global approach that aims to implement lifestyle therapies to reduce all risk factors simultaneously. It targets multiple risk factors together by striking at the underlying causes. Treating the underlying causes does not rule out the management of individual risk factors, but it may reinforce the control of multiple risk factors[43]. In practice, there is a tendency to switch from a vertical approach (by speciality) to a multidisciplinary horizontal approach, which enables early detection of the combination of risk factors, sometimes without obvious illness, as measure of effective prevention. So far, there is no proof that the lifestyle modification interventions targeting the metabolic syndrome are superior to those targeting the individual components[22], [48]. Recently, a new study published in 2010 analyzed data from the INTERHEART study, a case-control study of incident acute myocardial infarction that involved 12 297 cases and 14 606 controls from 52 countries. The results suggested that patients with metabolic syndrome are not at higher risk of future myocardial infarction than those with diabetes or hypertension alone[49]. The results strongly suggested that treating the individual risk factors is rather better than focusing on the metabolic syndrome, supporting therefore, the individual risk-factor approach.

3.5 Predictability of the metabolic syndrome to cardiovascular risk

One of the most important criticisms addressed to the concept of the metabolic syndrome was its efficiency to properly evaluate the global cardiovascular disease risk in clinical practice. The plethora of epidemiological, metabolic and clinical studies, published over the last 2 decades, have demonstrated that the different definitions of the metabolic syndrome were able to identify subgroups of patients at greater risk of type 2 diabetes[50] and at increased relative risk of coronary heart disease[51], [52]. Nevertheless, none of these definitions can properly assess global cardiovascular disease risk [32].

Many prospective studies documented the relation of metabolic syndrome to cardiovascular risk, particularly to cardiovascular morbidity, mortality as well as all-cause mortality. In the Kuopio Ischemic Heart Disease Risk Factor Study, a population-based, prospective cohort study of 1209 Finnish men aged 42 to 60 years, the 10-year cardiovascular disease risk was increased 2.1- and 2.5-fold with the ATP III and WHO definitions, respectively[3]. The same study found that the risk of death from cardiovascular disease was increased by 2.6–3 times, and the risk of all-cause mortality was increased 1.9–2.1 times with the presence of metabolic syndrome. The DECODE project, based on 11 prospective European cohort studies, comprising 6156 men and 5356 women, aged from 30 to 89 years reported that the overall hazard ratios for all-cause and cardiovascular mortality in non-diabetic persons with the metabolic syndrome were 1.44 and 2.26 in men and 1.38 and 2.78 in women, respectively[12]. In the WOSCOPS (West of Scotland Coronary Prevention) Study, a modified NCEP definition predicted CHD events, in the multivariate model incorporating conventional risk factors (hazard ratio=1.30). Men with 4 or 5 features of the metabolic syndrome had a 3.7-fold increase in risk for CHD and a 24.5-fold increase for diabetes compared with men without the syndrome [53]. In Botnia study, carried out on 4483 subjects, aged 35-70 years, followed for 7 years in Finland and Sweden, the risk for coronary heart disease and stroke was increased 3-fold in subjects with the WHO defined metabolic syndrome. Cardiovascular mortality was also markedly increased in subjects with the syndrome compared to those without it (12.0% vs. 2.2%, $P < 0.001$)[2].

In sum, the use of different definitions of the metabolic syndrome led to inconsistent results on its association with the risk of cardiovascular disease [51]. Systematic research reviews showed that the cardiovascular risk, conferred by the different definitions, varied between populations; in most studies, it was lower with the IDF definition as compared to other alternatives[54], [51]. In addition, two recent meta-analyses of longitudinal studies, showed that the relative risk of cardiovascular disease associated with the metabolic syndrome was higher in women compared to men[52], and higher in studies that used the WHO definition compared to studies that used the NCEP-ATP III definition[51].

3.6 Predictability of the metabolic syndrome to type 2 diabetes

The most important clinical dimension of the metabolic syndrome is its association with the risk of development of type 2 diabetes. Several prospective studies indicated that the metabolic syndrome predicts type 2 diabetes[24], [55], [56]. People with the syndrome were over 4 times as likely to develop type 2 diabetes compared with subjects who did not have it[1], although without excluding the diabetic subjects, this might not be surprising, since impaired fasting glucose (IFG) and impaired glucose tolerance (IGT) are components of the WHO definition[16]. In addition, neither the ATP III nor the IDF criteria excluded hyperglycaemia as 1 of the 5 criteria for the diagnosis of the metabolic syndrome. By these criteria, most patients with type 2 diabetes mellitus have the metabolic syndrome. In the San Antonio Heart Study, the NCEP definition of the metabolic syndrome predicted diabetes better than the WHO definition, independently of other factors. It was suggested therefore to lower the fasting glucose cut-off points to improve the diabetes prediction [55].

Despite the above data, there is an ongoing controversy as to whether the metabolic syndrome is associated with increased cardiovascular and diabetes risk or is simply a sum of the risk of the associated components: glucose tolerance, elevated blood pressure, dyslipidemia, and abdominal obesity[9]. According to a recent research review, aimed to examine the ability of the metabolic syndrome to predict vascular events and incident diabetes, the number of existing studies appeared limited to draw definite conclusions[54] and the metabolic syndrome predicts diabetes much more efficiently in non-diabetic individuals[57].

4. Evolution toward a new global "cardiometabolic risk" concept

The traditional risk assessment algorithms (Framingham, PROCAM or European SCORE, etc.) take into account classical risk factors such as age, sex, family history, blood pressure, smoking, cholesterol (both LDL and HDL), and diabetes. However, these risk assessment tools do not capture the risk of abdominal obesity and the related abnormalities of the metabolic syndrome. This is especially important with the recent sweeping epidemic of abdominal obesity, where many individuals are at increased risk of cardiovascular disease because of the presence of a constellation of metabolic abnormalities. It has been suggested that the cardiovascular disease risk of abdominal obesity and/or metabolic syndrome may be independent from or go beyond the risk predicted by traditional risk factors [32]. Moreover, the Framingham risk score does not assess properly lifetime risk particularly among young adults with abdominal obesity and metabolic syndrome who may not be considered at elevated risk of cardiovascular disease because of their young age[45]. Therefore, the existing cardiovascular disease risk assessment tools proved cumbersome in clinical practice and were not sufficient to adequately capture the additional risk related to the metabolic syndrome, such as the abdominal obesity, insulin resistance and related complications [32].

On the other hand, the metabolic syndrome as a clinical entity could not improve prediction of risk of cardiovascular disease [47], [22], because it did not incorporate important traditional risk factors, such as smoking, age and gender[45]. The current recommendations stress the need to focus on the assessment of the total burden of risk, the so-called global risk profile, rather than on individual or particular risk factor. This is because, the absolute risk of an acute coronary event depends on the totality of interacting risk determinants; some associated with adult lifestyle, others operating from early childhood[58].

On the whole, the presence of metabolic syndrome alone cannot predict global cardiovascular disease risk, nor do the available risk scores. Meanwhile, better risk assessment algorithms are needed to quantify diabetes and cardiovascular disease risk on a global scale[59]. This unremitting debate, as to whether the metabolic syndrome increases cardiovascular disease risk beyond the risk posed by traditional cardiovascular disease risk factors, has spurred the creation of a new concept named the global "cardiometabolic risk (CMR)". In order to move the field forward, a multidisciplinary International Chair on CMR was created, at the end of 2005, to provide a platform to discuss the concepts of abdominal obesity, metabolic syndrome, and global cardiovascular disease risk[32].

Global CMR is defined as the risk of cardiovascular disease resulting from the presence of traditional risk factors along with features of the metabolic syndrome [32], [59]. Under this model, CMR encompasses the overall cardiovascular disease risk, resulting from traditional risk factors (age, sex, smoking, hypertension, LDL cholesterol, HDL cholesterol, diabetes) and from the additional risks of intra-abdominal obesity or related features of the metabolic syndrome [32]. Under this working model, the metabolic syndrome is one of the potentially modifiable cardiovascular disease risk factors, besides smoking (Figure 1). It has been suggested that the cardiovascular risk of abdominal obesity/metabolic syndrome may be independent of or go beyond the risk predicted by traditional risk factors.

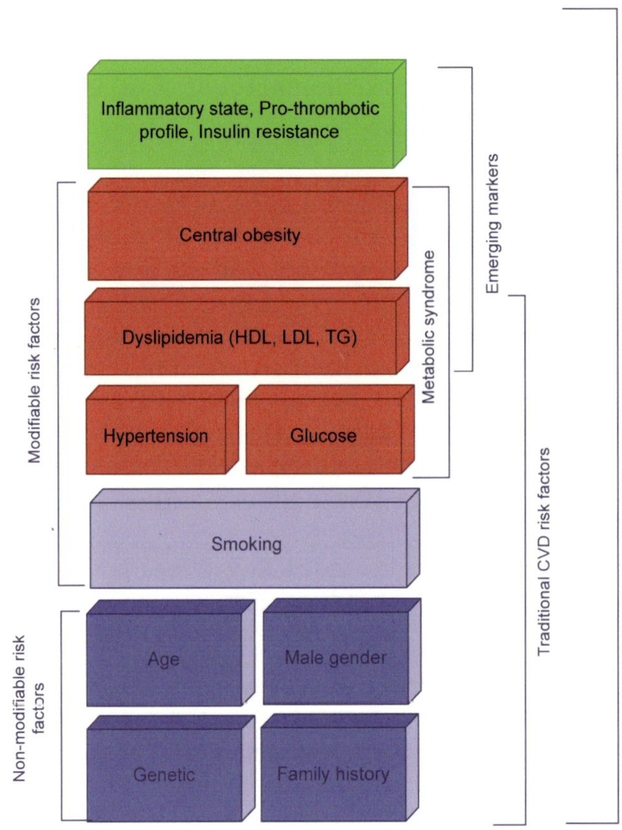

Fig. 1. The "building blocks" of global cardiometabolic risk, with adaptation from Desprès et al[32].

5. Epidemiology of metabolic syndrome

The metabolic syndrome is a cluster of cardiovascular risk factors associated with an increased risk of type 2 diabetes mellitus and cardiovascular morbidity and mortality[3]. This section aims to shed light on the current state-of-art with regards to the prevalence of the metabolic syndrome worldwide and its key determinants. Understanding the epidemiology of the metabolic syndrome, as regards the variation of its frequencies and its potential determinants, are essential pre-requisites to addressing public health needs.

5.1 Prevalence of metabolic syndrome

The multiplicity of prevalence data suggest that the metabolic syndrome is common worldwide, especially among older people and in certain ethnic populations[15]. The syndrome will undoubtedly become even more common over time, in parallel with the exploding epidemic of obesity and type 2 diabetes[60]. In addition, the worldwide increase in the prevalence of metabolic syndrome among children and adolescents[61], constitutes a greater public health concern, as emerging evidence has suggested that children with the metabolic syndrome increase their risk of developing adverse cardiovascular events later in life[62].

In this setting, the present section describes and compares the metabolic syndrome prevalence rates reported in different studies, carried out during the current decade, in various countries all over the world. A thorough literature search for publications, documenting the prevalence of the metabolic syndrome according to the existing definitions, was conducted with an emphasis on international prevalence comparison. The reported worldwide prevalence rates of the metabolic syndrome are depicted in Table 8 (A-D).

Globally, the prevalence of the metabolic syndrome was different across the countries in terms of gender, age groups and ethnicity, regardless of the definition used. In US population, the IDF definition led to a higher prevalence estimate (39%) than that based on the R-ATPIII criteria (34.5%)[63]. A spectacular increase in the prevalence was recorded among the same population, from 24% in 1988[63] to 34.5% in 2002[64], by using the NCEP-ATPIII definition. This raise was attributed to the increase in the prevalence of obesity between 1988 and 2000, as well as the aging of the population[65]. In European studies, the prevalence of the metabolic syndrome varied considerably between 18% in Italy[66] and 38% in Turkey[67]. The metabolic syndrome was also frequent in Middle Eastern countries[68] and India[69], although the lowest prevalence rates were recorded in Australia[70], and china[71]. Generally, the IDF criteria gave a higher prevalence rate as compared to the NCEP-ATPIII[60]. This was undoubtedly attributable to the lower waist circumference threshold to define the abdominal obesity criterion. The WHO criteria variably induced a higher prevalence rate when compared to the NCEP-ATPIII definition [60].

Irrespective of the criteria, studies were inconsistent regarding the gender-specific metabolic syndrome prevalence. While the metabolic syndrome was higher among men than women in France[72], [73], Germany[50], Ireland[74], Singapore[75], it was higher in Omani[68], Chinese[71] and Indian women[69]. In addition, accumulating evidence demonstrated that the prevalence of the metabolic syndrome was highly age-dependent, so as its individual components[15]. The prevalence increases with age through the sixth decade of life among men and seventh decade among women [76]. Race/ethnicity influenced also the prevalence of the metabolic syndrome. Some ethnic groups have a higher predisposition to central obesity than others: for example, the prevalence of central obesity is higher among South Asians than in Europeans. Asian populations have more metabolic abnormalities with the same obesity than do the Caucasians[71]. Thus, a modification of the waist circumference cut-off values of the NCEP-ATPIII definition has been proposed for Asian populations. By applying the European definition of waist circumference, the prevalence of metabolic syndrome was generally lower among Asian populations than among European populations, however, when modified Asian waist circumference criteria were used, the prevalence of metabolic syndrome increased and became similar (Korean population)[77] to or even higher (urban Indians)[69] than European populations. In USA, NCEP ATPIII-defined metabolic syndrome is more prevalent in Mexican Americans (31.9%) than in Caucasian (23.8%) and African American (21.6%)[7]. Ford et al reported that the metabolic syndrome was more common in Black and Hispanic women than in both counterpart men, which contrasted with the similar gender prevalence for Whites [7].

Country, year of publication	Acronym, setting and period of data collection	Study design	Age group and subjects number	Definition	subject's characteristics	Age-adjusted Prevalence of metabolic syndrome
USA, 2002[7]	Third National Health and Nutrition Examination Survey (NHANESIII), 1988-1994	Cross-sectional population-based sample	≥20years (8814 subjects)	NCEP ATPIII	White	23.8%*
					Mexican American	31.9%*
					African American	21.6%*
					Other	20.3%*
USA, 2004[84]	Dearborn, Michigan, 2004	Cross-sectional, random sample	20-75years, (542 subjects)	NCEP ATPIII	Arab Americans population	23% *
				WHO		28% *
USA, 2003[64]	Third National Health and Nutrition Examination Survey (NHANESIII), 1988-1994	Cross-sectional, representative sample	≥ 20 years, (8608 participants)	NCEP ATPIII	Total	23.9%*
					Men	24.2% *
					Women	23.5%*
				WHO	Total	25.1%*
					Men	27.9%*
					Women	22.6%*
USA, 2005[63]	National Health and Nutrition Examination Survey (NHANES), 1999-2002	Cross-sectional population-based sample	≥ 20years (3601 subjects)	NCEP ATPIII	Total	34.5%
					Men	33.7%
					Women	35.4%
				IDF	Total	39%
					Men	39.9%
					Women	38.1%

*Non age-adjusted prevalence rate
A Prevalence of the metabolic syndrome in USA

Table 8. Prevalence of the metabolic syndrome in different countries.

In fact, the cross-sectional and longitudinal epidemiological studies provided markedly different prevalence and incidence rates of the metabolic syndrome, because of the lack of internationally agreed-upon criteria to define the syndrome. The NHANES III surveys carried out in USA, aimed at comparing the prevalence of the metabolic syndrome according to the WHO and NCEP-ATPIII definitions, demonstrated a substantial discordance for gender and ethnicity[64]. The IDF definition, led generally to higher estimates of the prevalence, in all ethnic groups, especially among Mexican American men

[63]. An elevated IDF prevalence of the metabolic syndrome was similarly observed in other international studies[70], [78], [79], [66], [80], [67], [81]. In 8 European cohorts (DECODE Study), the metabolic syndrome prevalence rate defined according to the WHO, NCEP-ATPIII and EGIR varied widely among countries; the WHO definition showed particularly a wide gender-specific difference[82]. In Bruneck Italian Study, the prevalence of metabolic syndrome was significantly higher and almost doubled with the WHO criteria as compared to those of the NCEP (34.1% vs 17.8% respectively)[46].

Apart from definitions diversity, the wide variation of published data made direct international comparisons exceedingly difficult, because of important methodological differences with respect to the characteristics of target population, the study design, the sample selection, and the year of conduct.

In sum, the emerging prevalence data from population-based studies suggest that the metabolic syndrome is a quite common cardiometabolic disorder worldwide with a wide gender discrepancy. A very consistent finding was that the prevalence of the metabolic syndrome increased dramatically with age and varied considerably across ethnic groups. Racial/ethnic waist circumference component heterogeneity gave rise to substantial racial/ethnic variation in the prevalence of the metabolic syndrome itself. The use of different definitions in diverse populations resulted in wide ranging prevalence rates, thus highlighting the urgent need for a unified definition[83]. Moreover, only a few international studies reported age-adjusted prevalence rates, to enable meaningful comparison.

Australia, 2005[70]	Adelaide, south Australia study,	Random household sample	≥ 18 years, (4060 subjects)	NCEP ATPIII	Total	15%
					Men	15.7%
					Women	14.4%
				IDF	Total	22.8%
					Men	26.4%
					Women	19.4%

B Prevalence of the metabolic syndrome in Australia

Table 8. Prevalence of the metabolic syndrome in different countries.

Country, year of publication	Acronym, setting and period of data collection	Study design	Age group and subjects number	Definition	Subject's characteristics	Age-adjusted Prevalence rate
Europe, 2005[82]	The DECODE Study Group, 1991, except in Spain (1996-1997)	Seven cross-sectional European population-based studies	30-77years, (9140 subjects), Non-diabetic Europeans	WHO	Men	26.9%
					Women	19.5%
				EGIR	Men	17.9%
					Women	16.5%
				NCEP ATPIII	Men	22.7%
					Women	23.1%
Germany, 2008[50]	The European Prospective	Multi-centre, prospective cohort study	35-65years, (2796 subjects)	Revised NCEP ATPIII	Total	22.5% *
					Men	29.1%*
					Women	18.5%*

Country, year of publication	Acronym, setting and period of data collection	Study design	Age group and subjects number	Definition	Subject's characteristics	Age-adjusted Prevalence rate
	Investigation into Cancer and Nutrition-Potsdam Study (EPIC) Potsdam, 1994-1998			IDF	Total	28.3% *
					Men	33.2%*
					Women	25.2% *
France, 2006[72]	D.E.S.I.R Study, centre-western France, 1994-1996	Volunteered for health check-up	5446 subjects, 30-64 years	Revised NCEP ATPIII	Men	15%
					Women	10.1%
France, 2003[73]	Centre IPC (Investigation Préventives et Cliniques), Paris, 1999-2002	Volunteered for health check-up	62000 subjects, (mean age 53.2+/-9.1years)	Revised NCEP ATPIII	Men	11.8%*
					Women	7.6%*
Norway, 2007[78]	Nord-Trondelag Heart Study(HUNT 2), 1995-1997	Cross-sectional population-based sample	20-89 years, (10206 subjects	Revised NCEP ATPIII		25.9%*
				IDF		29.6%*
Finland, 2007[79]	The Cardiovascular risk in Yong Finns Study, 1986-2001	Population-based follow-up study	2182 subjects, 24-39 years	Revised NCEP ATPIII	Total	13%
				EGIR		9.8%
				IDF		14.3%
Ireland, 2003[74]	Primary care setting in the South of Ireland.	Random sample of attended subjects for screening from 17 general practice lists	50–69 years, (1,018 subjects)	WHO	Total	21%*
					Men	24.6%*
					Women	17.8%*
				NCEP-ATPIII	Total	20.7%*
					Men	21.8%*
					Women	21.5%*
Italy, 2003[46]	Bruneck Study, 1990	Prospective population-based survey	40–79 years, 888 subjects	WHO		34.1%*
				NCEP ATPIII		17.8%*
Italy, 2007[66]	FIBAR study,	Sample of individuals enrolled in a	2,945 subjects, mean age	Revised NCEP ATPIII	Total	16.6%*
				IDF		29.7%*

Country, year of publication	Acronym, setting and period of data collection	Study design	Age group and subjects number	Definition	Subject's characteristics	Age-adjusted Prevalence rate
		screening program for diabetes	55.2+/-11.5 years			
Spain, 2003[85]	Nutritional Survey of the Canary Islands (ENCA), 1997-1998)	Population-based study	18-74 years, 578 adults	NCEP ATPIII	Total	24.4%*
Spain, 2007	Province of Albacete	Cross-sectional, Population-based study	40-70 years, 425 subjects	Adapted NCEP ATPIII	Total	20.9%
Greece, 2007[86]	Greece	cross-sectional, a representative sample	adults, 9669 subjects	NCEP-ATP-III		23.3%
				Revised NCEP ATPIII		22.6%
				IDF		18.3%
Portugal, 2007[80]	Porto	Representative random sample, Population-based study	18-92 years,1433 subjects	WHO	adult residents	26.4%
				NCEP ATPIII 2001		24%
				IDF		41.9%
				AHA/NHLBI 2005		37.2%
Portugal, 2008[87]	VALSIM Study	Primary health care users	18-96 years, 16,856 subjects	NCEP ATPIII	total	27.5%
					Alentejo region	30.99%
					Algrave region	24.42%
Turkey, 2007[67]	Turkish Heart Study, 2003	Cross-sectional population-based sample	mean age 45± 13 years, (1568 subjects)	WHO	General adult population	19%
				EGIR		20%
				NCEP ATPIII		38%
				IDF		42%
Luxembourg, 2011[88]	ORISCAV-LUX survey, Luxembourg, 2007-2008	Cross-sectional population-based sample	18-69 years, 1432 subjects	R-ATP III	General adult population	24.7%*
				JIS (94/80cm)		28.0%*

C Prevalence of the metabolic syndrome in European countries

Table 8. Prevalence of the metabolic syndrome in different countries

Country, year of publication	Acronym, setting and period of data collection	Study design	Age group and subjects number	Definition	subject's characteristics	Age-adjusted Prevalence rate
Oman, 2003[68]	Nizwa study, 2001	Cross-sectional population-based sample	≥ 20years, (1419 subjects)	NCEP ATPIII	Total	21%
					Men	19.5%
					Women	23%
Chile, 2008[81]	Talca city study, year of data collection not mentioned	Probabilistic sample	18-74 years, (1007 subjects)	Revised NCEP ATPIII		29.5%
				IDF		36.4%
China, 2006[71]	The Chinese Multiprovincial Study, 1992	Prospective cohort study	35-64 years, (26972 subjects)	ATPIII according to Asian criteria of waist circumference	Men (≥ 90cm)	14.4%
					Women (≥ 80cm)	20%
				IDF according to Asian criteria of waist circumference	Men (≥ 90cm)	9.8%
					Women (≥ 80cm)	16.6%
South Korea, 2004[77]	Mokdong Study of Diabetes Prevalence, 1997	Random cluster sample	30-80 years, (1804 subjects)	ATPIII based on Asia-Pacific guidelines	Men (≥ 90cm)	29%*
					Women (≥ 80cm)	16.8%*
				ATPIII	Men (≥ 102 cm)	16%*
					Women ≥ 88cm)	10.7%*
South Korea, 2006[89]	Korean National Health and Nutrition Examination survey, 1998	Stratified multistage probability sampling design	20-80 years, (6824 subjects)	IDF (with specific waist circumference cut-off points)	Men (≥ 90cm)	13.5%
					Women (≥ 85cm)	15%
India, 2004[69]	Urban Indian population study	Population-based study	>20 years, (1123 subjects)	ATPIII	Total	24.9%
					Men	18.4%
					Women	30.9%
Seychelles (Indian Ocean, African region), 2008[90]	Seychelles Heart Study III, 2004	Cross-sectional, Population-based study	25-64 years, (1218 subjects)	WHO	Men	25%*
					Women	24.6%*
				ATPIII	Men	24%*
					Women	32.2%*
				IDF	Men	25.1%*
					Women	35.4%*
Singapore, 2004[75]	Singapore National Health Survey, 1998	Population-based study	18-69 years, (4723 subjects)	NCEP	Men (all races)	13.1%
					Chinese	10.8%
					Malays	17.3%
					Asian Indians	21.7%
					Women (all races)	11%
					Chinese	8.3%

Country, year of publication	Acronym, setting and period of data collection	Study design	Age group and subjects number	Definition	subject's characteristics	Age-adjusted Prevalence rate
					Malays	20%
					Asian Indians	19.3%
				NCEP-Asian criteria (Waist circumference 90 cm in men and 80 cm in women)	Men (all races)	20.9%
					Chinese	18.1%
					Malays	24.7%
					Asian Indians	32.4%
					Women (all races)	15.5%
					Chinese	12.5%
					Malays	23.8%
					Asian Indians	25.8%

D Prevalence of the metabolic syndrome in Asian countries

Table 8. Prevalence of the metabolic syndrome in different countries

5.2 Potential determinants of the metabolic syndrome

At every stage of life, health is determined by complex interactions between a multitude of factors that influence a person's disease or health status. With regards to the metabolic syndrome, the determinants which are centrally involved in its multi-factorial causation can be categorized as: biological or genetic susceptibility; socio-economic; environmental and behavioural factors.

5.2.1 Biological or genetic susceptibility

Although twin and family studies showed a high heritability for each of the individual components [91], the genetic basis of the metabolic syndrome, as a composite phenotype, has not yet been thoroughly investigated. A number of researches indicated a genetic susceptibility of the metabolic syndrome. However, the associations were weak and the replication of findings was poor[92], [93]. While the prevalence of the metabolic syndrome has increased markedly in the last decades, the human genome has not changed. At present, no single gene or cluster of genes has been consistently replicated for the expression of this phenotype (metabolic syndrome) among different populations[94], [95], probably due to the complex interactions between gene and environment.

The 'thrifty genotype' hypothesis was proposed to explain the emergence of insulin resistance and diabetes in populations, shifted from vigorous activity to provide subsistence nutrition to sedentary life style with food abundance. In urban societies, the modern abundant food environment may be responsible for the elevated insulin levels and excessive energy stores in some type 2 diabetic individuals, leading in consequence to insulin resistance and obesity[96].

Genetic background can interact with habitual dietary fat composition, thereby affecting predisposition to the metabolic syndrome, and may also determine the individual's responsiveness to altered dietary fat intake[97]. Recent research indicates that currently ineffective therapeutic dietary recommendations may require a 'personalised nutrition' approach, wherein the genetic profile may determine the responsiveness of patients to specific dietary fatty acid interventions[98].

5.2.2 Socio-economic determinants

Several prospective observational studies showed that low socio-economic position, measured as education level, income, or occupational class was associated with increased risk for type 2 diabetes[99] and coronary heart disease[100], [101]. Clinical features of the metabolic syndrome were more commonly observed among socio-economically disadvantaged individuals[102], in individuals with low education level[103], [104], and in those doing menial jobs[105]. There is increasing evidence that the distribution of the metabolic syndrome varies among different geographic and socioeconomic categories of the population, demonstrating notable health inequalities[106], [107], [108].

5.2.3 Behavioural or lifestyle determinants

Lifestyle choices imposed by modern civilization have been demonstrated to be centrally involved in the multi-factorial causation of severe atherosclerotic disease [108]. There has been an increasing body of evidence demonstrating that unhealthy behaviours were substantially responsible for epidemic prevalence and mortality of cardiovascular disease, diabetes and metabolic disorders[4], [5], [109]. In contrast, a healthy lifestyle including non-smoking, appropriate diet, satisfactory physical activity level and healthy weight provided substantial cardiovascular and metabolic benefits[110]. Among the major potentially modifiable risk factors for metabolic syndrome and its components are the following:

1. Smoking

Growing evidence pointed to smoking as an independent risk factor for metabolic syndrome and type 2 diabetes. Smoking is a strong risk factor for atherosclerotic cardiovascular disease, with a dose dependent relationship[111], [112]. Several population-based studies confirmed that cigarette smoking was independently associated with the metabolic syndrome [113], [114], [115], in particular in men[116]. The general belief is that insulin resistance or hyperinsulinemia is the main underlying mechanism. Increased insulin resistance may underlie the clustering of the metabolic and hemodynamic abnormalities that have potential atheroslerotic properties, designated the metabolic syndrome [14]. However, this hypothesis still needs to be tested in prospective studies.

2. Dietary habits

Although dietary intake has been linked to individual components of the metabolic syndrome [117], [118], [119], [97], the role of diet in its origin is not well understood[120]. Cross-sectional epidemiological studies demonstrated that dietary intake rich in whole-grain foods was linked to a lower prevalence of the metabolic syndrome [121], [122], although other study found no relation[123]. Dairy intake was inversely associated with the metabolic syndrome both prospectively and in cross-sectional studies [124,125]. Greater intakes of fruits and vegetables were associated with a lower prevalence of the metabolic syndrome [126]. Intakes of soft drinks were also positively associated with the prevalence of the metabolic syndrome, but the diet soda-metabolic syndrome incidence association was not yet hypothesized and needs further prospective studies [127].

Although various individual foods and nutrients were associated with the development or the progression of the metabolic syndrome, only a few studies examined the association with dietary patterns[128]. Prospective findings from Atherosclerosis Risk in Communities (ARIC) study suggested that consumption of a Western dietary pattern, meat, and fried foods promoted the incidence of the metabolic syndrome, whereas dairy consumption provided some protection[120].

Recently, dietary pattern analysis has emerged as an alternative and complementary approach to examine the relationship between diet and the risk of chronic diseases. Instead of looking at individual nutrients or foods, pattern analysis examines the effects of overall diet. Conceptually, dietary patterns address the effect of the diet as a whole and thus may provide a broader picture of food and nutrient consumption, and may thus be more predictive of disease risk than individual foods or nutrients[129], [130].

3. Alcohol consumption

Across the literature, the association between alcohol consumption and the metabolic syndrome is controversial and influenced by several factors, due to broad overlap of alcohol consumption with different components of metabolic syndrome. Protective and detrimental associations were reported between alcohol consumption and the metabolic syndrome, due to variations in drinking patterns and different alcohol effects on the metabolic syndrome components[131]. Mild to moderate alcohol consumption is associated with a lower prevalence of the metabolic syndrome, with a favourable influence on lipids, waist circumference, and fasting insulin. This association was strongest among whites and among beer and wine drinkers[132].

A recent meta-analysis study, aiming to support the evidence available regarding the relationship between alcohol consumption and the metabolic syndrome, as well as to identify the gender-specific dose-response, showed that alcohol consumption of less than 40 g/day in men and 20 g/day in women significantly reduced the prevalence of metabolic syndrome [133].

4. Physical activity

In agreement with the notion that physical inactivity is a risk factor of diabetes, obesity, dyslipidemia and hypertension[134], [135], [136], the prevalence of the metabolic syndrome was higher in subjects with poor physical activities[46], [137].

Sedentary behaviour is an important potential determinant of the metabolic syndrome. Several studies demonstrated that physical activity was inversely associated with the prevalence of the metabolic syndrome[138], [139], notably among those who spend much time in sedentary activity as watching television or video or using a computer[137]. The adverse effect of excess television watching on obesity and other cardiovascular risk factors is thought to be attributed, in part, to decreased energy expenditure and, in other pat, to increased energy intake. Therefore, understanding how sedentary behaviour relates to the metabolic syndrome may provide new opportunities for clinical and public health approaches in its prevention and control.

5. Psychosocial factors

Accumulating evidence implied that psychological mechanisms were possibly underlying the development of the metabolic syndrome. The syndrome appeared to be triggered by adverse psycho-social circumstances[140], certain chronic psychological pathologies[141,142] and chronic stress[102]. Individuals who had hostile personality and certain behaviour traits, were particularly predisposed to develop the metabolic syndrome [102]. Such factors might interact with others to encourage the development of metabolic syndrome. The stress is exacerbated by lack of social support and/or poor coping skills. As a vicious cycle, the negative psychological behaviours may induce unhealthy lifestyle and/or adverse social circumstances[143]. A large population study demonstrated a higher incidence of the metabolic syndrome among young women, but not in men, with a history of depression after controlling for other associated factors [141]. Features of the metabolic syndrome also appeared more common among women experiencing social anxiety [144]. These findings suggest the possibility of different gender-specific causal pathways to the metabolic syndrome development.

5.2.4 Environmental factors

Recently, the scientific evidence linking air pollution to heart attacks, strokes and cardiovascular death, has been substantially supported, especially for the fine particulate matter (PM). The major source of PM is fossil fuel combustion from industry, traffic, and power generation. Biomass burning, heating, cooking, indoor activities and forest fires may also be relevant sources, particularly in certain regions[145].

Several interrelated pathophysiologic mechanisms underlying the observed short-term and long-term [146]adverse cardiac effects of ambient air pollution have been elucidated[147], for instance, the pivotal role of vascular inflammation in pathogenesis and progression of atherosclerosis and coronary heart disease. Systemic inflammatory response to inhaled ambient particles has emerged as an important mediator of the PM-associated acute cardiac effects[148]. However, human data are still scant and conflicting with respect to the pathophysiologic mediators of cardiovascular disease associated with long-term exposure to fine PM. Researchers hypothesized that long-term exposure is associated with increased systemic inflammation, and that people with metabolic syndrome have a higher degree of inflammatory responses to PM.

5.2.5 Emergent factors

In a recent research study, a growing number of other factors, called "emerging or novel risk factors", have been described and linked with features of the metabolic syndrome. Several new bio-markers or candidate cardiovascular risk factors have been proposed as significant predictors of the atherosclerotic disease and its complications. These include inflammatory-, hemostasis or thrombosis-, lipid-related markers, oxidative stress, hormonal factors and infectious agents [149], [150], [151], [152], [153], [154]. Over the past few years, the concept of atherosclerosis as an inflammatory disorder has been substantially established[155]. However, the role of systematic inflammation needs further exploration. The novel bio-markers, psychological and environmental determinants are outside the scope of the present chapter and hence will not be further detailed.

6. Conclusion

The metabolic syndrome is a multi-factorial disorder and its development is the result of interactions between biological, behavioural and environmental factors. Despite disagreement over the relevance and clinical utility of the metabolic syndrome, most investigators agree that the clustering of metabolic risk factors is a real and relatively common phenomenon[60]. Around the world, the metabolic syndrome is now considered as one of the major public health challenges of the 21st century, associated with a 5-fold and 2- to 3-fold increase in type 2 diabetes and cardiovascular disease, respectively [32]. In consequence, the related premature morbidity and mortality could overcharge the health care system budgets of both developed and developing countries[16].

The introduction of the metabolic syndrome concept was a stimulus for a large number of epidemiological, metabolic, and genetic studies that moved up the scientific research field. In addition, the metabolic syndrome constitutes a comprehensive public health message and an easily educational tool for patients and health professionals, focusing on the multi-factorial nature of the atherosclerotic diseases. This approach recommends the same prevention and management strategies for both metabolic syndrome and its individual components (e.g., a healthy diet, regular physical activities, smoking cessation, weight loss and control, plus pharmacological intervention where necessary)[38].

7. References

[1] Meigs JB: Epidemiology of the metabolic syndrome, 2002. Am J Manag Care 2002;8:S283-292; quiz S293-286.

[2] Isomaa B, Almgren P, Tuomi T, Forsen B, Lahti K, Nissen M, Taskinen MR, Groop L: Cardiovascular morbidity and mortality associated with the metabolic syndrome. Diabetes Care 2001;24:683-689.

[3] Lakka HM, Laaksonen DE, Lakka TA, Niskanen LK, Kumpusalo E, Tuomilehto J, Salonen JT: The metabolic syndrome and total and cardiovascular disease mortality in middle-aged men. Jama 2002;288:2709-2716.

[4] Yarnell JW, Patterson CC, Bainton D, Sweetnam PM: Is metabolic syndrome a discrete entity in the general population? Evidence from the Caerphilly and Speedwell population studies. Heart 1998;79:248-252.

[5] Wilson PW, Kannel WB, Silbershatz H, D'Agostino RB: Clustering of metabolic factors and coronary heart disease. Arch Intern Med 1999;159:1104-1109.

[6] Trevisan M, Liu J, Bahsas FB, Menotti A: Syndrome X and mortality: a population-based study. Risk Factor and Life Expectancy Research Group. Am J Epidemiol 1998;148:958-966.

[7] Ford ES, Giles WH, Dietz WH: Prevalence of the metabolic syndrome among US adults: findings from the third National Health and Nutrition Examination Survey. Jama 2002;287:356-359.

[8] Schmidt MI, Watson RL, Duncan BB, Metcalf P, Brancati FL, Sharrett AR, Davis CE, Heiss G: Clustering of dyslipidemia, hyperuricemia, diabetes, and hypertension and its association with fasting insulin and central and overall obesity in a general population. Atherosclerosis Risk in Communities Study Investigators. Metabolism 1996;45:699-706.

[9] Grundy SM: Does the metabolic syndrome exist? Diabetes Care 2006;29:1689-1692; discussion 1693-1686.

[10] Grundy SM: Metabolic syndrome: connecting and reconciling cardiovascular and diabetes worlds. J Am Coll Cardiol 2006;47:1093-1100.

[11] Serrano Rios M, Caro JF, Carraro R, Gutiérrez Fuentes JA: The Metabolic Sndrome at the Begining of The XXIst Century: A Genetic and Molecular Approach. ed Elsevier, Madrid, Spain, 2005.
[12] Hu G, Qiao Q, Tuomilehto J, Balkau B, Borch-Johnsen K, Pyorala K: Prevalence of the metabolic syndrome and its relation to all-cause and cardiovascular mortality in nondiabetic European men and women. Arch Intern Med 2004;164:1066-1076.
[13] Reaven GM: Banting lecture 1988. Role of insulin resistance in human disease. Diabetes 1988;37:1595-1607.
[14] Liese AD, Mayer-Davis EJ, Haffner SM: Development of the multiple metabolic syndrome: an epidemiologic perspective. Epidemiol Rev 1998;20:157-172.
[15] Cameron AJ, Shaw JE, Zimmet PZ: The metabolic syndrome: prevalence in worldwide populations. Endocrinol Metab Clin North Am 2004;33:351-375, table of contents.
[16] Eckel RH, Grundy SM, Zimmet PZ: The metabolic syndrome. Lancet 2005;365:1415-1428.
[17] Vague J, Vague P, Tramoni M, Vialettes B, Mercier P: Obesity and diabetes. Acta Diabetol Lat 1980;17:87-99.
[18] Rader DJ: Effect of insulin resistance, dyslipidemia, and intra-abdominal adiposity on the development of cardiovascular disease and diabetes mellitus. Am J Med 2007;120:S12-18.
[19] Bansilal S, Farkouh ME, Fuster V: Role of insulin resistance and hyperglycemia in the development of atherosclerosis. Am J Cardiol 2007;99:6B-14B.
[20] Pouliot MC, Despres JP, Lemieux S, Moorjani S, Bouchard C, Tremblay A, Nadeau A, Lupien PJ: Waist circumference and abdominal sagittal diameter: best simple anthropometric indexes of abdominal visceral adipose tissue accumulation and related cardiovascular risk in men and women. Am J Cardiol 1994;73:460-468.
[21] Reaven G: The metabolic syndrome or the insulin resistance syndrome? Different names, different concepts, and different goals. Endocrinol Metab Clin North Am 2004;33:283-303.
[22] Kahn R, Buse J, Ferrannini E, Stern M: The metabolic syndrome: time for a critical appraisal: joint statement from the American Diabetes Association and the European Association for the Study of Diabetes. Diabetes Care 2005;28:2289-2304.
[23] Alberti KG, Zimmet PZ: Definition, diagnosis and classification of diabetes mellitus and its complications. Part 1: diagnosis and classification of diabetes mellitus provisional report of a WHO consultation. Diabet Med 1998;15:539-553.
[24] Laaksonen DE, Lakka HM, Niskanen LK, Kaplan GA, Salonen JT, Lakka TA: Metabolic syndrome and development of diabetes mellitus: application and validation of recently suggested definitions of the metabolic syndrome in a prospective cohort study. Am J Epidemiol 2002;156:1070-1077.
[25] Despres JP, Lemieux I, Prud'homme D: Treatment of obesity: need to focus on high risk abdominally obese patients. Bmj 2001;322:716-720.
[26] Balkau B, Charles MA: Comment on the provisional report from the WHO consultation. European Group for the Study of Insulin Resistance (EGIR). Diabet Med 1999;16:442-443.
[27] Balkau B, Charles MA, Drivsholm T, Borch-Johnsen K, Wareham N, Yudkin JS, Morris R, Zavaroni I, van Dam R, Feskins E, Gabriel R, Diet M, Nilsson P, Hedblad B: Frequency of the WHO metabolic syndrome in European cohorts, and an

alternative definition of an insulin resistance syndrome. In Diabetes Metab. 2002:364-376.
[28] Executive Summary of The Third Report of The National Cholesterol Education Program (NCEP) Expert Panel on Detection, Evaluation, And Treatment of High Blood Cholesterol In Adults (Adult Treatment Panel III). Jama 2001;285:2486-2497.
[29] Grundy SM, Cleeman JI, Daniels SR, Donato KA, Eckel RH, Franklin BA, Gordon DJ, Krauss RM, Savage PJ, Smith Jr SC, Spertus JA, Costa F: Diagnosis and management of the metabolic syndrome. An American Heart Association/National Heart, Lung, and Blood Institute Scientific Statement. Executive summary. Cardiol Rev 2005;13:322-327.
[30] Grundy SM, Brewer HB, Jr., Cleeman JI, Smith SC, Jr., Lenfant C: Definition of metabolic syndrome: Report of the National Heart, Lung, and Blood Institute/American Heart Association conference on scientific issues related to definition. Circulation 2004;109:433-438.
[31] Zimmet P, KG MMA, Serrano Rios M: [A new international diabetes federation worldwide definition of the metabolic syndrome: the rationale and the results]. Rev Esp Cardiol 2005;58:1371-1376.
[32] Despres JP, Lemieux I, Bergeron J, Pibarot P, Mathieu P, Larose E, Rodes-Cabau J, Bertrand OF, Poirier P: Abdominal obesity and the metabolic syndrome: contribution to global cardiometabolic risk. Arterioscler Thromb Vasc Biol 2008;28:1039-1049.
[33] Alberti KG, Eckel RH, Grundy SM, Zimmet PZ, Cleeman JI, Donato KA, Fruchart JC, James WP, Loria CM, Smith SC, Jr.: Harmonizing the metabolic syndrome: a joint interim statement of the International Diabetes Federation Task Force on Epidemiology and Prevention; National Heart, Lung, and Blood Institute; American Heart Association; World Heart Federation; International Atherosclerosis Society; and International Association for the Study of Obesity. Circulation 2009;120:1640-1645.
[34] Obesity: preventing and managing the global epidemic. Report of a WHO consultation. World Health Organ Tech Rep Ser 2000;894:i-xii, 1-253.
[35] Blaha M, Elasy TA: Clinical Use of the Metabolic Syndrome: Why the Confusion? Clinical Diabetes 2006;24:125-131.
[36] McLaughlin T, Allison G, Abbasi F, Lamendola C, Reaven G: Prevalence of insulin resistance and associated cardiovascular disease risk factors among normal weight, overweight, and obese individuals. Metabolism 2004;53:495-499.
[37] Ruderman N, Chisholm D, Pi-Sunyer X, Schneider S: The metabolically obese, normal-weight individual revisited. Diabetes 1998;47:699-713.
[38] Simmons RK, Alberti KG, Gale EA, Colagiuri S, Tuomilehto J, Qiao Q, Ramachandran A, Tajima N, Brajkovich Mirchov I, Ben-Nakhi A, Reaven G, Hama Sambo B, Mendis S, Roglic G: The metabolic syndrome: useful concept or clinical tool? Report of a WHO Expert Consultation. Diabetologia 2009.
[39] Grundy SM: What is the contribution of obesity to the metabolic syndrome? Endocrinol Metab Clin North Am 2004;33:267-282, table of contents.
[40] Grundy SM: Metabolic syndrome scientific statement by the American Heart Association and the National Heart, Lung, and Blood Institute. Arterioscler Thromb Vasc Biol 2005;25:2243-2244.

[41] Ferrannini E: Metabolic syndrome: a solution in search of a problem. J Clin Endocrinol Metab 2007;92:396-398.
[42] Ferrannini E, Balkau B: Insulin: in search of a syndrome. Diabet Med 2002;19:724-729.
[43] Grundy SM: Does a diagnosis of metabolic syndrome have value in clinical practice? Am J Clin Nutr 2006;83:1248-1251.
[44] Reaven GM: The metabolic syndrome: is this diagnosis necessary? Am J Clin Nutr 2006;83:1237-1247.
[45] Grundy SM: Metabolic syndrome: a multiplex cardiovascular risk factor. J Clin Endocrinol Metab 2007;92:399-404.
[46] Bonora E, Kiechl S, Willeit J, Oberhollenzer F, Egger G, Bonadonna RC, Muggeo M: Metabolic syndrome: epidemiology and more extensive phenotypic description. Cross-sectional data from the Bruneck Study. Int J Obes Relat Metab Disord 2003;27:1283-1289.
[47] Greenland P: Critical questions about the metabolic syndrome. Circulation 2005;112:3675-3676.
[48] Taslim S, Tai ES: The relevance of the metabolic syndrome. Ann Acad Med Singapore 2009;38:29-25.
[49] Mente A, Yusuf S, Islam S, McQueen MJ, Tanomsup S, Onen CL, Rangarajan S, Gerstein HC, Anand SS: Metabolic syndrome and risk of acute myocardial infarction a case-control study of 26,903 subjects from 52 countries. J Am Coll Cardiol 2010;55:2390-2398.
[50] Ford ES, Schulze MB, Pischon T, Bergmann MM, Joost HG, Boeing H: Metabolic syndrome and risk of incident diabetes: findings from the European Prospective Investigation into Cancer and Nutrition-Potsdam Study. Cardiovasc Diabetol 2008;7:35.
[51] Galassi A, Reynolds K, He J: Metabolic syndrome and risk of cardiovascular disease: a meta-analysis. Am J Med 2006;119:812-819.
[52] Gami AS, Witt BJ, Howard DE, Erwin PJ, Gami LA, Somers VK, Montori VM: Metabolic syndrome and risk of incident cardiovascular events and death: a systematic review and meta-analysis of longitudinal studies. J Am Coll Cardiol 2007;49:403-414.
[53] Sattar N, Gaw A, Scherbakova O, Ford I, O'Reilly DS, Haffner SM, Isles C, Macfarlane PW, Packard CJ, Cobbe SM, Shepherd J: Metabolic syndrome with and without C-reactive protein as a predictor of coronary heart disease and diabetes in the West of Scotland Coronary Prevention Study. Circulation 2003;108:414-419.
[54] Saely CH, Rein P, Drexel H: The metabolic syndrome and risk of cardiovascular disease and diabetes: experiences with the new diagnostic criteria from the International Diabetes Federation. Horm Metab Res 2007;39:642-650.
[55] Lorenzo C, Okoloise M, Williams K, Stern MP, Haffner SM: The metabolic syndrome as predictor of type 2 diabetes: the San Antonio heart study. Diabetes Care 2003;26:3153-3159.
[56] Wilson PW, D'Agostino RB, Parise H, Sullivan L, Meigs JB: Metabolic syndrome as a precursor of cardiovascular disease and type 2 diabetes mellitus. Circulation 2005;112:3066-3072.
[57] Vanuzzo D, Pilotto L, Mirolo R, Pirelli S: [Cardiovascular risk and cardiometabolic risk: an epidemiological evaluation]. G Ital Cardiol (Rome) 2008;9:6S-17S.

[58] Assmann G, Cullen P, Schulte H: Simple scoring scheme for calculating the risk of acute coronary events based on the 10-year follow-up of the prospective cardiovascular Munster (PROCAM) study. Circulation 2002;105:310-315.
[59] Despres JP, Lemieux I: Abdominal obesity and metabolic syndrome. Nature 2006;444:881-887.
[60] Grundy SM: Metabolic syndrome pandemic. Arterioscler Thromb Vasc Biol 2008;28:629-636.
[61] Ford ES, Li C, Zhao G, Pearson WS, Mokdad AH: Prevalence of the metabolic syndrome among U.S. adolescents using the definition from the International Diabetes Federation. Diabetes Care 2008;31:587-589.
[62] Morrison JA, Friedman LA, Wang P, Glueck CJ: Metabolic syndrome in childhood predicts adult metabolic syndrome and type 2 diabetes mellitus 25 to 30 years later. J Pediatr 2008;152:201-206.
[63] Ford ES: Prevalence of the metabolic syndrome defined by the International Diabetes Federation among adults in the U.S. Diabetes Care 2005;28:2745-2749.
[64] Ford ES, Giles WH: A comparison of the prevalence of the metabolic syndrome using two proposed definitions. Diabetes Care 2003;26:575-581.
[65] Alexander CM, Landsman PB, Grundy SM: The influence of age and body mass index on the metabolic syndrome and its components. Diabetes Obes Metab 2008;10:246-250.
[66] Mannucci E, Monami M, Bardini G, Ognibene A, Rotella CM: National Cholesterol Educational Program and International Diabetes Federation diagnostic criteria for metabolic syndrome in an Italian cohort: results from the FIBAR Study. J Endocrinol Invest 2007;30:925-930.
[67] Can AS, Bersot TP: Analysis of agreement among definitions of metabolic syndrome in nondiabetic Turkish adults: a methodological study. BMC Public Health 2007;7:353.
[68] Al-Lawati JA, Mohammed AJ, Al-Hinai HQ, Jousilahti P: Prevalence of the metabolic syndrome among Omani adults. Diabetes Care 2003;26:1781-1785.
[69] Gupta R, Deedwania PC, Gupta A, Rastogi S, Panwar RB, Kothari K: Prevalence of metabolic syndrome in an Indian urban population. Int J Cardiol 2004;97:257-261.
[70] Adams RJ, Appleton S, Wilson DH, Taylor AW, Dal Grande E, Chittleborough C, Gill T, Ruffin R: Population comparison of two clinical approaches to the metabolic syndrome: implications of the new International Diabetes Federation consensus definition. Diabetes Care 2005;28:2777-2779.
[71] Liu J, Grundy SM, Wang W, Smith SC, Jr., Vega GL, Wu Z, Zeng Z, Wang W, Zhao D: Ethnic-specific criteria for the metabolic syndrome: evidence from China. Diabetes Care 2006;29:1414-1416.
[72] Guize L, Thomas F, Pannier B, Bean K, Danchin N, Benetos A: [Metabolic syndrome: prevalence, risk factors and mortality in a French population of 62 000 subjects]. Bull Acad Natl Med 2006;190:685-697; discussion 697-700.
[73] Balkau B, Vernay M, Mhamdi L, Novak M, Arondel D, Vol S, Tichet J, Eschwege E: The incidence and persistence of the NCEP (National Cholesterol Education Program) metabolic syndrome. The French D.E.S.I.R. study. Diabetes Metab 2003;29:526-532.
[74] Villegas R, Perry IJ, Creagh D, Hinchion R, O'Halloran D: Prevalence of the metabolic syndrome in middle-aged men and women. Diabetes Care 2003;26:3198-3199.

[75] Tan CE, Ma S, Wai D, Chew SK, Tai ES: Can we apply the National Cholesterol Education Program Adult Treatment Panel definition of the metabolic syndrome to Asians? Diabetes Care 2004;27:1182-1186.

[76] Razzouk L, Muntner P: Ethnic, gender, and age-related differences in patients with the metabolic syndrome. Curr Hypertens Rep 2009;11:127-132.

[77] Oh JY, Hong YS, Sung YA, Barrett-Connor E: Prevalence and factor analysis of metabolic syndrome in an urban Korean population. Diabetes Care 2004;27:2027-2032.

[78] Hildrum B, Mykletun A, Hole T, Midthjell K, Dahl AA: Age-specific prevalence of the metabolic syndrome defined by the International Diabetes Federation and the National Cholesterol Education Program: the Norwegian HUNT 2 study. BMC Public Health 2007;7:220.

[79] Mattsson N, Ronnemaa T, Juonala M, Viikari JS, Raitakari OT: The prevalence of the metabolic syndrome in young adults. The Cardiovascular Risk in Young Finns Study. J Intern Med 2007;261:159-169.

[80] Santos AC, Barros H: Impact of metabolic syndrome definitions on prevalence estimates: a study in a Portuguese community. Diab Vasc Dis Res 2007;4:320-327.

[81] Mujica V, Leiva E, Icaza G, Diaz N, Arredondo M, Moore-Carrasco R, Orrego R, Vasquez M, Palomo I: Evaluation of metabolic syndrome in adults of Talca city, Chile. Nutr J 2008;7:14.

[82] The Decode Study G, Qiao Q: Comparison of three different definitions for the metabolic syndrome in non-diabetic Europeans. The British Journal of Diabetes & Vascular Disease 2005;5:161-168.

[83] Magliano DJ, Shaw JE, Zimmet PZ: How to best define the metabolic syndrome. Ann Med 2006;38:34-41.

[84] Jaber LA, Brown MB, Hammad A, Zhu Q, Herman WH: The prevalence of the metabolic syndrome among arab americans. Diabetes Care 2004;27:234-238.

[85] Alvarez Leon EE, Ribas Barba L, Serra Majem L: [Prevalence of the metabolic syndrome in the population of Canary Islands, Spain]. Med Clin (Barc) 2003;120:172-174.

[86] Athyros VG, Ganotakis ES, Elisaf MS, Liberopoulos EN, Goudevenos IA, Karagiannis A: Prevalence of vascular disease in metabolic syndrome using three proposed definitions. Int J Cardiol 2007;117:204-210.

[87] Fiuza M, Cortez-Dias N, Martins S, Belo A: Metabolic syndrome in Portugal: prevalence and implications for cardiovascular risk--results from the VALSIM Study. Rev Port Cardiol 2008;27:1495-1529.

[88] Alkerwi A, Donneau AF, Sauvageot N, Lair ML, Scheen A, Albert A, Guillaume M: Prevalence of the metabolic syndrome in Luxembourg according to the Joint Interim Statement definition estimated from the ORISCAV-LUX study. BMC Public Health 2011;11:4.

[89] Park HS, Lee SY, Kim SM, Han JH, Kim DJ: Prevalence of the metabolic syndrome among Korean adults according to the criteria of the International Diabetes Federation. Diabetes Care 2006;29:933-934.

[90] Kelliny C, William J, Riesen W, Paccaud F, Bovet P: Metabolic syndrome according to different definitions in a rapidly developing country of the African region. Cardiovasc Diabetol 2008;7:27.

[91] Groop L, Orho-Melander M: The dysmetabolic syndrome. J Intern Med 2001;250:105-120.
[92] Lin HF, Boden-Albala B, Juo SH, Park N, Rundek T, Sacco RL: Heritabilities of the metabolic syndrome and its components in the Northern Manhattan Family Study. Diabetologia 2005;48:2006-2012.
[93] Poulsen P, Vaag A, Kyvik K, Beck-Nielsen H: Genetic versus environmental aetiology of the metabolic syndrome among male and female twins. Diabetologia 2001;44:537-543.
[94] Joy T, Lahiry P, Pollex RL, Hegele RA: Genetics of metabolic syndrome. Curr Diab Rep 2008;8:141-148.
[95] Lahiry P, Pollex RL, Hegele RA: Uncloaking the genetic determinants of metabolic syndrome. J Nutrigenet Nutrigenomics 2008;1:118-125.
[96] King H: WHO and the International Diabetes Federation: regional partners. Bull World Health Organ 1999;77:954.
[97] Phillips C, Lopez-Miranda J, Perez-Jimenez F, McManus R, Roche HM: Genetic and nutrient determinants of the metabolic syndrome. Curr Opin Cardiol 2006;21:185-193.
[98] Phillips CM, Tierney AC, Roche HM: Gene-nutrient interactions in the metabolic syndrome. J Nutrigenet Nutrigenomics 2008;1:136-151.
[99] Agardh EE, Ahlbom A, Andersson T, Efendic S, Grill V, Hallqvist J, Ostenson CG: Explanations of socioeconomic differences in excess risk of type 2 diabetes in Swedish men and women. Diabetes Care 2004;27:716-721.
[100] Kaplan GA, Keil JE: Socioeconomic factors and cardiovascular disease: a review of the literature. Circulation 1993;88:1973-1998.
[101] Silventoinen K, Pankow J, Jousilahti P, Hu G, Tuomilehto J: Educational inequalities in the metabolic syndrome and coronary heart disease among middle-aged men and women. Int J Epidemiol 2005;34:327-334.
[102] Stewart-Knox BJ: Psychological underpinnings of metabolic syndrome. Proc Nutr Soc 2005;64:363-369.
[103] Wamala SP, Lynch J, Horsten M, Mittleman MA, Schenck-Gustafsson K, Orth-Gomer K: Education and the metabolic syndrome in women. Diabetes Care 1999;22:1999-2003.
[104] Lidfeldt J, Nyberg P, Nerbrand C, Samsioe G, Schersten B, Agardh CD: Socio-demographic and psychosocial factors are associated with features of the metabolic syndrome. The Women's Health in the Lund Area (WHILA) study. Diabetes Obes Metab 2003;5:106-112.
[105] Brunner EJ, Marmot MG, Nanchahal K, Shipley MJ, Stansfeld SA, Juneja M, Alberti KG: Social inequality in coronary risk: central obesity and the metabolic syndrome. Evidence from the Whitehall II study. Diabetologia 1997;40:1341-1349.
[106] Loucks EB, Rehkopf DH, Thurston RC, Kawachi I: Socioeconomic disparities in metabolic syndrome differ by gender: evidence from NHANES III. Ann Epidemiol 2007;17:19-26.
[107] Kim MH, Kim MK, Choi BY, Shin YJ: Educational disparities in the metabolic syndrome in a rapidly changing society--the case of South Korea. Int J Epidemiol 2005;34:1266-1273.
[108] Yarnell J, Yu S, McCrum E, Arveiler D, Hass B, Dallongeville J, Montaye M, Amouyel P, Ferrieres J, Ruidavets JB, Evans A, Bingham A, Ducimetiere P: Education,

socioeconomic and lifestyle factors, and risk of coronary heart disease: the PRIME Study. Int J Epidemiol 2005;34:268-275.

[109] Yoo S, Nicklas T, Baranowski T, Zakeri IF, Yang SJ, Srinivasan SR, Berenson GS: Comparison of dietary intakes associated with metabolic syndrome risk factors in young adults: the Bogalusa Heart Study. Am J Clin Nutr 2004;80:841-848.

[110] Fappa E, Yannakoulia M, Pitsavos C, Skoumas I, Valourdou S, Stefanadis C: Lifestyle intervention in the management of metabolic syndrome: could we improve adherence issues? Nutrition 2008;24:286-291.

[111] Kannel WB: Update on the role of cigarette smoking in coronary artery disease. Am Heart J 1981;101:319-328.

[112] Retnakaran R, Hanley AJ, Connelly PW, Harris SB, Zinman B: Cigarette smoking and cardiovascular risk factors among Aboriginal Canadian youths. Cmaj 2005;173:885-889.

[113] Oh SW, Yoon YS, Lee ES, Kim WK, Park C, Lee S, Jeong EK, Yoo T: Association between cigarette smoking and metabolic syndrome: the Korea National Health and Nutrition Examination Survey. Diabetes Care 2005;28:2064-2066.

[114] Masulli M, Vaccaro O: Association between cigarette smoking and metabolic syndrome. Diabetes Care 2006;29:482; author reply 482-483.

[115] Nakanishi N, Takatorige T, Suzuki K: Cigarette smoking and the risk of the metabolic syndrome in middle-aged Japanese male office workers. Ind Health 2005;43:295-301.

[116] Hong AR, Lee KS, Lee SY, Yu JH: [Association of current and past smoking with metabolic syndrome in men]. J Prev Med Public Health 2009;42:160-164.

[117] Appel LJ, Brands MW, Daniels SR, Karanja N, Elmer PJ, Sacks FM: Dietary approaches to prevent and treat hypertension: a scientific statement from the American Heart Association. Hypertension 2006;47:296-308.

[118] Parillo M, Riccardi G: Diet composition and the risk of type 2 diabetes: epidemiological and clinical evidence. Br J Nutr 2004;92:7-19.

[119] Jacobs DR, Jr., Gallaher DD: Whole grain intake and cardiovascular disease: a review. Curr Atheroscler Rep 2004;6:415-423.

[120] Lutsey PL, Steffen LM, Stevens J: Dietary intake and the development of the metabolic syndrome: the Atherosclerosis Risk in Communities study. Circulation 2008;117:754-761.

[121] Sahyoun NR, Jacques PF, Zhang XL, Juan W, McKeown NM: Whole-grain intake is inversely associated with the metabolic syndrome and mortality in older adults. Am J Clin Nutr 2006;83:124-131.

[122] Esmaillzadeh A, Mirmiran P, Azizi F: Whole-grain consumption and the metabolic syndrome: a favorable association in Tehranian adults. Eur J Clin Nutr 2005;59:353-362.

[123] McKeown NM, Meigs JB, Liu S, Saltzman E, Wilson PW, Jacques PF: Carbohydrate nutrition, insulin resistance, and the prevalence of the metabolic syndrome in the Framingham Offspring Cohort. Diabetes Care 2004;27:538-546.

[124] Pereira MA, Jacobs DR, Jr., Van Horn L, Slattery ML, Kartashov AI, Ludwig DS: Dairy consumption, obesity, and the insulin resistance syndrome in young adults: the CARDIA Study. JAMA 2002;287:2081-2089.

[125] Azadbakht L, Mirmiran P, Esmaillzadeh A, Azizi F: Dairy consumption is inversely associated with the prevalence of the metabolic syndrome in Tehranian adults. Am J Clin Nutr 2005;82:523-530.
[126] Esmaillzadeh A, Kimiagar M, Mehrabi Y, Azadbakht L, Hu FB, Willett WC: Fruit and vegetable intakes, C-reactive protein, and the metabolic syndrome. Am J Clin Nutr 2006;84:1489-1497.
[127] Dhingra R, Sullivan L, Jacques PF, Wang TJ, Fox CS, Meigs JB, D'Agostino RB, Gaziano JM, Vasan RS: Soft drink consumption and risk of developing cardiometabolic risk factors and the metabolic syndrome in middle-aged adults in the community. Circulation 2007;116:480-488.
[128] Esmaillzadeh A, Kimiagar M, Mehrabi Y, Azadbakht L, Hu FB, Willett WC: Dietary patterns, insulin resistance, and prevalence of the metabolic syndrome in women. Am J Clin Nutr 2007;85:910-918.
[129] Hu FB: Dietary pattern analysis: a new direction in nutritional epidemiology. Curr Opin Lipidol 2002;13:3-9.
[130] Kant AK: Dietary patterns and health outcomes. J Am Diet Assoc 2004;104:615-635.
[131] Fan AZ, Russell M, Naimi T, Li Y, Liao Y, Jiles R, Mokdad AH: Patterns of alcohol consumption and the metabolic syndrome. J Clin Endocrinol Metab 2008;93:3833-3838.
[132] Freiberg MS, Cabral HJ, Heeren TC, Vasan RS, Curtis Ellison R: Alcohol consumption and the prevalence of the Metabolic Syndrome in the US.: a cross-sectional analysis of data from the Third National Health and Nutrition Examination Survey. Diabetes Care 2004;27:2954-2959.
[133] Alkerwi A, Boutsen M, Vaillant M, Barre J, Lair ML, Albert A, Guillaume M, Dramaix M: Alcohol consumption and the prevalence of metabolic syndrome: a meta-analysis of observational studies. Atherosclerosis 2009;204:624-635.
[134] Helmrich SP, Ragland DR, Leung RW, Paffenbarger RS, Jr.: Physical activity and reduced occurrence of non-insulin-dependent diabetes mellitus. N Engl J Med 1991;325:147-152.
[135] Sallis JF, Patterson TL, Buono MJ, Nader PR: Relation of cardiovascular fitness and physical activity to cardiovascular disease risk factors in children and adults. Am J Epidemiol 1988;127:933-941.
[136] Blair SN, Goodyear NN, Gibbons LW, Cooper KH: Physical fitness and incidence of hypertension in healthy normotensive men and women. JAMA 1984;252:487-490.
[137] Ford ES, Kohl HW, 3rd, Mokdad AH, Ajani UA: Sedentary behavior, physical activity, and the metabolic syndrome among U.S. adults. Obes Res 2005;13:608-614.
[138] Irwin ML, Ainsworth BE, Mayer-Davis EJ, Addy CL, Pate RR, Durstine JL: Physical activity and the metabolic syndrome in a tri-ethnic sample of women. Obes Res 2002;10:1030-1037.
[139] Brien SE, Katzmarzyk PT: Physical activity and the metabolic syndrome in Canada. Appl Physiol Nutr Metab 2006;31:40-47.
[140] Horsten M, Mittleman MA, Wamala SP, Schenck-Gustafsson K, Orth-Gomer K: Social relations and the metabolic syndrome in middle-aged Swedish women. J Cardiovasc Risk 1999;6:391-397.

[141] Kinder LS, Carnethon MR, Palaniappan LP, King AC, Fortmann SP: Depression and the metabolic syndrome in young adults: findings from the Third National Health and Nutrition Examination Survey. Psychosom Med 2004;66:316-322.
[142] Raikkonen K, Matthews KA, Salomon K: Hostility predicts metabolic syndrome risk factors in children and adolescents. Health Psychol 2003;22:279-286.
[143] Vitaliano PP, Scanlan JM, Zhang J, Savage MV, Hirsch IB, Siegler IC: A path model of chronic stress, the metabolic syndrome, and coronary heart disease. Psychosom Med 2002;64:418-435.
[144] Landen M, Baghaei F, Rosmond R, Holm G, Bjorntorp P, Eriksson E: Dyslipidemia and high waist-hip ratio in women with self-reported social anxiety. Psychoneuroendocrinology 2004;29:1037-1046.
[145] Brook RD, Rajagopalan S, Pope CA, 3rd, Brook JR, Bhatnagar A, Diez-Roux AV, Holguin F, Hong Y, Luepker RV, Mittleman MA, Peters A, Siscovick D, Smith SC, Jr., Whitsel L, Kaufman JD: Particulate Matter Air Pollution and Cardiovascular Disease. An Update to the Scientific Statement From the American Heart Association. Circulation 2010.
[146] Gasparyan AY, Ayvazyan L, Mikhailidis DP, Kitas GD: Mean platelet volume: a link between thrombosis and inflammation? Current Pharmaceutical Design 2011;17:47-58.
[147] Chen JC, Schwartz J: Metabolic syndrome and inflammatory responses to long-term particulate air pollutants. Environ Health Perspect 2008;116:612-617.
[148] Pope CA, 3rd: What do epidemiologic findings tell us about health effects of environmental aerosols? J Aerosol Med 2000;13:335-354.
[149] Hackam DG, Anand SS: Emerging risk factors for atherosclerotic vascular disease: a critical review of the evidence. JAMA 2003;290:932-940.
[150] Kalayoglu MV, Libby P, Byrne GI: Chlamydia pneumoniae as an emerging risk factor in cardiovascular disease. JAMA 2002;288:2724-2731.
[151] Solenski NJ: Emerging risk factors for cerebrovascular disease. Curr Drug Targets 2007;8:802-816.
[152] Puig JG, Martinez MA: Hyperuricemia, gout and the metabolic syndrome. Curr Opin Rheumatol 2008;20:187-191.
[153] Imperatore G, Riccardi G, Iovine C, Rivellese AA, Vaccaro O: Plasma fibrinogen: a new factor of the metabolic syndrome. A population-based study. Diabetes Care 1998;21:649-654.
[154] Gasparyan AY, Stavropoulos-Kalinoglou A, Mikhailidis DP, Douglas KM, Kitas GD: Platelet function in rheumatoid arthritis: arthritic and cardiovascular implications. Rheumatology International 2011;31:153-164.
[155] Gasparyan AY: Inflammation, thrombosis and vascular biology: translating ideas into cardiovascular research and therapy. Open Cardiovasc Med J 2010;4:20-22.

8

Relationship Between Cardiovascular Risk Factors and Periodontal Disease: Current Knowledge

Sergio Granados-Principal[1], Nuri El-Azem[1], Jose L. Quiles[2], Patricia Perez-Lopez[2], Adrian Gonzalez[2] and MCarmen Ramirez-Tortosa[1]
[1]*Department of Biochemistry and Molecular Biology 2, Institute of Nutrition and Food Technology "José Mataix", Biomedical Research Center, University of Granada, Granada*
[2]*Department of Physiology, Institute of Nutrition and Food Technology "José Mataix", Biomedical Research Center, University of Granada, Granada, Spain*

1. Introduction

Periodontitis is a generally chronic disorder characterized by the breakdown of the tooth-supporting tissues and the impaired host inflammatory immune response. This condition is due fundamentally to an ecological imbalance between the normal microbial biofilm on teeth and the host tissues. There is increasing evidence linking periodontitis to systemic diseases, such as diabetes, rheumatoid arthritis, and, especially, CVD, hence the search for factors that may explain such relationships. A potential factor which could increase insulin resistance is the production of oxidative stress enhancing ROS in affected periodontal tissues (Bullon et al, 2009).

Metabolic syndrome as originally described is a combination of obesity, hypertension, impaired glucose tolerance or diabetes, hyperinsulinemia, and dyslipidemia (elevated triglycerides and decreased high-density lipoprotein-cholesterol [HDL-C] levels). These same features are also considered as risk factors for atherosclerosis, therefore leading to the deduction that metabolic syndrome constitutes a risk for coronary heart disease. In spite of extensive clinical research on metabolic syndrome, relatively little attention has been directed to its possible relationship to periodontitis. The available data come from epidemiological studies. In a group of 1315 affected individuals (30-92 yrs old), the prevalence of metabolic syndrome was higher among individuals with advanced periodontitis (66.7%) than in periodontally healthy individuals (48.8%) (Borges et al., 2007). Analysis of data from 13,710 participants in the NHANES III (Third National Health and Nutrition Examination Survey) showed a direct relationship between periodontitis and the prevalence of metabolic syndrome (37% in those with severe periodontitis *vs.* 18% in those with mild or no periodontitis), and, particularly, higher prevalence of obesity (48-54% *vs.* 31%), hypertension (51-56% *vs.* 27%), and high glucose levels (18-24% *vs.* 8%) were stated to be in the moderate to severe periodontitis group compared with the mild periodontitis or periodontally healthy group (D'Aiuto et al., 2008).

On the other hand, impaired glucose regulation disorders different from diabetes have been considered in periodontal research, and some encouraging findings have been obtained. Therefore, having deep pockets is significantly associated with impaired glucose tolerance in Japanese non-diabetic subjects and other study in an Israeli non-diabetic adult population revealed a higher occurrence of alveolar bone loss in subjects with elevated fasting glucose level of ≥ 100 mg/dL (Zadik et al, 2010).

A group of 5,632 participants in the Atherosclerosis Risk in Communities Study were examined in order to establish any relationship between periodontal status, interleukin 1-beta (IL-1β) levels in gingival crevicular fluid (GFC) and HOMA-IR index (Sutherland et al, 2002). An association between periodontal status and the 90th percentile of HOMA-IR was demonstrated, whenever coexisting high GCF IL-1β levels were present. This is an important finding, as IL-1β is related to the pathogenesis of insulin resistance, as well as tumor necrosis factor alpha (TNF-α) (Tilg and Moschen, 2008). Our study supports that a putative relationship between insulin resistance and periodontitis exists. When studied separately, diet can be related to both insulin resistance and periodontitis, nonetheless, we found out that dietary intake seems not to be a determining factor for insulin resistance when it is associated with periodontal disease (Granados-Principal et al, 2011).

Finally, in periodontitis, some perturbation in lipid biomarkers, for example increased total cholesterol in serum and lowdensity lipoprotein cholesterol, has been established. Thus, severe periodontitis is associated with a modest decrease in HDL and LDL cholesterol, and a more robust increase in plasma triacylglycerols. Intensive periodontal therapy results in reductions of total and LDL systemic cholesterols. Nevertheless, the relationship between fatty acids and periodontitis has been demonstrated in only a few studies. Some of these show that n-3 PUFA dietary supplementation modulates alveolar bone resorption following Porphyromonas gingivalis infection in rats and reduces the gingival tissue levels of prostaglandin E2, platelet-activation factor, and leukotriene B4, this being a useful adjunct in the treatment of CP. On the contrary, periodontitis patients with bone loss showed a higher n-6 PUFA plasma level than 27 control subjects. To clarify the situation, we investigated the potential linkage between periodontitis and plasma fatty acids profile, an established cardiovascular disease (CVD) risk factor. Our group has recently demonstrated in 35 years old patients that there is an inter-relationship between periodontitis, plasma fatty acids profile and the increase in metabolic risk factors for cardiovascular diseases (Ramirez-Tortosa et al, 2010). In that paper, the authors found that total plasma fatty acids, saturated, *n*-6 polyunsaturated and monounsaturated fatty acids, peroxidability index, soluble VCAM, TNF-α, cholesterol, triacylglycerols, and VLDL-c were significantly higher in the periodontitis group compared to the non-periodontitis group. The close association found between plasma triacylglycerols, LDL-c, saturated fatty acids, polyunsaturated fatty acids, total amount of fatty acids and coenzyme Q10 with some periodontal data such as periodontal probing depth, recession of the gingival margin and clinical attachment level (Pearson correlation between 0.3 and 0.6), leads to the conclusion that there is an inter-relationship between periodontitis, plasma fatty acids profile and the increase in metabolic risk factors for cardiovascular diseases.

Taking in account all above mentioned the aim of this chapter is to describe the cardiovascular risk factors related with periodontal disease and their relationship because perhaps an interaction between both diseases may result in a worse evolution of them.

2. Periodontitis

2.1 Introduction

Tooth structure consists of two different parts: crown, covered with enamel and root, under the gingival line. Dentin comprises most of the tooth parenchyma, and surrounds the pulp chamber, where there are lots of blood vessels and nerves.

Tooth is anchored firmly in the alveolus by the *periodontium*, a structure that is formed by gums, alveolar bone, tooth cementum and periodontal ligament. The periodontal ligament fixes the tooth concrete to the alveolar bone. Above the ligament, there is a gum fringe, just under the crown. Over the crown base; there is a few millimeters (1 to 3 mm) gap of gum that forms a superficial groove, in the border between the gum and the tooth.

Periodontitis is an inflammation and infection of bones and ligaments that act as holders of teeth. It appears when inflammation and infection of gums (gingivitis) is left without treatment or when this treatment is delayed so much time. This inflammation and infection disseminate from gums to ligaments and bones that holds teeth. Due to this loss of support, teeth finally fall out. This problem is infrequent in children, but it's the first cause of dental loss in adults and it affects between 10 % - 15 % of the world population (Baelum & Lopez, 2004).

Dental plaque and tartar accumulates on the basis of teeth. It can be prevented by adequate tooth cleaning methods and periodic cares from a professional. This inflammation makes that between the gum and teeth, cumulus of tartar and dental plaque are deposited. Continuous inflammation finally develops destruction of tissue and bones surrounding the teeth. Because dental plaque contains germs, it is probably to develop dental abscess, which also contributes to bone destruction. Microorganism at dental plaque releases inflammatory substances that provoke an inflammatory response by immune cells from the host. Leukocytes, mainly neutrophils are recruited by chemotactic stimuli, and they phagocyte and digest this bacteria, preventing them from releasing more inflammatory cytokines. Although this will prevent gingivitis to appear, when neutrophils are overloaded by an excess of bacteria, they degranulate, releasing lots of enzymes and cytokines, aggravating the inflammation and the gingivitis (Kinane, 2001).

It is to say that not all gingivitis progresses to periodontitis and that it does not have to affect every teeth at the same time. Not all periodontitis progress equally in each person, some are more resistant to the development of periodontitis and some are more given to it. Only a few people suffer from advanced tissue destruction around the teeth due to periodontitis and this disease passes with brief episodes of exacerbation and occasional remission. Most people who develop clinical signs of gingivitis do it after 10 - 20 days of plaque accumulation. It appears as redness, swelling and an increased tendency of the gingiva to bleed on gentle probing and it is still reversible to a normal status if the plaque is effectively removed. Periodontitis appears around 6 months before the establishment of gingivitis, but it depends on every single patient (Brecx et al, 1988).

There are several factors that modify the possibility of suffering periodontitis, besides a lack of dental care, such as smoking, drugs (calcium blockers as nifedipine, phenytoin or cyclosporines) hormonal status, stress, age, socioeconomic status and race, systemic diseases, genetics or individual immune response.

2.2 Immune response by host cells and inflammation

Inflammation at the periodontium begins when both bacteria and leukocytes start their fight releasing lots of pro inflammatory factors. The immune response is generated by cell wall components from the bacteria, including lipopolysaccharide (LPS) (Monteiro et al, 2009). Bacteria from the periodontium and some of its components are able to even reach other parts of the organism and produce an inflammatory response there (Tonetti, 2009).

It is now known some of those molecules implicated in the connective tissue destruction, although there are many pathways that correlates between them and participate in this process and we don´t know exactly which paper plays every molecule, but the most important involved players are: connective tissue metalloproteinases, reactive oxygen species (ROS) and phagocytosis of matrix components.

Matrix metalloproteinase activity is controlled in vivo through four separate mechanisms: First, they need to be activated by plasmin, trypsin or other proteinases. Second, interleukin-1 (IL-1) and transforming growth factor-β (TGF-β), induced in inflamed tissues, regulates metalloproteinase production. Third, an α2-macroglobulin serum inhibitor is able to inactivate matrix metalloproteinases and fourth, there is a group of protein inhibitors of matrix metalloproteinases (TIMP) that prevent the conversion of precursor forms of matrix metalloproteinases to their active forms.

Immune response to periodontitis is the key that opens the door to an oxidative stress status and ROS production in the host. Neutrophils are the first line of defense against this infection and one way to achieve their goal is through ROS and reactive nitrogen species (RNS) production by nicotinamide adenine dinucleotide phosphate-oxidase (NADPH oxidase) and nitric oxide synthase (NOS) respectively. Neutrophil NADPH oxidase is a proteic complex normally dissociated until stimulation by protein kinase C (PKC), which phosphorylate p47-*phox*, a protein that facilitates assembly of NADPH oxidase subunits. PKC is also activated by sn-1, 2-diacylglycerol (DAG). ROS produced then can also act as second messengers activating other pathways, included inflammation, immune response, cell proliferation or apoptosis (Fialkow et al, 2007).

T-cells and B-cells are involved in the defense against periodontitis. Their release products have been detected at the inflammation sites, such as interleukin-2 (IL-2), interleukin-12 (IL-12), tumor necrosis factor-α (TNF-α) and interferon-γ from lymphocyte T helper 1 (Th1); interleukin-4 (IL-4), interleukin-5 (IL-5), interleukin-6 (IL-6), interleukin-10 (IL-10) and interleukin-13 (IL-13) from lymphocyte T helper 2 (Th2) and TGF-β from lymphocyte T helper 3 (Th3). T-cells prevail in early stages of the disease while B-cells do it at later stages of periodontitis. It is thought to be a switch between them as the disease gets worse. There is also a great production of immunoglobulin G (IgG) and Immunoglobulin A (IgA) from B-cells (Kiane et al, 2007).

Other cells as macrophages, mononuclear antigen presenting cells, dendritic cells, endothelial cells or adipocytes participate in immune response. These cells possess surface receptors that recognize harmful molecules. Macrophages present a toll-like receptor that recognize lipopolysaccharide (toll-like receptor-4) produced by bacteria in periodontitis, and advanced glycation end products receptor (RAGE) for recognition of advanced glycation end products (AGEs) produced in diabetes. These receptors are able to activate nuclear factor kappa-beta (NF-κβ) pathway that promote the expression of inflammatory cytokines (Nassar et al, 2007).

NF- κβ pathway modulates a wide variety of gene expressions, but we are interested mostly in its capacity of modulating interleukin-8 (IL-8) expression, which regulates neutrophil migration. Activation of NF- κβ pathway will be an important contributor to inflammation whereas it is activated. TNF-α is one of the main activators of this pathway. If TNF-α is released, it is surely to have an enhanced NF- κβ pathway activation. Also IL-1β is able to activate NF- κβ pathway but in a lesser degree than TNF-α (Fitzgerald et al, 2007).

2.3 Periodontitis and ROS

ROS are chemically reactive molecules derived from oxygen that can damage lipids, proteins and DNA. They can also act as cell signaling molecules. ROS are produced every time at every single moment in every aerobic organism by the respiratory electron transport chain at the mitochondria, p450 cytochrome reactions, peroxisomal fatty acid metabolism and NADPH oxidase activity, but, normally, there is a balance between ROS and antioxidant molecules. It is when this balance is broken when ROS begin their harmful activity and an oxidative stress situation is established (Borges et al, 2007).

In mild and chronic periodontitis, ROS generation is enhanced and plasma antioxidant levels are depleted. This ROS generation at the site of periodontitis can also have systemic effects on other organs as ROS can diffuse into the blood stream and reach other places on the organism. This is specially worth investigating on it, because it is known that serious diseases as cardiovascular disease and diabetes are related with ROS generation at the organism.

People suffering from chronic periodontitis have higher C reactive protein (CRP) plasma levels. This is a powerful pro inflammatory molecule that also participates in other pathologies as obesity (D'Aiuto et al, 2010) and it is a good marker of the development of atherosclerosis and myocardial infarction (Tonetti, 2009).

As It has mentioned before, periodontitis appears as the result of all the cytokines, ROS and inflammatory molecules released from the microorganisms and the host immune cells at the site of the inflammation at the teeth. The presence of a high amount of neutrophils, as this is the main host response to bacterial invasions, give us the idea of the great amount of ROS that can be released from them to combat the infection. There is also systemic inflammation in periodontitis as assessed in some studies measuring plasma CRP (Paraskevas et al, 2008), which can influence the production or ROS all over the organism.

The most important ROS involved in periodontitis are:

Hydroxyl radical (*OH), very active in damaging DNA proteins and lipids. It is able to initiate the lipid peroxidation chain, leading to vasodilation and bone reabsorption. Its molecular mechanism of action is by stimulation of the NF-K B-IKB complex, activating then NK-κB, which helps nuclear translocation and downstream of proinflammatory cytokines as IL-2, IL-6, IL-8, β-interferon and TNF-α (Borges et al, 2007).

Hydrogen peroxide (H_2O_2), capable of crossing the nuclear membrane and damaging the DNA. DNA damage is measured by quantifying levels of 8-hydroxydeoxyguanosine (8-OHDG), that is increased in periodontal tissues in periodontitis (Ekundi et al, 2010).

Superoxide anion (O_2^{*-}), involved in bone reabsorption as many studies have corroborated by measuring the presence of this anion near the sites of bone reabsorption.

The most important cellular antioxidants are the enzymes superoxide dismutase (SOD), catalase, and glutathione peroxidase, glutathione-S transferases and aldehyde dehydrogenases. There are also non enzymatic antioxidants as carotenoids, vitamin E, C, coenzyme Q_{10}, α-lipoic acid, antioxidant minerals (selenium, zinc, copper, manganese), phenols, flavonoids, lycopene or hydroxytyrosol. When levels of these enzymes are lowered, the organism is unable to neutralize ROS and they can exert its harmful effect (Vicents & Taylor, 2006).

So, ROS are involved both in tissue destruction in periodontitis and in systemic inflammation. They are also involved in several systemic diseases as metabolic syndrome, diabetes, obesity or cardiovascular disease. This means that it can be a link between periodontitis and these diseases, which altogether are risk factors for cardiovascular disease. We are going to inquire in the relation of ROS, oxidative stress and these diseases to understand why the generation of ROS in periodontitis can be linked to the apparition or deterioration of these diseases that in the end lead to cardiovascular disease.

ROS sources

- Mitochondrial electron transport chain
- P450 cytochrome
- Peroxisomal fatty acid metabolism
- NADPH oxidase
- Xanthine oxidase
- Lipoxygenase
- Uncoupled NOS
- Myeloperoxidase
- Host immune cells

Fig. 1. ROS sources.

3. Cardiovascular disease

Cardiovascular diseases are the world's largest killers, claiming 17.1 million lives a year, representing 29% of all global deaths. Cardiovascular diseases (CVDs) are a group of disorders of the heart and blood vessels and include:

- Coronary heart disease
- Cerebrovascular disease
- Peripheral arterial disease
- Rheumatic heart disease
- Congenital heart disease
- Deep vein thrombosis and pulmonary embolism

Heart attacks and strokes are usually acute events and are mainly caused by a blockage that prevents blood from flowing to the heart or brain. The most common reason for this is a build-up of fatty deposits on the inner walls of the blood vessels that supply the heart or brain. Strokes can also be caused by bleeding from a blood vessel in the brain or from blood clots.

3.1 Cardiovascular disease and ROS

Although hypertension is the main cause for having a cardiovascular event, ROS can also affect and damage cardiac tissues directly, leaving heart more susceptible to any other damage. Sources of ROS in cardiac tissue are not already unknown for us. These sources are the mitochondrial respiratory chain, NADPH oxidases, xanthine oxidases, lipoxygenase, uncoupled NOS and myeloperoxidase. There are evidences that ROS production by these systems are involved in cardiac damage and the apparition of heart failure diseases as congestive heart failure, angiotensin II dependent cardiac hypertrophy or cardiac fibrosis ,inter alia.

It is known that ROS can harm cardiac tissue because after reperfusion injury, there is a great increase in ROS production, attributed to an overload of all the ROS sources mentioned above and to a high infiltration of neutrophils that release pro inflammatory citokynes. This will damage myocytes, impair contractile function and contribute to capillary leakage (Chang et al, 2010).

3.2 Cardiovascular disease and periodontitis

Nowadays, there are several studies linking periodontitis with cardiovascular diseases (Paquette et al, 2007). We have seen how periodontitis can lead to an oxidative stress status in the organisms that will promote the onset of other diseases as obesity, diabetes or hypertension that are risk factors for cardiovascular disease and the possible mechanisms of how this happens. There is also evidence of direct damage by ROS to cardiac tissue and even DNA from periodontal pathogens in atheroma plaques, suggesting that they can also spread from the periodontium and travel throughout the blood stream (Tonetti, 2009). But there is another one important fact about how periodontitis can affect cardiovascular health, and it is the formation of the atheroma plaque or atherosclerosis.

Atherosclerosis begins with stimuli from LDL or pro inflammatory proteins to endothelial cells which will express adhesion factors, chemokines and growth factors that attract monocytes from circulating blood. These monocytes can enter the intima and differentiate into macrophages. Macrophages then are able to uptake oxidized LDL and cholesterol and they transform in foam cells, damaging the intima. Then, activation of T lymphocytes, smooth muscle cells proliferation and migration and extracellular matrix deposition interact with molecules in the intima, promoting necrosis and forming fibrous plaques. These plaques are atheroma plaques and will grow and enlarge. Consequences of this could be occlusion of the artery where the atheroma plaque is formed or rupture of the plaque, releasing a plaque fragment that may be transformed into a thrombus that can obstruct blood flow anywhere on the body, with the risk of producing an acute cardiovascular event or stroke (Chang et al, 2010). ROS periodontitis production could be dangerous due to the oxidation of LDL and its pro atherogenic role. People with periodontitis have higher levels of plasma oxidized LDL levels, which means higher risk of developing atheroma plaque. Treatments directed to improve periodontitis achieved a lowering in oxidized LDL plasma levels (Tamaki et al, 2010). Platelets also contribute greatly to atheroma plaque formation. It is known that platelet activation is increased in people suffering from periodontitis, being greater this activation as periodontitis severity increases (Papapanagiotou et al, 2009). Furthermore, platelets are able to bind fibrinogen and form thrombi that can occlude any blood vessel by themselves without the need of an atheroma plaque. The reason of this platelet activation could be in the action of periodontitis associated bacteria. It is to say that platelets are activated by the vasodilator–stimulated phosphoprotein (VASP) whose mission is to regulate platelet activation. When phosphorylated, VASP inhibit platelet activation, but in periodontitis, there is a decrease in VASP phosphorylation due to direct interaction between these periodontitis associated bacteria and VASP, leading to higher platelet activation (Laky et al, 2011).

But atherogenesis is not the only risk factor involved in cardiovascular events. Mitochondria play an important part in heart damage. Mitochondria are the primary source of intracellular ROS. When damaged, mitochondria suffer a dysfunction in their activity making them to produce huge amounts of ROS and release pro apoptotic proteins into the cytosol that can trigger apoptosis in the cell. ROS are able to slowly damage mitochondria but the key is the damage to mitochondrial DNA (mtDNA) that is produced when, because of punctual mutations in mtDNA due to ROS action, mitochondria is unable to properly work and begins producing high amounts of ROS and these pro apoptotic proteins as cytochrome c or apoptosis inducing factor (AIF) that destroy the cell. People suffering from atherosclerosis have higher mtDNA damage (Humphrey et al, 2008).

High chain long fatty acids (FA) plasma concentration is also a common link between periodontitis, diabetes and cardiovascular risk. FA plasma concentrations are elevated in periodontitis (Ramirez-Tortosa et al, 2010) as they are in diabetes (Liu et al, 2010). Both elevations can together bring up a very high plasma fatty acids concentration. Normally, heart uses fatty acids as energy source generated by β-oxidation and also uses glucose in a lesser amount. This high plasma fatty acid concentration will force the heart to use almost only free fatty acids as substrate for energy production. Fatty acids get into the cell by passive diffusion (20% of fatty acids) and by active transport mediated by CD36 transporter (80% of fatty acids). Once inside the cell, fatty acids bind to a cytosolic fatty acid-binding protein and are transported to the outer mitochondrial membrane. There, fatty acids are sterified and get inside the mitochondrial matrix, where β-oxidation is performed. When the FA concentration is excessive, glycolytic intermediates and intracellular lipids accumulate because mitochondria are unable to β-oxidate all the FA. This FA excess will produce ROS inside the cardiomyocyte cytoplasm as a result of an increased FA oxidation. There will also be accumulation of DAG and ceramides. ROS and DAG will activate JNK, IKK kinases and PKC respectively. Together, they will downregulate insulin action through serine phosphorilation of insulin receptor substrate-1 (IRS-1), what will inactivate IRS-1 and stop the insulin pathway. Also, ceramides will inhibit Akt, what will also neutralize insulin action. It is still unknown why, but diabetes leads to heart hypertrophy and failure independently of atherosclerosis or hypertension. Experiments with rodents that lacked CD36 transporter showed that those rodents did not have any cardiac dysfunction. This could mean that an excessive FA intake and intramyocardial should be involved in cardiac failure somehow. A possible reason is the generation of ROS inside cardiomyocytes.

As it is known, ROS can activate NF-κβ with its consequent production of growth factors and pro inflammatory cytokines. ROS can also activate matrix metalloproteinases that have the capacity of remodeling the extracellular matrix and cleave sarcomeric proteins such as troponin-1 and myosin light chains-1 (MLC-1) what will cause deficiencies in heart contractility and even apoptosis if damage is too high. As important is the role of heart mitochondria in this process. ROS are able to damage mitochondria and make it produce even more ROS and loss of functionality. Damage to mitochondria will release pro apoptotic proteins such as cytochrome c, caspases 3 and 9 that will lead to cell death. If mitochrondrion is damaged and there is no apoptosis, loss of function will reduce β-oxidation rate and make FA accumulate, producing even more ROS and beginning the cycle (Dirkx et al, 2011).

Mitochondria have a key role in cardiac failure and remodeling. ROS generation is increased in failing myocardium as demonstrated by measurement of 8-iso-prostaglandin F2α. Heart is the main oxygen user in the body so ROS generation rate is higher in heart than in other organs. When heart is damaged, heart mitochondria ROS generation is enhanced, being able to damage myocytes, although, also NADPH oxidase and xanthine oxidase are able to produce ROS in heart and damage myocytes. Mitochondria have their own DNA (mtDNA), more susceptible to damage because:

1. It is less protected than nuclear DNA that possesses histones.
2. mtDNA is located in the mitochondrial matrix, where ROS production is constant by the electron transport chain activity.
3. mtDNA repair is not so effective as nuclear DNA repair.

There is also cardiac remodeling by activation of metalloproteinases by ROS. Cardiac metalloproteinases activity is increased in failing hearts possibly due to the high ROS generation in damaged cardiac tissue. Studies with metalloproteinases inhibitors show that inhibition limits early left ventricular dilatation in murine models (Tsutsui et al, 2009).

Periodontitis and cardiovascular disease

- ROS produced in periodontitis can damage cardiac tissue.
- ROS can also favour the atheroma plaque development.
- ROS damage mitochondria. Damaged mitochondrias produce even more ROS.
- ROS activate matrix metalloproteinases.
- High fatty acid concentrations in periodontitis produce more ROS.
- ROS activate NF-κβ, producing growth factors and pro-inflammatory cytokines.

Fig. 2. Periodontitis and cardiovascular disease

Metalloproteinases functions

- Participate in normal tissue remodelling.
- Regulate cell migration, invasion, proliferation and apoptosis.
- Regulate branching morphogenesis.
- Participate in angiogenesis.
- Participate in wound healing.
- Regulate extracelular matrix degradation.

Fig. 3. Metalloproteinases functions

Mitochondria and periodontitis are also well related. Bacterial lipopolysaccharide released during periodontitis by bacteria is able to damage mitochondria by decreasing mitochondria membrane potential, mitochondrial mass, CoQ_{10}, and protein expression. CoQ_{10} deficiency also makes a decrease in complex II + III, III and IV activities. This taken together raises ROS production inside the mitochondria. The next step before ROS damage is produced is liberation of cytochrome c, procaspase-9, caspase-3 and endonuclease G, resulting in DNA degradation and cell death.

4. Metabolic syndrome

Metabolic syndrome is a compound of afflictions that comprises hypertension, diabetes and dyslipidemia caused by abnormal obesity due to physical inactivity and overeating. According to the American Heart Association, metabolic syndrome comprises several risk factors as:

- Abdominal obesity (excessive fat tissue in and around the abdomen).
- Atherogenic dyslipidemia (blood fat disorders – high triglycerides, low high density lipoprotein (HDL) cholesterol and high low density lipoprotein (LDL) cholesterol – that foster plaque buildups in artery walls).
- Elevated blood pressure.
- Insulin resistance or glucose intolerance.
- Prothrombotic state (e.g., high fibrinogen or plasminogen activator inhibitor-1 in the blood).
- Proinflammatory state (e.g., elevated C-reactive protein in the blood).

Metabolic syndrome is associated with periodontitis as shown on epidemiological studies that demonstrate the relationship. In a group of 1315 patients, the prevalence of metabolic syndrome was higher in patients with advanced periodontitis (66.7 %) than in those periodontally healthy (48.8 %)(Borges et al, 2007). Another study from 13,710 participants in the NHANES III (Third National Health and Nutrition Examination Survey) showed a direct relationship between periodontitis and the prevalence of metabolic syndrome (37% in those with severe periodontitis vs. 18% in those with mild or no periodontitis) (D'Aiuto et al, 2008; Bullon et al, 2009).

People with the metabolic syndrome are at increased risk of coronary heart disease and other diseases related to plaque buildups in artery walls (e.g., stroke and peripheral vascular disease) and type II diabetes.

Abdominal obesity, insulin resistance and hypertension seem to be the most important of these risk factors in order to develop a cardiovascular disease. They are also influenced by oxidative stress as it will be described later.This syndrome is clinically important because of the associated cardiovascular risk accumulation, which exceeds that of the component parts. Thus, it is important to elucidate the pathophysiology of metabolic syndrome to prevent the development of the associated cardiovascular disease (CVD).

5. Obesity

Obesity is a state of fat mass excess. Adipose tissue is formed by adipose cells that store lipids and also preadipocites. Adipocites accumulate lipids and grow in number and shape. There is also a high number of infiltrating macrophages due to the expression of interleukins and a high rate of preadipocites differentiation into macrophages by *peroxisome proliferator-activated receptor gamma* (PPAR-γ) and TNF-α.

Adipocites release also many other molecules that have influence on other biological processes, for example, adiponectin, which favors insulin sensibility, lipid oxidation and has vascular protective properties but is downregulated in obesity, or angiotensinogen, that acts over blood pressure. This molecule concentration is reduced in metabolic syndrome and in diabetes.

5.1 Obesity, periodontitis and oxidative stress

Obesity is one of the most important parts of metabolic syndrome. It is known that there is systemic chronic inflammation and increased ROS generation in obesity, thus, leading to an oxidative stress situation. This is mainly due to the production of TNF-α, IL-6, non-esterified fatty acids, angiotensinogen and CRP (Ando & Fujita, 2009). Possible reasons why there is an increased ROS production in obesity can be: hyperglycemia, increased muscle activity to carry excessive weight, elevated tissue lipid levels, inadequate antioxidant defenses, chronic inflammation, endothelial ROS production and hyperleptinemia (D'Aiuto et al, 2008). We can see that many of these factors as hyperglycemia, inadequate antioxidant defenses, chronic inflammation and endothelial ROS production depends on other pathologies related to metabolic syndrome, and can be worsened if these pathologies are in an advance state of the disease, as diabetes or atherosclerosis.

Hyperglycemia and obesity are heavily linked, and therefore, obesity and diabetes. Obesity induces insulin resistance, suppress the expression of insulin receptors in fat tissue, causing glucose deregulation, hyperglycemia and later, β-cell destruction in pancreas, promoting diabetes. Due to the impossibility to catch glucose from cells because of this insulin resistance, glucose accumulates in the blood stream, leading to hyperglycemia. This leads to 3 different pathways that will end with the production of ROS:

- The first pathway is the polyol pathway where glucose is converted to sorbitol, which in excess produces oxidative damage. This pathway includes the participation of nicotinamide adenine dinucleotide phosphate (NADPH) oxidase activity, that produces O_2^{*-}, especially in the endothelium.

- The second pathway is the forming of advanced glycosylation end products (AGE) because of the reaction between glucose and proteins, lipids and nucleic acids. This AGEs binds to specific cell surface receptors (RAGE) and this promote the production of NF-κβ, which in turn activates PKC, sorbitol and transcription of vascular cell adhesion molecule-1 (VCAM-1) and intracellular adhesion molecule-1 (ICAM-1). All this molecules activation will raise ROS levels.
- The third pathway is just the glucose auto-oxidation with the generation of oxidants with similar reactivity as OH* and O_2^{*-} radicals.

All this three pathways together with an increased metabolic ROS production in obese people, inadequate antioxidant defenses due to an unsuitable diet and continuous antioxidant attrition will bring up an oxidative stress situation.

5.2 Obesity, periodontitis and fatty acids

It is important to talk about the lipid profile and changes in lipid peroxidation with ROS production in obesity because it could be linked with periodontitis and cardiovascular risk as Ramirez-Tortosa et al.(2010) found in one of their studies. Fat storage, excessive blood lipids and dyslipidemia are found in obesity with an increase in plasma saturated, monounsaturated and polyunsaturated fatty acids. Periodontitis is a systemic inflammation and ROS generator, what will contribute to the oxidation of LDL that are also elevated in obesity.

Dietary intake of lipids can also modify plasma lipid profile as people with high intake of saturated and n-6 polyunsaturated fatty acids, but not those with a higher intake of n-3 polyunsaturated fatty acids, have increased cardiovascular risk due to an increased oxidized lipoproteins and vascular inflammation. Total n-3 polyunsaturated fatty acids were associated with lower levels of pro inflammatory markers (IL-6, TNF-α, CRP), higher levels of anti-inflammatory markers (soluble IL-6r, IL-10, TGF-α) and lower levels of some markers of endothelial activation (sVCAM-1 and sICAM-1). This means that n-3 polyunsaturated fatty acids are cardio protective, but in periodontitis patients, n-6 polyunsaturated and saturated fatty acids predominate in plasma, a proatherogenic lipid profile that is responsible for the production of high levels of pro inflammatory TNF-α and proatherogenic sVCAM-1 and oxidized LDL (Ramirez-Tortosa et al, 2010).

There are many ways in which lipids can contribute to oxidative stress as uncoupling of mitochondria, susceptibility to ROS attack and production of PKC that also raise glucose levels. Also NADPH oxidase activity is increased in adipose tissue and there is a reduced activity of antioxidant enzymes as superoxide dismutase (SOD). All these reactions generate ROS, leading to lipid and protein oxidation and finally to oxidative stress.

As seen on this study, there are several changes in the lipid profile in common between periodontitis and obesity. These changes were in cholesterol, triacylglycerols, LDL, and very low density lipoproteins (VLDL) plasma levels that increased both in periodontitis groups as shown in this study and in obesity patients while HDL levels were decreased. As periodontitis and obesity are two diseases that share in common general systemic low grade inflammation, IL-6 is elevated in both diseases. One of IL-6 effects is to decrease lipoprotein lipase activity, a key enzyme involved in triglycerides catabolism and formation of adipose tissue. Reduction in its activity will produce hypertriglyceridemia (Monteiro et al, 2009).

While ROS have adverse effects on obesity development, and its production is increased in obesity, periodontitis ROS production may increment drastically ROS levels, worsening the oxidative stress situation in obese patients with periodontitis. Lots of studies link the relationship between obesity and oxidative stress (Vincent & Taylor, 2006) by measuring lipid peroxidation biomarkers as malondialdehyde (MDA), thiobarbituric reactive acid substances (TBARS), C reactive protein (CRP), lipid hydroperoxides, conjugated dienes, 4-hidroxynonenal (4HNE) and F_2isoprostanes (8-epiPGF$_2\alpha$).Those studies showed an increase in these biomarker levels in obese patients and also a decrease in antioxidant enzymes, showing that there is an increased oxidative stress in this situation. Plasma MDA levels are increased in obese patients and it is involved in systemic oxidative stress and in impairment of normal glucose metabolism in obese people, which will also contribute to the instauration of diabetes, another important risk factor in metabolic syndrome for the development of cardiovascular diseases. But not also MDA levels are increased in obesity. All the other obesity biomarkers mentioned above were increased.

Obesity and periodontitis

- Obesity leads to hyperglycemia what will lead to ROS production.
- There is an increased metabolic rate that produces high ROS levels.
- LDL and fatty acids are incremented both in obesity and periodontitis.
- There is a higher NADPH oxidase activity in obesity.
- Obesity and periodontitis ROS production together can cause an oxidative stress situation

Fig. 4. Obesity and periodontitis

It is evident the relation between the plasma lipid profile and the risk of developing atherogenesis. Specially, a high LDL concentration may lead to the development of the atherogenic plaque and subsequently raise the level of risk of suffering cardiovascular diseases. Now, there are evidences of an increase in these levels of plasma LDL in periodontitis (Ramirez-Tortosa et al, 2010). If we sum up this phenomenon with the rise of plasma LDL happening in obesity, we probably will have a high rise in plasma oxidized LDL and therefore a higher risk in developing atheroma plaque.

Another factor that promotes oxidative stress situations in obesity is the level of plasma leptin. Leptin is a polypeptide hormone that regulates food intake acting on hypothalamic centers. It is produced by adipose tissue. It is a cardiovascular risk factor in obese people. Leptin is chemically similar to IL-6 cytokine family and so it has pro inflammatory properties stimulating the proliferation of monocytes and macrophages and inflammatory cytokines. So, indirectly, it stimulates NADPH oxidase activity. It also stimulates directly H_2O_2 and OH* and reduces the activity of paranoxase (PON-1), and antioxidant enzyme and this reduction increases urinary and plasma 8-isoprostane and plasma MDA and hydroperoxides. Because PON-1 is involved in preventing the accumulation of peroxides in LDL, reduction in the activity of this enzyme could contribute to CAD development.

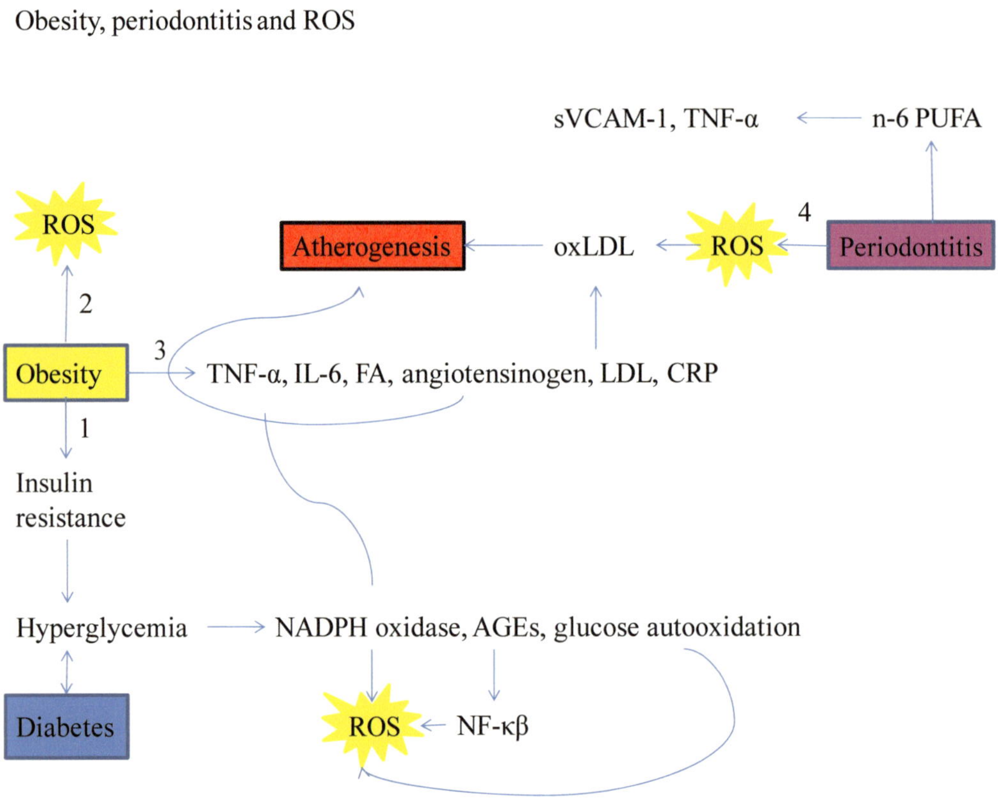

Fig. 5. Obesity, periodontitis and ROS. 1). Obesity is able to produce insulin resistance that will lead to hyperglycemia and diabetes. This hyperglycemia rises NADPH oxidase activity, favors the formation of AGEs and provoke glucose autooxidation. These three processes will generate ROS. 2). There is also a ROS generation by obesity due to a higher metabolism in obesity that will sum up to the produced by hyperglycemia. 3). There is an increased LDL and angiotensinogen plasma concentration in obesity that will support the formation of the atheroma plaque. 4). In addition, periodontitis is able to produce even more ROS to the organism, worsening the situation and leading to an oxidative stress status.

The last cardiovascular risk factor that obesity can modify is the endothelial function. Obese people also suffer from hypertension. Vascular endothelium presents some ROS sources that are deregulated in obesity because of the imbalance in rennin-angiotensin system as we saw before. Angiotensinogen converts to angiotensin II, leading to NADPH oxidase activity and xanthine oxidoreductase activity increase, LDL uptake by macrophages, nitric oxide synthase enzymatic uncoupling and the consequent formation of ROS, antioxidant depletion, lipid peroxidation and oxidative stress situation (Vicent & Taylor, 2006). Obesity is a risk factor for the development of glucose resistance, hypertension, diabetes, possibly due to the production of ROS and high plasma lipid levels.

6. Insulin resistance, glucose impairment, diabetes and periodontitis

Diabetes mellitus is a syndrome where carbohydrates, lipids and proteins metabolism is altered due to a lack of insulin secretion or to a decrease in tissues response to insulin. There are two kinds of diabetes:

- Diabetes mellitus type I: also called insulin dependent diabetes mellitus. In this diabetes, there is no production of insulin by pancreas.
- Diabetes mellitus type II: also called no insulin dependent diabetes mellitus. This diabetes presents a decrease in tissues response to insulin called insulin resistance.

The consequences of diabetes is that every cell, except encephalic cells, will not be able to properly use insulin, so plasma glucose levels raise and appears hyperglycemia.

Type II diabetes is strongly related to obesity. Almost every obese develop type II diabetes. The link between obesity and diabetes was unclear till the recent theory of ROS. As we saw before, obesity is an important factor in the development of diabetes because of the release of pro inflammatory cytokines and production of ROS that lead to an oxidative stress situation and the insulin resistance situation in obesity.

People with diabetes are at high risk of developing other health problems as macroangiopathies and microangiopathies. The first one consists on an accelerated atheromatosis that will have damaging effects over cardiovascular health. Microangiopathies affects to retina, kidney and peripheral nerves. Affliction of the kidney is an important fact in the instauration of a renal failure and diabetes is the first cause of chronic renal insufficiency. So, diabetes can cause accelerated atheromatosis with hypertension and chronic renal insufficiency, leaving the patient to a high cardiovascular disease risk situation.

Hyperglycemia produce decreased activity of vasodilators such as nitric oxide (NO), increased activity of angiotensin II, endothelin-1 and favors the production of permeability factors as vascular endothelial growth factor (VEGF). Later on, there is microvascular cell loss and capillary occlusion due to extracellular matrix overproduction by action of growth factors such as TGF-β and to deposition of extravasated acid-Schiff-positive plasma proteins. With respect to hypertension, these changes will produce glomerulosclerosis in the kidney, which will cause renal malfunction leading to hypertension.

Insulin resistance and hyperglycemia also provokes changes in blood lipid profile. Cholesterol enriched apolipoprotein B containing remnant particles levels, which is proatherogenic, is elevated in diabetes.

In diabetes, endothelial cells produce an excess of AGEs. Intracellular hyperglycemia originates autooxidation of glucose that ends with the formation of dicarbonyls that reacts with amino groups of intracellular and extracellular proteins to form AGEs. This AGEs importance keeps on the fact that, inter alia, they are able to react with macrophages and mesangial cells AGE receptors and to produce intracellular ROS that activates NF-κβ pathway with its consequent production of growth factors and pro inflammatory cytokines. AGE can also be formed on collagen to form very stable collagen macromolecules, resistant to normal enzymatic degradation. This AGE-modified collagen accumulates in the walls of blood vessels, narrowing the lumen. It also has affinity for LDL, so, AGE-modified collagen scavenges LDL and deposits them in the blood vessels walls, contributing to the formation of atheroma plaque and further cardiovascular problems. AGE-modified collagen has been shown to be found also in periodontal blood vessels.

AGE also promote the formation of VEGF that induces neovascularization and plays a major role in microvascular diabetes complications (Mealey & Oates, 2006). Another important molecule upregulated in diabetes is protein kinase C (PKC). This enzyme is activated by diacylglycerol, which levels are elevated in diabetes. PKC has several functions:

- Decrease eNOS activity and increase endothelin-1 activity, producing blood flow abnormalities.
- Increase VEGF levels, promoting vascular permeability and angiongenesis.
- Induce expression of TGF-β which promotes capillary occlusion.
- Induce overexpression of the fibrinolytic inhibitor PAI-1. By doing this, vascular occlusion is promoted.
- Activates NF-κβ pathway, releasing pro inflammatory cytokines.
- Activate NADPH oxidases that release ROS, leading to multiple effects in the organism.

Together with the formation of AGE and activation of PKC, in diabetes there is an increased flux in the polyol pathway and in the hexosamine pathway, both of them contributes to the progression of diabetes. But these four processes link together in a common pathway, the overproduction of superoxide by mitochondrial electron transport chain.

There is a value in the inner mitochondrial membrane proton gradient that when exceeded, superoxide production is highly increased. This limit is reached in diabetes, because of the overproduction of electron donors by the tricarboxilic acid cycle due to hyperglycemia. This is shown by measures of ROS that are elevated in mitochondria in diabetic patients. Overexpression of manganese superoxide dismutase (MnSOD) lowered these ROS levels and also lowered all the four factors that contribute to diabetes progression: formation of AGE, PCK, increased flux in polyol pathway and in hexosamine pathway. By inhibiting mitochondrial superoxide production, activation of NF-κβ is also inhibited. But not only MnSOD inhibits these processes, it also suppresses the increase in collagen synthesis in mesangial cells, decreases hyperglycemia induced apoptosis in dorsal root ganglion neurons, blocks hyperglycemia induced monocyte adhesion, prevents the inhibition of the anti atherogenic prostacyclin synthetase, PPAR-γ and endothelial nitric oxide synthase (eNOS).

This gives us an idea of how important is mitochondrial superoxide production and mitochondrial integrity in the development and progression of this disease. All damage done to mitochondria could affect its standard ROS production and transform the mitochondria in a potent ROS generator. This will not only affect progression of diabetes but also obesity, inflammation, hypertension, periodontitis, generating an oxidative stress situation (Brownlee, 2001).

6.1 Diabetes, periodontitis and oxidative stress

Diabetes and periodontitis are strongly related diseases. People suffering from diabetes have higher risk of developing periodontitis and people suffering from periodontitis have higher risk of developing diabetes. It is a positive feedback. Treatment of periodontal disease improves some diabetes complications as hyperglycemia or glycated hemoglobin. The way diabetes affects periodontitis may be as the result of the above mentioned processes that leads to release of pro inflammatory cytokines, activation of PKC that activates NADPH oxidase, accumulation of AGEs and deficiencies in tissue healing in diabetes. This would ease the damage produced in the periodontium and is associated with chronic periodontitis. Hyperglycemia produces inhibition of osteoblastic cell proliferation and collagen production so bone regeneration is attenuated and damage produced in the periodontium is this way higher, having mechanical diminished bone properties in the new formed teeth.

Studies have shown that specially TNF-α, IL-6 and IL-1β are markedly elevated in diabetes. Macrophages from diabetic patients release more TNF-α, PKC and O_2^- than macrophages from healthy patients (Karima et al, 2005), possibly due to a high glucose level and oxidative stress. Both diseases, periodontitis and diabetes are able to activate an immune host response with release of pro inflammatory cytokines and instauration of an oxidative stress situation. When both join together in the same patient, they can act synergistically (Nassar et al, 2007).

ROS can also be a final step in which some pathways converge to produce insulin resistance. It has been shown that TNF-α and dexamethasone are able to produce ROS. Although TNF-α is pro inflammatory and dexamethasone is an anti-inflammatory agent, both raise ROS levels and produce insulin resistance. Treatment with antioxidant molecules is able to decrease insulin resistance, measured as the defect in insulin mediated glucose uptake. Also, transgenic models of cell lines genetically modified to overexpress antioxidant enzymes and transgenic obese mice treated with antioxidants prevented insulin resistance after treatment with TNF-α and dexamethasone. This is indicative of the involvement of ROS in insulin resistance as antioxidant agents can prevent this process. Other evidences of ROS implicated in insulin resistance are the fact that in obesity, ROS are increased due to a constant inflammatory state, and this produce insulin resistance leading to diabetes. Also adipocytes treated with high doses of H_2O_2 or ROS inducers produce insulin resistance. The possible mechanism of ROS affecting insulin resistance can depend on the magnitude of ROS production, cell type affected, time of exposure, specific type of ROS or other factors that will activate any of the involved pathways as FoxO, MAPK, JAK/STAT, p53, phospholipase C, PI(3)K and other proteins encoded genes. A possible way is through activation of JNK by TNF-α. Antioxidant treatment reduces JNK insulin resistance mediated activity (Houstin et al, 2006). This could be the reason of how periodontitis could affect or worsen insulin resistance, by production of ROS that in the long term will produce diabetes as similarly happens in obesity. In periodontitis patients with type II diabetes, there is an increased C reactive protein level, which means there is increased IL-6 concentration that could exacerbate insulin resistance and contribute to diabetes worsening (Aspriello et al, 2011; Gomes-Filho et al, 2011).

It is important to have a good control of these diseases, preventing and if necessary, treating them. This is because as the worst the control of diabetes is the worst the effects on periodontitis severity and ROS production will be (Tsai et al, 2002; Lalla & Papapanou, 2011). As higher glycemic status, higher activity of PKC, NADPH oxidase and levels of DAG. DAG increases with hyperglycemia through the glycolytic /glycerol-3-phosphate acyltransferase pathway. This increase in DAG triggers activation of PKC. Also IL-1β levels are double in patients with poor glycemic control (>8 % glycohemoglobin test HbA1c) than in patients with good glycemic control. Periodontal treatment is able to reduce systemic inflammation, reduce serum TNF-α, C-reactive protein, IL-6, fibrinogen concentration, improves HbA1c levels and raise adiponectin concentration (Lalla and Papapanou, 2011).

Disease control consists on medication, healthy lifestyle and weight control for diabetes and proper oral hygiene for periodontitis. Avoid smoking for both diseases. It has been demonstrated that clinically treating periodontitis can reduce up to 48 % IL-6 levels in patients with periodontitis and type II diabetes (Tamaki et al, 2010) and also can reduce CRP levels (Marcaccini et al, 2009).

Diabetes is strongly related with hypertension and thus, cardiovascular disease. As mentioned above, one of the major complications of diabetes is the apparition of macroangiopathies and microangiopathies. These processes are favored by AGE products formed as a result of hyperglycemia and ROS production, protein kinase C and the renin angiotensin system activation.

AGEs products promote microangiopathies as seen by its apoptotic action over mesangial cells and the promotion of vascular endothelial growth factor (VEGF) which will contribute to glomerular hyperfiltration, an early renal dysfunction. Also, AGEs stimulate the production of insulin like growth factor-I, -II, PDGF and TGF-β in mesangial cells, which in turn produce type IV collagen, laminin and fibronectin. TGF-β is an important molecule that plays an important role in the pathogenesis of glomerulosclerosis and tubulointerstitial fibrosis. AGE-RAGE system is also related with the renin angiotensin system because angiotensin II produce ROS in renal cells and ROS are causative of AGEs. Then AGEs activate mesangial TGF-β-Smad system which activates production of angiotensin II (Yamagishi et al, 2011).

There are several ways for AGEs products to contribute to the development of macroangiopathies such as decrease in the elasticity of the vasculature, quenching of NO, decreasing vasodilation, increased oxidative stress that impairs NO synthase and produces peroxinitrite ($ONOO^-$), increase in plasma LDL or activation of atherosclerosis related genes by ROS generation as ICAM-1, VCAM-1, monocyte chemotactic protein-1(MCP-1), plasminogen activator inhibitor-1 (PAI-1), tissue factor, VEGF and RAGE. There is also a deficient tissue repair situation in diabetes because of a decrease in endothelial progenitor cells (EPCs) number, function and mobilization. These cells are capable of differentiate in endothelial cells. Deficit in endothelial repair may lead to accelerated atherosclerosis and higher risk of suffering from cardiovascular disease (Yamagishi et al, 2011).

As it has been mentioned before another important molecule with a protective paper against the formation of AGEs, is named PPAR-γ. This is a membrane receptor that acts as a transcription factor regulating the expression of genes. They participate in regulation of vascular tone, inflammation, hypertension, obesity and metabolic syndrome (Oyekan, 2011). PPAR-γ reduces blood pressure by reducing the expression of ATII type 1 receptor and inhibiting ATII signaling pathways, what will suppress the renin angiotensin system (RAS). Regulation of hypertension comes from the suppression of RAS and also of the thromboxane A_2 system. And by reducing hypertension, renal function is facilitated (Sugawara et al, 2010). PPAR-γ agonists could be a powerful tool to improve diabetes complications since its activation also inhibit nitrite, fibronectin and type IV collagen production by mesangial cells and attenuate AGE induced production of IL-8 and ICAM-1 in proximal tubular epithelial cells. PPAR-γ agonists also lower TNF-α by suppressing NF-κβ activation and downregulate RAGEs expression, what in the end leads to an avoidance of the release of ROS, MCP-1 or VCAM-1 (Yamagishi et al, 2011).

AGEs products are really harmful molecules produced in diabetes that can affect to oxidative stress by increasing ROS production and also raise the risk of cardiovascular disease by promoting renal failure and atherosclerosis and the develops of periodontitis.

Advanced glycation end products (AGEs) functions

- React with macrophages, mesangial cells and produce ROS.
- ROS activate NF-κβ.
- NF-κβ produce cytokines and growth factors (insulin like growth factor-I, platelet derived growth factor or TGF-β).
- AGEs forms modified collagen that accumulates in blood vessel walls.
- Scavenge LDL and deposit them in blood vessel walls.
- Promotes angiotensin II production.
- Quenching of NO.

Fig. 6. Advanced glycation end products (AGEs) functions

7. Conclusion

So, to summarize, periodontitis not also affects cardiac health in a direct manner by ROS production, but also in an indirect way by promoting the instauration of the metabolic syndrome (obesity, insulin resistance, atherogenic dyslipemia, hypertension, pro-inflammatory state and prothrombotic state). Even so, the common link between periodontitis and metabolic syndrome or cardiovascular disease is also the action of ROS either acting as a second messenger or directly damaging target molecules as proteins, lipids or DNA. We have seen that periodontitis is a process that generates a great amount of ROS, not only in the site of the infection, the periodontium, but also releases pro-inflammatory cytokines and ROS to the rest of the organism, leading to an oxidative stress situation and a depletion of anti-oxidant molecules over time. This will also contribute to aggravate any other illness that could be already present at the patient or simply help them to arise as any of the metabolic syndrome components. In fact, ROS are seen to participate in lots of organic processes and could be the reason of the instauration of certain afflictions as insulin resistance, hypertension or atheroma plaque development. ROS and oxidative stress are always present at every one of these illnesses that lead to cardiovascular disease, and they even participate directly in cardiovascular damage.

In obesity, hyperglycemia is able to produce ROS by 3 different ways as we saw before: AGEs formation and NF-κβ activation, conversion of glucose to sorbitol and activation of NADPH oxidase and glucose auto-oxidation. There is also a major metabolic rate in obese people and more NADPH oxidase activity that will produce more ROS than non-obese people. And this higher ROS generation together with the high plasma LDL and free fatty acids levels is able to damage the endothelium by promoting the formation of the atheroma plaque and lipid peroxidation.

In diabetes, AGEs formation produces ROS as in obesity. There is an increased flux in the polyol pathway that produces ROS. Also, diabetic macrophages release more TNF-α, IL-6 and IL-β, what will produce even more ROS. If this is not enough, in diabetes, angiotensin II levels are higher, and we have seen that it is able to produce ROS by stimulation of NADP oxidase.

In hypertension, angiotensin II, endothelin-1 and urotensin II levels are higher, so, they will stimulate NADPH oxidase with its consequents effects over ROS production. These ROS will also uncouple NO synthase and react with NO to form $ONOO^-$. In a hypertensive situation, mitochondria activity is elevated, and therefore, ROS generation will be higher, having higher risk for mitochondrial damage. ROS are also able to produce glomerulopathies and to oxidize LDL thus promoting the formation of atheroma plaque.

Finally, ROS can damage by themselves cardiomyocytes directly, leading to heart malfunction. They also activate matrix metalloproteinases that will remodel coronary blood vessels and arteries, leading to coronary insufficiency. As in hypertension, mitochondrion is also compromised by ROS action, with risk of releasing pro apoptotic molecules that will undergo cardiomyocyte apoptosis. Cardiomyocytes regeneration rate is scarce or even null, so cardiomyocyte loss is a very important event in heart damage and cardiovascular development.

All these processes implicate ROS production and an oxidative stress situation installed in the organism. We have seen that ROS are involved in lots of damaging mechanisms and they can ease the emergence of some of these afflictions that compromises cardiovascular health. Periodontitis, as a high ROS and pro inflammatory generator process can greatly contribute to aggravate all of these symptoms. It is not involved in cardiovascular failure by itself directly, but in an indirect manner, it can worsen the harmful effects exerted by metabolic syndrome. As we have seen, periodontal treatments decreased ROS generation and the risk of developing some of these illnesses. As these illnesses are risk factors for developing cardiovascular diseases, avoiding periodontitis also lowers the probability of developing these cardiovascular risk factors. This is a good trail that takes us to believe on the relationship between periodontitis and cardiovascular disease.

8. References

Ando K, Fujita T. (2009). Metabolic syndrome and oxidative stress. *Free Radic Biol Med.* 1; 47 (3): 213-8.

Aspriello SD, Zizzi A, Tirabassi G, Buldreghini E, Biscotti T, Faloia E, Stramazzotti D, Boscaro M, Piemontese M. (2011).Diabetes mellitus-associated periodontitis: differences between type 1 and type 2 diabetes mellitus. *J Periodontal Res.* 46(2): 164-9.

Baelum V, Lopez R. (2004). Periodontal epidemiology: towards social science or molecular biology?. *Community Dent Oral Epidemiol.* 32 (4): 239-49.

Borges I Jr, Moreira EA, Filho DW, de Oliveira TB, da Silva MB, Fröde TS. (2007). Proinflammatory and Oxidative Stress Markers in Patients with Periodontal Disease. *Mediators Inflamm.* 2007: 45794.

Borges PK, Gimeno SG, Tomita NE, Ferreira SR (2007). Prevalence and characteristics associated with metabolic syndrome in Japanese- Brazilians with and without periodontal disease. *Cad Saude Publica.* 23;657-668.

Brecx M, Frolicher I, Gehr P, Lang NP. (1998). Stereological observations on long term experimental gingivitis in man. *J ClinPeriodontol* 15: (621–627).

Brownlee M. (2001). Biochemistry and molecular cell biology of diabetic complications. *Nature.* 13; 414(6865): 813-20.

Bullon P, Morillo JM, Ramirez-Tortosa MC, Quiles JL, Newman HN, Battino M. (2009). Metabolic syndrome and periodontitis: is oxidative stress a common link?. *J Dent Res.* 88:503–18.

Bullon P, Cordero M, Quiles JL, Morillo JM, Ramirez-Tortosa MC, Battino M. (2011). Mitochondrial dysfunction promoted by Porphyromonas gingivalis lipolysaccharide as a possible link between cardiovascular disease and periodontitis. Free Radical in Medicine & Biology, in press.

Chang JC, Kou SJ, Lin WT, Liu CS. (2010). Regulatory role of mitochondria in oxidative stress and atherosclerosis. *World J Cardiol.* 26; 2 (6): 150-9.

D'Aiuto F, Sabbah W, Netuveli G, Donos N, Hingorani AD, Deanfield J, *et al.* (2008). Association of the metabolic syndrome with severe periodontitis in a large U.S. population-based survey. J *Clin Endocrin Metab.* 93;3989-3994.

D'Aiuto F, Nibali L, Parkar M, Patel K, Suvan J, Donos N. (2010). Oxidative Stress, Systemic Inflammation, and Severe Periodontitis. *J Dent Res.* 89 (11): 1241-6.

Dirkx E, Schwenk RW, Glatz JF, Luiken JJ, van Eys GJ. (2011). High fat diet induced diabetic cardiomyopathy. *Prostaglandins Leukot Essent Fatty Acids.* May 13. [Epub ahead of print] PMID: 21571515 [PubMed - as supplied by publisher]

Ekuni D, Endo Y, Irie K, Azuma T, Tamaki N, Tomofuji T, Morita M. (2010). Imbalance of oxidative/anti-oxidative status induced by periodontitis is involved in apoptosis of rat submandibular glands. *Arch Oral Biol.* 55 (2): 170-6.

Fialkow L, Wang Y, Downey GP. (2007). Reactive oxygen and nitrogen species as signaling molecules regulating neutrophil function. *Free RadicBiol Med.* 15; 42 (2): 153-64.

Fitzgerald DC, Meade KG, McEvoy AN, Lillis L, Murphy EP, MacHugh DE, Baird AW. (2007). Tumour necrosis factor-α (TNF-α) increases nuclear factor κB (NFκB) activity in and interleukin-8 (IL-8) release from bovine mammary epithelial cells. *Vet Immunol Immunopathol.* 15; 116 (1-2): 59-68.

Gomes-Filho IS, Freitas Coelho JM, Seixas da Cruz S, Passos JS, Teixeira de Freitas CO, AragãoFarias NS, Amorim da Silva R, Silva Pereira MN, Lima TL, Barreto ML. (2011). Chronic Periodontitis and C-reactive Protein Levels.*J Periodontol.* 82 (7): 969-78.

Houstis N, Rosen ED, Lander ES. (2006). Reactive oxygen species have a causal role in multiple forms of insulin resistance. *Nature.* 13; 440 (7086): 944-8.

Humphrey LL, Fu R, Buckley DI, Freeman M, Helfand M. (2008). Periodontal disease and coronary heart disease incidence: a systematic review and meta-analysis. *J Gen Intern Med.* 23 (12): 2079-86.

Karima M, Kantarci A, Ohira T, Hasturk H, Jones VL, Nam BH, Malabanan A, Trackman PC, Badwey JA, Van Dyke TE. (2005). Enhanced superoxide release and elevated protein kinase C activity in neutrophils from diabetic patients: association with periodontitis. *J Leukoc Biol.* 78 (4): 862-70.

Kinane DF, Mark Bartold P. (2007). Clinical relevance of the host responses of periodontitis. *Periodontol 2000.* 43: 278-93.

Kinane DF. (2001). Causation and pathogenesis of periodontal disease. *Periodontol 2000.* 25: 8–20.

Laky M, Assinger A, Esfandeyari A, Bertl K, Haririan H, Volf I. (2011). Decreased phosphorylation of platelet vasodilator-stimulated phosphoprotein in periodontitis--a role of periodontal pathogens. *Thromb Res.* 128 (2): 155-60.

Lalla E, Papapanou PN. (2011). Diabetes mellitus and periodontitis: a tale of two common interrelated diseases. *Nat Rev Endocrinol.* 28. doi: 10.1038/nrendo. 2011. 106.

Liu L, Li Y, Guan C, Li K, Wang C, Feng R, Sun C. (2010). Free fatty acid metabolic profile and biomarkers of isolated post-challenge diabetes and type 2 diabetes mellitus based on GC-MS and multivariate statistical analysis. *J Chromatogr B AnalytTechnol Biomed Life Sci.* 15; 878 (28): 2817-25.

Marcaccini AM, Meschiari CA, Sorgi CA, Saraiva MC, de Souza AM, Faccioli LH, Tanus-Santos JE, Novaes AB, Gerlach RF. (2009). Circulating interleukin-6 and high-sensitivity C-reactive protein decrease after periodontal therapy in otherwise healthy subjects. *J Periodontol.* 80 (4): 594-602.

Mealey BL, Oates TW. (2006). American Academy of Periodontology. Diabetes Mellitus and Periodontal Diseases. *J Periodontol.* 77 (8): 1289-303.

Monteiro AM, Jardini MA, Alves S, Giampaoli V, Aubin EC, FigueiredoNeto AM, Gidlund M. (2009). Cardiovascular disease parameters in periodontitis. *J Periodontol.* 80 (3): 378-88.

Nassar H, Kantarci A, van Dyke TE. (2007). Diabetic periodontitis: a model for activated innate immunity and impaired resolution of inflammation. *Periodontol 2000.* 43: 233-44.

Oyekan A. (2011). PPARs and their Effects on the Cardiovascular System. Clin Exp Hypertens. 33(5):287-93

Paquette DW, Brodala N, Nichols TC. (2007). Cardiovascular disease, inflammation, and periodontal infection. *Periodontol 2000.* 44: 113-26.

Papapanagiotou D, Nicu EA, Bizzarro S, Gerdes VE, Meijers JC, Nieuwland R, van der Velden U, Loos BG. (2009). Periodontitis is associated with platelet activation. Atherosclerosis. 202 (2): 605-11

Paraskevas S, Huizinga JD, Loos BG. (2008). A systematic review and meta-analyses on C-reactive protein in relation to periodontitis. *J Clin Periodontol.* 35 (4): 277-90.

Ramirez-Tortosa MC, Quiles JL, Battino M, Granados S, Morillo JM, Bompadre S, Newman HN, Bullon P. (2010).Periodontitis is associated with altered plasma fatty acids and cardiovascular risk markers. *Nutr Metab Cardiovasc Dis.* 20 (2): 133-9.

Sugawara A, Uruno A, Kudo M, Matsuda K, Yang CW, Ito S. (2010).Effects of PPARγ on hypertension, atherosclerosis, and chronic kidney disease. *Endocr J.* 57 (10): 847-52.

Sutherland WH, de Jong SA, Walker RJ, et al. (2002). Effect of meals rich in heated olive and safflower oils on oxidation of postprandial serum in healthy men. *Atherosclerosis* 160(1):195–203.

Tamaki N, Tomofuji T, Ekuni D, Yamanaka R, Morita M. (2010). Periodontal treatment decreases plasma oxidized LDL level and oxidative stress. *Clin Oral Investig.* 18 Aug 18.

Tonetti MS. (2009). Periodontitis and risk for atherosclerosis: an update on intervention trials. *J ClinPeriodontol.* 36; 10: 15-9.

Tsai C, Hayes C, Taylor GW. (2002). Glycemic control of type 2 diabetes and severe periodontal disease in the US adult population. *Community Dent Oral Epidemiol.* 30 (3): 182-92.

Tsutsui H, Kinugawa S, Matsushima S. (2009). Mitochondrial oxidative stress and dysfunction in myocardial remodelling. *Cardiovasc Res.* 15; 81 (3): 449-56.

Vincent HK, Taylor AG. (2006). Biomarkers and potential mechanisms of obesity-induced oxidant stress in humans. *Int J Obes (Lond).* 30 (3): 400-18.

Yamagishi SI, Maeda S, Matsui T, Ueda S, Fukami K, Okuda S. (2011). Role of advanced glycation end products (AGEs) and oxidative stress in vascular complications in diabetes. *Biochim Biophys Acta.* [Epub ahead of print] PMID: 21440603

Zadik Y, Bechor R, Galor S, Levin L. (2010). Periodontal disease might be associated even with impaired fasting glucose. *Br Dent J* 208. (10):E20.

9

Cardiovascular Risk Assessment in Diabetes and Chronic Kidney Diseases: A New Insight and Emerging Strategies

Ali Reza Khoshdel
AJA University of Medical Sciences, Tehran, Iran

1. Introduction

The post-millennium era witnesses a substantial epidemiologic transition in which cardiovascular disease (CVD) has taken more important role in mortality and morbidity in almost all parts of the world[1]. However, the natural history of CVD itself has also been evolving in parallel to changing life style and environmental risk factors. Nevertheless, despite a global movement for CVD control, the target points are still poorly achieved[2]. Therefore, a new look at the issue of CVD pathophysiology, CVD markers and risk assessment is necessary for a proper and effective care plan and targeting CVD prevention and control.

The classification of some elements to "*risk factors*" and "*risk markers*" has been controversial. There have been serious debates about the validity and impact of classic CVD risk factors. However, it is generally accepted that classic CVD risk factors cannot fully explain the epidemiology and natural history of the disease particularly in patients with co-morbidities. As a result several lists of emerging risk factors have been introduced with various clinical or research applications. Accordingly, several risk scores have been developed for risk assessment among various populations. Nevertheless, we face a network of associated risk factors with synergic effects, of which some factors play central roles and connect other factors together. For instance, central arterial pressure and arterial stiffness and also microalbuminuria have attracted more attention as summative CVD markers or risk factors and have been proposed as new targets for more efficient treatment.

Increasing evidence of cross-links among CVD, diabetes mellitus (DM) and chronic kidney disease (CKD) has been published in recent decades. DM and CKD are major comorbidities with CVD. In addition, several studies demonstrated greater frequency of CVD in DM and CKD, even in very early stages. On the other hand, our recent research revealed a significant impact of minimal heart dysfunction on further development of renal impairment[3]. Then, it seems that CVD, CKD and DM shares many risk factors and influences each other in various stages. This could be demonstrated as a pyramid with facets of presentations and a common pathophysiologic base. Considering this network of associations, we have introduced the concept of *circulatory (MARC) syndrome*, which facilitates understanding, evaluation, detection and interventions on the CVD risk factors earlier, easier and more effective. This concept preserves the positive features of the so called "*metabolic syndrome*" but prevents its weaknesses and improves its clinical applications. This leads to a novel paradigm in CVD management with new checking points, new targets and better achievements in the patients' care.

2. Epidemiologic trends in CVD risk factors

CVD has been evolving through 4 epidemiologic transition periods[1] with increasing frequency of proportion of death due to CVD during the first 3 stages and a slight decrease in the disease rate in the 4th stage, possibly due to controlling CV risk factors. However, it seems that a 5th stage is being developed due to epidemic diabetes, hypertension, obesity and chronic kidney disease as well as leveling off the smoking session rate in combination to social and economic instability in many countries. Consequently, epidemiologic trends in CVD and CV risk factors have been changing during the past decades both in developed and in developing countries. Developing countries, in particular, experience a substantial rise in CVD and younger age at onset of the disease, which is partially attributed to their demographic remodeling including a high population growth rate and inverted population pyramid with a majority of young individuals [1]. Furthermore, these countries face to a "*dual epidemiology*" of contrasting an undernourished and poor population against a significant proportion of overweight and obese groups. The last World Health Organization report on global burden of disease and risk factors demonstrated that the highest rates of CV death were in Eastern Europe, Central Asia, Middle East and North Africa. Also six out of 10 countries with highest rate of diabetes were in Eastern Mediterranean and Middle East region. However, there was a considerable heterogeneity in other regions which reflects different stages of epidemiologic transitions even in a single country like China[1, 4].

Eight risk factors (alcohol use, tobacco use, high blood pressure, high body mass index, high cholesterol, high blood glucose, low fruit and vegetable intake, and physical inactivity) account for 61% of cardiovascular deaths[4]. Moreover, air pollution, climate change, psychosocial stressors and maternal-foetal metabolic adaptation are also introduced as important CV risk factors[1]. However the pattern of the risk factors differs in subgroups of age, gender and patient groups while some factors loses their impact in parallel to homogeneity of the factor in the group[5]. It also evolves as a population passes through epidemiologic transitions from traditional to emerging risk factors.

From a practical perspective, primary and secondary prevention must be arranged for modifiable risk factors. The Framingham Study and subsequently the INTERHEART study have identified the important risk factors and targets for modification. Moreover, an analysis of 10 studies across the world in which there has been a decline in CVD mortality, demonstrated that risk factor modification was associated with 44% of the decline in the Netherlands, 50–54% in the USA, and 76% in North Karelia, Finland. New treatments are responsible for 23–47% of the decline in mortality[1]. Although, economic, cultural and logistic conditions have various impacts on preventive strategies in different population; *risk assessment* is a fundamental step for any CV preventive strategy.

2.1 CV risk in diabetes mellitus

CVD is the leading cause of mortality among DM patients [6, 7] with the prevalence of, incidence of, and mortality from all forms of CVD being 2-8 fold higher in diabetics when compared to a non-diabetic population. DM is accompanied with various cardiovascular abnormalities including endothelial dysfunction, increased oxidative stress and micro- and macrovascular consequences leading to coronary artery disease, left ventricular dysfunction (particularly diastolic dysfunction), hypertensive heart disease and reduced cardiac reserve[8]. A different trend in CV risk factors has been reported in patients with and without DM in Framingham Study from 1970 to 2005. This study demonstrated a greater increase in BMI, greater decrease in cholesterol and similar reduction in hypertension in DM when compared to non-DM[2].

The special writing group for the *American Heart Association* established that the goal of risk assessment would be to identify subclinical CVD in patients with DM which would lead to better management and improvement in disease morbidity and mortality. Furthermore they also designated DM as a "coronary risk equivalent" and indicated that DM patients belong in the same risk category as patients with known CVD[9]. This risk increases with age (>35 yrs), younger age at onset of DM, duration of DM (>10 yrs), presence of microvascular complications and other CV risk factors [10, 11]. Screening and CV risk assessment of DM patients is also strongly recommended in many guidelines including a French guideline which recommended screening for silent myocardial ischemia (including exercise stress testing) in DM patients with one additional risk factor [9]. However, the *American Heart Association* recommended exercise testing in this group when individuals plan moderate to high intensity exercise[11]. Furthermore, while the hemodynamic response to increased physical activity is a predictor of future hypertension [12] and is helpful in the early diagnosis of heart failure[13], it might also provide further information about the factors contributing to impaired cardiovascular control even in DM patients without additional risk. Accordingly, we demonstrated in a study of more than 17000 patients (including 1722 DM pts) an impaired hemodynamic response to exercise stress testing in DM group compared to non-diabetics and most importantly showed that the responses predicts the development of ESRD in diabetic patients[3, 14-16]. (Figure 1) Furthermore, in an outpatient setting of patients with diabetes and hypertension; we reported a substantial proportion of patients being non-dipper for nocturnal blood pressure. This study also showed an inverse relationship between white coat hypertension and arterial stiffness or microalbuminuria[17]. A comparison between normal individuals, patients with impaired fasting glucose, and diabetic patients did also demonstrate an increment of arterial stiffness in these groups[18]. In conclusion, all above evidence indicate subclinical arterial changes early in DM.

2.2 CV risk in diabetic kidney disease

About 10-40% of patients with diabetes mellitus (DM) develop nephropathy. Consequently with an increasing DM global prevalence and an aging population, DM has become the leading single cause of ESRD in many developed and developing countries [19-24]. Moreover, it is now proven that even a mild reduction in kidney function is accompanied by an increased cardiovascular (CV) risk [25, 26]. In addition, cardiac and renal DM complications share many risk factors and markers including microalbuminuria (mA), atherosclerosis and arteriosclerosis [27-29]. Therefore, evaluation and treatment of renal risk factors should not only prevent progression to End-Stage Renal Disease (ESRD), but also reduce CV risk.

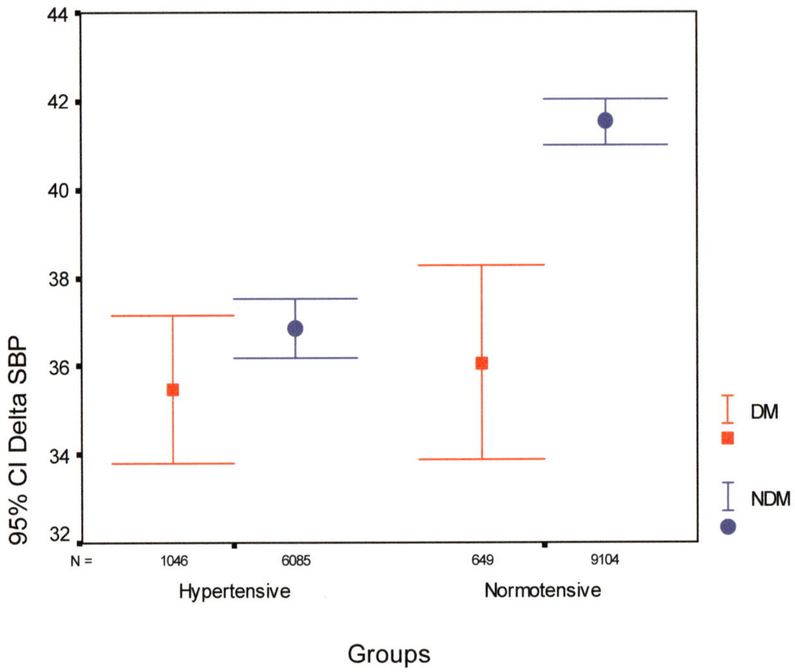

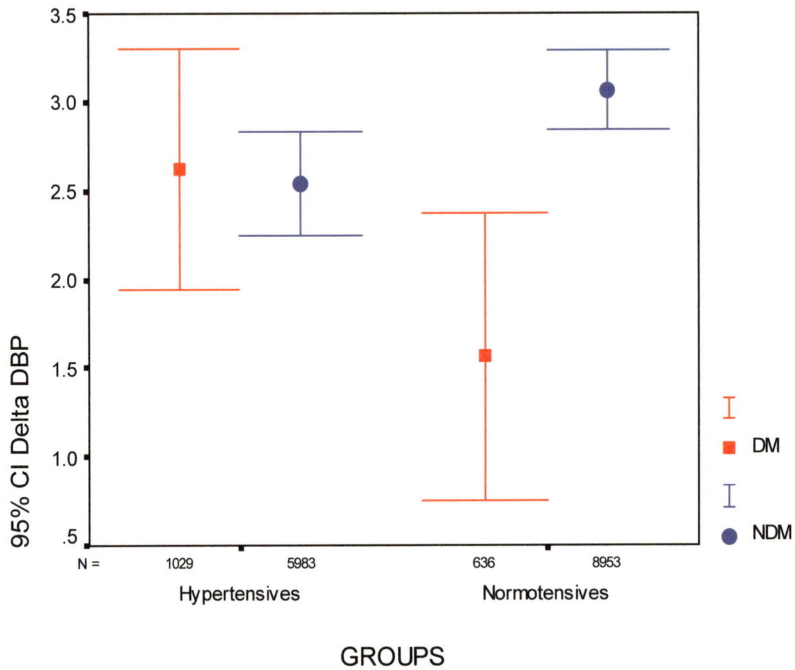

Fig. 1. Differential response of DM and NDM to the exercise test in hypertensive and normotensive subgroups

While the development and progression of renal damage in DM occurs very slowly, it often remains subclinical and undiagnosed for years [30], which inhibits effective prevention and intervention at a time when renal damage may be reversible. Therefore, early identification of diabetic nephropathy (DN) is a medical priority [31, 32]. Although mA is currently regarded as an early marker of DN, it is now preferably considered as a marker of a generalized endotheliopathy and then a CV risk marker. However, irreversible damage has often occurred when mA is detected [30, 33]. Furthermore, mA may not accurately represent the severity of renal damage, absent in marked renal dysfunction [34, 35] or may regress or fluctuate during the disease [34, 36]. Consequently, other markers, preferably in their early stages, should also be investigated as a potential guide to the progression of ESRD [31]. Arterial compliance changes occur early in DM and since arterial stiffness is an established independent predictor of mortality in the later stages of nephropathy [37-39], it should also correlate with renal function and BP profile in the earlier stages of DM.

Based on the above understanding, we made a large study including several subsets with various range of kidney function and compared CV risk factors in DM and non-DM, focusing on early stages in particular. The findings indicated that even in early stages of renal impairment without clinical presentation, DM patients had a greater level of arterial stiffness compared to non-DM. As a result, indices of arterial stiffness could be applied for a better CV risk management particularly in DM[40]. (Figure2). Multivariant analysis revealed arterial stiffness, hemoglobin, systolic blood pressure and triglyceride as the main determinants of renal function in DM (Table 1). Application of artificial neural network for analysis of major predictors of kidney function also determined arterial stiffness, hemoglobin, triglyceride, diabetes and blood pressure profile among major determinants of renal function.

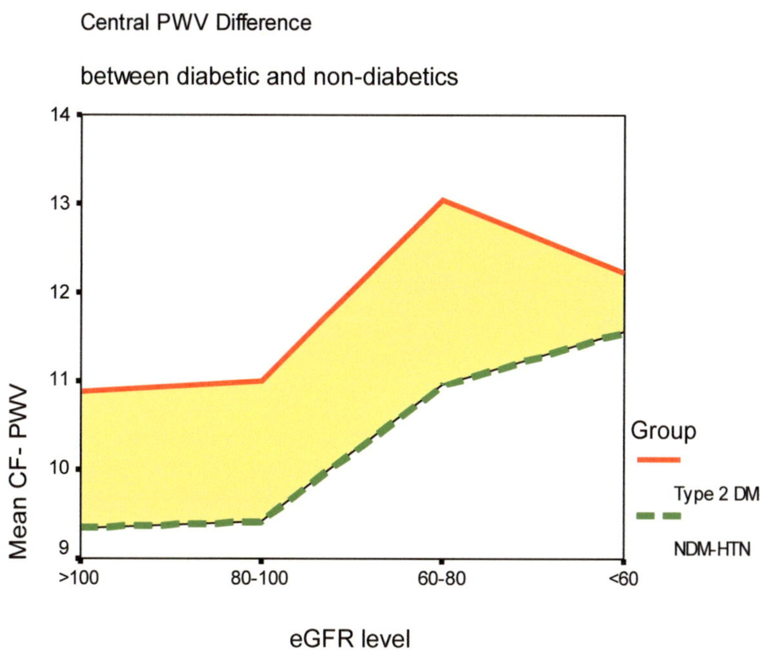

Fig. 2. Difference in the central arterial stiffness (as measured with CF-PWV) between type 2DM and NDM groups across levels of eGFR

Adj.R^2	Model 1 48%	Model 2 49%	Model 3 50%	Model 4 51%	Model 5 52%	Model 6 52%	Model 7 53%	Model 8 52%
rTr	0.397 0.259	0.403 0.245	0.393 0.249	0.411 0.222	0.410 0.219	0.202 0.116	0.202 0.115	**0.298** **0.009**
Male Gender	-0.279 0.038	-0.278 0.036	-0.263 0.033	-0.282 0.015	-0.288 0.012	-0.275 0.014	-0.269 0.015	**-0.281** **0.012**
CV disease	-0.273 0.040	-0.275 0.037	-0.269 0.037	-0.287 0.018	-0.280 0.020	-0.283 0.018	-0.282 0.017	**-0.277** **0.021**
Hb	0.352 0.010	0.342 0.009	0.329 0.008	0.351 0.002	0.351 0.002	0.356 0.002	0.355 0.001	**0.361** **0.001**
HbA1c	-0.152 0.217	-0.163 0.161	-0.153 0.168	-0.158 0.150	-0.155 0.154	-0.149 0.165	-0.164 0.122	**-0.186** **0.082**
TG	-0.304 0.014	-0.294 0.013	-0.287 0.013	-0.293 0.010	-0.288 0.010	-0.299 0.007	-0.300 0.006	**-0.273** **0.012**
Peripheral DBP	0.087 0.597	0.101 0.516	0.129 0.323	0.149 0.225	0.148 0.222	0.158 0.187	0.173 0.142	
ACE-I	0.099 0.396	0.105 0.354	0.109 0.328	0.094 0.372	0.089 0.394	0.079 0.440		
HR	-0.199 0.540	-0.207 0.517	-0.207 0.513	-0.207 0.508	-0.211 0.496			
ARB	0.057 0.597	0.056 0.598	0.065 0.532	0.062 0.541				
Age	-0.075 0.635	-0.071 0.649	-0.072 0.642					
Peripheral SBP	0.060 0.689	0.048 0.739						
Insulin	**-0.040** **0.748**							

Table 1. Regression models for determinants of eGFR in the DM group, Values are ß (upper line) and P value (lower line)

2.3 CV risk in ESRD

Cardiovascular disease (CVD) is a common complication in end-stage renal disease (ESRD) with a 10 to 30 times greater CVD mortality compared to the general population[41]. Traditional CV risk factors while more prevalent, cannot fully explain this increased CV event rate in ESRD[28] and other factors including increased lipoprotein-a (lipo-a), adipokines, asymmetric dimethylarginine (ADMA), hyperhomocysteinemia, hyperparathyroidism and arterial stiffness have been implicated [27, 42-46]. In turn, arterial stiffness is affected by several hemodynamic and metabolic factors.

Diabetes mellitus (DM) is the leading cause of ESRD [43]. It is also a major CV risk. Despite medications and attempts to control these CV risk factors, CV events still remain the most common cause of mortality both in DM and in ESRD [47-49]. While a greater risk of CV events is expected in DM compared to non-DM patients with ESRD , the available reports regarding the risk profile in DM and non-DM patients with ESRD are conflicting [42, 43, 50-53]. Likewise interactions between ESRD and DM in the development and progression of arterial stiffness are not completely clear [54, 55]. As a result of several metabolic factors which contribute in arterial stiffening, vascular calcification is proposed as the fundamental phenomena in arterial stiffness and is certainly a frequent finding in ESRD and DM [56-58]. However the mechanisms for the development of vascular calcification are not completely understood. In particular, reports of its relationship with calcium homeostatic mechanisms including parathyroid hormone (PTH), phosphate and the calcium-phosphate product (Ca×P) and vitamin D are inconsistent[58-62].

In an attempt to clarify classic and emerging risk factors in ESRD, we conducted a study of 100 diabetic and non-diabetic (paired matched for age and gender) individuals with ESRD and demonstrated blood pressure, heart rate, height and renal function as well as metabolic profiles, including cholesterol, homocystein, lipo(a) and CRP were comparable. However, carotid-femoral PWV (12.3 ±0.5 vs 10.3± 0.2; $P<0.001$) and pulse pressure (71.2± 2.2 vs 64.2 ±2.4) were significantly greater in the DM group, despite a comparable AIx and waveform reflection time. Multivariate analysis demonstrated PTH to be a significant PWV determinant after adjustment for DM, renal function and BP ($P=0.038$). As a particular novel finding, calcium-phosphate product had a u-shape association with central and peripheral PWV ($P<0.05$), that is both low and high levels of calcium-phosphate product increases the CV risk in this group which was similar to its relationship with mortality, reported by Block et al. In conclusion, arterial stiffness as an established, independent and strong predictor of mortality in ESRD patients [63, 64] is possibly the factor that links cardiac and renal disease (Figure 3)[25]. Consequently, we proposed a model that can explain association of the factors (Figure 4).

2.4 CV risk in kidney transplanted patients

Kidney transplant patients have a lower risk of CVD compared to dialysis patients, even after controlling important source of selection bias including age[65]. However, CVD is still a common cause of post-transplant death [19]. Nevertheless, classic risk factors cannot fully explain the CV risk in this population. It is reported that the Framingham CV risk score significantly underestimates the risk of ischemic heart disease in transplant patients [66] and therefore, non-classic risk factors including C-reactive protein, homocystein and renal function as well as arterial stiffness may contribute in CV risk in this population [67, 68].

In support to the previously demonstrated findings our group studied 100 kidney transplanted patients (including 33 DM) and reported with a comparable classic CV risk factors, homocystein and renal function had a greater arterial stiffness when compared to non-DM. Also an improvement in central arterial stiffness was observed after a year of follow-up[69, 70]. This is in line with the other evidence that cardiac function in DM transplant candidates is carefully evaluated prior to transplantation and LV systolic, diastolic function and arterial compliance improves shortly after a successful renal transplant [71-75]. It was also concluded that assessment of arterial stiffness may improve pre-transplantation risk assessment both in donors and recipients[70].

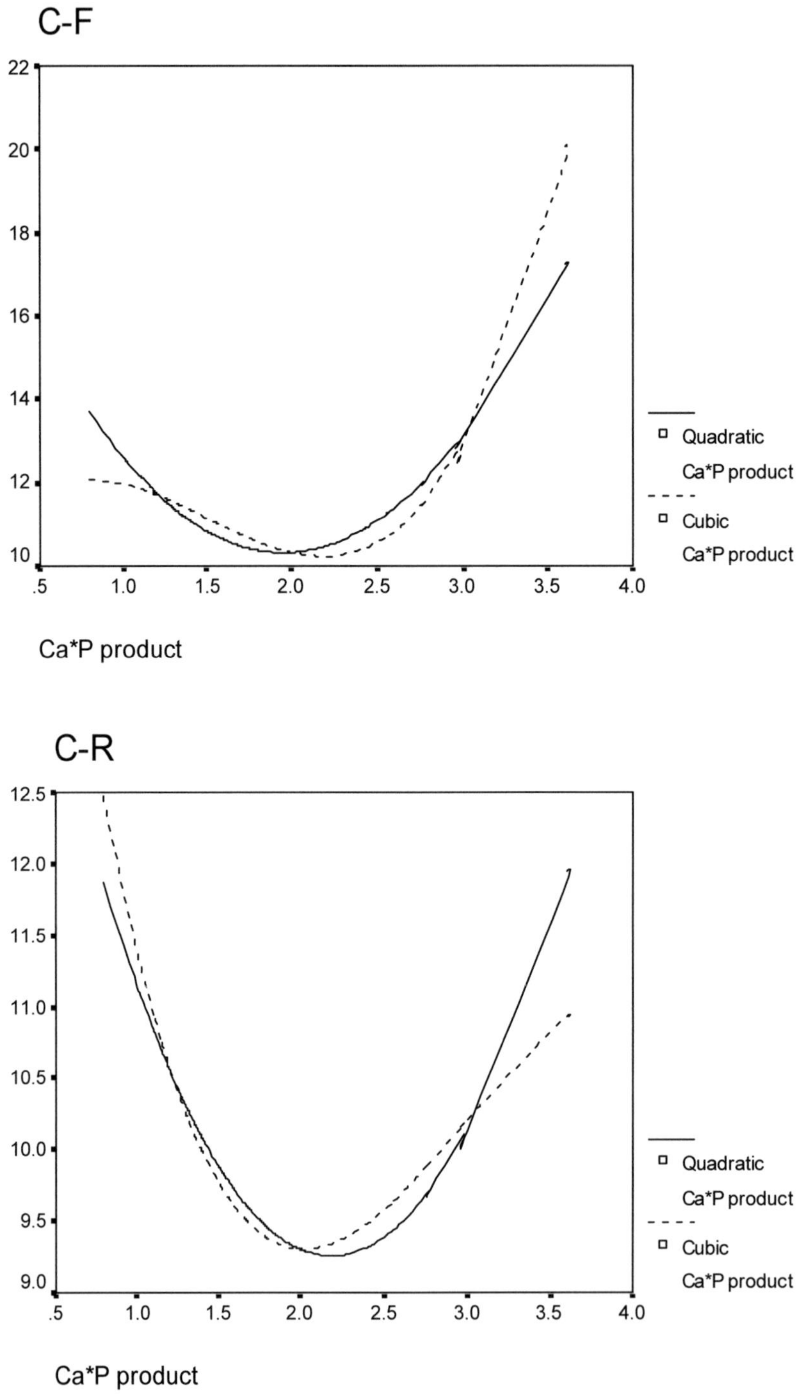

Fig. 3. Non-linear relationship between central (left) and peripheral (right) pulse wave velocity with calcium-phosphorus product in ESRD

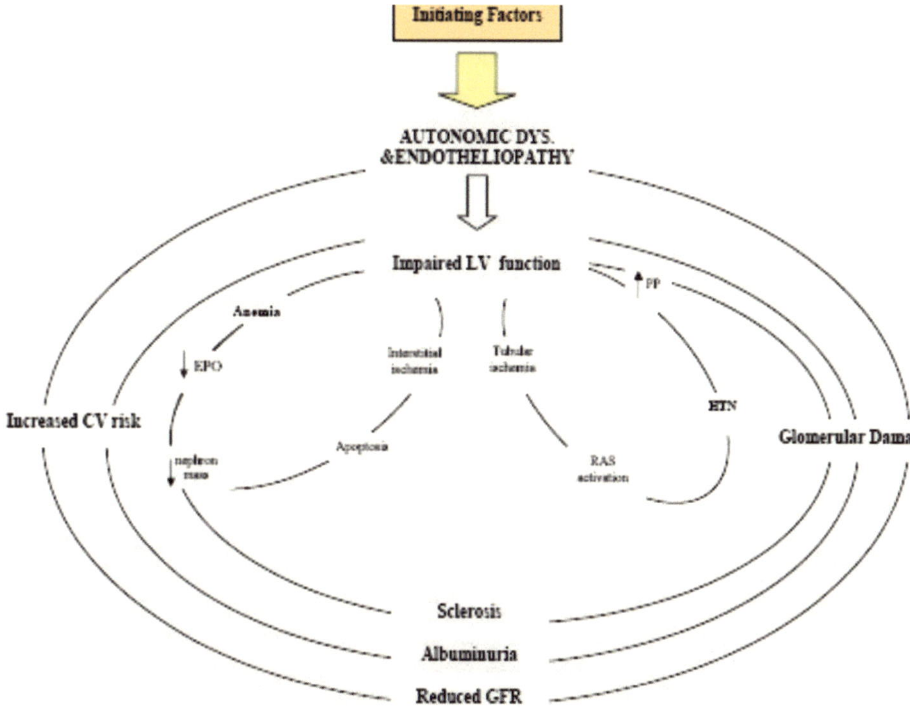

Fig. 4. Hypothetical model for explaining Renal-Cardiac Cross talk

3. Fundamentals in CVD risk assessment

The global epidemic of diabetes and chronic kidney diseases and their effect on the increased incidence of CVD, stresses on undeniable requirement for a timely effective CVD risk assessment in order to implement prevention strategies.

Risk assessment is a fundamental component of primary and secondary preventive strategies and an important skill in clinical epidemiology in particular for chronic diseases such as diabetes mellitus (DM) with potentially preventable multi-organ involvement. Although many risk factors have been identified as promoting DM complications, the presence of a risk factor only demonstrates the "risk" or the "possibility" of the given outcome since not all patients with the factor develop an adverse outcome and vice versa. However from a preventive point of view the medical approach is the attempted reduction of all risks factors so as to decrease this possibility. Nevertheless, decision thresholds are important determinants of risk factor management.

Traditionally, patients are assessed and managed based on the presence or absence of individual risk factors with a target point for each risk factor being determined and medical interventions (commonly by separate specialties) applied to achieve these targets. However, these risk factors also interact and can augment or diminish each others effect. In other words, patients with a particular risk factor might be more prone or more susceptible to be influenced by another risk factor. Moreover risk factors may have a *synergistic effect* thereby producing a greater impact beyond a summation of their individual risk. Accordingly, different target points have been assigned for various patient subgroups. For instance, recent practice guidelines suggested different target blood pressures for DM patients with and without proteinuria [76, 77]. Nevertheless, most risk factors such as BP have a linear relationship with the adverse outcome (i.e. CV events or mortality), even when levels are below the arbitrarily defined cut-off points[78, 79]. In an attempt to overcome this problem, new definitions such as pre-hypertension, pre-DM and pre-microalbuminuria have been added to recent practice guidelines [76, 77, 80], although they may have enhanced uncertainty and confusion rather than improve patient care.

While the target point approach appears to be straightforward, there may be a substantial risk of unnecessary treatment or neglect when treating certain patients. Consequently, a *multifactorial risk assessment* approach whereby a planned therapy is based on an individual's absolute risk is now encouraged [81]. This multidisciplinary approach is expected to be more effective, both medically and economically.

The simplest way to estimate a multifactorial global risk is to use the number of the present risk factors. For instance the number of present components of the metabolic syndrome associated with the risk of CV disease in DM or the development of renal impairment [82, 83]. Alternatively, each factor can be graded in an individual patient and scored (e.g. using the GCS in comatose diabetic patients) and then the total score is considered as representative of the severity of the condition and predictive for the outcome [84]. A more scientific approach would be to sort the factors according to their importance or the strength of their association and calculate a total risk or a "*risk score*" by summation of the weighted utilities of the factors. The appointed weight could be based on expert opinion or better still on more objective criteria. This technique should simulate the medical decision making process by a medical practitioner where the better the weighting the more accurate the diagnosis. Statistical methods including inferential analysis, discriminating analysis and probabilistic methods should facilitate this process. While multivariate analyses, including linear and logistic regression, are commonly used for this purpose, factor selection and modeling is the back bone of risk score development. Inappropriate modeling substantially damages the risk score performance [85]. Moreover, while the developed risk score can be ideally used in a similar population, it should not be extrapolated to other populations or even in the same population after a few years due to life style and risk factors changes, available medications or advanced diagnostic methods for the given outcome. Therefore, they must be repeatedly validated in the target population and re-evaluated to remain applicable in clinical practice. This process would yield an equation that would predict the outcome [86]. Although linear models are relatively simple and powerful methods for prediction, their essential assumptions including normality, independence and uniformity of variance must be fulfilled to be applicable [87]. Therefore, non-linear transformation is occasionally required and regression techniques can then be used to find the best discriminant function or decision boundary. However in most clinical situations many factors have equivocal discriminatory power and risk factors have interactions and clusters overlap. As a result the data space is multidimentional [86]. In these cases, intelligent systems including artificial neural networks can improve modeling and prediction. They provide a framework by selecting the most important discriminant items and appropriate form of boundaries [86, 88, 89]. Many [85] but not all [90, 91] studies have reported that neural networks outperform conventional statistical methods. There are a few experiments of ANN application in clinical practice, including our innovative system for chronic kidney insufficiency that is already mentioned in this chapter.

4. Clustering CV risk factors: A critical appraisal

In medical science, a "*syndrome*" is defined as an "aggregate of symptoms and signs or several conditions associated with any morbid process and constituted together they produce the picture of the disease"[92]. These components are usually caused by a unifying underlying pathology and their combination confers a risk that is different from the sum of the parts. The main purpose of such a description is to help in the diagnosis, treatment and prognosis of the disease.

The Metabolic Syndrome has been a useful construct in clinical practice as well as a valuable model to understand the interactions of diverse CV risk factors. However the concept has been critically appraised for its limited validity and clinical usefulness. This necessitates a novel model for a better and more effective risk assessment in clinical practice.

The metabolic syndrome was first described by *G.M. Reaven* in 1988 to describe a cluster of risk factors contributing to the incidence of diabetes mellitus (DM), cardiovascular (CV) events and also mortality[93]. The definition of this syndrome remains a matter of debate and has been revised on several occasions by different organisations[94-99]. Despite some diversity, obesity, hyperglycemia, dyslipidemia and hypertension have been constant syndrome components and the central concept of such descriptions is the unity of the background pathophysiologic process and the interaction between the elements. Several epidemiologic studies have illustrated the relationship between the metabolic syndrome, CV events and mortality[100-107]; however the syndrome was recently criticised by the American Diabetes Association for its modest consistency and limited clinical application[102] and the use of the term metabolic syndrome was discouraged. Furthermore, its clinical use has recently been described as artificial, confusing and ambiguous recast of traditional risk factors [108-111], with no advantage [110] and even more false positive rate in predicting diabetes and CV disease [112] compared to the usual Framingham risk assessment. In contrast, INTERHEART, a large worldwide prospective study demonstrated that the impact of risk factor clustering is much more than simply multiplying the risk of individual factors for acute myocardial infarction[113]. Although the general clinical strategy against the presence of each risk factor (either single or in combination with others) remains constant, the threshold of interventions may differ by accepting or denying the metabolic syndrome[114]. Hence, while the current definitions are controversial, evidence-based syndrome improvement must target better clinical applicability and higher predictive power of the modifiable outcomes.

Insulin resistance is presumed to be the common pathway for all features of the metabolic syndrome[115]; yet insulin related measurements are not standardized and vary widely [116, 117]. Furthermore, despite the widespread assumption among clinicians, hyperinsulinemia and insulin resistance are not equivalent terms[102]. Besides, while 78% of individuals with metabolic syndrome have insulin resistance, only 48% of patients with insulin resistance manifest the metabolic syndrome[118]. Consequently, Leptin resistance has been suggested as an alternative mechanism which also leads to hyperinsulinemia and other metabolic syndrome features [119].Therefore the association of hyperinsulinemia and other elements of this syndrome are not constant and many other factors may also play important roles as underlying mechanisms in clustering the risk factors. In other words, the metabolic syndrome is beyond insulin resistance, the phenomena which may simply be one of many abnormalities linked to a more fundamental, truly unifying pathophysiology [102,

120]. Likewise, the metabolic syndrome diagnosis is not always associated with a higher CV risk, for example an increased risk was not observed in elderly diabetic and non-diabetic American Indians as well as women with suspected CV disease but normal angiography[121-123]. In addition the application of different syndrome definitions can cause a 15-20% disagreement in patient classification [102] thereby changing the predictive value of the syndrome diagnosis for CV disease and mortality [101, 106, 124]. This accumulating evidence demonstrates that the association of the current syndrome components with CV disease and with each other is uncertain. Even reports supporting the metabolic syndrome state that "detecting the metabolic syndrome is only one part of the overall CV risk assessment and is not an adequate tool to estimate the 10-year risk for coronary heart disease"[125]. This is probably due to the many other related factors not included as syndrome criteria. In fact, residual analysis of many longitudinal studies demonstrates a high unexplained variance (as much as 47%) when metabolic syndrome components were considered as independent variables[102]. By and large, the current body of evidence strongly suggests that the metabolic syndrome definition needs to be standardized and additional factors included[114]. For example, despite several epidemiologic studies demonstrating the relationship between the metabolic syndrome and microalbuminuria, this factor was only incorporated into the World Health Organisation syndrome criteria in 1998 [126] which was not expressed in any other descriptions. Likewise renal failure, now accepted as an independent CV risk factor, as well as anaemia, have not been considered as a part of the metabolic syndrome. Moreover, the impact of endothelioarterial pathology has been overlooked and cardiac disease has been considered simply as an outcome and not an interacting part of the syndrome.

We have introduced the term of "*circulatory syndrome*" as a more refined clinical construct which is composed of many disease markers including **M**etabolic, **A**rterial, **R**enal and **c**ardiac components (simply abbreviated as: "**MARC**")

5. Circulatory (MARC) syndrome

Circulatory syndrome is a cluster of *risk markers* with synergic effects. The proposed syndrome consists of eight major components (Figure 5), as follows (in the "MARC" order):

- Abnormal glucose metabolism
- Dyslipidemia
- Hypertension
- Arterial stiffness
- Microalbuminuria
- Renal impairment
- Anaemia
- Left ventricular dysfunction

All of these "markers" occur on a background of oxidative stress, inflammation, hypercoagulability and endotheliopathy *(underlying factors)* and can be accelerated by factors such as aging, obesity, smoking and physical inactivity *(predisposing factors)*. Furthermore they can be simply and non-invasively assessed in outpatient clinical settings. While the mechanisms underlying the circulatory syndrome are poorly understood, it must be strongly stated that *vascular-endothelial pathways* link all and are of pathological significance. Activation of the renin-angiotensin system, insulin resistance and increased sympathetic activation are all by-products of the underlying pathogenic process. Since these markers represent the extent of the underlying disease process, they could also manifest as risk factors for other components and thereby enhance their development. Considering the interrelationships, the final outcome in this model can be considered to be CV events, stroke or renal failure; all of which are associated with general circulatory health. Consequently the condition of the circulatory system and these markers is directly related to the mortality rate.

Primordial studies demonstrate a robust and valid utility of the "MARC" syndrome concept and a useful risk assessment approach in chronic kidney disease and diabetes mellitus. However, larger prospective cohorts are required for further validation of the concept.

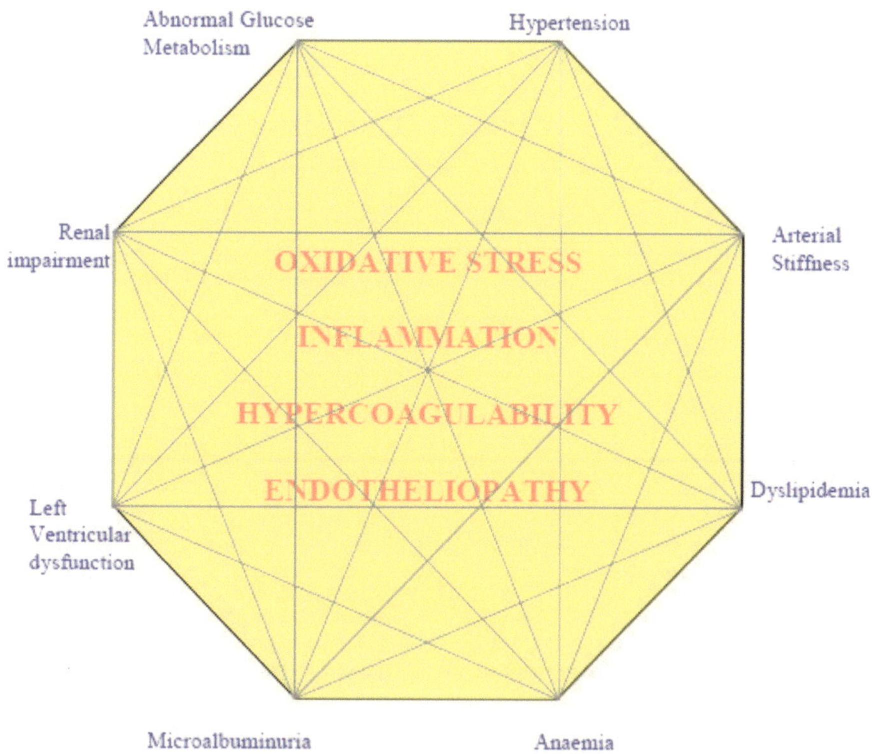

Fig. 5. An illustrative **Circulatory Syndrome**; A cluster of cardiac, renal, arterial and circulatory markers of disease that are interconnected through the endothelium; the common media (**underlying factors**) include oxidative stress, inflammation, hypercoagulability state and endotheliopathy which contribute in the main mechanisms of the phenomena; the third dimension (**precipitating factors**) include age, obesity, physical inactivity and smoking which accelerate the phenomena.

Rationale For Inclusion Of The Components

The Circulatory Syndrome shares some elements with the metabolic syndrome. However it includes additional metabolic and non-metabolic factors (Table2).

Abnormal Glucose Metabolism Fasting Plasma Glucose >6.1 mmol/l ; or 2hr post prandial >7.8 mmol/l
Hypertension SBP≥130 mmHg; and/or DBP≥ 85 mmHg
GFR MDRD eGFR <90 ml/min/1.73 m^2
Microalbuminuria Urinary Albumin creatinine ratio (ACR) [two occasions] >2.5 (male) >3.5 (female)
Arterial Stiffness Upper quartile for PWV, AI or ambulatory PP in the population
Left ventricular dysfunction Any evidence of systolic or diastolic; Imaging techniques or Exercise test (MET <6, impaired systolic BP response) or BNP> 100 pg/ml Previous myocardial infarction
Anemia Hb< 12 female HB<13 male
Dyslipidemia Triglyceride ≥ 1.7 mmol/l or HDL<1 (male) or <1.3 (female) mmol/l or Elevated Apolipoprotein B

GFR: Glomerular Filtration Rate, PWV: Pulse Wave Velocity, AI: Augmentation Index, PP: Pulse Pressure, SBP: Systolic Blood Pressure, DBP: Diastolic Blood Pressure, MET: Estimated multiples of resting oxygen uptake, BNP: Brain Natriuretic Peptide, HDL: High Density Lipoprotein

Table 2. Preliminary Diagnostic Criteria for Circulatory Syndrome;

(1) Abnormal glucose metabolism: Diabetes and abnormalities in glucose metabolism are well known risk factors for cardiac, arterial and renal disease as well as anemia [127, 128]. Although insulin resistance and hyperinsulinemia can be attributed to these complications, they may occur with or without insulin resistance because several other mechanisms including advanced glycation end products, autonomic nervous instability, imbalance between the renin-angiotensin system and nitric oxide, hemodynamic changes and endothelial dysfunction with subsequent ADMA accumulation (an inhibitor for nitric oxide synthesis) and adiponectin deficiency also contribute in the process [120, 129, 130]. Furthermore, albuminuria, arterial stiffness and intima media thickness increase with the increasing number of metabolic syndrome components even before fulfilling the diagnostic criteria for the syndrome, particularly amongst subjects with type 2 DM [131]. In addition, alterations in BP circadian rhythm and BP profile including non-dipper nocturnal BP is now considered as a manifestation of arterial remodelling and is associated with other manifestation of endothelial dysfunction including mA and arterial stiffness.

(2) Lipid abnormalities: Dyslipidemia including increased LDL and TG as well as low HDL is a major risk in patients with chronic renal disease, hypertension and diabetes[105, 132-134]. Genetic variants of lipoprotein lipase correlate with the presence and degree of albuminuria [135]. Dyslipidemia is an independent determinant of progression toward chronic kidney disease and is a known cardiac risk factor [28, 44]. It also contributes to arterial micro-inflammation and atherosclerosis[136]. From different perspective, the correction of lipid abnormalities can reduce albuminuria in subjects with the metabolic syndrome [137], decrease inflammatory markers[138], improve renal function[139], increase arterial compliance[140], improve left ventricular function [138] and prevent CV events[136]. It is noteworthy that obesity was not incorporated into our criteria since there is an opposite relationship between BMI and survival in CKD (reverse epidemiology) [108] and therefore less obese patients with CKD reach to ESRD.

(3) Blood pressure abnormalities: Hypertension is introduced as the leading risk factor of death according to WHO report of global health [4].Hypertension and altered blood pressure circadian rhythm are common co-morbidities with diabetes and pre-diabetic states as well as kidney disease[141]. BP is strongly associated with arterial stiffness and promotes left ventricular dysfunction[29] . In the setting of insulin resistance the vasodilatory effect of insulin can be lost but its renal sodium reabsorption stimulation is preserved. In addition, insulin-induced sympathetic activity increases the prevalence of hypertension in the metabolic syndrome [120]. Furthermore, while salt sensitivity is associated with impaired glucose metabolism, oxidative stress, dyslipidemia and insulin resistance [142, 143] ,it also increases efferent glomerular arteriolar tone and thereby raises glomerular capillary pressure and proteinuria [144] as well as inducing blood pressure abnormalities via renal sodium reabsorption and sympathetic overactivity[145].

(4) Arterial stiffness: Decreased arterial compliance is influenced by both atherosclerosis and arteriosclerosis, as well as functional arterial abnormalities [29, 146]. It occurs very early in the process of kidney disease and DM [147, 148], even preceding microalbuminuria [149] and has also been observed in normal individuals with a close family history of DM [148]. Recent studies have illustrated that increased central arterial stiffness in hypercholesterolemia, even in newly diagnosed individuals, is associated with low-grade systemic inflammation [150, 151]. Arterial stiffness in turn increases LV load and leads to ventricular stiffness and diastolic dysfunction [152, 153]. It has also been suggested as the linking factor between renal impairment and CV diseases [25]. Of great importance, decreased arterial compliance predicts mortality in variant patient groups, independently from other risk factors [38, 154-156].

(5) Microalbuminuria is now accepted as a marker of renal, cardiac and arterial damage being predictive for the further development of CV events, renal failure and DM [25, 134]. It is also closely associated with the prevalence of anaemia [128] , hypertension [157] and metabolic syndrome components [131]. Microalbuminuria commonly occurs early in subjects with abnormal glucose metabolism [147, 158] and is correlated with dyslipidemia [159], arterial stiffness[160, 161] and increased coagulability[162] as well as inflammatory markers[163, 164]. Furthermore the presence of microalbuminuria predicts ventricular dysfunction, coronary heart disease and exercise intolerance[165, 166].

(6) Renal impairment: Kidney function can not be isolated from the health of the heart and arteries and is also associated with the metabolic syndrome components. Alterations in glomerular structure are seen very early in the obesity-mediated metabolic syndrome[82] . Renal hemodynamic reserve is already impaired in patients with asymptomatic left ventricular dysfunction [167]. In addition, the kidney has an important role in insulin and glucose metabolism [168]and insulin resistance has a predictive value for chronic kidney disease [82, 95]. Renal function has been called the Cinderella shoe of CV risk profile [169] and the impact of even minor renal dysfunction on CV function is now well established [25] with endothelial cell dysfunction is likely to be the linking factor between renal and cardiac disease[25, 134, 170]. However endothelial dysfunction in turn is a consequence of inflammation and oxidative stress and is accelerated by these phenomena[171] and is also correlated with a number of the metabolic syndrome components [131]. Decreased arterial compliance increases ventricular wall tension and stiffness and consequently diastolic dysfunction[153]. This in turn may lead to partial renal ischemia, followed by activation of the renin-angiotensin system and tubulointerstitial damage[170]. On the other hand, hyperfiltration which is observed in the early stages of diabetic nephropathy and hypertension [172, 173], leads to increased glomerular pressure and resultant sclerosis which in turn accelerates hypertension[141].

(7) Anemia: Anemia is a common finding in DM and has multifactorial mechanisms[128]. Early tubulointerstitial occurs which disease decreases EPO production and moreover inflammatory cytokines reduce EPO responsiveness leading to anaemia[174]. It is also associated with the level of albuminuria[128] .Anaemia in turn, increases the progression toward CKD, oxidative stress, tissue ischemia, ventricular stress and mortality[175-177]. Of interest, a recent study demonstrated the contribution of anemia to the frequent diastolic dysfunction in DM, as well as its association with brain natriuretic peptide (BNP) and suggested using this factor to identify diabetic patients at increased risk of cardiac dysfunction [175]. Therefore, accumulating evidence has introduced anemia as an important risk factor for the circulatory system. On the other hand, correction of anemia improves the prognosis in chronic kidney disease, heart failure and DM and its complications as well as decreasing mortality [177-179]

(8) Left Ventricular dysfunction: In contrast to the metabolic syndrome, ventricular function is proposed as an interactive part of the circulatory syndrome. This idea is supported by reports of a lack of a relationship between the metabolic syndrome and mortality in individuals who have good cardiorespiratory fitness [180]. On the other hand even a mild stage of ventricular failure, as manifested by impaired exercise response is predictive for mortality[181, 182].Ventricular function determines blood pressure and renal perfusion and in turn is influenced by kidney function, anemia and arterial stiffness and microalbuminuria [153, 183]. Diastolic dysfunction occurs early in DM, is correlated with arterial stiffness and affects exercise response [184]. Furthermore, it has been reported that asymptomatic patients with type 2 DM have subclinical ventricular dysfunction which is related to glycated hemoglubin and LDL cholesterol [185]. Also a recent in vitro study demonstrated that myocyte relaxation and Ca^{2+} handling are abnormal in early uremia, leading to uremic cardiomyopathy [186].

Additional evidence: It is of great interest that some hypoglycaemic agents reduce blood pressure via suppression of the renin-angiotensin system and some ACE inhibitors can reduce insulin resistance in addition to reducing microalbuminuria and arterial stiffness, which raises the possibility of the presence of a common pathway for the adverse effects of hyperglycemia and hypertension[187-189]. Likewise, some lipid lowering agents may exhibit mild anticoagulant and hypotensive effects [190] and angiotensin inhibitors have anti-inflammatory actions [191] which also indicate a possible common source of these abnormalities.

It could be expected that genetic predisposition including nephron underdosing, ACE gene polymorphism, congenital tubular defects and also some other factors such as aging, obesity and smoking produce organ damage susceptibility [133, 192-194].

The above evidence suggests that a genetic profile or a common pathologic process induces a network of metabolic (including alterations in glucose, salt, insulin and lipid metabolism) and hemodynamic abnormalities (due to renin-angiotensin system stimulation, sympathetic overactivity and decreased nitric oxide bioavailability) which are followed by anaemia, hypercoagulability, tissue ischemia, arterial stiffness, hypertension, renal and cardiac dysfunction, the other features of the circulatory syndrome (figure 5).

Underlying Pathology

It is proposed that inflammation is the fuel that "burns" the circulatory syndrome. The association between inflammatory markers and both DM and hypertension is so strong that these diseases has recently been redefined as inflammatory diseases, as has atheroma[195-198]. Advanced glycation end products (AGEs) which accumulate in DM activate inflammatory cells[195]. Likewise, insulin resistance has a strong link with inflammation, although additional mechanisms including genetic factors may influence this relationship[199]. In addition, high LDL cholesterol induces oxidative stress and increases inflammation[200]. On the other hand HDL and apolipoprotein A1 have anti-inflammatory and anti-oxidant properties[201]. Hence, metabolic elements of the syndrome are correlated with inflammation.

Inflammation is known to be a modifier of the relationship between microalbuminuria and hypertension [163, 202]. Hence, CRP has been frequently promoted as a part of the metabolic syndrome [102, 125, 203]. Moreover, inflammatory markers such as CRP are now considered to be independent predictors of DM [195] and its complications including left ventricular hypertrophy, endothelial dysfunction, albuminuria and renal failure [25, 171, 204, 205].

There is a close relationship between inflammation and hypercoagulability [164, 206]. Furthermore, hypercoagulability is also linked to the metabolic syndrome, dyslipidemia, anaemia and even the hemodynamic response to exercise [201, 207-209]. It is also associated with a poorer outcome in coronary artery disease, heart failure and is correlated with the severity of target-organ damage including renal impairment [210-212]. Consequently, diabetic and metabolic syndrome patients are at high risk for thrombotic events [213-215] and have an increased level of clotting factors including tissue plasminogen activator (tPA) and von Willenbrand Factor (vWF) and D-dimer when compared to the controls[216]. Additionally, insulin and lipids may have direct inhibitory effects on coagulation and platelet function through nitric oxide, a pathway that is impaired in DM patients [217].

By and large, this interlinking mesh of inflammatory mediators, oxidative stress, endotheliopathy and hypercoagulability makes a common soil for development of the circulatory (MARC) syndrome.

6. New targets and novel approache to CVD risk modification

The above description of the "circulatory syndrome" clearly has clinical applications. The identification of commonly evaluated markers such as blood pressure, glucose and lipids in a patient should also prompt a search for other markers which make up the circulatory syndrome. A suspected circulatory syndrome should facilitate decision making for diagnostic procedures in asymptomatic but high risk patients. Also treatment of each syndrome component should be accompanied by management of the other components. Furthermore, any difficulty in treating one circulatory syndrome marker should probably leads to a more aggressive treatment program for other components as is currently proposed in patients with renal disease, diabetes and associated hypertension. Hence, management of the proposed "Circulatory Syndrome" would need an interdisciplinary approach with the collaboration of different medical subspecialties.

7. A novel approach to diabetic nephropathy (DN)

The evidence of the close relationship of DM, hypertension, renal function, cardiac function, arterial compliance and metabolic factors have already been discussed. Accordingly the proposed concept of the "*Circulatory Syndrome*" could be applied as a novel approach to DN. This approach should overcome the potential barriers to achieving target points in DM and enhance medications efficacy. According to this new perspective, the treatment of co-morbidities in DM including heart failure, renal failure, arterial stiffness, anemia and the hypercoagulability state as well as reducing any potential inflammation source (e.g. chronic infections, immunology-mediated disease and sensitivities) should enhance adherence to the target points and disease control. This needs a "*multidisciplinary approach*" to CV risk management in DM, in which a clinical epidemiologist or a care plan manager must have a central role. Additionally a global risk score is preferred to the current target points for each risk factor so that the threshold of intervention is clearly defined based on several potential risk factors and assessment of adherence to the guideline is estimated by risk score alterations.

8. New markers

Given the serious limitations of using mA as a single disease marker in screening [31], a multifactorial approach is required to boost screening efficacy and allow reliable risk estimation in DN. The Japanese Society of Nephrology is the only professional organization that has formally added renal hypertrophy and urinary type IV collagen to their guideline as early markers of the existence of DN [218]. There is also evidence for other potential markers including glomerular, tubular, interstitial, endothelioarterial, genetic and cellular markers. However their applicability, validity and reliability must be investigated in a parallel test with mA.

These markers help risk stratification for patients without mA or with fluctuating proteinuria. Furthermore, they facilitate diagnosis of other facets of diabetic kidney damage and also explain the link between cardiac and renal complications of DM.

9. New strategies

The threshold of action for screening, intervention and assessment must be revised based on current DN knowledge and should be followed by altered strategies to define high risk patients. It should also include all pathological aspects of DN including those proposed in the "Circulatory Syndrome", although these will need to be refined, particularly in asymptomatic patients.

In terms of treatment, research findings about renal benefits of the renin-angiotensin-aldosterone system (RAAS) blocking irrespective of blood pressure and albuminuria [219] have not fully integrated into Clinical practice guidelines. Likewise, while recent research has demonstrated advantages of lipid lowering agents even in patients with normal lipid levels [220], the threshold for action remains at higher levels. Similarly, treating anemia has a significant impact on renal function preservation even in early stages of renal disease and erythropoietin therapy has potential advantages for cardiac, neural, endothelial and renal protection [221] as well as a general benefits due to reduction in the oxidative stress, insulin resistance and cytokine accumulation in DM patients (as mentioned in our recently published paper [222]); yet decision criteria are not completely clear in this regard. With accumulating evidence, the threshold for anemia correction is expected to be reduced in a near future.

Regarding follow-up, recent reliable and practical assessments should be considered including central and/or ambulatory BP. Also for renal function, eGFR (based on the MDRD or the Cockcroft-Gault formula) is superior to plasma creatinine [223].

10. New treatment targets

It might be argued that with considering the circulatory syndrome concept and increasing number of the action sites, the number of medication is ought to be increased. Then since increased number of medications usually leads to reduced patients' compliance, such an approach may not only fail to improve disease control, but also make the problem more complex. While possibly true, there are potential solutions. For instance many experts encourage *"poly-pills"* which include a combination of the required agents. Although it may have better patients' acceptance, it cannot reduce the potential adverse effect of polypharmacy. Alternatively and ideally, the type of treatment must be revised in order to meet multiple targets using a single medication (*"super-pills"*).

New treatment options: The marked advantages of using ACE-I and ARB has been appreciated with a 60-70% risk reduction the risk of progression to overt nephropathy in several large clinical trials [224-226]. However this optimistic result would not be completely achieved in routine practice and they can not abrogate the progression of kidney disease. This may suggest incomplete blockage of the RAAS by current medication dose which allow "aldosterone synthesis escape"[227]. Although a recent meta-analysis of randomized trials with ACE-Is and ARBs yielded only a small renoprotection benefit (and no benefit in DM) and demonstrated a smaller benefit in large studies [228], it contradicts previous meta-analysis [229, 230] and seems to be biased by the accessory results from the Antihypertensive and Lipid Lowering treatment to prevent Heart attack Trial (ALLHAT) which was not originally designed for renal outcome evaluation [231].

A combination with beta blockers or calcium channel blockers or a diuretic was previously recommended in the practice guidelines, newer combinations of ACE-I and indapamide, ACE-I and spirinolactone and a double blockage of RAAS (ACE-I and ARB) have been demonstrated promising in terms of lowering BP and mA, which is also supported by the new understanding of ACE-2 enzyme, angiotensin recptor-2 and the role of aldosterone in CKD progression [232] In addition, using pioglitazone or rosiglitazone in combination with sulphonylurea with or without metformine has also been suggested by experts as an effective combination; however the available clinical data is still limited. Finally, it is noteworthy that while identification and management of hypertensive patients with elevated heart rate (with beta-blockers or calcium antagonists)is recommended by expert consensus [233], non-selective beta blockers (e.g. propranolol) generally decrease GFR by lowering cardiac output. In contrast, the ß1-selective agents (e.g. metoprolol and atenolol) may have a beneficial effect on declining GFR as well as protecting heart against heart failure. However these may also have adverse effect on plasma glucose and atenolol must be adjusted in renal failure due to its impaired renal clearance. On the other hand non-selective vasodilating beta blockers (Carvedilol and Labetalol) not only reduce BP but also have antioxidant and renoprotective effects [234]. Finally, considering of erythropoietine (EPO) in medical management of diabetes is expected to improve CV health in DM [222, 235].

New agents: Several animal models have suggested many potential candidates for prevention and treatment of DN. Renoprotective effect of ALT-711 (a cross link breaker of the advance glycosylation end product), ruboxistaurin (an inhibitor for protein kinase C), eplerenone (a new aldosterone antagonist), thiamine and a modified heparin glycosaminoglycan have been reported, as being effective in reducing albuminuria and renal lesions [232, 236, 237]. However, very few human studies have been conducted in human of which the combination of ACE-I and omepatrilat (an endopeptidase inhibitor), sulodexide (a glycosaminoglycan), Pirfenidone (TGF-ß inhibitor) and pimagedine (a second generation inhibitor of advanced glycation end product) have had dramatic beneficial effects in DM patients [232, 236, 238]. There are also some evidence of the efficacy of folic acid on endothelial function improvement in different groups of patients including type 2 DM [239].

Developing novel drugs opposing the action of TGF-ß, connective tissue growth factors, cytokines and reactive oxygen species is the next step. Also by recognizing the role of relaxin [240], urotensin II [241] and vascular calcification contributors, additional medication might one day be available.

Multipotential agents: Accumulating evidence demonstrates the polydimentional action of some medications on glycaemic and BP control, reducing lipid and mA and improvement in arterial compliance. For instance, blocking of the renin-angiotensin system has anti-diabetic and anti-inflammatory effects as well as antihypertensive actions and improves mA and arterial stiffness at the same time [187, 189, 191]. This also applies to some lipid lowering agents [190, 220]. Likewise, insulin-sensitizing thiazolidinediones (TZDs) ameliorate mA and are antihypertensive [242]. Also metformin improves both endothelial function and the metabolic syndrome [243]. From a different point of view, treating anemia with erythropoietin may also have cardiac, renal, neurohormonal and metabolic benefits due to anemia correction of anemia and the cytoprotective effects of erythropoietin *perse* [221, 222, 244]. Several researches are being conducted to introduce and develop novel EPO replacement therapies such as synthetic erythropoietic proteins, continuous EPO receptor activators (CERA), EPO gene transfer using retroviral vectors and implementation of EPO producing cells in A-V fistula graft which will create a revolution in related therapies [222].

With the axial role of RAAS in the pathogenesis of DN, non-hemodynamic effects of ACE-I and ARB including their action on TGF-ß, extracellular matrix and cytokines have the focus of several studies in recent years [237]. According to a recent study Losartan improves resistance artery lesions and prevents TGF-ß production in untreated hypertensive patients [245]. In addition, ACE-I agents potentiate bradykinin-induced tissue plasminogen activator (t-PA) release leading to endothelial fibrinolytic function [246, 247]. Consequently several studies have indicated that the renoprotective of these drugs is independent of their antihypertensive effect [229].

The recognition of a new class of nuclear receptors named "peroxisome proliferators-activated receptor" (PPAR) has provided an additional field for action against DN and consequently its CV complications. Rosiglitazone is a PPAR-γ agonist which was demonstrated as being effective in lowering blood pressure and reversing insulin resistance [248]. Likewise, several studies have verified the multipotential action of PPAR-α agonists including Fenofibrate in reducing fasting blood glucose, ameliorating insulin resistance, decreasing mA, correction of lipid metabolism, suppressing collagen by mesangeal cells, preventing glomerulosclerosis as well as antihypertensive [242, 249]. This body of evidence supports the potential impact of multipotential drugs in the future treatment of DN.

11. Conclusion

Early diagnosis and management of CV risk, particularly in diabetes and chronic kidney disease requires a new insight and subsequently a novel approach to the disease is mandatory. While our studies demonstrated various facets of the interactions between renal, cardiac, arterial and metabolic factors, the proposed *"Circulatory Syndrome"* can facilitate formulation of new strategies for the better diagnosis and management of CV risk. Accordingly, a multidisciplinary evaluation of glycemic control, lipids, anemia, blood pressure profile, albuminuria, GFR and ventricular function as well as an assessment of arterial compliance (as an axial element) provides adequate information for early and effective identification of high risk patients for progression toward CVD. The proposed concept of the **"*Circulatory (MARC) Syndrome*"** is expected to facilitate this revolution by a multidisciplinary approach.

12. References

[1] Gersh, B., K. Sliwa, B. Mayosi, et al., *The epidemic of cardiovascular disease in the developing world: global implications.* Eur Heart J, 2010. 31: p. 642-648.

[2] Preis, S., M. Pencina, S. Hwang, et al., *Trends in Cardiovascular Disease Risk Factors in Individuals With and Without Diabetes Mellitus in the Framingham Heart Study.* Circulation, 2009. 120: p. 212-20.

[3] Khoshdel, A.R. *Hemodynamic response to exercise predicts the development of severe renal failure.* in *International Society of Nephrology.* 2007. Rio, Brazil.

[4] *Global Health Risks: Morbidity and burden of disease attributable to selected major risks.* WHO Global Reports. 2009. 70.

[5] Mukamal, K., R. Kronmal, R. Tracy, et al., *Traditional and novel risk factors in older adults: cardiovascular risk assessment late in life.* Am J Geriatr Cardiol, 2004. 13(2): p. 69-80.

[6] Gu, K., C.C. Cowie, and M.I. Harris, *Diabetes and decline in heart disease mortality in US adults.* Jama, 1999. 281(14): p. 1291-7.

[7] Gu, K., C.C. Cowie, and M.I. Harris, *Mortality in adults with and without diabetes in a national cohort of the U.S. population, 1971-1993.* Diabetes Care, 1998. 21(7): p. 1138-45.

[8] Shange, Q. and G. Yip, *Diabetic heart disease: the story continues.* Journal of Human Hypertension, 2011. 25: p. 141-143.

[9] Grundy, S.M., B. Howard, S. Smith, Jr., et al., *Prevention Conference VI: Diabetes and Cardiovascular Disease: executive summary: conference proceeding for healthcare professionals from a special writing group of the American Heart Association.* Circulation, 2002. 105(18): p. 2231-9.

[10] *Impact of diabetes on cardiovascular disease risk and all-cause mortality in older men: influence of age at onset, diabetes duation and established and novel risk factors.* Arch Intern Med, 2011. 171(5): p. 404-10.

[11] Gibbons, R.J. and E.M. Antman, *ACC/AHA 2002 Guideline Update For Exercise Testing,* in *ACC/AHA Practice Guidelines.* 2002, American College of Cardiology; American Heart Association: Bethesda, USA.

[12] Stewart, K.J., J. Sung, H.A. Silber, et al., *Exaggerated Exercise Blood Pressure is related to impaired endothelial vasodilator function.* American Journal of Hypertension, 2004. 17: p. 314-320.

[13] Bell, D.S.H., *Heart Failure: A serious and common comorbidity of diabetes.* Clinical Diabetes, 2004. 22(2): p. 61-5.

[14] Khoshdel, A., S. Carney, and s. White. *Disturbed Hemodynamic Cardiac Exercise Stress Test Reponse in non-smoking, Normolipidemic, Normotensive Diabetic Subjects.* in *Cardiovascular disease in the 21st century: Shaping the future.* 2006. Sydney.

[15] Khoshdel, A.R., S.L. Carney, and S. White, *Disturbed hemodynamic cardiac exercise stress test response in non-smoking, normolipidemic, normotensive, diabetic subjects.* Diabetes Res Clin Pract, 2007. 75(2): p. 193-9.

[16] Khoshdel, A.R. and S.L. Carney. *HEMODYNAMIC RESPONSE TO EXERCISE PREDICTS THE DEVELOPMENT OF SEVERE RENAL FAILURE.* in *14th World Congress on Heart Disease.* 2008. Toronto, CANADA, July 2008: American Heart Association.

[17] Khoshdel, A. and S. Carney, *Wrist cuff blood pressure self-measurement in diabetic patients: comparable to ambulatory blood pressure monitoring.* Hypertension, 2006. 49(6): p. 1470.

[18] Khoshdel, A.R., *Circulatory syndrome a new insight into the early diagnosis and management of renal-cardiovascular risk in diabetes mellitus,* in *School of Medicine and Public Health.* 2007, University of Newcastle (N.S.W.). Newcastle. p. 356.

[19] McDonald, S. and L. Excell, *Australia and New Zealand Dialysis and Transplant Registry (28th report),* ed. K.H.A. Commonwealth Department of Health and Ageing, New Zealand Ministry of Health. 2005.

[20] Haghighi, A.N., B. Broumand, M. D'Amico, et al., *The epidemiology of end-stage renal disease in Iran in an international perspective.* Nephrol Dial Transplant, 2002. 17(1): p. 28-32.

[21] Feest, T.G., J. Rajamahesh, C. Byrne, et al., *Trends in adult renal replacement therapy in the UK: 1982-2002.* Qjm, 2005. 98(1): p. 21-8.

[22] Barsoum, R.S., *Chronic kidney disease in the developing world.* N Engl J Med, 2006. 354(10): p. 997-9.
[23] Rutkowski, B., *Changing pattern of end-stage renal disease in central and eastern Europe.* Nephrol Dial Transplant, 2000. 15(2): p. 156-60.
[24] Friedman, E.A., *ESRD in diabetic persons.* Kidney International, 2006. 70: p. S51-54.
[25] Ritz, E., *Heart and kidney: fatal twins?* Am J Med, 2006. 119(5 Suppl 1): p. S31-9.
[26] London, G., *Cardiovascular disease in end-stage renal failure: role of calcium-phosphate disturbances and hyperparathyroidism.* J Nephrol, 2002. 15(2): p. 209-10.
[27] Zoccali, C., *Traditional and emerging cardiovascular and renal risk factors: an epidemiologic perspective.* Kidney Int, 2006. 70(1): p. 26-33.
[28] Zoccali, C., *Cardiorenal risk as a new frontier of nephrology: research needs and areas for intervention.* Nephrol Dial Transplant, 2002. 17 Suppl 11: p. 50-4.
[29] Vlachopoulos, C. and M. O'Rourke, *Genesis of the normal and abnormal arterial pulse.* Curr Probl Cardiol, 2000. 25(5): p. 303-67.
[30] Massry, S.G. and R.J. Glassock, *Textbook of Nephrology.* 2001, Philadelphia: Lippincott Williams. 876.
[31] Caramori, M.L., P. Fioretto, and M. Mauer, *The need for early predictors of diabetic nephropathy risk: is albumin excretion rate sufficient?* Diabetes, 2000. 49(9): p. 1399-408.
[32] Taal, M.W. and B.M. Brenner, *Predicting initiation and progression of chronic kidney disease: Developing renal risk scores.* Kidney Int, 2006. 70(10): p. 1694-705.
[33] MacIsaac, R.J., S. Panagiotopoulos, K.J. McNeil, et al., *Is nonalbuminuric renal insufficiency in type 2 diabetes related to an increase in intrarenal vascular disease?* Diabetes Care, 2006. 29(7): p. 1560-6.
[34] Tabaei, B.P., A.S. Al-Kassab, L.L. Ilag, et al., *Does microalbuminuria predict diabetic nephropathy?* Diabetes Care, 2001. 24(9): p. 1560-6.
[35] Kramer, H.J., Q.D. Nguyen, G. Curhan, et al., *Renal insufficiency in the absence of albuminuria and retinopathy among adults with type 2 diabetes mellitus.* Jama, 2003. 289(24): p. 3273-7.
[36] Perkins, B.A., L.H. Ficociello, K.H. Silva, et al., *Regression of microalbuminuria in type 1 diabetes.* N Engl J Med, 2003. 348(23): p. 2285-93.
[37] Guerin, A.P., J. Blacher, B. Pannier, et al., *Impact of aortic stiffness attenuation on survivial of patients in end-stage renal failure.* Circulation, 2001. 20: p. 987-92.
[38] London, G.M., J. Blacher, B. Pannier, et al., *Arterial wave reflections and survival in end-stage renal failure.* Hypertension, 2001. 38(3): p. 434-8.
[39] London, G.M. and J.N. Cohn, *Prognostic application of arterial stiffness: task forces.* Am J Hypertens, 2002. 15(8): p. 754-8.
[40] Khoshdel, A.R., S.L. Carney, B.R. Nair, et al., *Better management of cardiovascular diseases by pulse wave velocity: combining clinical practice with clinical research using evidence-based medicine.* Clin Med Res, 2007. 5(1): p. 45-52.
[41] Sarnak, M.J., A.S. Levey, A.C. Schoolwerth, et al., *Kidney disease as a risk factor for development of cardiovascular disease: a statement from the American Heart Association Councils on Kidney in Cardiovascular Disease, High Blood Pressure Research, Clinical Cardiology, and Epidemiology and Prevention.* Circulation, 2003. 108(17): p. 2154-69.
[42] Cheung, A.K., M.J. Sarnak, G. Yan, et al., *Atherosclerotic cardiovascular disease risks in chronic hemodialysis patients.* Kidney Int, 2000. 58(1): p. 353-62.
[43] Sasso, F.C., L. De Nicola, O. Carbonara, et al., *Cardiovascular risk factors and disease management in type 2 diabetic patients with diabetic nephropathy.* Diabetes Care, 2006. 29(3): p. 498-503.

[44] Locatelli, F., J. Bommer, G.M. London, et al., *Cardiovascular disease determinants in chronic renal failure: clinical approach and treatment.* Nephrol Dial Transplant, 2001. 16(3): p. 459-68.

[45] Thomas, S.M. and G.C. Viberti, *Cardiovascular risk in diabetic kidney disease: a model of chronic renal disease.* Kidney Int Suppl, 2005(98): p. S18-20.

[46] *Metabolic syndrome, chronic kidney and cardiovascular diseases: role of adipokines.* Cardiol Res Prac, 2011.

[47] Morrish, N.J., S.L. Wang, L.K. Stevens, et al., *Mortality and causes of death in the WHO Multinational Study of Vascular Disease in Diabetes.* Diabetologia, 2001. 44 Suppl 2: p. S14-21.

[48] Racki, S., L. Zaputovic, B. Vujicic, et al., *Comparison of survival between diabetic and non-diabetic patients on maintenance hemodialysis: A single-centre experience.* Diabetes Res Clin Pract, 2006.

[49] Rossing, K., P.K. Christensen, P. Hovind, et al., *Progression of nephropathy in type 2 diabetic patients.* Kidney Int, 2004. 66(4): p. 1596-605.

[50] Wheeler, D.C., J.N. Townend, and M.J. Landray, *Cardiovascular risk factors in predialysis patients: baseline data from the Chronic Renal Impairment in Birmingham (CRIB) study.* Kidney Int Suppl, 2003(84): p. S201-3.

[51] Shinohara, K., T. Shoji, Y. Tsujimoto, et al., *Arterial stiffness in predialysis patients with uremia.* Kidney Int, 2004. 65(3): p. 936-43.

[52] Blacher, J., K. Demuth, A.P. Guerin, et al., *Influence of biochemical alterations on arterial stiffness in patients with end-stage renal disease.* Arterioscler Thromb Vasc Biol, 1998. 18(4): p. 535-41.

[53] Ishimura, E., S. Okuno, K. Kitatani, et al., *Different risk factors for peripheral vascular calcification between diabetic and non-diabetic haemodialysis patients--importance of glycaemic control.* Diabetologia, 2002. 45(10): p. 1446-8.

[54] Shoji, T., M. Emoto, K. Shinohara, et al., *Diabetes Mellitus, Aortic Stiffness, and Cardiovascular mortality in End-Stage Renal disease.* J Am Soc Nephrol, 2001. 12: p. 2117-24.

[55] Aoun, S., J. Blacher, M.E. Safar, et al., *Diabetes mellitus and renal failure: effects on large artery stiffness.* J Hum Hypertens, 2001. 15(10): p. 693-700.

[56] Floege, J. and M. Ketteler, *Vascular calcification in patients with end-stage renal disease.* Nephrol Dial Transplant, 2004. 19 Suppl 5: p. V59-66.

[57] Goodman, W.G., *Vascular calcification in chronic renal failure.* Lancet, 2001. 358(9288): p. 1115-6.

[58] London, G.M., A.P. Guerin, S.J. Marchais, et al., *Arterial media calcification in end-stage renal disease: impact on all-cause and cardiovascular mortality.* Nephrol Dial Transplant, 2003. 18(9): p. 1731-40.

[59] Smith, J.C., M.D. Page, R. John, et al., *Augmentation of central arterial pressure in mild primary hyperparathyroidism.* J Clin Endocrinol Metab, 2000. 85(10): p. 3515-9.

[60] Rubin, M.R., M.S. Maurer, D.J. McMahon, et al., *Arterial stiffness in mild primary hyperparathyroidism.* J Clin Endocrinol Metab, 2005. 90(6): p. 3326-30.

[61] Chow, K.M., C.C. Szeto, and P.K. Li, *Parathyroid hormone and mineral metabolism do not have significant impact on pulse pressure in patients undergoing peritoneal dialysis.* Clin Nephrol, 2003. 60(4): p. 266-9.

[62] Suzuki, T., K. Yonemura, Y. Maruyama, et al., *Impact of serum parathyroid hormone concentration and its regulatory factors on arterial stiffness in patients undergoing maintenance hemodialysis.* Blood Purif, 2004. 22(3): p. 293-7.

[63] Blacher, J., M.E. Safar, A.P. Guerin, et al., *Aortic pulse wave velocity index and mortality in end-stage renal disease.* Kidney Int, 2003. 63(5): p. 1852-60.

[64] Safar, M.E., J. Blacher, B. Pannier, et al., *Central pulse pressure and mortality in end-stage renal disease.* Hypertension, 2002. 39: p. 735-8.

[65] Wolfe, R.A., V.B. Ashby, E.L. Milford, et al., *Comparison of mortality in all patients on dialysis, patients on dialysis awaiting transplantation, and recipients of a first cadaveric transplant.* N Engl J Med, 1999. 341(23): p. 1725-30.

[66] Kasiske, B.L., H.A. Chakkera, and J. Roel, *Explained and unexplained ischemic heart disease risk after renal transplantation.* J Am Soc Nephrol, 2000. 11(9): p. 1735-43.

[67] Barenbrock, M., M. Kosch, E. Joster, et al., *Reduced arterial distensibility is a predictor of cardiovascular disease in patients after renal transplantation.* J Hypertens, 2002. 20(1): p. 79-84.

[68] Marcen, R., *Cardiovascular risk factors in renal transplantation--current controversies.* Nephrol Dial Transplant, 2006. 21 Suppl 3: p. iii3-8.

[69] Khoshdel, A.R. and S.L. Carney, *Arterial stiffness in kidney transplant recipients: an overview of methodology and applications.* Urol J, 2008. 5(1): p. 3-14.

[70] Khoshdel, A.R., S.L. Carney, P. Trevillian, et al., *Evaluation of arterial stiffness and pulse wave reflection for cardiovascular risk assessment in diabetic and nondiabetic kidney transplant recipients.* Iran J Kidney Dis, 2010. 4(3): p. 237-43.

[71] Dudziak, M., A. Debska-Slizien, and B. Rutkowski, *Cardiovascular effects of successful renal transplantation: a 30-month study on left ventricular morphology, systolic and diastolic functions.* Transplant Proc, 2005. 37(2): p. 1039-43.

[72] Nakajima, K., T. Ochiai, T. Suzuki, et al., *Beneficial effects of renal transplantation on cardiovascular disorders in dialysis patients.* Surg Today, 1998. 28(8): p. 811-5.

[73] Ferreira, S.R., V.A. Moises, A. Tavares, et al., *Cardiovascular effects of successful renal transplantation: a 1-year sequential study of left ventricular morphology and function, and 24-hour blood pressure profile.* Transplantation, 2002. 74(11): p. 1580-7.

[74] Kocak, H., K. Ceken, A. Yavuz, et al., *Effect of renal transplantation on endothelial function in haemodialysis patients.* Nephrol Dial Transplant, 2006. 21(1): p. 203-7.

[75] Zoungas, S., P.G. Kerr, S. Chadban, et al., *Arterial function after successful renal transplantation.* Kidney Int, 2004. 65(5): p. 1882-9.

[76] Chobanian, A.V., G.L. Bakris, H.R. Black, et al., *The Seventh Report of the Joint National Committee on Prevention, Detection, Evaluation, and Treatment of High Blood Pressure: The JNC 7 Report 10.1001/jama.289.19.2560.* JAMA, 2003: p. 289.19.2560.

[77] *Standards of medical care in diabetes.* Diabetes Care, 2004. 27 Suppl 1: p. S15-35.

[78] Chobanian, A.V., G.L. Bakris, H.R. Black, et al., *The Seventh Report of the Joint National Committee on Prevention, Detection, Evaluation, and Treatment of High Blood Pressure: the JNC 7 report.* Jama, 2003. 289(19): p. 2560-72.

[79] Lewington, S., R. Clarke, N. Qizilbash, et al., *Age-specific relevance of usual blood pressure to vascular mortality: a meta-analysis of individual data for one million adults in 61 prospective studies.* Lancet, 2002. 360(9349): p. 1903-13.

[80] Brantsma, A.H., S.J. Bakker, H.L. Hillege, et al., *Urinary albumin excretion and its relation with C-reactive protein and the metabolic syndrome in the prediction of type 2 diabetes.* Diabetes Care, 2005. 28(10): p. 2525-30.

[81] Campbell, N.R., N.A. Khan, and S.A. Grover, *Barriers and remaining questions on assessment of absolute cardiovascular risk as a starting point for interventions to reduce cardiovascular risk.* J Hypertens, 2006. 24(9): p. 1683-5.
[82] Peralta, C.A., M. Kurella, J.C. Lo, et al., *The metabolic syndrome and chronic kidney disease.* Curr Opin Nephrol Hypertens, 2006. 15(4): p. 361-5.
[83] Yokoyama, H., M. Kuramitsu, S. Kanno, et al., *Relationship between metabolic syndrome components and vascular properties in Japanese type 2 diabetic patients without cardiovascular disease or nephropathy.* Diabetes Res Clin Pract, 2007. 75(2): p. 200-6.
[84] Jennett, B., *Epidemiology of head injury.* J Neurol Neurosurg Psychiatry, 1996. 60(4): p. 362-9.
[85] Sargent, D.J., *Comparison of artificial neural networks with other statistical approaches: results from medical data sets.* Cancer, 2001. 91(8 Suppl): p. 1636-42.
[86] Cross, S.S., R.F. Harrison, and R.L. Kennedy, *Introduction to neural networks.* Lancet, 1995. 346(8982): p. 1075-9.
[87] Goldfarb-Rumyantzev, A.S. and L. Pappas, *Prediction of renal insufficiency in Pima Indians with nephropathy of type 2 diabetes mellitus.* Am J Kidney Dis, 2002. 40(2): p. 252-64.
[88] West, D. and V. West, *Model selection for a medical diagnostic decision support system: a breast cancer detection case.* Artif Intell Med, 2000. 20(3): p. 183-204.
[89] Baxt, W.G., *Application of artificial neural networks to clinical medicine.* Lancet, 1995. 346(8983): p. 1135-8.
[90] Sherriff, A. and J. Ott, *Artificial neural networks as statistical tools in epidemiological studies: analysis of risk factors for early infant wheeze.* Paediatr Perinat Epidemiol, 2004. 18(6): p. 456-63.
[91] Schwarzer, G., W. Vach, and M. Schumacher, *On the misuses of artificial neural networks for prognostic and diagnostic classification in oncology.* Stat Med, 2000. 19(4): p. 541-61.
[92] *Stedman's Medical Dictionary.* 27th edition ed. 2000, Baltimore: Lippincott, Williams and Wilkins. p.1746.
[93] Reaven, G.M., *Banting lecture 1988. Role of insulin resistance in human disease.* Diabetes, 1988. 37(12): p. 1595-607.
[94] Ormezzano, O., J.P. Baguet, P. Francois, et al., *Is there any real target organ damage associated with white-coat normotension?* Clin Auton Res, 2004. 14(3): p. 160-6.
[95] Balkau, B. and M.A. Charles, *Comment on the provisional report from the WHO consultation. European Group for the Study of Insulin Resistance (EGIR).* Diabet Med, 1999. 16(5): p. 442-3.
[96] Einhorn, D., G.M. Reaven, R.H. Cobin, et al., *American College of Endocrinology position statement on the insulin resistance syndrome.* Endocr Pract, 2003. 9(3): p. 237-52.
[97] Grundy, S.M., H.B. Brewer, Jr., J.I. Cleeman, et al., *Definition of metabolic syndrome: Report of the National Heart, Lung, and Blood Institute/American Heart Association conference on scientific issues related to definition.* Circulation, 2004. 109(3): p. 433-8.
[98] *Executive Summary of The Third Report of The National Cholesterol Education Program (NCEP) Expert Panel on Detection, Evaluation, And Treatment of High Blood Cholesterol In Adults (Adult Treatment Panel III).* Jama, 2001. 285(19): p. 2486-97.
[99] *Third Report of the National Cholesterol Education Program (NCEP) Expert Panel on Detection, Evaluation, and Treatment of High Blood Cholesterol in Adults (Adult Treatment Panel III) final report.* Circulation, 2002. 106(25): p. 3143-421.

[100] Alexander, C.M., P.B. Landsman, S.M. Teutsch, et al., *NCEP-defined metabolic syndrome, diabetes, and prevalence of coronary heart disease among NHANES III participants age 50 years and older.* Diabetes, 2003. 52(5): p. 1210-4.

[101] Athyros, V.G., E.S. Ganotakis, M.S. Elisaf, et al., *Prevalence of vascular disease in metabolic syndrome using three proposed definitions.* Int J Cardiol, 2006.

[102] Kahn, R., J. Buse, E. Ferrannini, et al., *The metabolic syndrome: time for a critical appraisal: joint statement from the American Diabetes Association and the European Association for the Study of Diabetes.* Diabetes Care, 2005. 28(9): p. 2289-304.

[103] Malik, S., N.D. Wong, S.S. Franklin, et al., *Impact of the metabolic syndrome on mortality from coronary heart disease, cardiovascular disease, and all causes in United States adults.* Circulation, 2004. 110(10): p. 1245-50.

[104] Girman, C.J., T. Rhodes, M. Mercuri, et al., *The metabolic syndrome and risk of major coronary events in the Scandinavian Simvastatin Survival Study (4S) and the Air Force/Texas Coronary Atherosclerosis Prevention Study (AFCAPS/TexCAPS).* Am J Cardiol, 2004. 93(2): p. 136-41.

[105] Ford, E.S., *The metabolic syndrome and mortality from cardiovascular disease and all-causes: findings from the National Health and Nutrition Examination Survey II Mortality Study.* Atherosclerosis, 2004. 173(2): p. 309-14.

[106] Hunt, K.J., R.G. Resendez, K. Williams, et al., *National Cholesterol Education Program versus World Health Organization metabolic syndrome in relation to all-cause and cardiovascular mortality in the San Antonio Heart Study.* Circulation, 2004. 110(10): p. 1251-7.

[107] Scuteri, A., S.S. Najjar, C.H. Morrell, et al., *The metabolic syndrome in older individuals: prevalence and prediction of cardiovascular events: the Cardiovascular Health Study.* Diabetes Care, 2005. 28(4): p. 882-7.

[108] Bakker, S.J., R.T. Gansevoort, and D. de Zeeuw, *Metabolic syndrome: a fata morgana?* Nephrol Dial Transplant, 2007. 22(1): p. 15-20.

[109] Blaha, M. and T.A. Elasy, *Clinical use of metabolic syndrome: Why the confusion?* Clinical Diabetes, 2006. 24(3): p. 125-131.

[110] Mitka, M., *Metabolic syndrome recasts old cardiac, diabetes risk factors as a "new" entity.* Jama, 2004. 291(17): p. 2062-3.

[111] Alberti, K.G., P. Zimmet, and J. Shaw, *The metabolic syndrome--a new worldwide definition.* Lancet, 2005. 366(9491): p. 1059-62.

[112] Stern, M.P., K. Williams, C. Gonzalez-Villalpando, et al., *Does the metabolic syndrome improve identification of individuals at risk of type 2 diabetes and/or cardiovascular disease?* Diabetes Care, 2004. 27(11): p. 2676-81.

[113] Yusuf, S., S. Hawken, S. Ounpuu, et al., *Effect of potentially modifiable risk factors associated with myocardial infarction in 52 countries (the INTERHEART study): case-control study.* Lancet, 2004. 364(9438): p. 937-52.

[114] Khoshdel, A.R., *Metabolic syndrome: Erasing the problem or constructing a better answer.* BMJ rapid response at www.bmj.com, 2008. 27th March 2008.

[115] Reaven, G., *The metabolic syndrome or the insulin resistance syndrome? Different names, different concepts, and different goals.* Endocrinol Metab Clin North Am, 2004. 33(2): p. 283-303.

[116] Robbins, D.C., L. Andersen, R. Bowsher, et al., *Report of the American Diabetes Association's Task Force on standardization of the insulin assay.* Diabetes, 1996. 45(2): p. 242-56.

[117] Wallace, T.M., J.C. Levy, and D.R. Matthews, *Use and abuse of HOMA modeling.* Diabetes Care, 2004. 27(6): p. 1487-95.
[118] Liao, Y., S. Kwon, S. Shaughnessy, et al., *Critical evaluation of adult treatment panel III criteria in identifying insulin resistance with dyslipidemia.* Diabetes Care, 2004. 27(4): p. 978-83.
[119] Unger, R.H., *Lipid overload and overflow: metabolic trauma and the metabolic syndrome.* Trends Endocrinol Metab, 2003. 14(9): p. 398-403.
[120] Eckel, R.H., S.M. Grundy, and P.Z. Zimmet, *The metabolic syndrome.* Lancet, 2005. 365(9468): p. 1415-28.
[121] Bruno, G., F. Merletti, A. Biggeri, et al., *Metabolic syndrome as a predictor of all-cause and cardiovascular mortality in type 2 diabetes: the Casale Monferrato Study.* Diabetes Care, 2004. 27(11): p. 2689-94.
[122] Resnick, H.E., K. Jones, G. Ruotolo, et al., *Insulin resistance, the metabolic syndrome, and risk of incident cardiovascular disease in nondiabetic american indians: the Strong Heart Study.* Diabetes Care, 2003. 26(3): p. 861-7.
[123] Marroquin, O.C., K.E. Kip, D.E. Kelley, et al., *Metabolic syndrome modifies the cardiovascular risk associated with angiographic coronary artery disease in women: a report from the Women's Ischemia Syndrome Evaluation.* Circulation, 2004. 109(6): p. 714-21.
[124] Lakka, H.M., D.E. Laaksonen, T.A. Lakka, et al., *The metabolic syndrome and total and cardiovascular disease mortality in middle-aged men.* Jama, 2002. 288(21): p. 2709-16.
[125] Grundy, S.M., J.I. Cleeman, S.R. Daniels, et al., *Diagnosis and management of the metabolic syndrome: an American Heart Association/National Heart, Lung, and Blood Institute Scientific Statement.* Circulation, 2005. 112(17): p. 2735-52.
[126] Alberti, K.G. and P.Z. Zimmet, *Definition, diagnosis and classification of diabetes mellitus and its complications. Part 1: diagnosis and classification of diabetes mellitus provisional report of a WHO consultation.* Diabet Med, 1998. 15(7): p. 539-53.
[127] Knudsen, S.T., P.L. Poulsen, K.W. Hansen, et al., *Pulse pressure and diurnal blood pressure variation: association with micro- and macrovascular complications in type 2 diabetes.* Am J Hypertens, 2002. 15(3): p. 244-50.
[128] Thomas, M.C., R.J. MacIsaac, C. Tsalamandris, et al., *Anemia in patients with type 1 diabetes.* J Clin Endocrinol Metab, 2004. 89(9): p. 4359-63.
[129] Bongartz, L.G., M.J. Cramer, P.A. Doevendans, et al., *The severe cardiorenal syndrome: 'Guyton revisited'.* Eur Heart J, 2005. 26(1): p. 11-7.
[130] Becker, B., F. Kronenberg, J.T. Kielstein, et al., *Renal insulin resistance syndrome, adiponectin and cardiovascular events in patients with kidney disease: the mild and moderate kidney disease study.* J Am Soc Nephrol, 2005. 16(4): p. 1091-8.
[131] Yokoyama, H., M. Kuramitsu, S. Kanno, et al., *Relationship between metabolic syndrome components and vascular properties in Japanese type 2 diabetic patients without cardiovascular disease or nephropathy.* Diabetes Res Clin Pract, 2006.
[132] Saydah, S.H., J. Fradkin, and C.C. Cowie, *Poor control of risk factors for vascular disease among adults with previously diagnosed diabetes.* Jama, 2004. 291(3): p. 335-42.
[133] Fox, C.S., M.G. Larson, E.P. Leip, et al., *Predictors of new-onset kidney disease in a community-based population.* Jama, 2004. 291(7): p. 844-50.
[134] Amann, K., C. Wanner, and E. Ritz, *Cross-Talk between the Kidney and the Cardiovascular System.* J Am Soc Nephrol, 2006. 17(8): p. 2112-9.
[135] Mattu, R.K., J. Trevelyan, E.W. Needham, et al., *Lipoprotein lipase gene variants relate to presence and degree of microalbuminuria in Type II diabetes.* Diabetologia, 2002. 45(6): p. 905-13.

[136] Colhoun, H.M., D.J. Betteridge, P.N. Durrington, et al., *Primary prevention of cardiovascular disease with atorvastatin in type 2 diabetes in the Collaborative Atorvastatin Diabetes Study (CARDS): multicentre randomised placebo-controlled trial.* Lancet, 2004. 364(9435): p. 685-96.
[137] Geluk, C.A., F.W. Asselbergs, H.L. Hillege, et al., *Impact of statins in microalbuminuric subjects with the metabolic syndrome: a substudy of the PREVEND Intervention Trial.* Eur Heart J, 2005. 26(13): p. 1314-20.
[138] Sola, S., M.Q. Mir, S. Lerakis, et al., *Atorvastatin improves left ventricular systolic function and serum markers of inflammation in nonischemic heart failure.* J Am Coll Cardiol, 2006. 47(2): p. 332-7.
[139] Elisaf, M. and D.P. Mikhailidis, *Statins and renal function.* Angiology, 2002. 53(5): p. 493-502.
[140] Dogra, G.K., G.F. Watts, D.C. Chan, et al., *Statin therapy improves brachial artery vasodilator function in patients with Type 1 diabetes and microalbuminuria.* Diabet Med, 2005. 22(3): p. 239-42.
[141] Zandi-Nejad, K., V.A. Luyckx, and B.M. Brenner, *Adult hypertension and kidney disease: the role of fetal programming.* Hypertension, 2006. 47(3): p. 502-8.
[142] Fuenmayor, N., E. Moreira, and L.X. Cubeddu, *Salt sensitivity is associated with insulin resistance in essential hypertension.* Am J Hypertens, 1998. 11(4 Pt 1): p. 397-402.
[143] Sharma, A.M., U. Schorr, and A. Distler, *Insulin resistance in young salt-sensitive normotensive subjects.* Hypertension, 1993. 21(3): p. 273-9.
[144] Weir, M.R., *Impact of salt intake on blood pressure and proteinuria in diabetes: importance of the renin-angiotensin system.* Miner Electrolyte Metab, 1998. 24(6): p. 438-45.
[145] Resnick, L.M., *Ionic basis of hypertension, insulin resistance, vascular disease, and related disorders. The mechanism of "syndrome X".* Am J Hypertens, 1993. 6(4): p. 123S-134S.
[146] Cohn, J.N., A.A. Quyyumi, N.K. Hollenberg, et al., *Surrogate markers for cardiovascular disease: functional markers.* Circulation, 2004. 109(25 Suppl 1): p. IV31-46.
[147] Kimoto, E., T. Shoji, K. Shinohara, et al., *Preferential stiffening of central over peripheral arteries in type 2 diabetes.* Diabetes, 2003. 52(2): p. 448-52.
[148] Hopkins, K.D., E.D. Lehmann, R.L. Jones, et al., *A family history of NIDDM is associated with decreased aortic distensibility in normal healthy young adult subjects.* Diabetes Care, 1996. 19(5): p. 501-3.
[149] Ratto, E., G. Leoncini, F. Viazzi, et al., *Ambulatory arterial stiffness index and renal abnormalities in primary hypertension.* J Hypertens, 2006. 24(10): p. 2033-8.
[150] Pirro, M., G. Schillaci, G. Savarese, et al., *Low-grade systemic inflammation impairs arterial stiffness in newly diagnosed hypercholesterolaemia.* Eur J Clin Invest, 2004. 34(5): p. 335-41.
[151] Wilkinson, I. and J.R. Cockcroft, *Cholesterol, lipids and arterial stiffness.* Adv Cardiol, 2007. 44: p. 261-77.
[152] Mottram, P.M., B.A. Haluska, R. Leano, et al., *Relation of arterial stiffness to diastolic dysfunction in hypertensive heart disease.* Heart, 2005. 91(12): p. 1551-6.
[153] Gates, P.E., H. Tanaka, J. Graves, et al., *Left ventricular structure and diastolic function with human ageing. Relation to habitual exercise and arterial stiffness.* Eur Heart J, 2003. 24(24): p. 2213-20.
[154] Cruickshank, K., L. Riste, S.G. Anderson, et al., *Aortic Pulse-Wave Velocity and its relationship to Mortality in Diabetes and Glucose intolerance.* Circulation, 2002. 106: p. 2085-90.

[155] Laurent, S., P. Boutouyrie, R. Asmar, et al., *Aortic stiffness is an independent predictor of all-cause and cardiovascular mortality in hypertensive patients.* Hypertension, 2001. 37: p. 1236-41.

[156] Meaume, S., A. Rudnichi, A. Lynch, et al., *Aortic pulse wave velocity as a marker of cardiovascular disease in subjects over 70 years old.* J Hypertens, 2001. 19(5): p. 871-7.

[157] Cerasola, G., S. Cottone, G. Mule, et al., *Microalbuminuria, renal dysfunction and cardiovascular complication in essential hypertension.* J Hypertens, 1996. 14(7): p. 915-20.

[158] Cruickshank, K., L. Riste, S.G. Anderson, et al., *Aortic pulse-wave velocity and its relationship to mortality in diabetes and glucose intolerance: an integrated index of vascular function?* Circulation, 2002. 106(16): p. 2085-90.

[159] Niskanen, L., M. Uusitupa, H. Sarlund, et al., *Microalbuminuria predicts the development of serum lipoprotein abnormalities favouring atherogenesis in newly diagnosed type 2 (non-insulin-dependent) diabetic patients.* Diabetologia, 1990. 33(4): p. 237-43.

[160] Smith, A., J. Karalliedde, L. De Angelis, et al., *Aortic pulse wave velocity and albuminuria in patients with type 2 diabetes.* J Am Soc Nephrol, 2005. 16(4): p. 1069-75.

[161] Kohara, K., Y. Tabara, R. Tachibana, et al., *Microalbuminuria and arterial stiffness in a general population: the Shimanami Health Promoting Program (J-SHIPP) study.* Hypertens Res, 2004. 27(7): p. 471-7.

[162] Peppa-Patrikiou, M., M. Dracopoulou, and C. Dacou-Voutetakis, *Urinary endothelin in adolescents and young adults with insulin-dependent diabetes mellitus: relation to urinary albumin, blood pressure, and other factors.* Metabolism, 1998. 47(11): p. 1408-12.

[163] Pedrinelli, R., G. Dell'Omo, V. Di Bello, et al., *Low-grade inflammation and microalbuminuria in hypertension.* Arterioscler Thromb Vasc Biol, 2004. 24(12): p. 2414-9.

[164] Aso, Y., N. Yoshida, K. Okumura, et al., *Coagulation and inflammation in overt diabetic nephropathy: association with hyperhomocysteinemia.* Clin Chim Acta, 2004. 348(1-2): p. 139-45.

[165] Kelbaek, H., T. Jensen, B. Feldt-Rasmussen, et al., *Impaired left-ventricular function in insulin-dependent diabetic patients with increased urinary albumin excretion.* Scand J Clin Lab Invest, 1991. 51(5): p. 467-73.

[166] Estacio, R.O., J.G. Regensteiner, E.E. Wolfel, et al., *The association between diabetic complications and exercise capacity in NIDDM patients.* Diabetes Care, 1998. 21(2): p. 291-5.

[167] Magri, P., M.A. Rao, S. Cangianiello, et al., *Early impairment of renal hemodynamic reserve in patients with asymptomatic heart failure is restored by angiotensin II antagonism.* Circulation, 1998. 98(25): p. 2849-54.

[168] Sarafidis, P.A. and L.M. Ruilope, *Insulin resistance, hyperinsulinemia, and renal injury: mechanisms and implications.* Am J Nephrol, 2006. 26(3): p. 232-44.

[169] Ruilope, L.M., D.J. van Veldhuisen, E. Ritz, et al., *Renal function: the Cinderella of cardiovascular risk profile.* J Am Coll Cardiol, 2001. 38(7): p. 1782-7.

[170] Safar, M.E., G.M. London, and G.E. Plante, *Arterial stiffness and kidney function.* Hypertension, 2004. 43(2): p. 163-8.

[171] Zoccali, C., R. Maio, G. Tripepi, et al., *Inflammation as a mediator of the link between mild to moderate renal insufficiency and endothelial dysfunction in essential hypertension.* J Am Soc Nephrol, 2006. 17(4 Suppl 2): p. S64-8.

[172] Levine, D.Z., *Hyperfiltration, nitric oxide, and diabetic nephropathy.* Curr Hypertens Rep, 2006. 8(2): p. 153-7.

[173] Palatini, P., P. Mormino, F. Dorigatti, et al., *Glomerular hyperfiltration predicts the development of microalbuminuria in stage 1 hypertension: the HARVEST.* Kidney Int, 2006. 70(3): p. 578-84.
[174] Weiss, G. and L.T. Goodnough, *Anemia of chronic disease.* N Engl J Med, 2005. 352(10): p. 1011-23.
[175] Srivastava, P.M., M.C. Thomas, P. Calafiore, et al., *Diastolic dysfunction is associated with anaemia in patients with Type II diabetes.* Clin Sci (Lond), 2006. 110(1): p. 109-16.
[176] Smith, K.J., A.J. Bleyer, W.C. Little, et al., *The cardiovascular effects of erythropoietin.* Cardiovasc Res, 2003. 59(3): p. 538-48.
[177] Ritz, E., *Managing anaemia and diabetes: a future challenge for nephrologists.* Nephrol Dial Transplant, 2005. 20 Suppl 6: p. vi21-5.
[178] Kovesdy, C.P., B.K. Trivedi, K. Kalantar-Zadeh, et al., *Association of anemia with outcomes in men with moderate and severe chronic kidney disease.* Kidney Int, 2006. 69(3): p. 560-4.
[179] Streeter, R.P. and D. Mancini, *Treatment of anemia in the patient with heart failure.* Curr Treat Options Cardiovasc Med, 2005. 7(4): p. 327-32.
[180] Katzmarzyk, P.T., T.S. Church, and S.N. Blair, *Cardiorespiratory fitness attenuates the effects of the metabolic syndrome on all-cause and cardiovascular disease mortality in men.* Arch Intern Med, 2004. 164(10): p. 1092-7.
[181] Jouven, X., J.P. Empana, P.J. Schwartz, et al., *Heart-rate profile during exercise as a predictor of sudden death.* N Engl J Med, 2005. 352(19): p. 1951-8.
[182] Williams, S.G., M. Jackson, L.L. Ng, et al., *Exercise duration and peak systolic blood pressure are predictive of mortality in ambulatory patients with mild-moderate chronic heart failure.* Cardiology, 2005. 104(4): p. 221-6.
[183] Bonapace, S., A. Rossi, M. Cicoira, et al., *Aortic distensibility independently affects exercise tolerance in patients with dilated cardiomyopathy.* Circulation, 2003. 107(12): p. 1603-8.
[184] Boyer, J.K., S. Thanigaraj, K.B. Schechtman, et al., *Prevalence of ventricular diastolic dysfunction in asymptomatic, normotensive patients with diabetes mellitus.* Am J Cardiol, 2004. 93(7): p. 870-5.
[185] Vinereanu, D., E. Nicolaides, A.C. Tweddel, et al., *Subclinical left ventricular dysfunction in asymptomatic patients with Type II diabetes mellitus, related to serum lipids and glycated haemoglobin.* Clin Sci (Lond), 2003. 105(5): p. 591-9.
[186] McMahon, A.C., R.U. Naqvi, M.J. Hurst, et al., *Diastolic dysfunction and abnormality of the Na+/Ca2+ exchanger in single uremic cardiac myocytes.* Kidney Int, 2006. 69(5): p. 846-51.
[187] Ando, K. and T. Fujita, *Anti-diabetic effect of blockade of the renin-angiotensin system.* Diabetes Obes Metab, 2006. 8(4): p. 396-403.
[188] Derosa, G., A.F. Cicero, A. Dangelo, et al., *Thiazolidinedione effects on blood pressure in diabetic patients with metabolic syndrome treated with glimepiride.* Hypertens Res, 2005. 28(11): p. 917-24.
[189] Raji, A. and J. Plutzky, *Insulin resistance, diabetes, and atherosclerosis: thiazolidinediones as therapeutic interventions.* Curr Cardiol Rep, 2002. 4(6): p. 514-21.
[190] Undas, A., K.E. Brummel-Ziedins, and K.G. Mann, *Statins and blood coagulation.* Arterioscler Thromb Vasc Biol, 2005. 25(2): p. 287-94.
[191] Fliser, D., K. Buchholz, and H. Haller, *Antiinflammatory effects of angiotensin II subtype 1 receptor blockade in hypertensive patients with microinflammation.* Circulation, 2004. 110(9): p. 1103-7.

[192] Gross, M.L., K. Amann, and E. Ritz, *Nephron number and renal risk in hypertension and diabetes.* J Am Soc Nephrol, 2005. 16 Suppl 1: p. S27-9.

[193] Hobson, A., P.A. Kalra, and P.R. Kalra, *Cardiology and nephrology: time for a more integrated approach to patient care?* Eur Heart J, 2005. 26(16): p. 1576-8.

[194] Lee, Y.J. and J.C. Tsai, *ACE gene insertion/deletion polymorphism associated with 1998 World Health Organization definition of metabolic syndrome in Chinese type 2 diabetic patients.* Diabetes Care, 2002. 25(6): p. 1002-8.

[195] Zozulinska, D. and B. Wierusz-Wysocka, *Type 2 diabetes mellitus as inflammatory disease.* Diabetes Res Clin Pract, 2006.

[196] Li, J.J., C.H. Fang, and R.T. Hui, *Is hypertension an inflammatory disease?* Med Hypotheses, 2005. 64(2): p. 236-40.

[197] Li, J.J. and J.L. Chen, *Inflammation may be a bridge connecting hypertension and atherosclerosis.* Med Hypotheses, 2005. 64(5): p. 925-9.

[198] Lind, L., *Circulating markers of inflammation and atherosclerosis.* Atherosclerosis, 2003. 169(2): p. 203-214.

[199] Shoelson, S.E., J. Lee, and A.B. Goldfine, *Inflammation and insulin resistance.* J Clin Invest, 2006. 116(7): p. 1793-801.

[200] Ridker, P.M., N. Rifai, N.R. Cook, et al., *Non-HDL cholesterol, apolipoproteins A-I and B100, standard lipid measures, lipid ratios, and CRP as risk factors for cardiovascular disease in women.* Jama, 2005. 294(3): p. 326-33.

[201] Sagastagoitia, J.D., Y. Saez, M. Vacas, et al., *Association between inflammation, lipid and hemostatic factors in patients with stable angina.* Thromb Res, 2006.

[202] Stuveling, E.M., S.J. Bakker, H.L. Hillege, et al., *C-reactive protein modifies the relationship between blood pressure and microalbuminuria.* Hypertension, 2004. 43(4): p. 791-6.

[203] Ridker, P.M., P.W. Wilson, and S.M. Grundy, *Should C-reactive protein be added to metabolic syndrome and to assessment of global cardiovascular risk?* Circulation, 2004. 109(23): p. 2818-25.

[204] Stehouwer, C.D., M.A. Gall, J.W. Twisk, et al., *Increased urinary albumin excretion, endothelial dysfunction, and chronic low-grade inflammation in type 2 diabetes: progressive, interrelated, and independently associated with risk of death.* Diabetes, 2002. 51(4): p. 1157-65.

[205] Palmieri, V., R.P. Tracy, M.J. Roman, et al., *Relation of left ventricular hypertrophy to inflammation and albuminuria in adults with type 2 diabetes: the strong heart study.* Diabetes Care, 2003. 26(10): p. 2764-9.

[206] Devaraj, S., R.S. Rosenson, and I. Jialal, *Metabolic syndrome: an appraisal of the pro-inflammatory and procoagulant status.* Endocrinol Metab Clin North Am, 2004. 33(2): p. 431-53, table of contents.

[207] Matteucci, E., J. Rosada, M. Pinelli, et al., *Systolic blood pressure response to exercise in type 1 diabetes families compared with healthy control individuals.* J Hypertens, 2006. 24(9): p. 1745-51.

[208] Keung, Y.K. and J. Owen, *Iron deficiency and thrombosis: literature review.* Clin Appl Thromb Hemost, 2004. 10(4): p. 387-91.

[209] Nieuwdorp, M., E.S. Stroes, J.C. Meijers, et al., *Hypercoagulability in the metabolic syndrome.* Curr Opin Pharmacol, 2005. 5(2): p. 155-9.

[210] Sechi, L.A., L. Zingaro, C. Catena, et al., *Relationship of fibrinogen levels and hemostatic abnormalities with organ damage in hypertension.* Hypertension, 2000. 36(6): p. 978-85.

[211] Danesh, J., S. Lewington, S.G. Thompson, et al., *Plasma fibrinogen level and the risk of major cardiovascular diseases and nonvascular mortality: an individual participant meta-analysis.* Jama, 2005. 294(14): p. 1799-809.

[212] Marcucci, R., A.M. Gori, F. Giannotti, et al., *Markers of hypercoagulability and inflammation predict mortality in patients with heart failure.* J Thromb Haemost, 2006. 4(5): p. 1017-22.

[213] Vicari, A.M., M.V. Taglietti, F. Pellegatta, et al., *Deranged platelet calcium homeostasis in diabetic patients with end-stage renal failure. A possible link to increased cardiovascular mortality?* Diabetes Care, 1996. 19(10): p. 1062-6.

[214] Haffner, S.M., L. Mykkanen, A. Festa, et al., *Insulin-resistant prediabetic subjects have more atherogenic risk factors than insulin-sensitive prediabetic subjects: implications for preventing coronary heart disease during the prediabetic state.* Circulation, 2000. 101(9): p. 975-80.

[215] Isomaa, B., P. Almgren, T. Tuomi, et al., *Cardiovascular morbidity and mortality associated with the metabolic syndrome.* Diabetes Care, 2001. 24(4): p. 683-9.

[216] Bloomgarden, Z.T., *Third Annual World Congress on the Insulin Resistance Syndrome: Atherothrombotic disease.* Diabetes Care, 2006. 29(8): p. 1973-80.

[217] Juhan-Vague, I., M.C. Alessi, A. Mavri, et al., *Plasminogen activator inhibitor-1, inflammation, obesity, insulin resistance and vascular risk.* J Thromb Haemost, 2003. 1(7): p. 1575-9.

[218] Inomat, S., M. Haneda, T. Moriya, et al., *[Revised criteria for the early diagnosis of diabetic nephropathy].* Nippon Jinzo Gakkai Shi, 2005. 47(7): p. 767-9.

[219] Deferrari, G., M. Ravera, and V. Berruti, *Treatment of diabetic nephropathy in its early stages.* Diabetes Metab Res Rev, 2003. 19(2): p. 101-14.

[220] Ferrier, K.E., M.H. Muhlmann, J.P. Baguest, et al., *Intensive Cholesterol Reduction lowers blood pressure and large artery stiffness in isolated systolic hypertension.* Journal of American College of Cardiology, 2002. 39(6): p. 1020-5.

[221] Maiese, K., F. Li, and Z.Z. Chong, *New avenues of exploration for erythropoietin.* Jama, 2005. 293(1): p. 90-5.

[222] Khoshdel, A., S. Carney, A. Gillies, et al., *Potential roles of erythropoietin in the management of anaemia and other complications diabetes.* Diabetes Obes Metab, 2007.

[223] Levey, A.S., J. Coresh, E. Balk, et al., *National Kidney Foundation practice guidelines for chronic kidney disease: evaluation, classification, and stratification.* Ann Intern Med, 2003. 139(2): p. 137-47.

[224] Fox, K.M., *Efficacy of perindopril in reduction of cardiovascular events among patients with stable coronary artery disease: randomised, double-blind, placebo-controlled, multicentre trial (the EUROPA study).* Lancet, 2003. 362(9386): p. 782-8.

[225] *Randomised trial of a perindopril-based blood-pressure-lowering regimen among 6,105 individuals with previous stroke or transient ischaemic attack.* Lancet, 2001. 358(9287): p. 1033-41.

[226] Yusuf, S., P. Sleight, J. Pogue, et al., *Effects of an angiotensin-converting-enzyme inhibitor, ramipril, on cardiovascular events in high-risk patients. The Heart Outcomes Prevention Evaluation Study Investigators.* N Engl J Med, 2000. 342(3): p. 145-53.

[227] Bianchi, S., R. Bigazzi, and V.M. Campese, *Long-term effects of spironolactone on proteinuria and kidney function in patients with chronic kidney disease.* Kidney Int, 2006. 70(12): p. 2116-23.

[228] Casas, J.P., W. Chua, S. Loukogeorgakis, et al., *Effect of inhibitors of the renin-angiotensin system and other antihypertensive drugs on renal outcomes: systematic review and meta-analysis.* Lancet, 2005. 366(9502): p. 2026-33.

[229] Jafar, T.H., P.C. Stark, C.H. Schmid, et al., *Progression of chronic kidney disease: the role of blood pressure control, proteinuria, and angiotensin-converting enzyme inhibition: a patient-level meta-analysis.* Ann Intern Med, 2003. 139(4): p. 244-52.
[230] Jafar, T.H., C.H. Schmid, M. Landa, et al., *Angiotensin-converting enzyme inhibitors and progression of nondiabetic renal disease. A meta-analysis of patient-level data.* Ann Intern Med, 2001. 135(2): p. 73-87.
[231] Mann, J.F., W.M. McClellan, R. Kunz, et al., *Progression of renal disease--can we forget about inhibition of the renin-angiotensin system?* Nephrol Dial Transplant, 2006. 21(9): p. 2348-51; discussion 2352-3.
[232] Bilous, R.W., *Treatment strategies for early nephropathy,* in *Issues in nephrology.* accessed 2004, www.medscape.com.
[233] Palatini, P., A. Benetos, G. Grassi, et al., *Identification and management of the hypertensive patient with elevated heart rate: statement of a European Society of Hypertension Consensus Meeting.* J Hypertens, 2006. 24(4): p. 603-10.
[234] Bakris, G.L., P. Hart, and E. Ritz, *Beta blockers in the management of chronic kidney disease.* Kidney Int, 2006. 70(11): p. 1905-13.
[235] Khoshdel, A., S. Carney, A. Gillies, et al., *Potential roles of erythropoietin in the management of anaemia and other complications diabetes.* Diabetes Obes Metab, 2008. 10(1): p. 1-9.
[236] Gross, J.L., M.J. de Azevedo, S.P. Silveiro, et al., *Diabetic nephropathy: diagnosis, prevention, and treatment.* Diabetes Care, 2005. 28(1): p. 164-76.
[237] Bloomgarden, Z.T., *Diabetic nephropathy.* Diabetes Care, 2005. 28(3): p. 745-51.
[238] McGowan, T.A., Y. Zhu, and K. Sharma, *Transforming growth factor-beta: a clinical target for the treatment of diabetic nephropathy.* Curr Diab Rep, 2004. 4(6): p. 447-54.
[239] Mangoni, A.A., R.A. Sherwood, B. Asonganyi, et al., *Short-term oral folic acid supplementation enhances endothelial function in patients with type 2 diabetes.* Am J Hypertens, 2005. 18(2 Pt 1): p. 220-6.
[240] Samuel, C.S. and T.D. Hewitson, *Relaxin in cardiovascular and renal disease.* Kidney Int, 2006. 69(9): p. 1498-502.
[241] Ashton, N., *Renal and vascular actions of urotensin II.* Kidney Int, 2006. 70(4): p. 624-9.
[242] Varghese, Z., J.F. Moorhead, and X.Z. Ruan, *The PPARalpha ligand fenofibrate: meeting multiple targets in diabetic nephropathy.* Kidney Int, 2006. 69(9): p. 1490-1.
[243] Vitale, C., G. Mercuro, A. Cornoldi, et al., *Metformin improves endothelial function in patients with metabolic syndrome.* J Intern Med, 2005. 258(3): p. 250-6.
[244] Lipton, S.A., *Erythropoietin for neurologic protection and diabetic neuropathy.* N Engl J Med, 2004. 350(24): p. 2516-7.
[245] Gomez-Garre, D., J.L. Martin-Ventura, R. Granados, et al., *Losartan improves resistance artery lesions and prevents CTGF and TGF-beta production in mild hypertensive patients.* Kidney Int, 2006. 69(7): p. 1237-44.
[246] Oliver, J.J. and D.E. Newby, *Endothelial fibrinolytic function in hypertension: the expanding story.* J Hypertens, 2005. 23(8): p. 1471-2.
[247] Roldan, V. and F. Marin, *Are we content with lowering blood pressure alone, or should we be asking something more from the antihypertensive drugs we use?: effects of antihypertensive agents on fibrinolytic function.* J Hum Hypertens, 2004. 18(10): p. 681-3.
[248] Ritz, E., *PPARgamma agonists: killing two birds with one stone?* J Hypertens, 2004. 22(9): p. 1673-4.
[249] Park, C.W., Y. Zhang, X. Zhang, et al., *PPARalpha agonist fenofibrate improves diabetic nephropathy in db/db mice.* Kidney Int, 2006. 69(9): p. 1511-7.

10

Non Invasive Assessment of Cardiovascular Risk Profile: The Role of the Ultrasound Markers

Marco Matteo Ciccone*, Michele Gesualdo, Annapaola Zito, Cosimo Mandurino, Manuela Locorotondo and Pietro Scicchitano

Cardiovascular Diseases Section, Department of Emergency and Organ Transplantation (DETO), University of Bari, Bari, Italy

1. Introduction

Atherosclerosis, with its complications, is the most frequent cause of death all over the world, and it is the underlying cause of about 50% of all deaths in developed countries (1).

Recent studies showed the key role played by inflammation and immune responses in development, progression, and rupture of atherosclerotic plaque (2,3,4). The presence of an immune reaction and/or infective antigens as potential triggers of atherogenesis (5,6) makes atherosclerosis be considered as an autoimmune disease in which the adaptive immune system is targeted against self-antigens modified by biochemical factors such as oxidative stress and hypercholesterolemia (7). These give rise to plaque birth (8,9) and the inflammatory status of the plaque makes the lesions unstable, inducing their abruption and acute thrombotic obstruction. Therefore, it induces impairment in endothelial function in bioactive antiatherogenic or proatherogenic molecules production (10), although other factors could increase such an imbalance: age (11), sex (12), hypertension (13), obesity (14), smoking (15), dyslipidemia (16), diabetes (17), all able to increase oxidative stress and vascular inflammation (18), morphological wall alterations and subsequently progression of atheromatous lesions.

The initial atherosclerosis stages silently and symptom free occur since childhood (19); the clinical expressions (i.e., sudden cardiac death, myocardial infarction, angina pectoris, stroke, aortic aneurysm, renovascular hypertension, and intermittent claudication) involve 2 over 3 men and 1 over 2 women after age 40, and almost 60% of deaths are due to a cardiovascular disease cause (20). Thus, there has been an increase in recognition of the importance of subclinical atherosclerosis, and early detection of this insidious process must be the goal for improving cardiovascular health through prevention, and treatment of risk factors.

Currently, non-invasive risk profile assessments can be evaluated not only with some laboratory parameters, (lipids and systemic inflammation markers as white blood cells,

---

* Corresponding Author

reactive C protein and erythrocyte segmentation rate), but also with ultrasonographic methods that detect subclinical atherosclerosis. Three internationally validated methods had been adopted in order to evaluate endothelium function: brachial artery flow-mediated vasodilation (FMD) (21,22), antero-posterior abdominal aorta diameter (APAO) (23) and intima-media thickness of the common carotid artery (CCA-IMT) (24,25). Cause of their non-invasiveness, feasibility and cheap cost, these techniques are the best tools for the physicians to assess functional and morphological alterations of the arteries before a cardiovascular event occurs and the feasibility of therapies to reduce atherosclerosis burden (26).

2. FMD technique

The endothelium is a real "organ", endowed with autocrine and paracrine properties and playing an essential role in controlling vasomotion by producing molecules able to modulate blood, such as nitric oxide (NO), the most important vasodilator molecule produced by endothelial cells) (27). Shear stress is the main element able to determine increasing in NO production, its action being exerted perpendicularly to the long axis of the vessel.

Nevertheless, endothelial cells can also produce substances with vasoconstrictor action, as endothelin-1, (27) above all in case of increased age, hyperhomocysteinemia, smoking, diabetes, hypercholesterolemia, and hypertension (28): in these case it could be detected the presence of reduced vasodilating response to endothelial stimuli. Instead, diet and exercise can improve endothelial function (29). Lipid-lowering therapy (30,31), antioxidants (32), estrogen replacement (33) and treatment with angiotensin-converting enzyme inhibition or receptor blockade (34) improve this response.

Thus, endothelial dysfunction is considered the basic pathogenic mechanism of cardiovascular disease (35) and therefore can be considered as an early marker of cardiovascular risk.

In fact, the endothelial dysfunction seems to be the earliest event in the process of atherosclerotic plaque formation, appearing even before structural lesion of the vessel wall (36); for this reason the evaluation of endothelial function could be a useful tool for early stratification of patients at risk for cardiovascular events.

Studies in postmenopausal women suggest that endothelial dysfunction may be a predisposing factor for the development of hypertension (37) and diabetes (38), thus being not only a consequence of risk factors but also a pathogenetic mechanism for their onset.

Moreover, impaired endothelium-dependent vasomotion may contribute to the genesis of cardiovascular events by modulating the stability of plaque and coronary vasospasm. In fact, the analysis of Lerman and Zeiher (39) showed that endothelial dysfunction, assessed both at coronary and peripheral level, is significantly predictive of cardiovascular events independently of the presence of traditional cardiovascular risk factors.

3. Procedure description

A non-invasive method to assess endothelium-dependent flow-mediated vasodilation (FMD) was developed in the 1990s: it consisted in inducing endothelial cells to release NO

(40,41) through mechanical stimulation originating from increasing in vessel wall "shear stress". It is usually performed at brachial artery level by high-frequency ultrasonographic imaging (21).

It is performed in a quiet, temperature-controlled (22–24°C) room, early in the morning and it adopts a high resolution ultrasonograph connected to an image analysis system and a sphygmomanometer cuff applied around the forearm to create a flow stimulus in the brachial artery. The examination requires the patients to be supine, at rest, fast for at least 8 to 12 hours before the study; all vasoactive medications (calcium channel blockers, ß-adrenergic blocking agents, nitrates and converting enzyme inhibitors) should be withheld for at least 4 half-lives, if possible. Moreover, subjects should avoid substances that might impair FMD such as caffeine, high-fat foods, and vitamin C or use tobacco for at least 4 to 6 hours before the study (table 1).

FACTORS	COMMENTS
Hours	The examination should be performed at the same time of day
Temperature	Ultrasonographic evaluation should be performed at constant temperature, in an environment equipped with air conditioning
Drugs	All vasoactive drugs should be discontinued the night before the exam
Coffee and The	The day of the examination, the patient should refrain from taking coffee or tea
Smoking	Patients should abstain from smoking
Influence of food	Patients should not take copious meals or high in fat
Brachial artery diameter	It must be between 2.5 and 5 mm

Table 1. Prerequisites and factors that influence the flow-mediated dilation

The 7,5 MHz electronic probe is positioned 4–5 cm above ante-cubital fossa to obtain longitudinal B-mode vascular scanning of the brachial artery with clear anterior and posterior intimal-lumen interfaces, and once the optimal artery image is achieved, the probe can be maintained in the right position using a mechanical arm. A pulsed wave Doppler recording is obtained from the midartery.

The procedure lasts 9 minutes: the first minute evaluate baseline diameter, measured at the onset of the R-wave on the electrocardiogram.

At the end of the first minute, the cuff is inflated 200-250 mmHg in order to close arterial inflow of the forearm (42). This causes ischemia and, consequentially, dilation of downstream resistance vessels by autoregulatory mechanisms.

After the sixth minute, the cuff is rapidly deflated: a brief high-flow state through the brachial artery to accommodate the dilated resistance vessels happens, and this reactive hyperemia produces a shear stress stimulus that induces the endothelium to release nitric oxide with subsequent vasodilation of the brachial artery between the 6th and 9th minute.

The software calculates FMD value as percentage of increasing of diameter value from baseline:

$$FMD = [(\text{postiperemia diameter} - \text{baseline diameter}) / \text{baseline diameter}] \times 100$$

The maximal increase in diameter occurs approximately 60 to 90 seconds after cuff release. FMD values greater than 5-10% are considered "normal" (21). A schematic overview of this imaging technique could be observed in figure 1a.

This reactive hyperemia phase is confirmed by measuring the arterial blood flow using pulse-wave Doppler. The peak blood flow in the brachial artery is obtained with the sample volume in the centre of the artery and a correction angle of 70°. It is estimated at rest and during the first 15 s after cuff deflation, taking the average of the pulsed Doppler velocity signal of 3 measurements. The maximum speeds considered normal is 50–70 cm/s. Reactive hyperemia is calculated as the ratio of the maximal velocity divided by the maximal velocity at baseline.

Because of its low reproducibility and accuracy (43,44), the technique requires very high methodology accuracy and a mechanical support for the probe with micrometer adjustment to prevent movement of the vascular probe, and specific software ("FMD Studio") to measure second to second changes in artery caliber (21). The variations in caliber measured are small (from 0 to 15%), so the FMD represents a stimulus-type "on / off" poorly modulated.

Therefore, in order to obtain results that have a clinical validity, it is necessary to study a large number of patients. In support of the role of endothelial function as marker of cardiovascular risk and of the validity of the FMD method, there is also correlation with the invasive test data of coronary endothelial function (45) and with the severity and extent of atherosclerosis coronary (46).

Moreover, the noninvasive nature of the technique allows repeated measurements over time to study the effectiveness of various interventions that may affect vascular health.

4. APAO

Up to now the infrarenal anteroposterior diameter of abdominal aorta (APAO) has been always related to the abdominal aortic aneurysms (AAAs), as a measurement to be used in the diagnostic and follow-up phase of this disease and for surgical intervention planning.

An abdominal aortic aneurysm is defined by some authors as an infrarenal aortic diameter ≥ 3.0 cm, or a ratio between infrarenal and suprarenal aorta diameters greater than 1.2, all measured by ultrasound B-mode (47). As coronary heart disease and stroke continue to be the leading causes of death and disability among adults in developed countries, an early detection of vascular damage and, consequently, adequate cardiovascular risk stratification has received an intense attention in the last years in order to decrease the impact of cardiovascular disease.

To detect the "primum movens" of atherosclerotic disease, several studies have been conducted in the last years for identify new ultrasonographic markers (48).

Intima-media thickness of abdominal aorta has been firstly suggested as cardiovascular risk marker in patients stratification risk profile (49).

Recently, in addition to arterial wall thickening, attention has been paid on APAO as a possible early marker of atherosclerosis (before clinical manifestations have become evident). Indeed, arterial dilatation is a well-known age-related manifestation, and some of the molecular events causing this alterations are involved in the pathogenesis of cardiovascular disease (50,51).

There is a relationship between APAO in the non-aneurysmal range (<30 mm in diameter) and all-cause mortality: in a cohort of 12203 men aged 65 years and older infrarenal aortic diameter is turned out to be an independent predictor of all-cause mortality, particularly cardiovascular mortality (52). In another study on 4734 participants > 65 years old underwent to abdominal aortic ultrasound evaluation, has been demonstrated that for those with an infrarenal aortic diameters >2.0 cm, there was a significantly higher risk of future cardiovascular events and total mortality, suggesting a value of infrarenal aortic diameters between 2.0 and 3.0 cm as another manifestation of subclinical atherosclerosis (53).

Furtheremore, Allison et al (54) showed that age, gender, body mass index, and the presence and extent of calcified atherosclerosis in both the abdominal aorta and iliac arteries are significantly associated with increasing aortic diameter independently of other cardiovascular risk factors. A study by Ciccone et al. involving women with polycystic ovary syndrome PCOS (55) showed that the increase in APAO is the earliest arterial alteration in women with PCOS, thus preceding the IMT of other arteries such as common carotid arteries and common femoral arteries. This identifies APAO as an early marker of atherosclerosis.

However, this alteration seems to be due to body weight secondary to PCOS and not to PCOS *per se*. In fact, Gorter PM et al (56) showed that intra-abdominal fat accumulation and metabolic syndrome are associated with larger infrarenal aortic diameter in patients with clinically evident arterial disease, indicating a role for intra-abdominal fat in the development of larger aortic diameters.

To explain these findings it can be hypothesized that APAO may represent a measure of cumulative exposure to genetic and environmental risk factors implicated in atherosclerosis development. For these reasons, APAO can be considered as an early marker of cardiovascular risk, and because of its noninvasive measurement and feasibility might be used to investigate determinants of atherosclerosis at an early stage of the process and to assess modifiers of atherosclerosis disease progression, such as lifestyle and pharmacological interventions.

5. Procedure description

Wilmink and colleagues (57,58) showed that the use of ultrasounds to measure the infrarenal aortic diameter is attractive as it is rapid, cheap, and noninvasive. The good accuracy of infrarenal aortic diameter measurements by ultrasound makes this method acceptable for clinical decision-making.

With the patient in supine position, the examination is carried out with a 3.5 MHz electronic probe placed one centimetre left of the umbilicus. The longitudinal ultrasound scans allow the study of the aorta and the best image in long axis projection of the abdominal aorta is used for the measurement. To improve the image acquisition, subjects are asked to keep fasting for at least 6-8 hours and follow a fiber diet for the two days prior to the examination to reduce intestinal bloating (diet preparation). To reduce the bias and interobserver variability the study of infrarenal abdominal aorta should be performed by same physician (59,60).

In the study of Ciccone et al.(55) the anteroposterior diameter of the aorta was defined as the maximal external cross-sectional measurement. It was calculated as the distance between the near and the far walls of the abdominal aorta on images that were frozen in systole. All the measurements were performed at 0.5, 1, and 2 cm above the umbilicus and were expressed in centimetres (see also Figure 1c and 1d).

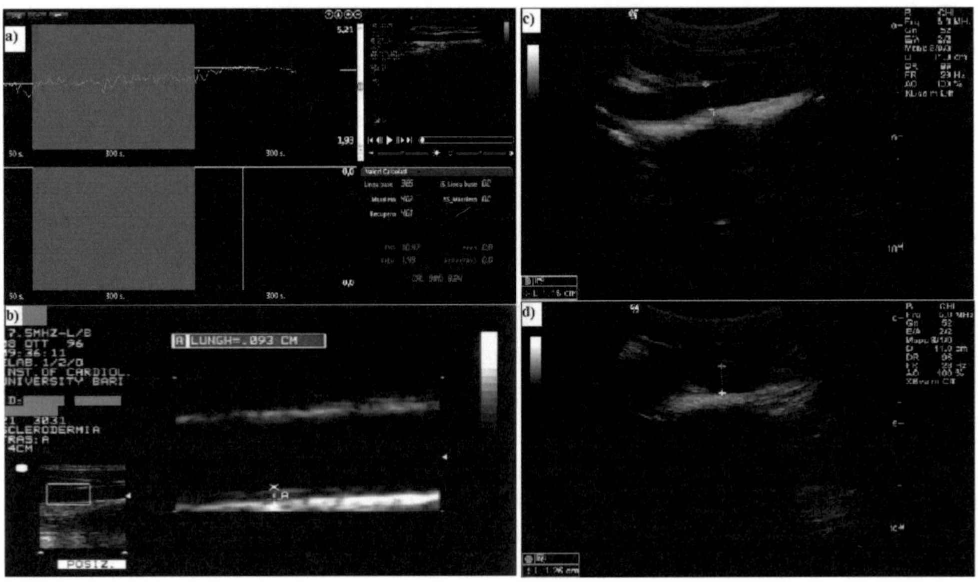

Fig. 1. a) Flow-mediated vasodilation (FMD) technique image. **b)** Ultrasound evaluation of common carotid artery intima-media thickness. **c)** Antero-posterior abdominal aorta diameter in long axis views. **d)** Antero-posterior abdominal aorta diameter in short axis views

However, in several studies the position of the probe and the part of abdominal aorta evaluated may be different.

van den Bosch et al. (61) studied distal aortic diameter to assess the relationship between abdominal aortic diameter and peripheral arterial occlusive disease. They demonstrated that both patients with an aortic diameter too large and patients with an aortic diameter too small are prone to peripheral arterial occlusive disease.

The study of Norman P. et al. (52) was carried out using a 3.75 mol/L Hz probe to measure the maximum transverse and antero-posterior diameter of the infrarenal aorta. The largest measurement was recorded as the aortic diameter.

Pleumeekers et al. (62) evaluated the observer variability of ultrasound measurements of proximal and distal part of the abdominal aorta. Their results were that ultrasound measurements are more accurate for the distal than for the proximal aorta measurement and the definition of the aortic diameter based on a combination of both distal and proximal measurement may be more accurate.

6. IMT

Atherosclerosis is a disease with a slowly progressive course and a long asymptomatic period. The clinical manifestations generally appear in middle age (63), and the first event triggered by atherosclerosis can be fatal.

Since the atherosclerotic disease is a multidistrict and multifocal process, identifying the changes of the vascular wall at subclinical stages of atherosclerosis is essential in assessing global cardiovascular risk (64) and in promoting the use of preventive strategies, as well as optimization of preventive and protective care.

Among imaging techniques for detection of early preclinical stages of atherosclerosis, the best is the measurement of the carotid intima-media thickness (CCA-IMT) using ultrasound high-resolution B-mode; the evaluation of this parameter is a noninvasive and reproducible method for identifying and quantifying subclinical vascular disease.

It is a well-validated research tool that has been translated increasingly into clinical practice as a cardiovascular risk marker (65,66).

Many studies demonstrated the role of CCA-IMT in the early evaluation of atherosclerosis disease. In fact, this parameter was found to be associated with the presence of cardiovascular risk factors (67,68,69) and with atherosclerotic lesions in other vascular districts, such as coronary and lower extremity arteries (70,71,72). Gasparyan (73) already put on evidence the importance of carotid ultrasound assessment in the clinical practice. Apart from CCA-IMT evaluation, the ultrasound evaluation should consider all the characteristics of carotid wall: it is necessary to evaluate IMT and, at the same time, morphological aspects of carotid wall.

Prospective epidemiological studies showed that individuals with elevated carotid IMT are more likely to suffer from cardiovascular or cerebrovascular events, suggesting that thickened carotid IMT is a powerful and independent indicator of the likelihood of general arteriosclerosis (74,75). The predictive power of carotid IMT is maintained even after adjustment for major cardiovascular risk factors. Thus, measurement of IMT may provide informations in addition to traditional risk factors during assessment of global cardiovascular risk profile in asymptomatic subjects (76).

SSeveral works in the last decade confirmed the role of this parameter in the early detection of atherosclerosis and in measure of its severity (77,78).

Moreover, changes in carotid IMT may be used as a measure of efficacy of pharmacologic intervention.

7. Procedure description

Carotid ultrasound can be performed using vascular echographic apparatus equipped with high-frequency transducers (usually 3-10 MHz and linear array) and appropriate software.

The patient should be positioned supine with slight (45°) hyperextension and rotation of the neck in the direction opposite the probe.

CCA-IMT is defined as the distance between the lumen-intima interface and the media-adventitia interface, which corresponds to the inner and outer echogenic lines seen on the B-mode ultrasound image [see figure 1b] (24,79).

Measurement of carotid IMT (c-IMT) is traditionally performed with the image of the carotid artery in the longitudinal axis, revealing the common carotid artery, the carotid bifurcation, and the internal and external carotid arteries.

Although these measurements have been performed for years, significant variability exists when measuring the near wall due to technical and acoustic difficulties encountered when imaging the c-IMT of the near wall (80). Due to these technical limitations, clinical measurement of c-IMT using B-mode ultrasound is often applied to the far (posterior) wall of the common carotid artery.

IMT is measured at about 2 cm proximal to the dilation of the bulb of the common carotid artery.

Three measurements coming from three different sites [according to the method described by Pignoli et al. (79): about 2 cm above the flow-divider, about ½ cm above the flow-divider and in middle zone] are considered for IMT evaluation. An average of all these values would be calculated at the end of the measures.

Mean IMT (m-IMT) and maximum IMT (M-IMT) are measured. m-IMT represents the mean value of all measurements at each common carotid artery, averaging the left and right sides. M-IMT represents the mean value of the single highest IMT measurements at each common carotid artery, averaging the left and right sides. Carotid plaque is defined as the presence of a greater than 1.5 mm c-IMT measurement or an area within the carotid artery that is at least 50% greater than the size of the surrounding vessel wall.

The same physician should perform the evaluation in order to reduce bias and improve the results.

A problem associated with the ultrasonographic IMT measurement is the variation in the readings, which leads to different results of repeated measurements from the same observer. In general, the inter- and intra-observer errors are acceptable and the technique has a good reproducibility (81,82).

8. References

[1] Lusis AJ. Atherosclerosis. *Nature* 2000;407:233–41.

[2] Ross R. Atherosclerosis: an inflammatory disease. *N Engl J Med* 1999; 340: 115-126.

[3] Jan M, Meng S, Chen NC, Mai J, Wang H, Yang XF. Inflammatory and autoimmune reactions in atherosclerosis and vaccine design informatics. J Biomed Biotechnol. 2010;2010:459798. Epub 2010 Apr 15.

[4] Libby P, Okamoto Y, Rocha VZ, Folco E. Inflammation in atherosclerosis: transition from theory to practice. *Circulation Journal.* 2010;74(2):213–220.

[5] Guan XR, Jiang LX, Ma XH, Wang LF, Quan H, Li HY. Respiratory syncytial virus infection and risk of acute myocardial infarction. *Am J Med Sci.* 2010;340(5):356-9.

[6] Makris GC, Makris MC, Wilmot VV, Geroulakos G, Falagas ME. The role of infection in carotid plaque pathogenesis and stability: the clinical evidence. *Curr Vasc Pharmacol.* 2010;8(6):861-72. Review.

[7] Nilsson J, Hansson GK. Autoimmunity in atherosclerosis: a protective response losing control? *Journal of Internal Medicine.* 2008;263(5):464–478.

[8] Nilsson J, Wigren M, Shah PK. Regulatory T cells and the control of modified lipoprotein autoimmunity-driven atherosclerosis. *Trends in Cardiovascular Medicine.* 2009;19(8):272–276.

[9] Hansson GK. Mechanisms of disease: inflammation, atherosclerosis, and coronary artery disease. *New England Journal of Medicine.* 2005;352(16):1685–1626.

[10] Vanhoutte PM, Shimokawa H, Tang EH, Feletou M. Endothelial dysfunction and vascular disease. *Acta Physiol.* 2009;196(2):193–222.

[11] Juonala M, Magnussen CG, Venn A, Dwyer T, Burns TL, Davis PH, Chen W, Srinivasan SR, Daniels SR, Khnen M, Laitinen T, Taittonen L, Berenson GS, Viikari JS, Raitakari OT. Influence of Age on Associations Between Childhood Risk Factors and Carotid Intima-Media Thickness in Adulthood: The Cardiovascular Risk in Young Finns Study, the Childhood Determinants of Adult Health Study, the Bogalusa Heart Study, and the Muscatine Study for the International Childhood Cardiovascular Cohort (i3C) Consortium. Circulation. 2010;122(24):2514-20.

[12] Vaccarino V, Badimon L, Corti R, de Wit C, Dorobantu M, Hall A, Koller A, Marzilli M, Pries A, Bugiardini R. Ischemic Heart Disease in Women: Are There Sex Differences in Pathophysiology and Risk Factors?: Position Paper from the Working Group on Coronary Pathophysiology & Microcirculation of the European Society of Cardiology. Cardiovasc Res. 2010 Dec 14. [Epub ahead of print]

[13] Dzau VJ. Atherosclerosis and hypertension: mechanisms and interrelationships. *Journal of Cardiovascular Pharmacology.* 1990;15(supplement 5):S59–S64.

[14] Mangge H, Almer G, Truschnig-Wilders M, Schmidt A, Gasser R, Fuchs D. Inflammation, adiponectin, obesity and cardiovascular risk. Curr Med Chem. 2010;17(36):4511-20.

[15] Lloyd-Jones DM, Wilson PWF, Larson MG, Beiser A, Leip EP, D'Agostino RB, Levy D. Framingham risk score and prediction of lifetime risk for coronary heart disease. *The American Journal of Cardiology.* 2004;94(1):20–24. doi: 10.1016/j.amjcard.2004.03.023.

[16] Ishigaki Y, Oka Y, Katagiri H. Circulating oxidized LDL: a biomarker and a pathogenic factor. *Curr Opin Lipidol.* 2009;20(5):363-9.

[17] Almdal T, Scharling H, Jensen JS, Vestergaard H. The independent effect of type 2 diabetes mellitus on ischemic heart disease, stroke, and death: a population-based study of 13,000 men and women with 20 years of follow-up. *Arch Intern Med.* 2004;164(13):1422-6

[18] Deanfield JE, Halcox JP, Rabelink TJ. Endothelial function and dysfunction: testing and clinical relevance. *Circulation.* 2007;115(10):1285–1295.

[19] Toth PP. Subclinical atherosclerosis: what it is, what it means and what we can do about it. *Int J Clin Prac* 2008, 62:1246-1254.

[20] Rosamond W, Flegal K, Furie K, Go A, Greenlund K, Haase N, Hailpern SM, Ho M, Howard V, Kissela B, Kittner S, Lloyd-Jones D, McDermott M, Meigs J, Moy C, Nichol G, O'Donnell C, Roger V, Sorlie P, Steinberger J, Thom T, Wilson M, Hong Y, for the American Heart Association Statistics Committee and Stroke Statistics Subcommittee: Heart Disease and Stroke Statistics--2008 Update: A Report From the American Heart Association Statistics Committee and Stroke Statistics Subcommittee. *Circulation* 2008, 117:e25-e146.

[21] Corretti MC, Anderson TJ, Benjamin EJ, et al. Guidelines for the ultrasound assessment of endothelial-dependent flow-mediated vasodilation of the brachial artery: a report of the International Brachial Artery Reactivity Task Force. *J Am Coll Cardiol* 2002; 39: 257-65.

[22] Tomiyama H, Yamashina A. Non-invasive vascular function tests: their pathophysiological background and clinical application. *Circ J*. 2010;74(1):24-33.

[23] Leite CC, Wajchenberg BL, Radominski R, Matsuda D, Cerri GG, Halpern A. Intra-abdominal thickness by ultrasonography to predict risk factors for cardiovascular disease and its correlation with anthropometric measurements. Metabolism. 2002 Aug;51(8):1034-40.

[24] Touboul PJ, Hennerici MG, Meairs S, Adams H, Amarenco P, Bornstein N, Csiba L, Desvarieux M, Ebrahim S, Fatar M, Hernandez Hernandez R, Jaff M, Kownator S, Prati P, Rundek T, Sitzer M, Schminke U, Tardif JC, Taylor A, Vicaut E, Woo KS, Zannad F, Zureik M. Mannheim Carotid Intima-Media Thickness Consensus (2004–2006). *Cerebrovasc Dis* 2007;23(1):75-80.

[25] Ciccone MM, Balbarini A, Porcelli MT, Santoro D, Cortese F, Scicchitano P, Favale S, Butitta F, De Pergola G, Gullace G, Novo S. Carotid artery intima-media thickness: normal and percentile values in the italian population (CAMP study). *EJCPR* 2010 [in press].

[26] Ciccone MM, Favale S, Scicchitano P, Mangini F, Mitacchione G, Gadaleta F, Longo D, Iacoviello M, Forleo C, Quistelli G, Taddei S, Resta O, Carratù P. Reversibility of the endothelial dysfunction after CPAP therapy in OSAS patients. *Int J Cardiol.* 2011 Feb 24. [Epub ahead of print].

[27] Luscher TF, Vanhoutte PM. The endothelium: modulator of cardiovascular function. Boca Raton, FL: CRC Press, 1990.

[28] Brunner H, Cockcroft JR, Deanfield J, Donald A, Ferrannini E, Halcox J, Kiowski W, Luscher TF, Mancia G, Natali A, Oliver JJ, Pessina AC, Rizzoni D, Rossi GP, Salvetti A, Spieker LE, Taddei S, Webb DJ. Endothelial function and dysfunction. Part II: Association with cardiovascular risk factors and diseases: a statement by the Working Group on Endothelins and Endothelial Factors of the European Society of Hypertension. *J Hypertens* 2005; 23:233–246.

[29] Sowers JR, Lester MA. Diabetes and cardiovascular disease. *Diabetes Care.* 1999;22(suppl 3):C14-C20.

[30] Megnien JL, Simon A, Andriani A, Segond P, Jeannin S, Levenson J. Cholesterol lowering therapy inhibits the lowflow mediated vasoconstriction of the brachial artery in hypercholesterolemic subjects. *Br J Clin Pharmacol* 1996;42: 187-93.

[31] Cohen JD, Drury JH, Ostdiek J, Finn J, Babu BR, Flaker G, et al. Benefits of lipid lowering on vascular reactivity in patients with coronary artery disease and

average cholesterol levels: a mechanism for reducing clinical events? *Am Heart J* 2000; 139:734-8.

[32] Plotnick GD, Corretti MC, Vogel RA. Effect of antioxidant vitamins on the transient impairment of endothelium-dependent brachial artery vasoactivity following a single high-fat meal. *JAMA* 1997;278:1682-6.

[33] Koh KK, Cardillo C, Bui MN, et al. Vascular effects of estrogen and cholesterol-lowering therapies in hypercholesterolemic postmenopausal women. *Circulation* 1999;99: 354-60.

[34] Wilmink HW, Banga JD, Hijmering M, Erkelens WD, Stroes ES, Rabelink TJ. Effect of angiotensin-converting enzyme inhibition and angiotensin II type 1 receptor antagonism on postprandial endothelial function. *J Am Coll Cardiol* 1999; 34:140-5.

[35] Toborek M, Kaiser S. Endothelial cell functions. Relationship to atherogenesis. *Basic Res Cardiol* 1999,94:295–314.

[36] Ludmer PL, Selwyn AP, Shook TL, et al. Paradoxical vasoconstriction induced by acetylcholine in atherosclerotic coronary arteries. *N Engl J Med* 1986; 315: 1046-1051.

[37] Rossi R, Chiurlia E, Nuzzo A, Cioni E, Origliani G, Modena MG. Flow-mediated vasodilation and the risk of developing hypertension in healthy postmenopausal women. *J Am Coll Cardiol* 2004;44:1636–1640.

[38] Rossi R, Cioni E, Nuzzo A, Origliani G, Modena MG. Endothelial-dependent vasodilation and incidence of type 2 diabetes in a population of healthy postmenopausal women. *Diabetes Care* 2005; 28:702–707.

[39] Lerman A, Zeiher AM. Endothelial function: cardiac events. *Circulation* 2005; 111: 363-8.

[40] Joannides R, Haefeli WE, Linder L, et al. Nitric oxide is responsible for flow-dependent dilatation of human peripheral conduit arteries in vivo. *Circulation* 1995;91:1314-19.

[41] Agewall S, Hulthe J, Fagerberg B, et al. Post-occlusion brachial artery vasodilatation after ischaemic handgrip exercise is nitric oxide mediated. *Clin Physiol Funct Imaging* 2002;22:18-23.

[42] Pyke KE, Tschakovsky ME. The relationship between shear stress and flow-mediated dilatation: implications for the assessment of endothelial function. *J Physiol* 2005;568:357-369.

[43] O'Rourke MF, Nichols WW. Shear stress and flow-mediated dilation. *Hypertension* 2004; 44: 119-120.

[44] Sonka M, Liang W, Lauer RM. Automated analysis of brachial ultrasound image sequences: early detection of cardiovascular disease via surrogates of endothelial function. *IEEE Trans Med Imaging* 2002;21:1271- 1279.

[45] Takase B, Uehata A, Akima T, et al. Endothelium-dependent flow-mediated vasodilation in coronary and brachial arteries in suspected coronary artery disease. *Am J Cardiol* 1998;82:1535-39.

[46] Neunteufl T, Katzenschlager R, Hassan A, et al. Systemic endothelial dysfunction is related to the extent and severity of coronary artery disease. *Atherosclerosis* 1997;129:111-18.

[47] Hirsch AT, Haskal ZJ, Hertzer NR, Bakal CW, Creager MA, Halperin JL, Hiratzka LF, Murphy WR, Olin JW, Puschett JB, Rosenfield KA, Sacks D, Stanley JC, Taylor LM, Jr, White CJ, White J, White RA, Antman EM, Smith SC, Jr, Adams CD, Anderson JL, Faxon DP, Fuster V, Gibbons RJ, Hunt SA, Jacobs AK, Nishimura R, Ornato JP,

Page RL, Riegel B. ACC/AHA 2005 Practice Guidelines for the management of patients with peripheral arterial disease (lower extremity, renal, mesenteric, and abdominal aortic): a collaborative report from the American Association for Vascular Surgery/Society for Vascular Surgery, Society for Cardiovascular Angiography and Interventions, Society for Vascular Medicine and Biology, Society of Interventional Radiology, and the ACC/AHA Task Force on Practice Guidelines (Writing Committee to Develop Guidelines for the Management of Patients With Peripheral Arterial Disease): endorsed by the American Association of Cardiovascular and Pulmonary Rehabilitation; National Heart, Lung, and Blood Institute; Society for Vascular Nursing; Trans Atlantic Inter-Society Consensus; and Vascular Disease Foundation. *Circulation.* 2006;113(11):e463–654.

[48] Simon A, Gariepy J, Levenson J. Ultrasonographic study of the arterial walls: application to the detection of preclinical atherosclerosis. Arch Mal Coeur Vaiss. 1997;90 Spec No 2:7-10.

[49] Astrand H, Sandgren T, Ahlgren AR, Länne T. Noninvasive ultrasound measurements of aortic intima-media thickness: implications for in vivo study of aortic wall stress. J Vasc Surg. 2003 Jun;37(6):1270-6.

[50] Grimshaw G, Thompson J. Changes in diameter of the abdominal aorta with age: an epidemiological study. *J Clin Ultrasound.* 1997;25:7–13.

[51] Lakatta E. Arterial and cardiac aging: major shareholders in cardiovascular disease enterprises. Part 3: Cellular and molecular clues to heart and arterial aging. *Circulation.* 2003;107:490–497.

[52] Norman P, Le M, Pearce C, Jamrozik K. Infrarenal aortic diameter predicts all-cause mortality. Arterioscler Thromb Vasc Biol. 2004 Jul;24(7):1278-82.

[53] Freiberg MS, Arnold AM, Newman AB, Edwards MS, Kraemer KL, Kuller LH. Abdominal aortic aneurysms, increasing infrarenal aortic diameter, and risk of total mortality and incident cardiovascular disease events: 10-year follow-up data from the Cardiovascular Health Study. Circulation. 2008 Feb 26;117(8):1010-7.

[54] Allison MA, Kwan K, Di Tomasso D, Wright CM, Criqui MH. The epidemiology of abdominal aortic diameter. *J Vasc Surg.* 2008;48(1): 121–127.

[55] Ciccone MM, Favale S, Bhuva A, Scicchitano P, Caragnano V, Lavopa C, De Pergola G, Loverro G. Anteroposterior diameter of the infrarenal abdominal aorta is higher in women with polycystic ovary syndrome. *Vasc Health Risk Manag.* 2009;5(3):561-6.

[56] Gorter PM, Visseren FL, Moll FL, van der Graaf Y; SMART Study Group. Intra-abdominal fat and metabolic syndrome are associated with larger infrarenal aortic diameters in patients with clinically evident arterial disease. J Vasc Surg. 2008 Jul;48(1):114-20.

[57] Wilmink AB, Quick CR, Hubbard CS, Day NE. Effectiveness and cost of screening for abdominal aortic aneurysm: results of a population screening program. J Vasc Surg. 2003 Jul;38(1):72-7.

[58] Wilmink AB, Forshaw M, Quick CR, Hubbard CS, Day NE. Accuracy of serial screening for abdominal aortic aneurysms by ultrasound. J Med Screen. 2002;9(3):125-7.

[59] Lederle FA, Walker JM, Reinke DB. Selective screening for abdominal aortic aneurysms with physical examination and ultrasound. *Arch Intern Med.* 1988;148(8):1753–1756.

[60] Brady AR, Gerald F, Fowkes R, Thompson SG, Powell JT. Aortic aneurysm diameter and risk of cardiovascular mortality. *Arterioscler Thromb Vasc Biol.* 2001;21(7):1203–1207.

[61] van den Bosch MA, van der Graaf Y, Eikelboom BC, Algra A, Mali WP; SMART Study Group. Second Manifestations of ARTerial Disease. Distal aortic diameter and peripheral arterial occlusive disease. J Vasc Surg. 2001;34(6):1085-9.

[62] Pleumeekers HJ, Hoes AW, Mulder PG, van der Does E, Hofman A, Laméris JS, Grobbee DE. Differences in observer variability of ultrasound measurements of the proximal and distal abdominal aorta. J Med Screen. 1998;5(2):104-8.

[63] Pathobiological Determinants of Atherosclerosis in Youth (PDAY) Research Group. Relationship of atherosclerosis in young men to serum lipoprotein cholesterol concentration and smoking. A preliminary report from the PDAY. *J Am Med Ass.*1990;264:3018-24.

[64] Mary J., Roman MJ, Naqvi TZ, Gardin JM, et al. Clinical application of noninvasive vascular ultrasound in cardiovascular risk stratification: a report from the American Society of Echocardiography and the Society for Vascular Medicine and Biology. American Society of Echocardiography Report. *Vasc.med.* 2006; 11: 201-211.

[65] Gepner AD, Keevil JG, Wyman RA, Korcarz CE, Aeschlimann SE, Busse KL, et al. Use of carotid intima-media thickness and vascular age to modify cardiovascular risk prediction. *J Am Soc Echocardiogr* 2006;19: 1170-4.

[66] Ali YS, Rembold KE, Weaver B, Wills MB, Tatar S, Ayers CR, et al. Prediction of major adverse cardiovascular events by age-normalized carotid intimal medial thickness. *Atherosclerosis* 2006;187:186-90.

[67] Heiss G, Sharrett AR, Barnes R, Chambless LE, Szklo M, Alzola C. Carotid atherosclerosis measured by B-mode ultrasound in populations: associations with cardiovascular risk factors in the ARIC study. Am J Epidemiol 1991; 134: 250-6.

[68] De Pergola G, Ciccone M, Pannacciulli N, Modugno M, Sciaraffia M, Minenna A, Rizzon P, Giorgino R. Lower insulin sensitivity as an independent risk factor for carotid wall thickening in normotensive, non-diabetic, non-smoking normal weight and obese premenopausal women. *Int J Obes Relat Metab Disord.* 2000;24:825-9.

[69] Pannacciulli N, De Pergola G, Ciccone M, Rizzon P, Giorgino F, Giorgino R Effect of family history of type 2 diabetes on the intima-media thickness of the common carotid artery in normal-weight, overweight, and obese glucose-tolerant young adults. *Diabetes Care.* 2003;26:1230-4.

[70] Nagai Y, Metter J, Earley CJ, et al. Increased carotid artery intimal-medial thickness in asymptomatic older subjects with exercise-induced myocardial ischemia. *Circulation* 1998; 98: 1504-9.

[71] Bots ML, Hofman A, Grobbee DE. Common carotid intima- media thickness and lower extremity arterial atherosclerosis. The Rotterdam Study. *Arterioscler Thromb* 1994; 14: 1885-91.

[72] Balbarini A, Buttitta F, Limbruno U, Petronio AS, Baglini R, Strata G, Mariotti R, Ciccone M, Mariani M. Usefulness of carotid intima-media thickness measurement and peripheral B-mode ultrasound scan in the clinical screening of patients with coronary artery disease. *Angiology.* 2000;51:269-79.

[73] Gasparyan AY. The Use of Carotid Artery Ultrasonography in Different Clinical Conditions. *The Open Cardiovascular Medicine Journal* 2009, 3, 78-80

[74] Chambless LE, Folsom AR, Clegg LX. Carotid wall thickness is predictive of incident clinical stroke: the Atherosclerosis Risk in Communities (ARIC) Study. *Am J Epidemiol* 2000; 151: 478-87.

[75] O'Leary DH, Polak JF, Kronmal RA, Manolio TA, Burke GL, Wolfson SK Jr. Carotid-artery intima and media thickness as a risk factor for myocardial infarction and stroke in older adults. Cardiovascular Health Study Collaborative Research Group. *N Engl J Med* 1999; 340: 14-22.

[76] Greenland P, Abrams J, Aurigemma GP, et al. Prevention Conference V: Beyond secondary prevention. Identifying the high-risk patient for primary prevention: noninvasive tests of atherosclerotic burden. Writing Group III. *Circulation* 2000; 101: E16-E22.

[77] Kablak-Ziembicka A, Tracz W, Przewlocki T, Pieniazek P, Sokolowski A, Konieczynska M. Association of increased carotid intima-media thickness with the extent of coronary artery disease. *Heart* 2004;90:1286 –90.

[78] Iglesias del Sol A, Bots ML, Grobbee DE, Hofman A, Witteman JC. Carotid intimamedia thickness at different sites: relation to incident myocardial infarction; the Rotterdam Study. *Eur Heart J* 2002;23:934–40.

[79] Pignoli P, Tremoli E, Poli A, Oreste P, Paoletti R. Intimal plus medial thickness of the arterial wall: a direct measurement with ultrasound imaging. *Circulation.* 1986;74(6):1399-406.

[80] van Swijndregt ADM. An in-vitro evaluation of the line pattern of the near and far walls of carotid arteries using B-mode ultrasound. *Ultrasound Med Biol.* 1996; 22(8):1007-1015.

[81] Tang R, Hennig M, Thomasson B, et al. Baseline reproducibility of B-mode ultrasonic measurement of carotid artery intima-media thickness: the European Lacidipine Study on Atherosclerosis (ELSA). *J. Hypertens* 2000;18:197-2018.

[82] Touboul, P. J.; Vicaut, E.; Labreuche, J.; Belliard, J. P.; Cohen, S.; Kownator, S. Pithois-Merli Design, Baseline Characteristics and Carotid Intima-Media Thickness Reproducibility in the PARC Study. *Cerebrovascular Diseases.* 19:57-63, 2005.

11

Endothelial Progenitor Cell Number: A Convergence of Cardiovascular Risk Factors

Michel R. Hoenig[1] and Frank W. Sellke[2]
[1]*Department of Surgery, The Alfred Hospital, Melbourne*
[2]*Department of Cardiothoracic Surgery, Rhode Island Hospital and Brown Medical School, Providence,*
[1]*Australia*
[2]*USA*

1. Introduction

The bone marrow of adult humans is a source of endothelial progenitor cells (EPCs) that circulate in the blood and repair damaged endothelium. The number and function of EPCs is predictive of endothelial function and cardiovascular events. Herein we discuss the impact of individual risk factors on EPC numbers and discuss the potential utility of EPC number as a cardiovascular risk-assessment tool that integrates traditional and emerging cardiovascular risk factors.

2. The systemic basis of cardiovascular disease

Cardiovascular disease the leading cause of mortality in the Western world and manifests as coronary disease, peripheral vascular disease, or ischemic stroke depending on the vascular territory affected. The ageing population and projected increases in prevalence and costs of care have highlighted the need for more effective prevention of cardiovascular disease (Heidenreich, Trogdon et al. 2011). These manifestations of cardiovascular disease share common risk factors of age, hypertension, diabetes, hypercholesterolemia and smoking (Roger, Go et al. 2011). Endothelial dysfunction is the precursor lesion to atherosclerosis and reflects depressed nitric oxide (NO) release from the endothelium (Furchgott 1996; Valgimigli, Merli et al. 2003). Basal release of NO from the endothelium regulates vascular tone and antagonizes the actions of vasoconstrictor substances. Further, NO possesses anti-platelet actions and down-regulates adhesion molecules that attract inflammatory cells to the endothelium (Deanfield, Halcox et al. 2007). The degree of endothelial dysfunction shows a graded response to the number of cardiac risk factors present (Bonetti, Lerman et al. 2003; Davignon and Ganz 2004) and is predictive of clinical events (Bonetti, Lerman et al. 2003; Davignon and Ganz 2004; Deanfield, Halcox et al. 2007). Since endothelial dysfunction occurs systemically, the atherosclerotic process involves a large portion of the arterial tree before it becomes clinically manifest (Deanfield, Halcox et al. 2007). Patient presentations to a cardiologist, cardiac surgeon, vascular surgeon or stroke neurologist with clinically manifest atherosclerosis are typically preceded by decades of endothelial dysfunction and depressed vascular repair throughout the entire arterial bed (Ross 1993). The systemic nature of atherosclerosis is highlighted by the fact that >50% of patients with stroke or peripheral vascular disease have co-morbid atherosclerotic coronary disease (Hirsch, Haskal et al. 2006; Brott, Halperin et al. 2011) and patients with manifest disease in multiple arterial beds are at an increased risk of cardiovascular death and recurrent events (Steg, Bhatt et al. 2007). Since the description of circulating marrow cells that repair the endogenous arterial bed, "endothelial progenitor cells" (EPCs), an increasing research interest has been focused on how risk factors impact on the numbers of these cells and their ability to repair the vasculature and maintain endothelial function.

3. Endothelial progenitor cells and atherosclerosis

The modern concept that circulating marrow cells, EPCs, circulate in adult animals and repair the vasculature originates stems from the observation in the late 90s that marrow-derived mononuclear cells circulate in adult animals and directly contribute to neovascularization in animal models of hindlimb ischemia, myocardial infarct remodeling and post-stroke neovascularization (Asahara, Murohara et al. 1997; Asahara, Masuda et al. 1999; Zhang, Zhang et al. 2002; Metharom and Caplice 2007). The clinical relevance of EPC numbers was brought to the forefront cardiovascular risk prognostication when EPC numbers were shown to correlate positively with flow mediated brachial artery reactivity (a measure of endothelial function) and inversely with the Framingham risk score (Hill, Zalos et al. 2003; Ghani, Shuaib et al. 2005; Chironi, Walch et al. 2007). Endothelial dysfunction observed in patients with cardiovascular disease or its risk factors may reflect a depressed ability to "renew" the endothelium from the circulating pool of EPCs which act to restore endothelial function. Indeed, patients with coronary artery disease (CAD) and stroke were shown to have EPC numbers that are reduced when compared to *age-matched* healthy volunteers (Vasa, Fichtlscherer et al. 2001; Lambiase, Edwards et al. 2004; Ghani, Shuaib et al. 2005). EPC numbers, which are usually assessed by flow cytometry for CD34+KDR+ cells, carry prognostic significance in patients with and without cardiovascular disease. EPC numbers predict clinical events in patients with established CAD. Amongst patients with CAD, lower EPC numbers were associated with increased severity of CAD and higher risks of death from cardiovascular causes, major cardiovascular events, revascularization or hospitalization (Schmidt-Lucke, Rossig et al. 2005; Werner, Kosiol et al. 2005; Kunz, Liang et al. 2006; Wang, Gao et al. 2007). In asymptomatic individuals, EPC numbers correlate with the number of vascular beds with subclinical disease. In a study using ultrasound to characterize disease in the carotid artery, abdominal aorta and femoral artery, the number of EPCs cells was shown to be decreased stepwise in patients with plaque in 0, 1, 2 and 3 of the sites (Chironi, Walch et al. 2007). Further, EPC numbers correlate with cardiovascular disease surrogates such as carotid intima-media thickness even after correction for the Framingham risk score and C-reactive protein (Fadini, Coracina et al. 2006).

In addition to absolute EPC numbers, the functional capacity of EPCs in repairing the vasculature is impaired by cardiac risk factors. EPCs harvested from the marrow of human patients with ischemic cardiomyopathy show an impaired capacity to effect neovascularization and incorporate into the vasculature in a mouse hindlimb ischemia model (Heeschen, Lehmann et al. 2004). In a human trial testing the efficacy of EPCs in repairing the coronary vasculature after a re-perfused myocardial infarction, the migratory capacity of EPCs to chemotaxins was the strongest multivariate predictor of reduction in infarct size (Britten, Abolmaali et al. 2003). Reduced EPC migration to chemotaxins and reduced ability of human EPCs to effect neovascularization in animal hindlimbs has also been related to individual cardiovascular risk factors such as increasing age, hypertension, hypercholesterolemia, family history of CAD, smoking and high Framingham risk scores (Vasa, Fichtlscherer et al. 2001; Hill, Zalos et al. 2003; Heeschen, Lehmann et al. 2004; Schmidt-Lucke, Rossig et al. 2005; Wang, Gao et al. 2007). While EPCs can be harvested from bone marrow to treat myocardial ischemia (Britten, Abolmaali et al. 2003) or threatened limb ischemia (Comerota, Link et al. 2010) on an investigational basis, herein we focus on the impact of cardiovascular risk factors on EPCs and the potential utility of measuring EPC numbers for risk assessment in primary and secondary prevention. We discuss the impact of individual risk factors on EPC number with a focus on studies undertaken in human subjects and describe how risk factor control boosts EPC numbers. Each of the discussed risk factors individually suppresses EPC mobilization from the marrow and decreases peripheral survival making EPC number a universal risk factor (Hoenig, Bianchi et al. 2008).

4. Insulin resistance, the metabolic syndrome and diabetes

Diabetes is a risk factor associated with heightened cardiovascular risk and endothelial dysfunction (De Vriese, Verbeuren et al. 2000; III 2002). In some series, diabetes has been associated with the same coronary risk as established coronary disease thereby making it a "coronary artery disease risk-equivalent" (Haffner, Lehto et al. 1998). Diabetics without manifest cardiovascular disease have decreased EPC numbers compared to age-matched controls (Tepper, Galiano et al. 2002) and diabetics with manifest macrovascular disease such as CAD, peripheral vascular disease or stroke have further reduced EPC numbers (Fadini, Miorin et al. 2005; Brunner, Hoellerl et al. 2011). Further, EPCs in diabetics are dysfunctional when compared to EPCs from non-diabetic subjects. The depressed EPC numbers in diabetes are thought to contribute to impaired collateralization of vascular ischemic beds (Waltenberger 2001) and may predispose this group to developing non-healing diabetic ulcers which may be ameliorated by injecting EPCs into ischemic lower limb muscles (Huang, Li et al. 2005). Indeed, among diabetic patients with peripheral vascular disease, EPC numbers correlated negatively with the ankle brachial index and patients with ischemic ulcers had the lowest EPC numbers (Fadini, Miorin et al. 2005). Blood sugar levels are inversely correlated with EPC numbers implying a direct relationship between hyperglycemia and depressed EPC numbers (Fadini, Miorin et al. 2005). In the laboratory, hyperglycemia directly impairs EPC function by impairing the ability of these cells to migrate (Krankel, Adams et al. 2005). Diabetics with good glucose control have higher EPC numbers and more functional EPCs when compared to diabetics with poorly controlled glucose (Churdchomjan, Kheolamai et al. 2010) and treating newly-diagnosed diabetics with secretagogues increases EPC numbers and is associated with a concordant improvement in endothelial function (Kusuyama, Omura et al. 2006; Liao, Chen et al. 2010). Likewise, insulin-sensitizing agents such as pioglitazone or rosiglitazone boost EPC numbers and the increase in EPCs is correlated with the reduction in C-reactive protein and increase in adiponectin (Kusuyama, Omura et al. 2006; Makino, Okada et al. 2008). The inverse relationship between EPC numbers and HbA1c and insulin resistance indices implies that EPC numbers decline in pre-diabetic states such as the metabolic syndrome and insulin resistance (Tepper, Galiano et al. 2002; Penno, Pucci et al. 2011). Indeed, EPC numbers decrease as more metabolic syndrome criteria are met (Fadini, de Kreutzenberg et al. 2006; Jialal, Devaraj et al. 2010) and are also decreased in other pre-diabetic states such as gestational diabetes (Penno, Pucci et al. 2011) or the polycystic ovarian syndrome (Dessapt-Baradez, Reza et al. 2011). Given that EPC numbers repair the vasculature and maintain endothelial dysfunction, this decreased capacity for repair of the vasculature may provide a mechanism for the increased risk of cardiovascular events observed in patients with the metabolic syndrome (Mottillo, Filion et al. 2010).

5. Gender and age

Age and male gender are irreversible cardiovascular risk factors. Healthy middle-aged women have higher EPC numbers than men (Hoetzer, MacEneaney et al. 2007). Young men have similar EPC numbers as post-menopausal women and this may explain why men are prone to cardiovascular disease at a younger age. Women, on average tend to develop cardiovascular disease after menopause with an incidence that equals that of age-matched men 10 years after the menopause. This time in a woman's life, 10 years after the menopause, is associated with a decrease in EPC numbers and EPC function (Bulut, Albrecht et al. 2007; Rousseau, Ayoubi et al. 2010). This decline in EPC numbers may be due to the lack of estrogen since hyper-estrogenic states (e.g. during ovarian stimulation) have been shown to be associated with an increase in EPC numbers and there is a normal variation with the ovarian cycle (Rousseau, Ayoubi et al. 2010). Hormone replacement therapy can boost EPC numbers in post-menopausal females by 25% (Bulut, Albrecht et al. 2007) and enhance endothelial function (Sanada, Higashi et al. 2003; Kalantaridou, Naka et al. 2006).

Ageing is associated with endothelial dysfunction and dysfunctional EPCs that are more prone to apoptosis and have reduced proliferative capacity (Heiss, Keymel et al. 2005; Kushner, Maceneaney et al. 2011). Further, the elderly are less able to mobilize EPCs in response to ischemic stimuli (Scheubel, Zorn et al. 2003). With ageing, the endothelial progenitor cells have shortened telomeres, which are the repetitive DNA at the ends of chromosomes that protect DNA integrity (Kushner, Van Guilder et al. 2009). Telomere shortening has been described in patients with CAD compared to healthy controls (Ogami, Ikura et al. 2004). Hence, this may provide a mechanism whereby EPCs from elderly individuals are more likely to undergo proliferative senescence and an increased susceptibility to apoptosis which can contribute to decreased EPC numbers. This generally occurs around the age of 55 which is temporally associated with the increased period of cardiovascular risk within a human's lifetime (Kushner, Van Guilder et al. 2009). Hence, the ability to generate functional EPCs, to rejuvenate the endothelium lining the arteries and maintain endothelial function may be key in the pathogenesis of cardiovascular disease with aging.

6. Hypertension

Hypertension is associated with a doubling in the risk for cardiovascular disease with every 20/10 mmHg increment (Chobanian, Bakris et al. 2003). Hypertension is associated with endothelial dysfunction and decreased EPC numbers and reduced EPC function (Vasa, Fichtlscherer et al. 2001; Umemura, Soga et al. 2008; Schulz, Gori et al. 2011). The treatment of hypertension, specifically with drugs inhibiting the renin-angiotensin system, is associated with increased EPCs whereas the use of other classes of drugs such as calcium antagonists, diuretics, and beta-blockers has not been associated with such effects

(Umemura, Soga et al. 2008). Similarly, treatment of diabetics with angiogentinsin receptor blockers boosts EPC numbers (Bahlmann, de Groot et al. 2005). Treating patients with an angiotensin-converting enzyme (ACE) inhibitor such as ramipril has similar effects (Bahlmann, de Groot et al. 2005). Angiotensin II reduces the proliferative capacity of cultured EPCs and induces cell death (Imanishi, Hano et al. 2005). Such observations may explain why drugs such as ACE inhibitors may have beneficial effects that are greater than the observed reduction in blood pressure (Yusuf, Sleight et al. 2000).

7. Dyslipidemia

Hypercholesterolemia is a pivotal cardiovascular risk factor and much there is much focus on treating this risk factor (ATP III 2002). Low density lipoprotein cholesterol (LDL-C) is the primary treatment target in both primary and secondary prevention of cardiovascular disease and there is a log-linear relationship between LDL-C level and CAD risk (ATP III 2002). LDL-C is inversely correlated with EPC number and function in human patients (Chen, Zhang et al. 2004). Statin therapy has been shown to increase EPC numbers and function (Fadini, Albiero et al. 2010; Jaumdally, Goon et al. 2010) and to enhance EPC numbers in response to ischemic stimuli (Spadaccio, Pollari et al. 2010; Hibbert, Ma et al. 2011). The improvement of endothelial function associated with statin use is directly correlated with the increase in EPC numbers and measures of EPC function (Higashi, Matsuoka et al. 2010). Similarly, lipid apheresis for resistant hypercholesterolemia improves EPC function and mobilization (Patschan, Patschan et al. 2009; Ramunni, Brescia et al. 2010). Low high density lipoprotein cholesterol (HDL-C) has been identified as secondary therapeutic target and reconstituted HDL-C infusion improves endothelial function and raises EPC numbers (Nieuwdorp, Vergeer et al. 2008).

8. Inflammatory conditions

Inflammatory conditions such as rheumatoid arthritis (RA) have, relative to traditional risk factors, been only recently associated with an increased cardiovascular risk. Like other cardiovascular risk factors, RA is associated with endothelial dysfunction (Herbrig, Haensel et al. 2006). Patients with RA have a life expectancy that is reduced by 5-10 years and the excess mortality is from cardiovascular disease which is increased roughly 4-fold (Wrigley, Lip et al. 2010). RA is particularly associated with a virulent form of coronary atherosclerosis characterized by high coronary artery calcium scores. However, the patients with RA that are at particular cardiovascular risk are those with active disease and high disease activity scores (Grisar, Aletaha et al. 2005). EPC numbers and EPC proliferative capacity show an inverse correlation with disease activity scores (Grisar, Aletaha et al. 2005; Herbrig, Haensel et al. 2006; Egan, Caporali et al. 2008). The increased risk of cardiovascular events is not limited to RA and has been described in other inflammatory states such as systemic lupus erythematosus (SLE) (Urowitz, Bookman et al. 1976; Roman, Shanker et al. 2003), human immunodeficiency virus (HIV) infection (van Leuven, Sankatsing et al. 2007), inflammatory bowel disease (Danese and Fiocchi 2003) or periodontitis (Mattila, Nieminen et al. 1989). Pre-menopausal women with SLE have a risk of myocardial infarction that is increased a staggering 50-fold compared to healthy controls (Manzi, Meilahn et al. 1997). SLE is associated with impaired EPC function and hence a decreased capacity to repair the endothelium (Deng, Li et al. 2010; Ablin, Boguslavski et al. 2011). Inflammatory conditions are almost universally associated with increased inflammatory markers such as C-reactive protein (CRP) and cytokines such as tumor necrosis factor alpha (TNF-α) which is primarily made by macrophages and inhibits proliferation of repair cells in the body. CRP and TNF- α are directly toxic to EPCs; reducing survival and impairing function (Verma, Kuliszewski et al. 2004; Chen, Zhong et al. 2011). The number of EPCs in patients with inflammatory diseases such as Kawasaki's disease is inversely correlated with plasma CRP and TNF- α (Xu, Men et al. 2010). Treating inflammatory disease such as RA with steroids or anti-TNF-α therapies boosts EPC numbers and may thus have salutary effects on cardiovascular health (Ablin, Boguslavski et al. 2006; Grisar, Aletaha et al. 2007).

9. Physical activity

A recent meta-analysis has shown that individuals exercising ~150 minutes at moderate intensity have a 14% lower risk of CAD compared to sedentary individuals (Sattelmair, Pertman et al. 2011). There was a dose-response relationship with higher grades of physical activity associated with proportional reductions in incident CAD. In patients with CAD, exercise-based rehabilitation is associated with a 20% reduction in mortality and a 26% reduction in cardiac mortality (Taylor, Brown et al. 2004). Exercise enhances endothelial function and increases NO bioavailability (Hambrecht, Adams et al. 2003; Green, Maiorana et al. 2004; Higashi and Yoshizumi 2004). Since EPC number is a fundamental determinant of endothelial function, it would be expected that exercise mobilizes EPCs. Indeed, a three month exercise prescription in humans increases EPC numbers and this independent of the effects of exercise on body mass, adiposity, blood pressure or lipids (Hoetzer, Van Guilder et al. 2007). Importantly, the improvement in endothelial function correlated with the increase in the number of circulating EPCs ($r=0.81$, $p<0.001$) and the increase in NO synthesis (Steiner, Niessner et al. 2005). This suggests that exercise-induced EPC mobilization enhances vascular repair. Exercise may also halt atherosclerotic disease progression as ascertained in both the coronary and carotid beds (Belardinelli, Paolini et al. 2001; Hambrecht, Walther et al. 2004; Rauramaa, Halonen et al. 2004). While multiple studies have shown exercise to mobilize EPCs, the total amount of physical activity has been associated directly with EPC numbers which is consistent with a dose-response (Adams, Lenk et al. 2004; Sandri, Adams et al. 2005; Luk, Dai et al. 2009). Of great interest is the intensity of exercise required to mobilize EPCs. Most protocols have described symptom-limited exercise testing that is of a vigorous nature (Adams, Lenk et al. 2004; Rehman, Li et al. 2004; Sandri, Adams et al. 2005). While 10 minutes of moderate (~70% of VO2 max) exercise did not increased circulating EPC numbers, 30 minutes of moderate or intense (~80% VO2 max) exercise increased EPC numbers (Laufs, Urhausen et al. 2005). This level of intensity is approximately consistent with guideline recommendations for the secondary prevention of CAD (Smith, Allen et al. 2006).

10. Conclusion: A paradigm for cardiovascular risk assessment

From the above discussion, it is clear that cardiovascular risk factors individually and collectively decrease EPC number and function. This includes traditional risk factors such as age, gender, lipids, hypertension and smoking as well as emerging risk factors such as inflammatory diseases and risk factors that are difficult to quantify such as a family history of vascular disease. Moreover, EPC numbers respond to risk factor modification and thus may provide a dynamic assessment of cardiovascular risk. EPC numbers correlate directly with endothelial function and inversely with Framingham risk score in asymptomatic individuals (Hill, Zalos et al. 2003; Ghani, Shuaib et al. 2005; Chironi, Walch et al. 2007). EPC numbers correlate inversely with the number of vascular beds with subclinical disease in asymptomatic patients (Chironi, Walch et al. 2007) and with cardiovascular disease surrogates such as carotid intima-media thickness after correction for the Framingham risk score and CRP (Fadini, Coracina et al. 2006). We believe that the measurement of EPCs represents a unique opportunity for cardiovascular risk assessment in the primary prevention setting. While patients in the low risk category by traditional risk factors are unlikely to have their risk category altered by EPC measurement, EPC measurement could be of great utility in the asymptomatic patient at intermediate risk of cardiovascular disease. Such a patient could be re-categorized into a low risk category if their EPC count is high or could deemed suitable for the commencement of medications for risk factor control if the EPC count is low and categorizes the patient at higher risk. Patients who are at high risk by traditional risk-assessment tools or who have established cardiovascular disease would need treatment and would be unlikely to have high EPC counts. This proposed paradigm is illustrated in Figure 1.

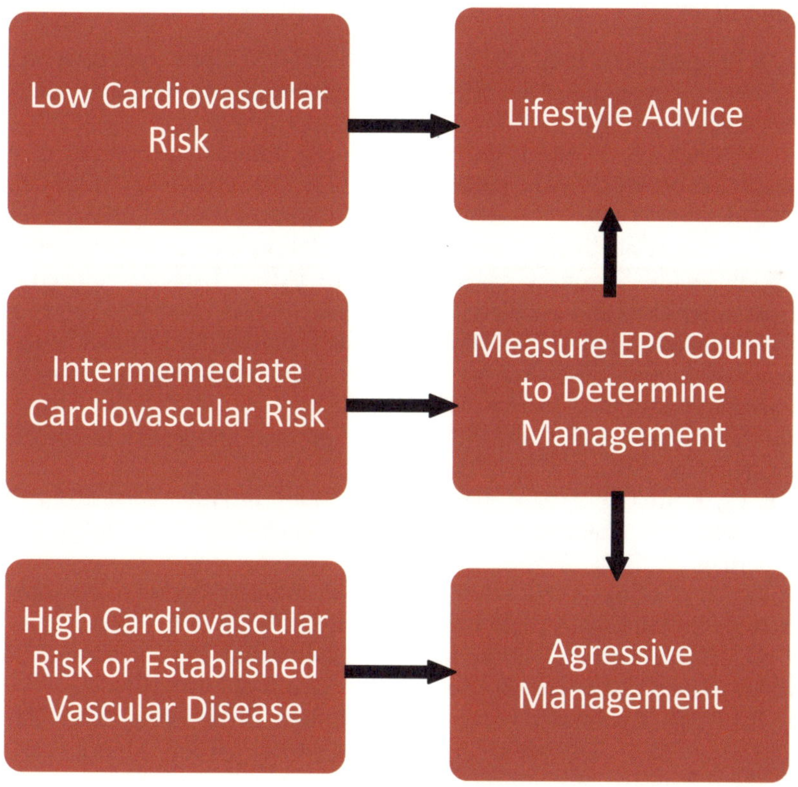

Fig. 1. A Proposed Paradigm for the Prevention of Cardiovascular Disease Utilizing EPCs

The measurement of EPC utilizes flow cytometry which is available in many metropolitan hospitals. The cost of a single EPC count is relatively low costing ~35AUD (30€ or $40USD)

if EPCs are defined as CD34+KDR+ cells. However, there are several barriers to the implementation of EPC number as a cardiovascular risk prognosticator. Firstly, there is lack of universal agreement on the surface markers that define EPCs. While most studies define EPCs as CD34+KDR+ cells, others also utilize the AC133 surface marker. We propose that the CD34+KDR+ definition should be utilized since EPC number measured in this way have predicted cardiovascular events (Schmidt-Lucke, Rossig et al. 2005; Werner, Kosiol et al. 2005; Kunz, Liang et al. 2006; Wang, Gao et al. 2007). The second major barrier to the implementation of EPC number in routine cardiovascular risk assessment is the lack of established "normal" and "at risk" levels. These need to be established from primary prevention cohorts and can be measured retrospectively in one cohort and then validated in another. Thirdly, a set of standards for the measurement of EPC numbers will be required. This would include studies on the normal biological variability of EPC numbers and accepted standards for acceptable intra-measurement and inter-measurement coefficients of variation. However, this marker of cardiovascular risk has many advantages which include integrating cardiovascular risk in a single measurement and followed serially to assess the impact of risk factor modification on cardiovascular risk.

11. References

Ablin, J. N., V. Boguslavski, et al. (2006). "Effect of anti-TNFalpha treatment on circulating endothelial progenitor cells (EPCs) in rheumatoid arthritis." Life sciences 79(25): 2364-2369.

Ablin, J. N., V. Boguslavski, et al. (2011). "Enhanced adhesive properties of endothelial progenitor cells (EPCs) in patients with SLE." Rheumatology international 31(6): 773-778.

Adams, V., K. Lenk, et al. (2004). "Increase of Circulating Endothelial Progenitor Cells in Patients with Coronary Artery Disease After Exercise-Induced Ischemia." Arterioscler Thromb Vasc Biol 24(4): 684-690.

Asahara, T., H. Masuda, et al. (1999). "Bone Marrow Origin of Endothelial Progenitor Cells Responsible for Postnatal Vasculogenesis in Physiological and Pathological Neovascularization." Circ Res 85(3): 221-228.

Asahara, T., T. Murohara, et al. (1997). "Isolation of putative progenitor endothelial cells for angiogenesis." Science 275(5302): 964-967.

Bahlmann, F. H., K. de Groot, et al. (2005). "Stimulation of endothelial progenitor cells: a new putative therapeutic effect of angiotensin II receptor antagonists." Hypertension 45(4): 526-529.

Belardinelli, R., I. Paolini, et al. (2001). "Exercise training intervention after coronary angioplasty: the ETICA trial." J Am Coll Cardiol 37(7): 1891-1900.

Bonetti, P. O., L. O. Lerman, et al. (2003). "Endothelial Dysfunction: A Marker of Atherosclerotic Risk." Arterioscler Thromb Vasc Biol 23(2): 168-175.

Britten, M. B., N. D. Abolmaali, et al. (2003). "Infarct Remodeling After Intracoronary Progenitor Cell Treatment in Patients With Acute Myocardial Infarction (TOPCARE-AMI): Mechanistic Insights From Serial Contrast-Enhanced Magnetic Resonance Imaging." Circulation 108(18): 2212-2218.

Brott, T. G., J. L. Halperin, et al. (2011). "2011 ASA/ACCF/AHA/AANN/AANS /ACR/ASNR/CNS/SAIP/SCAI/SIR/SNIS/SVM/SVS Guideline on the Management of Patients With Extracranial Carotid and Vertebral Artery Disease: A

Report of the American College of Cardiology Foundation/American Heart Association Task Force on Practice Guidelines, and the American Stroke Association, American Association of Neuroscience Nurses, American Association of Neurological Surgeons, American College of Radiology, American Society of Neuroradiology, Congress of Neurological Surgeons, Society of Atherosclerosis Imaging and Prevention, Society for Cardiovascular Angiography and Interventions, Society of Interventional Radiology, Society of NeuroInterventional Surgery, Society for Vascular Medicine, and Society for Vascular Surgery." Circulation.

Brunner, S., F. Hoellerl, et al. (2011). "Circulating Angiopoietic Cells and Diabetic Retinopathy in Type 2 Diabetes Mellitus, with or without Macrovascular Disease." Investigative ophthalmology & visual science 52(7): 4655-4662.

Bulut, D., N. Albrecht, et al. (2007). "Hormonal status modulates circulating endothelial progenitor cells." Clinical research in cardiology : official journal of the German Cardiac Society 96(5): 258-263.

Chen, J. Z., F. R. Zhang, et al. (2004). "Number and activity of endothelial progenitor cells from peripheral blood in patients with hypercholesterolaemia." Clinical science 107(3): 273-280.

Chen, T. G., Z. Y. Zhong, et al. (2011). "Effects of tumour necrosis factor-alpha on activity and nitric oxide synthase of endothelial progenitor cells from peripheral blood." Cell proliferation 44(4): 352-359.

Chironi, G., L. Walch, et al. (2007). "Decreased number of circulating CD34+KDR+ cells in asymptomatic subjects with preclinical atherosclerosis." Atherosclerosis 191(1): 115-120.

Chobanian, A. V., G. L. Bakris, et al. (2003). "Seventh report of the Joint National Committee on Prevention, Detection, Evaluation, and Treatment of High Blood Pressure." Hypertension 42(6): 1206-1252.

Churdchomjan, W., P. Kheolamai, et al. (2010). "Comparison of endothelial progenitor cell function in type 2 diabetes with good and poor glycemic control." BMC endocrine disorders 10: 5.

Comerota, A. J., A. Link, et al. (2010). "Upper extremity ischemia treated with tissue repair cells from adult bone marrow." Journal of vascular surgery : official publication, the Society for Vascular Surgery [and] International Society for Cardiovascular Surgery, North American Chapter 52(3): 723-729.

Danese, S. and C. Fiocchi (2003). "Atherosclerosis and inflammatory bowel disease: sharing a common pathogenic pathway?" Circulation 107(7): e52.

Davignon, J. and P. Ganz (2004). "Role of Endothelial Dysfunction in Atherosclerosis." Circulation 109(23_suppl_1): III-27-32.

De Vriese, A. S., T. J. Verbeuren, et al. (2000). "Endothelial dysfunction in diabetes." British journal of pharmacology 130(5): 963-974.

Deanfield, J. E., J. P. Halcox, et al. (2007). "Endothelial Function and Dysfunction: Testing and Clinical Relevance." Circulation 115(10): 1285-1295.

Deanfield, J. E., J. P. Halcox, et al. (2007). "Endothelial function and dysfunction: testing and clinical relevance." Circulation 115(10): 1285-1295.

Deng, X. L., X. X. Li, et al. (2010). "Comparative study on circulating endothelial progenitor cells in systemic lupus erythematosus patients at active stage." Rheumatology international 30(11): 1429-1436.

Dessapt-Baradez, C., M. Reza, et al. (2011). "Circulating vascular progenitor cells and central arterial stiffness in polycystic ovary syndrome." PloS one 6(5): e20317.

Egan, C. G., F. Caporali, et al. (2008). "Endothelial progenitor cells and colony-forming units in rheumatoid arthritis: association with clinical characteristics." Rheumatology 47(10): 1484-1488.

Fadini, G. P., M. Albiero, et al. (2010). "Rosuvastatin stimulates clonogenic potential and anti-inflammatory properties of endothelial progenitor cells." Cell biology international 34(7): 709-715.

Fadini, G. P., A. Coracina, et al. (2006). "Peripheral Blood CD34+KDR+ Endothelial Progenitor Cells Are Determinants of Subclinical Atherosclerosis in a Middle-Aged General Population." Stroke 37(9): 2277-2282.

Fadini, G. P., S. V. de Kreutzenberg, et al. (2006). "Circulating CD34+ cells, metabolic syndrome, and cardiovascular risk." Eur Heart J 27(18): 2247-2255.

Fadini, G. P., M. Miorin, et al. (2005). "Circulating endothelial progenitor cells are reduced in peripheral vascular complications of type 2 diabetes mellitus." Journal of the American College of Cardiology 45(9): 1449-1457.

Furchgott, R. F. (1996). "The 1996 Albert Lasker Medical Research Awards. The discovery of endothelium-derived relaxing factor and its importance in the identification of nitric oxide." Jama 276(14): 1186-1188.

Ghani, U., A. Shuaib, et al. (2005). "Endothelial Progenitor Cells During Cerebrovascular Disease." Stroke 36(1): 151-153.

Green, D. J., A. Maiorana, et al. (2004). "Effect of exercise training on endothelium-derived nitric oxide function in humans." J Physiol 561(Pt 1): 1-25.

Grisar, J., D. Aletaha, et al. (2007). "Endothelial progenitor cells in active rheumatoid arthritis: effects of tumour necrosis factor and glucocorticoid therapy." Annals of the rheumatic diseases 66(10): 1284-1288.

Grisar, J., D. Aletaha, et al. (2005). "Depletion of endothelial progenitor cells in the peripheral blood of patients with rheumatoid arthritis." Circulation 111(2): 204-211.

Haffner, S. M., S. Lehto, et al. (1998). "Mortality from coronary heart disease in subjects with type 2 diabetes and in nondiabetic subjects with and without prior myocardial infarction." The New England journal of medicine 339(4): 229-234.

Hambrecht, R., V. Adams, et al. (2003). "Regular physical activity improves endothelial function in patients with coronary artery disease by increasing phosphorylation of endothelial nitric oxide synthase." Circulation 107(25): 3152-3158.

Hambrecht, R., C. Walther, et al. (2004). "Percutaneous Coronary Angioplasty Compared With Exercise Training in Patients With Stable Coronary Artery Disease: A Randomized Trial." Circulation 109(11): 1371-1378.

Heeschen, C., R. Lehmann, et al. (2004). "Profoundly Reduced Neovascularization Capacity of Bone Marrow Mononuclear Cells Derived From Patients With Chronic Ischemic Heart Disease." Circulation 109(13): 1615-1622.

Heidenreich, P. A., J. G. Trogdon, et al. (2011). "Forecasting the Future of Cardiovascular Disease in the United States: A Policy Statement From the American Heart Association." Circulation 123(8): 933-944.

Heiss, C., S. Keymel, et al. (2005). "Impaired progenitor cell activity in age-related endothelial dysfunction." Journal of the American College of Cardiology 45(9): 1441-1448.

Herbrig, K., S. Haensel, et al. (2006). "Endothelial dysfunction in patients with rheumatoid arthritis is associated with a reduced number and impaired function of endothelial progenitor cells." Annals of the rheumatic diseases 65(2): 157-163.

Hibbert, B., X. Ma, et al. (2011). "Pre-procedural atorvastatin mobilizes endothelial progenitor cells: clues to the salutary effects of statins on healing of stented human arteries." PloS one 6(1): e16413.
Higashi, Y., H. Matsuoka, et al. (2010). "Endothelial function in subjects with isolated low HDL cholesterol: role of nitric oxide and circulating progenitor cells." American journal of physiology. Endocrinology and metabolism 298(2): E202-209.
Higashi, Y. and M. Yoshizumi (2004). "Exercise and endothelial function: role of endothelium-derived nitric oxide and oxidative stress in healthy subjects and hypertensive patients." Pharmacol Ther 102(1): 87-96.
Hill, J. M., G. Zalos, et al. (2003). "Circulating Endothelial Progenitor Cells, Vascular Function, and Cardiovascular Risk." N Engl J Med 348(7): 593-600.
Hirsch, A. T., Z. J. Haskal, et al. (2006). "ACC/AHA 2005 Practice Guidelines for the management of patients with peripheral arterial disease (lower extremity, renal, mesenteric, and abdominal aortic): a collaborative report from the American Association for Vascular Surgery/Society for Vascular Surgery, Society for Cardiovascular Angiography and Interventions, Society for Vascular Medicine and Biology, Society of Interventional Radiology, and the ACC/AHA Task Force on Practice Guidelines (Writing Committee to Develop Guidelines for the Management of Patients With Peripheral Arterial Disease): endorsed by the American Association of Cardiovascular and Pulmonary Rehabilitation; National Heart, Lung, and Blood Institute; Society for Vascular Nursing; TransAtlantic Inter-Society Consensus; and Vascular Disease Foundation." Circulation 113(11): e463-654.
Hoenig, M. R., C. Bianchi, et al. (2008). "Hypoxia inducible factor-1 alpha, endothelial progenitor cells, monocytes, cardiovascular risk, wound healing, cobalt and hydralazine: a unifying hypothesis." Current drug targets 9(5): 422-435.
Hoetzer, G. L., O. J. MacEneaney, et al. (2007). "Gender differences in circulating endothelial progenitor cell colony-forming capacity and migratory activity in middle-aged adults." The American journal of cardiology 99(1): 46-48.
Hoetzer, G. L., G. P. Van Guilder, et al. (2007). "Aging, exercise, and endothelial progenitor cell clonogenic and migratory capacity in men." J Appl Physiol 102(3): 847-852.
Huang, P., S. Li, et al. (2005). "Autologous transplantation of granulocyte colony-stimulating factor-mobilized peripheral blood mononuclear cells improves critical limb ischemia in diabetes." Diabetes care 28(9): 2155-2160.
III, A. T. P. (2002). "Third Report of the National Cholesterol Education Program (NCEP) Expert Panel on Detection, Evaluation, and Treatment of High Blood Cholesterol in Adults (Adult Treatment Panel III) final report." Circulation 106(25): 3143-3421.
Imanishi, T., T. Hano, et al. (2005). "Angiotensin II accelerates endothelial progenitor cell senescence through induction of oxidative stress." Journal of hypertension 23(1): 97-104.
Jaumdally, R. J., P. K. Goon, et al. (2010). "Effects of atorvastatin on circulating CD34+/CD133+/ CD45- progenitor cells and indices of angiogenesis (vascular endothelial growth factor and the angiopoietins 1 and 2) in atherosclerotic vascular disease and diabetes mellitus." Journal of internal medicine 267(4): 385-393.
Jialal, I., S. Devaraj, et al. (2010). "Decreased number and impaired functionality of endothelial progenitor cells in subjects with metabolic syndrome: implications for increased cardiovascular risk." Atherosclerosis 211(1): 297-302.
Kalantaridou, S. N., K. K. Naka, et al. (2006). "Premature ovarian failure, endothelial dysfunction and estrogen-progestogen replacement." Trends in endocrinology and metabolism: TEM 17(3): 101-109.

Krankel, N., V. Adams, et al. (2005). "Hyperglycemia reduces survival and impairs function of circulating blood-derived progenitor cells." Arteriosclerosis, thrombosis, and vascular biology 25(4): 698-703.

Kunz, G. A., G. Liang, et al. (2006). "Circulating endothelial progenitor cells predict coronary artery disease severity." American heart journal 152(1): 190-195.

Kushner, E. J., O. J. Maceneaney, et al. (2011). "Aging Is Associated with a Proapoptotic Endothelial Progenitor Cell Phenotype." Journal of vascular research 48(5): 408-414.

Kushner, E. J., G. P. Van Guilder, et al. (2009). "Aging and endothelial progenitor cell telomere length in healthy men." Clinical chemistry and laboratory medicine : CCLM / FESCC 47(1): 47-50.

Kusuyama, T., T. Omura, et al. (2006). "Effects of treatment for diabetes mellitus on circulating vascular progenitor cells." Journal of pharmacological sciences 102(1): 96-102.

Lambiase, P. D., R. J. Edwards, et al. (2004). "Circulating Humoral Factors and Endothelial Progenitor Cells in Patients With Differing Coronary Collateral Support." Circulation 109(24): 2986-2992.

Laufs, U., A. Urhausen, et al. (2005). "Running exercise of different duration and intensity: effect on endothelial progenitor cells in healthy subjects." Eur J Cardiovasc Prev Rehabil 12(4): 407-414.

Liao, Y. F., L. L. Chen, et al. (2010). "Number of circulating endothelial progenitor cells as a marker of vascular endothelial function for type 2 diabetes." Vascular medicine 15(4): 279-285.

Luk, T. H., Y. L. Dai, et al. (2009). "Habitual physical activity is associated with endothelial function and endothelial progenitor cells in patients with stable coronary artery disease." European journal of cardiovascular prevention and rehabilitation : official journal of the European Society of Cardiology, Working Groups on Epidemiology & Prevention and Cardiac Rehabilitation and Exercise Physiology 16(4): 464-471.

Makino, H., S. Okada, et al. (2008). "Pioglitazone treatment stimulates circulating CD34-positive cells in type 2 diabetes patients." Diabetes research and clinical practice 81(3): 327-330.

Manzi, S., E. N. Meilahn, et al. (1997). "Age-specific incidence rates of myocardial infarction and angina in women with systemic lupus erythematosus: comparison with the Framingham Study." American journal of epidemiology 145(5): 408-415.

Mattila, K. J., M. S. Nieminen, et al. (1989). "Association between dental health and acute myocardial infarction." BMJ 298(6676): 779-781.

Metharom, P. and N. M. Caplice (2007). "Vascular disease: a new progenitor biology." Current vascular pharmacology 5(1): 61-68.

Mottillo, S., K. B. Filion, et al. (2010). "The metabolic syndrome and cardiovascular risk a systematic review and meta-analysis." Journal of the American College of Cardiology 56(14): 1113-1132.

Nieuwdorp, M., M. Vergeer, et al. (2008). "Reconstituted HDL infusion restores endothelial function in patients with type 2 diabetes mellitus." Diabetologia 51(6): 1081-1084.

Ogami, M., Y. Ikura, et al. (2004). "Telomere shortening in human coronary artery diseases." Arteriosclerosis, thrombosis, and vascular biology 24(3): 546-550.

Patschan, D., S. Patschan, et al. (2009). "LDL lipid apheresis rapidly increases peripheral endothelial progenitor cell competence." Journal of clinical apheresis 24(5): 180-185.

Penno, G., L. Pucci, et al. (2011). "Circulating endothelial progenitor cells in women with gestational alterations of glucose tolerance." Diabetes & vascular disease research : official journal of the International Society of Diabetes and Vascular Disease.

Ramunni, A., P. Brescia, et al. (2010). "Effect of low-density lipoprotein apheresis on circulating endothelial progenitor cells in familial hypercholesterolemia." Blood purification 29(4): 383-389.
Rauramaa, R., P. Halonen, et al. (2004). "Effects of Aerobic Physical Exercise on Inflammation and Atherosclerosis in Men: The DNASCO Study: A Six-Year Randomized, Controlled Trial." Ann Intern Med 140(12): 1007-1014.
Rehman, J., J. Li, et al. (2004). "Exercise acutely increases circulating endothelial progenitor cells and monocyte-/macrophage-derived angiogenic cells." J Am Coll Cardiol 43(12): 2314-2318.
Roger, V. L., A. S. Go, et al. (2011). "Heart disease and stroke statistics--2011 update: a report from the American Heart Association." Circulation 123(4): e18-e209.
Roman, M. J., B. A. Shanker, et al. (2003). "Prevalence and correlates of accelerated atherosclerosis in systemic lupus erythematosus." The New England journal of medicine 349(25): 2399-2406.
Ross, R. (1993). "The pathogenesis of atherosclerosis: a perspective for the 1990s." Nature 362(6423): 801-809.
Rousseau, A., F. Ayoubi, et al. (2010). "Impact of age and gender interaction on circulating endothelial progenitor cells in healthy subjects." Fertility and sterility 93(3): 843-846.
Sanada, M., Y. Higashi, et al. (2003). "A comparison of low-dose and standard-dose oral estrogen on forearm endothelial function in early postmenopausal women." The Journal of clinical endocrinology and metabolism 88(3): 1303-1309.
Sandri, M., V. Adams, et al. (2005). "Effects of Exercise and Ischemia on Mobilization and Functional Activation of Blood-Derived Progenitor Cells in Patients With Ischemic Syndromes: Results of 3 Randomized Studies." Circulation 111(25): 3391-3399.
Sattelmair, J., J. Pertman, et al. (2011). "Dose Response Between Physical Activity and Risk of Coronary Heart Disease." Circulation.
Scheubel, R. J., H. Zorn, et al. (2003). "Age-dependent depression in circulating endothelial progenitor cells in patients undergoing coronary artery bypass grafting." Journal of the American College of Cardiology 42(12): 2073-2080.
Schmidt-Lucke, C., L. Rossig, et al. (2005). "Reduced Number of Circulating Endothelial Progenitor Cells Predicts Future Cardiovascular Events: Proof of Concept for the Clinical Importance of Endogenous Vascular Repair." Circulation 111(22): 2981-2987.
Schulz, E., T. Gori, et al. (2011). "Oxidative stress and endothelial dysfunction in hypertension." Hypertension research : official journal of the Japanese Society of Hypertension 34(6): 665-673.
Smith, S. C., Jr., J. Allen, et al. (2006). "AHA/ACC guidelines for secondary prevention for patients with coronary and other atherosclerotic vascular disease: 2006 update: endorsed by the National Heart, Lung, and Blood Institute." Circulation 113(19): 2363-2372.
Spadaccio, C., F. Pollari, et al. (2010). "Atorvastatin increases the number of endothelial progenitor cells after cardiac surgery: a randomized control study." Journal of cardiovascular pharmacology 55(1): 30-38.
Steg, P. G., D. L. Bhatt, et al. (2007). "One-year cardiovascular event rates in outpatients with atherothrombosis." Jama 297(11): 1197-1206.
Steiner, S., A. Niessner, et al. (2005). "Endurance training increases the number of endothelial progenitor cells in patients with cardiovascular risk and coronary artery disease." Atherosclerosis 181(2): 305-310.

Taylor, R. S., A. Brown, et al. (2004). "Exercise-based rehabilitation for patients with coronary heart disease: systematic review and meta-analysis of randomized controlled trials." Am J Med 116(10): 682-692.

Tepper, O. M., R. D. Galiano, et al. (2002). "Human endothelial progenitor cells from type II diabetics exhibit impaired proliferation, adhesion, and incorporation into vascular structures." Circulation 106(22): 2781-2786.

Umemura, T., J. Soga, et al. (2008). "Aging and hypertension are independent risk factors for reduced number of circulating endothelial progenitor cells." American journal of hypertension 21(11): 1203-1209.

Urowitz, M. B., A. A. Bookman, et al. (1976). "The bimodal mortality pattern of systemic lupus erythematosus." The American journal of medicine 60(2): 221-225.

Valgimigli, M., E. Merli, et al. (2003). "Endothelial dysfunction in acute and chronic coronary syndromes: evidence for a pathogenetic role of oxidative stress." Archives of Biochemistry and Biophysics Cardiac Ischemia/Reperfusion and Free Radicals 420(2): 255-261.

van Leuven, S. I., R. R. Sankatsing, et al. (2007). "Atherosclerotic vascular disease in HIV: it is not just antiretroviral therapy that hurts the heart!" Current opinion in HIV and AIDS 2(4): 324-331.

Vasa, M., S. Fichtlscherer, et al. (2001). "Number and Migratory Activity of Circulating Endothelial Progenitor Cells Inversely Correlate With Risk Factors for Coronary Artery Disease." Circ Res 89(1): 1e-7.

Verma, S., M. A. Kuliszewski, et al. (2004). "C-reactive protein attenuates endothelial progenitor cell survival, differentiation, and function: further evidence of a mechanistic link between C-reactive protein and cardiovascular disease." Circulation 109(17): 2058-2067.

Waltenberger, J. (2001). "Impaired collateral vessel development in diabetes: potential cellular mechanisms and therapeutic implications." Cardiovascular research 49(3): 554-560.

Wang, H. Y., P. J. Gao, et al. (2007). "Circulating endothelial progenitor cells, C-reactive protein and severity of coronary stenosis in Chinese patients with coronary artery disease." Hypertension research : official journal of the Japanese Society of Hypertension 30(2): 133-141.

Werner, N., S. Kosiol, et al. (2005). "Circulating Endothelial Progenitor Cells and Cardiovascular Outcomes." N Engl J Med 353(10): 999-1007.

Wrigley, B. J., G. Y. Lip, et al. (2010). "Coronary atherosclerosis in rheumatoid arthritis: could endothelial progenitor cells be the missing link?" The Journal of rheumatology 37(3): 479-481.

Xu, M. G., L. N. Men, et al. (2010). "The number and function of circulating endothelial progenitor cells in patients with Kawasaki disease." European journal of pediatrics 169(3): 289-296.

Yusuf, S., P. Sleight, et al. (2000). "Effects of an angiotensin-converting-enzyme inhibitor, ramipril, on cardiovascular events in high-risk patients. The Heart Outcomes Prevention Evaluation Study Investigators." The New England journal of medicine 342(3): 145-153.

Zhang, Z. G., L. Zhang, et al. (2002). "Bone Marrow-Derived Endothelial Progenitor Cells Participate in Cerebral Neovascularization After Focal Cerebral Ischemia in the Adult Mouse." Circ Res 90(3): 284-288.

12

Nitric Oxide Signalling in Vascular Control and Cardiovascular Risk

Annette Schmidt
Leibniz-Institute of Arteriosclerosis Research at the University of Muenster, Germany

1. Introduction

Nitric oxide - a free radical molecule - has been known for many decades, but only since its recognition as endothelium-derived relaxing factor (EDRF) the interest in the molecule has exponentially increased (Moncada, 1991). At the present time NO is an important messenger that regulates numerous functions and also participates in the pathogenesis of various diseases (Lloyd-Jones & Block, 1996). NO is generated from the conversion of arginine to citrulline in a multistep oxidation process by the NO-synthase (NOS), a NADPH-dependent enzyme that requires Calcium-Calmodulin, Flavinadeninedinucleotide, Flavinmononcleotide and Tetrahydro-L-biopterin as cofactors (Förstermann et al., 1994). Three isoforms of NOS have been identified. All isoenzymes, the neuronal NOS (nNOS), the inducible NOS (iNOS) and the endothelial NOS (eNOS) (Liu & Huang, 2008), are homodimers with subunits of 130 - 160 kDa. As major signalling molecule of the vascular system NO is generated by the constitutively expressed eNOS.

2. Endothelial nitric oxide synthase (eNOS) and nitric oxide (NO) function

2.1 eNOS

The endothelium maintains the balance between vasodilation and vasoconstriction. NO generated by eNOS acts via cGMP-dependent pathway in a paracrine manner on neighbouring smooth muscle cells (SMC) diffusing radially from the production site. NO has a half-life of only a few milliseconds *in vivo* (**Tab. 1**) and rapidly reacts with iron of the heme moiety in the active site of the enzyme guanylate cyclase, stimulating it to produce the intracellular cGMP that in turn enhances the release of neurotransmitters resulting in SMC relaxation and vasodilation (**Fig. 1**). Acting via cGMP-independent pathways it is used in part to S-nitrosylation of intracellular or extracellular proteins (Castel & Vaudry, 2001; Mallis et al., 2001; Sun et al., 2001) or by inhibiting intraendothelial generated superoxide anions (Clancy et al., 1992).

2.2 NO functions

Beside its role as vasodilator various other activities of NO have been described: **(I)** NO prevents the expression of cell adhesion molecules thereby preventing leukocytes/monocytes adhering to vascular endothelium and their immigration into the

Compound	Blood/Plasma Levels, nmol/L	T1/2
Nitrate	20 000 - 50 000	5 - 8 hours
Nitrite	100 - 500	1 - 5 minutes
NO	<1	1- 2 milliseconds
Hb-NO	<1 - 200	15 minutes
S-nitroso-Hb	<1 - 200	--
S-nitroso-albumin	1 - 200	--

Table 1. Basal blood/plasma levels and half-lifes of some NO-related compounds. Values are approximated from studies in human. For Hb-NO, S-nitroso-Hb and S-nitroso-albumin, no firm agreement about normal values has been reached, and reported values vary greatly. T1/2 for Hb-NO is from pig experiments, values for S-nitroso-Hb and S-nitroso-albumin are unknown (from J.O. Lundberg and E. Weitzberg, Arterioscler Thromb Vasc Biol, 2005;25:915-922).

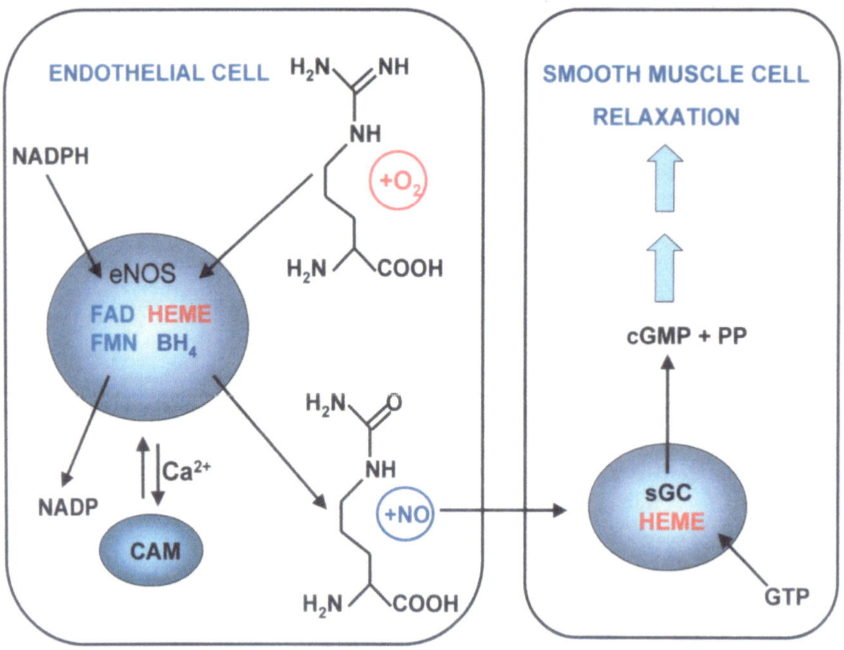

Fig. 1. Nitric oxide signalling axis as therapeutic target in cardiac and vascular disorders. The endothelial eNOS catalyses the formation of NO from L-arginine through two sequential monooxygenation steps. The nitrogen atom of NO is derived from the guanodinogroup of the L-arginine side chain and the oxygen atom of NO derived from molecular oxygen. The cGMP generation in the vascular smooth muscle cell is catalysed by the soluble guanylate cyclase stimulated by the nitric oxide generated by the adjacent endothelial cell.

arterial wall. The monocytes accumulated in the arterial wall can promote local expression or activation of matrixmetalloproteases, which decrease the strength of the cap by degrading collagen and other extracellular matrix components. Furthermore, activated macrophages kill neighbouring SMC by lytic damage leading to necrosis or by inducing apoptosis (Kockx et al., 1996, 1998). **(II)** NO reduces the influx of lipoproteins into the vascular wall and inhibits LDL oxidation. **(III)** NO inhibits DNA synthesis (Förstermann et al., 1994) and proliferation of SMC (Li & Förstermann, 2000; Li et al., 2002a). **(IV)** NO released towards the vascular lumen is a potent inhibitor of platelet aggregation and adhesion (Busse et al., 1987; Radomski et al., 1987). **(V)** NO can react with superoxide anion $O_2^{-\cdot}$ forming the potent peroxynitrite ($ONOO^-$), which causes oxidative damage, nitration and S-nitrosylation of biomolecules. Furthermore, $ONOO^-$ oxidizes the NOS cofactor 5,6,7,8-tetrahydrobiopterin with the consequence of uncoupling NOS from NO synthesis thereby leading NOS to a superoxide producing proarteriosclerotic enzyme (Förstermann, 2006). **(VI)** Exogenous NO released from DETA/NONOate causes overexpression of TGF-beta and extracellular matrix in cultured human coronary smooth muscle cells (A. Schmidt et al., 2003).

2.3 eNOS-independent sources of NO

The generation of NO is not restricted to NO-synthases. An endothelium-independent source of bioactive NO is the ingestion of dietary (inorganic) nitrate. Naturally occurring dietary nitrate (celery, cress, chervil, beetroot, spinach, rucula contain up to 250 mg NO/100 g fresh weight) elevate the tissue und blood plasma level of nitrite via bioconversion in the entero-salivary circulation. When nitrite is acidified, it yields HNO_2, which decomposes to NO and other nitrogen oxides

$$NO_2^- + H^+ \rightleftharpoons HNO_2 \quad (1)$$

$$2\,HNO_2 \rightarrow N_2O_2 + H_2O \quad (2)$$

$$N_2O_2 \rightarrow NO + NO_2 \quad (3)$$

Studies have indicated that acid-catalysed nitrite reduction to NO can also take place in blood vessels and tissues already at a moderately low pH and within nitrite concentrations normally present *in vivo.*

The NO generated by eNOS has a half-life ($T^1/_2$) of 1-2 milliseconds and rapidly oxidizes to nitrate (NO_2^-). Nitrate however is not a final end product of NO metabolism but can be a substrate for NOS-independent regeneration to NO (Benjamin et al., 1994; Lundberg et al., 1994). Therefore other sources of nitrate in mammalians can contribute to the formation of NO such as nitrate generated from commensal bacteria in the digestive tract or nitrate present in foodstuff. Thus, in a study of Milkowski (Milkowski et al., 2010) it was shown that the consumption of nitrite- and nitrate-rich food such as fruits, leafy vegetables, and cured meals along with antioxidants can compensate for any disturbance in endogenous NO. Regular intake of nitrate-containing food such as green leafy vegetables may ensure that blood and tissue levels of nitrite and NO pools are maintained at a level sufficient to compensate for any disturbances in endogenous NO synthesis. In several studies (Kapil et al., 2010a, 2010b; Tang et al., 2011) it was shown that nitrate supplementation or vegetable intake (such as beetroot juice) causes dose-dependent elevation in plasma nitrite concentration, elevation of cGMP concentration with a consequent decrease in blood pressure and reduction the risk of ischaemic stroke. The collective body of evidence suggests that food enriched with nitrate and nitrite provide significant health benefits with very little risk. The weak and inconclusive data on the cancer risk of nitrite/nitrate and processed meats are far outweighed by the health benefit of restoring NO homeostasis via dietary nitrite and nitrate (Tang et al., 2011).

3. Regulation of eNOS activity

3.1 Phosphorylation

eNOS synthesizes NO in a pulsatile Ca^{2+}/calmodulin-dependent manner with eNOS activity markedly increasing when intracellular Ca^{2+} increases. Ca^{2+} induces the binding of calmodulin to the enzyme thus increasing the rate of electron transfer from NADPH to heme center (Hemmens & Mayer, 1998). However, eNOS can be activated by other stimuli as increased intracellular Ca^{2+}. The best-established stimulus is the shear stress of flowing blood, which can increase enzyme activity. This activation is mediated by phosphorylation of the enzyme (**Fig. 2**). The eNOS protein can be phosphorylated on several Ser, Thr and Tyr residues. Two main changes in enzyme function have been found. Phosphorylation of Ser^{1177} stimulates the flux of electrons within the reductase domain and increases the Ca^{2+} sensitivity of the enzyme (Fleming & Busse, 2003). Several protein kinases participate in phosphorylation of eNOS at Ser^{1177}. These kinases include Akt, protein kinase A, 5'-AMP activated protein kinase and calmodulin-dependent kinase II. A negative regulatory site for phosphorylation is Thr^{495} under non-stimulated conditions probably by protein kinase C. Thr^{495} interferes with the binding of calmodulin to the calmodulin-binding domain. Dephosphorylation of Thr^{495} is associated with stimuli such as histamine and bradykinine both elevating intracellular Ca^{2+} concentration. Dephosphorylation of Thr^{495} has also been shown to favour eNOS uncoupling (Lin et al., 2003). Other phosphorylation sites including Ser^{114}, Ser^{633} and some Tyr residues are not known to have major consequences for enzyme activity (Fleming & Busse, 2003; Fleming, 2010).

eNOS-associated proteins such as caveolin, heat shock protein 90 or eNOS interacting proteins provide the scaffold for the formation of the eNOS protein complex and its intracellular location (Fleming & Busse, 2003).

eNOS levels in endothelial cells can be regulated by changes in eNOS mRNA stability.

3.2 Enhancers of NO availability

Statins. Statins are a group of compounds which lower LDL-cholesterol, are inhibiting the enzyme 3-hydroxy-3-methylglutaryl coenzyme A. Beside their lipid lowering property statins improve vascular relaxation, reduce vascular inflammation, reduce oxidative stress, decrease thrombosis and platelet aggregation (E. Schulz et al., 2004; Sowers, 2003). These beneficial effects of statins are in part mediated by an effect on eNOS because they can be blocked by L-NMMA (L-NG-monomethylarginine), an inhibitor of eNOS (John, et al., 1998; Rosenson & Tangney, 1998). Statins increase the expression of eNOS via Rho isoprenylation (Laufs et al., 1998) or posttranslational mechanism (Kureishi et al., 2000).

Superoxide dismutase (SOD). Superoxide dismutase has a key antioxidant role by dismutation of $O_2^{\cdot-}$ into oxygen and hydrogen peroxide. In humans, three forms of the enzyme are present (SOD1, SOD2 and SOD3). In the cardiovascular system, the action of extracellular SOD3 (Cu-Zn-SOD) lowers $O_2^{\cdot-}$ and maintains vascular NO levels (Jung et al., 2007).

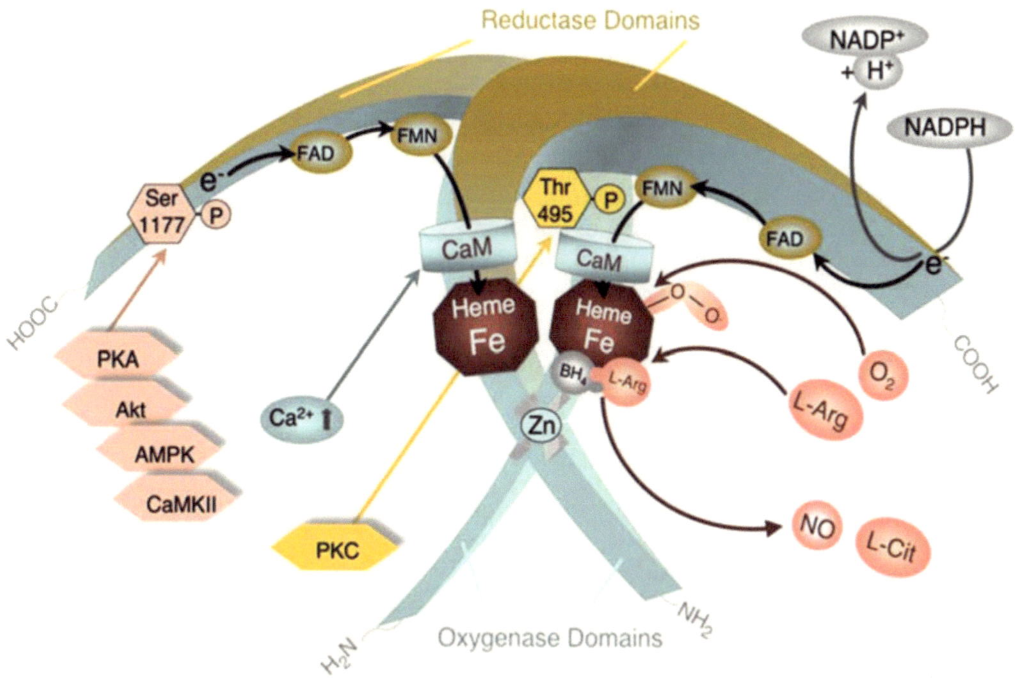

Fig. 2. Regulation of eNOS activity by intracellular Ca^{2+} and phosphorylation. An increase in intracellular Ca^{2+} (as produced by agonists such as histamine or bradykinin) leads to an enhanced binding of CaM (calmodulin) to the enzyme, which in turn displaces an auto-inhibitory loop and facilitates the flow of electrons from NADPH in the reductase domain to the heme in the oxygenase domain. There are several potential phosphorylation sites in eNOS, but most is known about the functional consequences of phosphorylation of Ser^{1177} (human eNOS sequence) in the reductase domain and Thr^{495} (human eNOS sequence) within the CaM-binding domain. In resting endothelial cells, Ser^{1177} is usually not phosphorylated. Phosphorylation is induced when the cells are exposed to fluid shear stress, estrogens, VEGF, insulin, or bradykinin. The kinases responsible for phosphorylation depend on the primary stimulus. Shear stress elicits the phosphorylation of Ser^{1177} by activating protein kinase A (PKA), estrogen and VEGF phosphorylate eNOS mainly via Akt, insulin probably activates both Akt and the AMP-activated protein kinase (AMPK), and the bradykinin-induced phosphorylation of Ser^{1177} is mediated by CaMKII. Phosphorylation of the Ser^{1177} residue increases the flux of electrons through the reductase domain and thus enzyme activity. The Thr^{495} residue of human eNOS tends to be constitutively phosphorylated in endothelial cells. Thr^{495} is a negative regulatory site, and its phosphorylation is associated with a decrease in enzyme activity. The constitutively active kinase that phosphorylates eNOS Thr^{495} is most probably protein kinase C (PKC). The phosphatase that dephosphorylates Thr^{495} appears to be protein phosphatase1. (Figure and legend from U. Förstermann, Pflügers Arch - Eur J Physiol, 2010;459:923-933)

Catalase. Catalase decomposes hydrogen peroxide to water and oxygen. Overexpression of catalase has protective effects in the cardiovascular system such as delayed development of arteriosclerosis (Yang et al., 2004) and inhibition of angiotensin II-induced aortic wall hypertrophy (Zhang et al., 2005).

Glutathion peroxidase (GPx). Several isoenzymes of GPx were found in mammals, the isoenzyme 1 being most abundant. In patients with coronary artery disease the activity of red blood cell GPx1 is inversely associated with the risk of cardiovascular events (Blankenberg et al., 2003). In ApoE-deficient mice, the deficiency of GPx1 leads to arteriosclerotic lesion progression (Torzewski et al., 2007).

Heme oxygenase (HO). In break down of heme CO, biliverdin and free ferrous iron are formed. The biliverdin is converted to bilirubin, which has radical-scavenging properties (Jiang et al., 2006). The carbon monoxide has antiproliferative and anti-inflammatory as well as vasodilatory properties (Morita, 2005).

Thioredoxin (Trx). Thioredoxin seems to exert most of its ROS-scavenging properties through Trx peroxidase (peroxiredoxin), which uses endogenous SH groups as reducing equivalents. Thioredoxin is present in endothelial- and vascular smooth muscle cells. It exerts its ROS-scavenging properties through Trx peroxidase. Trx scavens ROS and nitric peroxide, $ONOO^-$ (Yamawaki et al., 2003).

Paraoxonase (PON). The PON family of enzymes acts as vascular antioxidant defense and protects against coronary artery disease (Aviram et al., 1998). The PON1 and PON3 enzymes are synthesized in the liver and circulate in plasma associated with the high-density lipoprotein (HDL) fraction. The capacity of HDL in decreasing HDL and LDL lipid peroxidation largely depends on its PON1 content (Aviram et al., 1998). Deletion of the PON1 gene increases oxidative stress in mouse macrophages and aortae (Rozenberg et al., 2005). The enzyme has been shown to reduce ROS in human endothelial cells, vascular smooth muscle cells, and fibroblasts (Horke et al., 2007).

4. eNOS – A multiple cofactors-dependent enzyme

eNOS is a homodimer protein and consists of two subunits: **(I)** the alpha reductase domain which is able to transfer electrons from NADPH to FAD and FMN and can bind calmodulin for stimulation of electron transfer. It has a limited capacity to reduce molecular oxygen to superoxide ($O_2^{\cdot-}$) (Stuehr et al., 2001). **(II)** The oxygenase domain of eNOS is unable to bind the cofactor 5,6,7,8-tetrahydrobiopterin or L-arginine and can not catalyse NO production. The presence of heme allows for NOS dimerization and is the only cofactor that is essential for NOS for the interaction and coupling reductase and oxygenase domains. eNOS monomers are unable to bind the 5,6,7,8-tetrahydrobiopterin or the L-arginine and can not catalyse NO production. Under pathological conditions the molecular oxygen is no longer coupled to L-arginine reduction but results in the production of superoxide. This phenomenon is referred to eNOS uncoupling (Förstermann & Münzel, 2006; Li et al., 2002b).

5. eNOS uncoupling

5.1 Molecular mechanisms leading to eNOS uncoupling

Various mechanisms can contribute to eNOS uncoupling (**Fig. 3**). Their inbalance causes eNOS dysfunction and cardiovascular risk. This has been shown by numerous clinical studies and for experimental animals. **(I)** Inhibition of eNOS activity. A lack or deficiency of eNOS disrupted at the calmodulin binding site resulted in enhanced arteriosclerosis or peripheral coronary arteriosclerosis and aortic aneurism in ApoE/eNOS double knock out mice (Chen et al., 2001; Hodgin et al., 2002; Knowles et al., 2000; Kuhlencordt et al., 2001).

(II) eNOS uncoupling factors such as hypercholesterolemia, diabetes, smoking, hypertension are associated with endothelial dysfunction. Evidence for uncoupling of eNOS has been obtained in endothelial cells treated with LDL (Pritchard et al., 1995) in peroxynitrite-treated rat aorta (Laursen et al., 2001) and in spontaneously hypertensive rats (Li et al., 2006), in human diabetes (Heitzer et al., 2000) and streptozotocin-induced diabetic rats (Hink et al., 2001). **(III)** Arginine deficiency. L-arginine - the physiological substrate of eNOS - is a constituent amino acid and present in human blood plasma in a concentration of 113.6±14.6 µM (Psychogios et al., 2011). A decrease of L-arginine induced in hypercholesterolemia below physiological levels favours eNOS uncoupling and formation of ROS. Beside L-arginine the asymmetric dimethylated form of arginine (ADMA) is a major

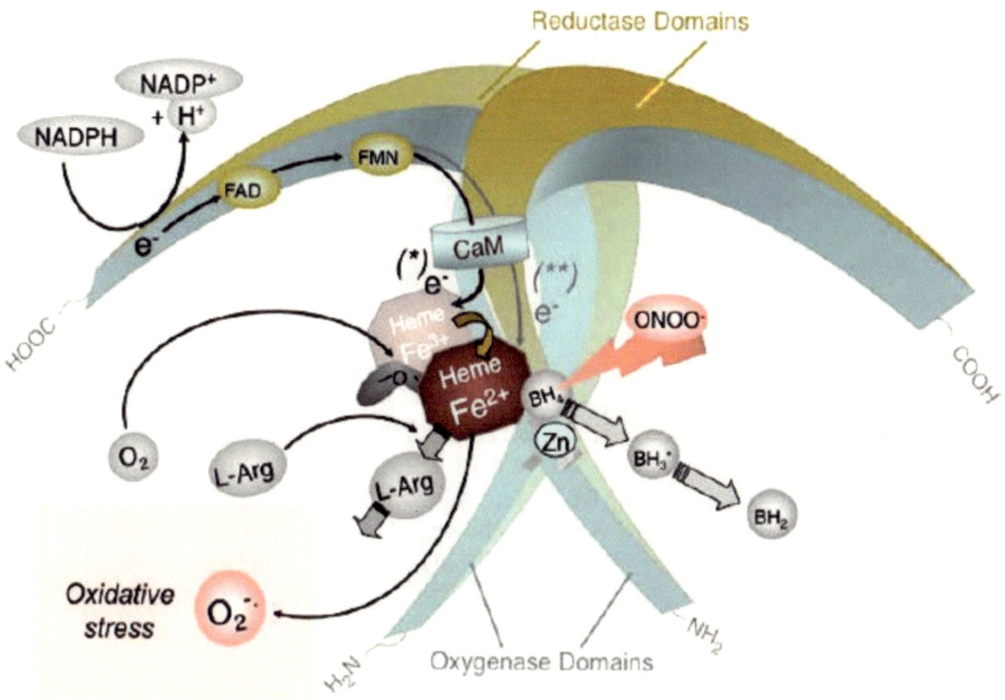

Fig. 3. Scheme of an endothelial NO synthase (eNOS) whose oxygen reduction is uncoupled from NO synthesis. Oxidative stress is associated with endothelial dysfunction. ONOO− can oxidize BH_4 to biologically inactive products such as trihydrobiopterin radical ($BH_3\cdot$) or trihydrobiopterin radical cation protonated at N5 ($BH_3\cdot H^+$). The $BH_3\cdot$ radical can be converted to the quinonoid 6,7-[8H]-H2-biopterin (BH_2), which also lacks biological activity. When ONOO− overwhelms the cell's capacity to re-reduce these products to BH_4, eNOS "uncouples" and reduces oxygen to $O_2-\cdot$, but does not synthesize NO anymore. eNOS then contributes to oxidative stress in the cell. (Figure and legend from U. Förstermann, Pflügers Arch - Eur J Physiol, 2010;459:923-933)

component of blood plasma in a concentration of 0.4-0.8 μM (Billecke et al., 2009) and acts as an endogenous inhibitor of eNOS. ADMA is formed by dimethylation of protein-bound L-arginine and released by proteolysis. ADMA acts as a local competitor of L-arginine (Cooke, 2004; Maas, 2005). Arginase is an ubiquitous enzyme which catalyses the degradation of arginine to ornithine and urea. Two isoenzymes are found in mammals. Arginase I catalyses the final step of the urea cycle in liver. Arginase II is a mitochondrial enzyme that functions in L-arginine homeostasis and can be dysregulated by ox LDL (Ryoo et al., 2006) resulting in eNOS uncoupling. **(IV)** 5,6,7,8-tetrahydrobiopterin deficiency. 5,6,7,8-tetrahydrobiopterin deficiency causes eNOS dysfunction and uncoupling (Moens & Kass, 2006), if the primary function of 5,6,7,8-tetrahydrobiopterin such as both allosteric and redox function, the improvement, the binding affinity of L-arginine for eNOS and providing the second electron to the heme of eNOS are missing. These alterations have the consequence that the reduction of molecular oxygen still occurs at the heme site of eNOS but oxidation of the guanidine nitrogen of L-arginine is prevented so that the reduced oxygen is converted by the uncoupled eNOS to superoxide instead of NO and citrulline (Gao et al., 2007; Xia et al. 1998). Even the partially oxidized 5,6,7,8-tetrahydrobiopterin - the 7,8-tetrahydrobiopterin (BH_2) - has no eNOS cofactor activity and is unable to prevent superoxide formation of eNOS (Gao et al., 2007). In addition, BH_2 probably competes with BH_4 for eNOS binding. Therefore the ratio BH_4/BH_2 is important for eNOS activity (Shinozaki et al., 1999; Vasquez-Vivar et al., 2002). Apparently a diminished BH_4/BH_2 level rather than BH_4 deficiency is a molecular trigger for eNOS uncoupling (Crabtree et al., 2008). Normally the majority of BH_4 is present in vascular endothelial cells (Antoniades et al., 2007; Katusic, 2001) in a concentration of 1.40 pM/10^6 cells. Intracellular BH_4 concentration has been found under hypercholesterolemic conditions thus aortic BH_4 levels are decreased by 50% in hypercholesterolemic ApoE knockout mice compared with wild-type mice (Ozaki et al., 2002), but also discrepant results are described (d'Uscio et al. 2003; d'Uscio & Katusic, 2006) apparently depending on the degree of hypercholesterolemia and differences in the level of oxidative stress. The tissue level of BH_4 is determined by the balance of biosynthesis from GTP via de novo synthesis by GTP cyclo hydrolase (GCH-1) or by the salvage pathway from BH_2 back to BH_4 and degradation by oxidation of BH_4 to BH_2 (T.S. Schmidt & Alp, 2007) – a process that can be rapidly accelerated by peroxynitrite (Landmesser et al., 2003; Laursen et al., 2001; Zou et al. 2002).

The oxidase-mediated stress of BH_4 can be increased by several ROS producing enzyme systems such as NADPH oxidase that plays a major role in vascular cells (Förstermann, 2008; Harrison et al., 2003; Schnabel & Blankenberg, 2007), by xanthine oxidase, cytochrome P450 monooxygenase and enzymes of the respiratory chain. Xanthine oxidase is generated from xanthine dehydrogenase by proteolysis. This enzyme is another potential source of ROS in vascular disease. The enzyme readily donates electrons to molecular oxygen, thereby producing $O_2^{-\cdot}$ and hydrogen peroxide. Oxypurinol, an inhibitor of xanthine oxidase decreases $O_2^{-\cdot}$ production and improves endothelium-dependent vascular relaxation to acetylcholine in blood vessels from hyperlipidemic animals (Ohara et al., 1993). This suggests a contribution of xanthine oxidase to endothelial dysfunction in early hypercholesterolemia. Experimental evidence suggests that endothelial cells themselves can express xanthine dehydrogenase (xanthine oxidase) and that this expression is regulated in a redox sensitive way depending on endothelial NADPH oxidase (McNally et al., 2003).

All these cited cofactors required for regulation eNOS activity depend on the physiological transcription and translation of the corresponding genes. These processes, however, are regulated by epigenetics. Epigentics refer to chromatin-based pathways including three distinct but highly interrelated mechanisms: DNA methylation, Histone density and posttranslational modifications. These factors together offer new perspectives on transcriptional control paradigm in vascular endothelial cells and provide a molecular basis for understanding how the environment impacts the genome to modified function and disease susceptibility (Yan et al., 2010).

5.2 Mechanisms leading to a loss of function of eNOS

Oxidative stress is associated with endothelial dysfunction. Mechanistically, superoxide derived from NADPH oxidases and/or xanthine oxidase may combine with NO formed by a still functional eNOS. This would lead to increased formation of peroxinitrite (Laursen et al., 2001). Peroxynitrite has been shown to oxidize BH_4 to biological inactive products. Significant $O_2^{-\cdot}$ production also occurs when concentrations of L-arginine fall below the levels required to saturate the enzyme. In these circumstances eNOS catalysis the uncoupled reduction to O_2 leading to the production of $O_2^{-\cdot}$ and/or H_2O_2. Whether L-arginine concentration ever becomes critical as a substrate *in vivo* appears questionable since the K_m of eNOS for L-arginine is ~3 μM while the L-arginine plasma concentration is ~100 μM and a ~10-fold accumulation of L-arginine within cells (Closs et al., 2000).

5.3 eNOS uncoupling in arteriosclerosis

Under cardiovascular risk factors such as diabetes, hypertension, smoking, the enzymatic reduction of molecular oxygen by eNOS is no longer used for L-arginine conversion to citrulline and NO, but the uncoupling of oxidase and reductase chain of eNOS produced ROS via the NADPH domains. The cardiovascular risk factors initiate the eNOS uncoupling and this can occur before arteriosclerotic lesions can be detected. The eNOS uncoupling can be triggered by various mechanisms which include BH_4 deficiency, shortage of L-arginine or HSP 90, inhibitory phosphorylation of eNOS on Thr^{495} (see above) eNOS redistribution to the cytosolic fraction of the cell, oxidation of the zinc-thiolate cluster in eNOS or elevated ADMA levels (Sud et al. 2008). Among all of these mechanisms the reaction BH_4 to BH_2 is probably a dominant factor, and BH_4 deficiency seems to be the primary cause for eNOS uncoupling in pathophysiology. Some researchers have postulated that eNOS may exist in two separate pools: a coupled form and an uncoupled form. The coupled enzyme is associated with the membrane and is readily accessible to the "signalome" for activation and NO production, whereas the uncoupled enzyme may reside in the cytosol and produces superoxide (Gharavi et al., 2006; Sullivan et al., 2006). In eNOS overexpressing mice for example, there is clear evidence for eNOS uncoupling (i.e. eNOS-mediated ROS production). In the same mice, however, NO-generating activity is elevated 2-fold when compared with wild-type mice (the total eNOS protein levels are elevated 8-fold) (Bendall et al., 2005). Thus, it is possible that coupled eNOS and uncoupled eNOS may exist in the same tissue at the same time.

The principle mechanisms of vascular protection by eNOS-derived NO and the consequences of endothelial dysfunction and the concomitant eNOS uncoupling are listed in **Tab. 2.**

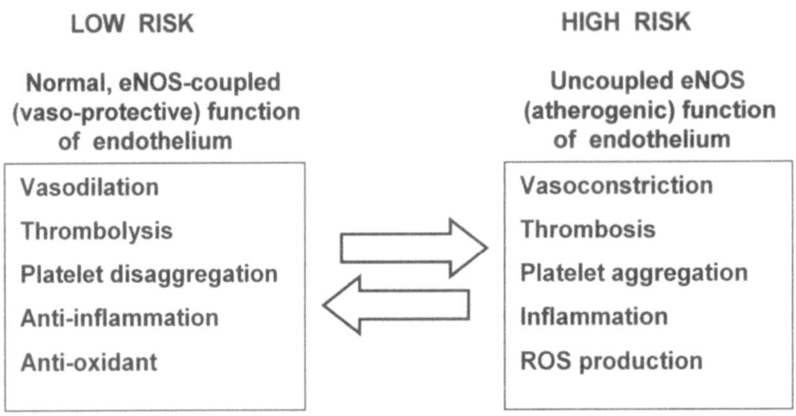

Table 2. The vaso-protective effect of eNOS is not restricted to the control of arterial dilation and constriction. The NO released towards the vascular lumen is a potent inhibitor of platelet aggregation and adhesion. The expression and formation of the alpha and beta component of various integrins including the cell adhesion molecules ICAM and VCAM can also be inhibited and reduce the transendothelial migration of macrophages and T-lymphocytes known to be an early event in the development of arteriosclerosis and characteristic for its inflammatory phases. The uncoupled eNOS leads to an excessive production of superoxide ($O_2^{\cdot -}$) and in turn to the formation of highly toxic peroxynitrite (Förstermann & Münzel, 2006).

6. eNOS-independent production of reactive oxygen species in vascular disease

Beside the eNOS there are several enzymes that can produce ROS in the endothelial cells: NADPH oxidase, xanthine oxidase, and enzymes of the mitochondrial respiratory chain are of major importance.

NADPH oxidases. Several isoforms of ROS producing NADPH oxidase are present and active in the vascular wall. In arteriosclerotic arteries the NADPH oxidase subunits NOX 2 and NOX 4 (Sorescu et al., 2002) have been identified.

Xanthine oxidase (XO). Increased cholesterol levels have been shown to stimulate the release of xanthine oxidase from the liver into the circulation. The circulating xanthine oxidase than can associate with endothelial glycosaminoglycans (White et al., 1996) however endothelial cells themselves can express xanthine oxidase and the expression is regulated in a redox sensitive pathway depending on endothelial NADPH oxidase (McNally et al., 2003) (**Fig. 4**).

Respiratory chain of the mitochondria. The molecular oxygen is consumed by mitochondria thereby forming $O_2^{\cdot -}$. Evidence has been provided that some cardiovascular diseases are associated with mitochondrial dysfunction (Ramachandran et al., 2002) and the mitochondrial production of ROS may be linked to the development of early arteriosclerotic lesions.

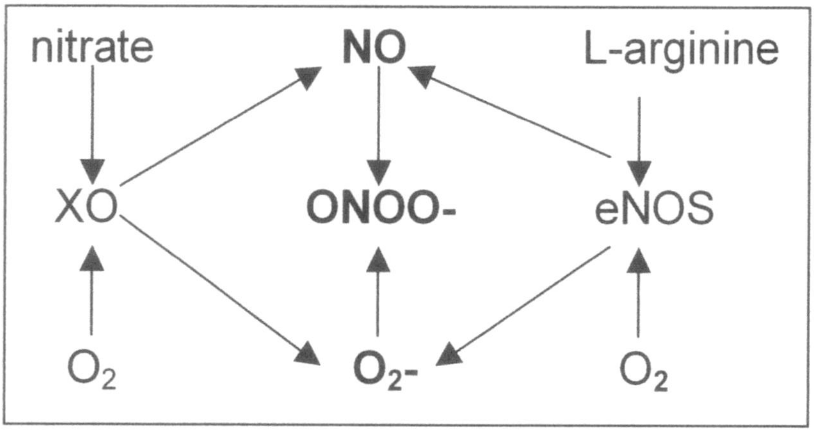

Fig. 4. XO and NOS are capable of generating either NO or superoxide (O_2) depending on the conditions. When the supply of L-arginine and oxygen is good, NOS makes NO, whereas the same enzyme may generate considerable amounts of superoxide when L-arginine or cofactors are limited. XO generates superoxide, for example, during reperfusion after ischemia, whereas nitrite reduction to NO occurs preferentially during hypoxia. NO generation from XO can be beneficial and works as a backup system to supply NO during hypoxia when NO synthesis from NOS is compromised. Detrimental effects of these 2 enzyme systems can also be foreseen, for example, in a situation in which NO and superoxide are generated simultaneously and react to form potentially harmful peroxynitrite. (Figure and legend from J.O. Lundberg and E. Weitzberg, Arterioscler Thromb Vasc Biol, 2005;25:915 - 922)

7. Factors protecting against eNOS uncoupling and oxidative stress

7.1 Nitric oxide donors

NO-delivering drugs (NO donors) are used for their potential therapeutic benefit in coronary heart disease risk patients (D.J. Lefer & A.M. Lefer, 1988) by increasing coronary blood flow and dilating coronary arteries. Several studies have described the action of NO donors on vascular smooth muscle cells (Sarkar et al., 1997; A. Schmidt et al. 2003; Young et al., 2000). The pathway leading to NO formation differs among individual NO donor classes: indirect NO donors such as organic nitrates (nitroglycerol, isosorbide mononitrate, isosorbide dinitrate) require enzymatic catalysis, other NO donors require interaction with thiols to release NO, some have to undergo oxidation or reduction. In contrast, direct NO donors generate NO non-enzymatically. Examples are nicorandil, SIN-1 (the active metabolite of molsidomine) and the group of 1-substituted diazen-1-ium-1,2-diolates that releases NO spontaneously with a half-life from minutes to hours (Mooradian et al., 1995).

7.2 The NO donor DETA/NONOate

The compound (Z)-1-[2-Aminoethyl)-N-(2-ammonioethyl) amino] diazen-1-ium-1,2-diolate (in the following detNO) belongs to the class of direct NO donors. Under cell culture conditions detNO releases spontaneously NO with a half-life of about 20 h at 37° C in a strictly first order reaction (Hrabie et al., 1993; Keefer et al., 1996; Mooradian et al., 1995), thereby disintegrating to two NO and diethylentriamine. Diethylentriamine, the byproduct of detNO disintegration, is known to be effectiveless (Mooradian et al., 1995; Sarkar et al., 1997). detNO has been successful used (Boyle et al., 2002; Ishimaru et al., 2001; A. Schmidt et al., 2003). In experimental studies (A. Schmidt et al., 2008) on cultured endothelial cells exogenously applied NO released from the NO donor detNO has a dual function in the regulation of eNOS expression. During short-term exposure of endothelial cells, exogenous detNO enhances the phosphorylation of the protein kinase Akt that in turn activates eNOS of endothelial cells by increasing its phosphorylation leading to a higher release of endogenous NO.

Phosphorylation can be achieved by exposure of human vascular endothelial cells to 150 µmol/L detNO. In short-term experiments in Western blot analysis detNO shows a clear increase of eNOS phosphorylation at Ser^{1177} after a short lag phase, detectable 20 min after detNO addition. The phosphorylation is mediated by the protein kinase Akt that is converted into p-Akt within 10 min after addition of detNO in a concentration-dependent manner. The phosphorylated Akt increases in turn Ser^{1177} phosphorylation of eNOS. This phosphorylation cascade could be reverted by preincubation of the cells with the PI-3 kinase inhibitor LY294002 that prevents phosphorylation of both Akt and eNOS. Thr^{495} is constitutively phosphorylated in all endothelial cells (Fleming & Busse, 2003) and is a negative regulatory site, i.e. phosphorylation leads to a decrease of eNOS activity. The release of endogenous NO in response to exogenous detNO was confirmed by L-[2,3,4,5-^{3}H]arginine as indicator. The eNOS-mediated conversion of [^{3}H]arginine to NO and [^{3}H]citrulline was measured and the results are given in [^{3}H]citrulline equivalents. A statistically significant increase of endogenous NO production after 20 and 30 min exposure to detNO is shown. N-nitro-L-arginine methyl ester HCl (NAME), a competitive NOS inhibitor, verifies the reaction conditions of the assay. Taking this reaction sequence into account, the effect of the NO donor could be considered partially a trigger for the acceleration of endogenous NO production that finally effects vasodilation via the physiologic pathway. This leads to the hypothesis of a potential switch from an exogenously applied to an endogenously generated NO stimulation (**Fig. 5**).

7.3 Long-term application of detNO and other NO donors

In contrast an exposure of endothelial cells to detNO for 24 and 48 h reduces the eNOS protein content as compared with controls. Densitometry revealed a reduced eNOS protein content after 24 h and 48 h. Real-time RT-PCR confirmed the reduced transcription of eNOS-specific mRNA. For direct determination of the reduced eNOS enzyme activity after long-term exposure to detNO, [2,3,4,5-^{3}H]arginine was added to the culture medium. The radioactivity of [^{3}H]citrulline formed by the NADPH-dependent NOS oxidoreductase is direct proportional to the NO produced and released by the endothelial cells. Under these conditions the results show a significant reduction of NO production expressed as [^{3}H]citrulline equivalents in accordance to the reduced Ser^{1177} phosphorylation of eNOS. Taken together, these results emphasize a limitation of NO donors as long-term therapeutics owing to the inhibition of eNOS synthesis. However, whether exogenous NO donors are operative and effective in a similar way also in humans is still uncertain. In numerous clinical studies the outcome of repeated administration of indirect or direct NO donors to patients with coronary artery disease were ambiguous and the potential benefit of long-acting nitrates has remained controversial. Pathways leading to NO formation differ significantly among individual NO donor classes. In the Fourth International Study of

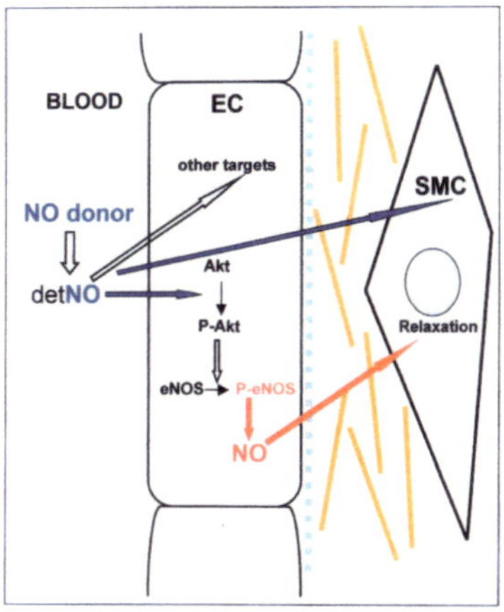

Fig. 5. Scheme of the new mechanism of action of the NO-donor DETA/NONOate in cultured human vascular endothelial cells. During short-term exposure the exogenous NO donor enhances the phosphorylation of the protein kinase Akt (PKB) that in turn activates eNOS of the endothelial cells by increasing its phosphorylation of Ser^{1177} leading to a higher release of the physiological endogenous NO as judged by the conversion of [^{3}H]arginine to [^{3}H]citrulline. The NOS-released NO reaches the smooth muscle cell and effects vasodilation.

Infarct Survival (ISIS-4), there was no significant reduction in five-week mortality and no survival advantage (ISIS-4 (Fourth International Study of Infarct Survival) Collaborative Group, 1995). Chronic administration of long acting nitrates in patients with healed myocardial infarction resulted in an increased number of patients with cardiac events (Ishikawa et al., 1996) and an increased risk of cardiac deaths occurred in CAD patients with long acting nitrates (Nakamura et al., 1999). Furthermore, a study on 19 healthy volunteers documented that isosorbide mononitrate given over 7 days impaired endothelial function due to formation of free radicals (Thomas et al., 2007). In total, epidemiological evidence indicates that chronic administration of long acting nitrates increase rather than decreases fatal and non-fatal events (Ishikawa et al., 1996; Nakamura et al., 1999). This view is confirmed by experiments on human vascular endothelial cells, which show detNO-induced cell cycle arrest and hypertrophy. Cultured quiescent EC released from the G_o-phase by seeding at a low density re-enter the cell cycle and proliferate up to confluence. In this phase detNO causes a dose-dependent suppression of proliferation of EC indicated by a decreased incorporation of [^{3}H]thymidine and a cell cycle arrest. The antiproliferative effect of detNO was associated with a remarkable increase of cell protein content that continued up to a 2-3-fold amount of control cells within 3 days while the cell number indicates an inhibition of cell proliferation and shows neither increase nor decrease. The elevated total cell protein was the result of *de novo* synthesis indicated by measurements of [^{3}H]leucine incorporation into total cellular protein. After 48 h incubation of subconfluent cultures in the presence of [4,5-^{3}H]leucine the incorporated radioactivity was 24.8 x 10^3 dpm/10^5 control cells and 34.6 x 10^3 dpm/10^5 cells exposed to detNO. The concomitant upregulation of p21 refers to a block at the G_1-phase of the cell cycle. The detNO-induced metabolic alterations convert the cells into a hypertrophic phenotype. Measurements of cell volume show an increase from 2.49 ± 0.18 up to 3.38 ± 0.36 (200 µmol/L detNO) fL /cell.

The inhibition of proliferation is cytostatic but not cytotoxic as evaluated by cell death determination and is reversible. A quantitative determination of mono- and oligonucleosomes revealed no significant apoptotic cell death in detNO-pretreated cells. When the medium of detNO-induced growth-arrested cells is replaced by a standard medium, cell proliferation recovers within the following 48 h with continuous increase of cell number.

7.4 Antioxidant compounds potentially protecting against vascular oxidative stress

Important antioxidant enzymes include superoxide dismutase (SOD), glutathione peroxidase (GPx), catalase, heme oxygenase (HO), and the thioredoxin (Trx) peroxidase and perhaps also paraoxonases (PON) (see Chapter 3.2).

Pentaerythritol tetranitrate (PETN) is a NO donor that does not induce significant nitrate tolerance and reduces oxidative stress (probably by inducing heme oxygenase). **Sepiapterin** can be reduced in cells by sepiapterin reductase (SR) to 7,8-BH_2, sepiapterin reductase catalyses the following reaction

$$\text{7,8-dihydrobiopterin} + NADP^+ \rightleftharpoons \text{tetrahydrobiopterin} + NADPH + H^+$$

Midostaurin, betulinic acid and ursolic acid upregulate eNOS and concomitantly decrease NADPH oxidase expression (Li & Förstermann, 2009).

AVE9488 and AVE3085, a new class of eNOS enhancers, upregulated the promotor activity of eNOS *in vitro* and *in vivo*. Application to wild type and ApoE-knockout mice over 12 weeks enhanced vascular eNOS expression at mRNA and protein level (Xue et al., 2010). The hybrid NO-releasing prodrug PABA/NO can be stabilized as nanoparticle with significant stability in mice circulation over 24h (Kumar et al., 2010).

Nebivolol - a NO-releasing beta-blocker induced a consistent increase of aortic eNOS expression rabbits receiving high-cholesterol diet (de Nigris et al., 2008). NO-releasing S-nitrosothiol-modified xerogels are capable of generating NO for up to 2 weeks (Riccio et al., 2009). These new generation of NO donors might be a rational approach to develop a new generation of antiatherogenic and anti-inflammatory NO donors. AVE9488 and AVE3085 are eNOS transcription enhancers that reverse eNOS uncoupling and preserve eNOS functionality.

Angiotensin II type 1-receptor blockers (ARBs), estrogens and erythropoietin (EPO) enhance (6R)-5,6,7,8-BH_4 synthesis by stimulating GCH1 expression or activity (Li & Förstermann, 2009.)

Angiotensin-converting enzyme (ACE) inhibitors, the aldosterone antagonist eplerenone and the renin inhibitor aliskiren prevent (6R)-5,6,7,8-BH_4 oxidation by decreasing the expression and/or activity of NADPH oxidase.

8. Clinical implications

Cardiovascular risk factors cause oxidative stress that alters the endothelial cells capacity and leads to endothelial dysfunction. The term „endothelial dysfunction" is used to refer to an incompetence of endothelial cell-dependent vasorelaxation resulting from eNOS uncoupling but a molecular or biochemical basis for biomarkers indicating uncoupled eNOS has not been established. A biomarker is a characteristic that is objectively measured and evaluated as an indicator for normal or pathogenic processes or pharmacological response to a therapeutic intervention. As biomarkers for cardiovascular diseases oxLDL, CRP, IL-6, fibrinogen, TNF-alpha, MMP-9, MPO and cell adhesion molecules have been proposed (Vasan, 2006). Indirect biomarkers for eNOS uncoupling are a number of pharmaceuticals that have been shown to act as vaso-protective agents. Such agents listed by Förstermann (Förstermann, 2010) are: pentaerythritol tetranitrate, a NO donor that does not induce significant nitrate tolerance and reduces oxidative stress probably by inducing heme oxygenase 1, L-arginine stimulates NO release from eNOS, folic acid may improve eNOS functionality by stabilising BH_4 and stimulating the endogenous regeneration of BH_2 back to BH_4, sepiapterin can be reduced in cells by sepiapterin reductase to BH_2 and further dihydrofolate reductase to form BH_4, midostaurin, betulinic acid and ursolic acid upregulate eNOS and concomitantly decrease NADPH oxidase expression, AVE9488 and AVE3085 are eNOS transcription enhancers that reverse eNOS uncoupling and preserve eNOS functionality, statins, angiotensin II type 1-receptor blockers, estrogens and erythropoietin enhance BH_4 synthesis by stimulating GTP cyclohydrolase1 expression or activities. Statins, angiotensin converting enzyme inhibitors, the aldosterone antagonist eplerenone and the renin inhibitor prevent BH_4 oxidation by decreasing the expression and/or activity of NADPH oxidase. All these compounds are secondary biomarkers indicating a pharmacological response to a therapeutic intervention.

Clinically, endothelial function can be assessed by invasive or non-invasive techniques (for review see Esper et al., 2006). These techniques evaluate the endothelial functional capacity depending on the amount of NO produced and the resulting vasodilation effect. The percentage of vasodilation with respect to the basal value represents the endothelial functional capacity. A non-invasive technique most often used is the transient flow-modulate endothelium-dependent post-ischemic vasodilation performed on conductance arteries such as the brachial, radial or femoral arteries. This vasodilation is compared with the vasodilation produced by NO donors. The vasodilation is quantified by measuring the arterial diameter with high-resolution ultrasonography. Laser-Doppler techniques are used to consider tissue perfusion. There is no doubt that endothelial dysfunction contributes to the initiation and progression of arteriosclerosis and could be considered an independent vascular risk factor.

9. Conclusion

Nitric oxide produced in vascular endothelial cells by the nitric oxide synthase is a major signalling molecule for maintaining vascular homeostasis. The nitric oxide synthase - constitutionally expressed by endothelial cells – is a dimeric enzyme molecule depending on multiple cofactors for its physiological activity and optimal endothelial function. Any imbalance of reductase and NADPH oxygenase or deficient supply of the enzyme substrate L-arginine or of cofactors leads to an upregulation of endothelial nitric oxide synthase and oxygenase activity with the consequence of an uncoupling of the nitric oxide synthase and production of detrimental reactive oxygen species and/or highly toxic peroxinitrate instead of nitric oxide. The resulting endothelial dysfunction implies a high cardiovascular risk. Several drugs reverting endothelial nitric oxide synthase uncoupling and/or improving endothelial dysfunction are in clinical use. Nitric oxide delivering drugs (NO donors) show potential therapeutical benefit and are used to relief or prevent acute episodes of angina pectoris by activating the endothelial nitric oxide synthase – a new mechanism found for the NO donor DETA/NONOate. However, a long-term administration of NO donors has been found to reduce endothelial nitric oxide synthase of endothelial cells drastically (in cell culture experiments). This could be the basis for development of a new generation of NO donors that mimics the low continuous pulsatile stress-induced release of endogenous nitric oxide.

10. Acknowledgment

The author wishes to thank Prof. Dr. E. Buddecke, Muenster, for critical discussion and revising the manuscript.

11. References

Antoniades, C., Shirodaria, C., Crabtree, M., Rinze, R., Alp, N., Cunnington, C., Diesch, J., Tousoulis, D., Stefanadis, C., Leeson, P., Ratnatunga, C., Pillai, R., & Channon, K.M. (2007). Altered plasma versus vascular biopterins in human atherosclerosis reveal relationships between endothelial nitric oxide synthase coupling, endothelial function, and inflammation. *Circulation,* 116(24):2851-2859

Aviram, M., Rosenblat, M., Bisgaier, C.L., Newton, R.S., Primo-Parmo, S.L., & La Du, B.N. (1998). Paraoxonase inhibits high-density lipoprotein oxidation and preserves its functions. A possible peroxidative role for paraoxonase. *J Clin Invest,* 101:1581–1590

Bendall, J.K., Alp, N.J., Warrick, N., Cai, S., Adlam, D., Rockett, K., Yokoyama, M., Kawashima, S., & Channon, K.M. (2005). Stoichiometric relationships between endothelial tetrahydrobiopterin, endothelial NO synthase (eNOS) activity, and eNOS coupling in vivo: insights from transgenic mice with endothelialtargeted GTP cyclohydrolase 1 and eNOS overexpression. *Circ Res,* 97(9):864-871

Benjamin, N., O'Driscoll, F., Dougall, H., Duncan, C., Smith, L., Golden, M., & McKenzie, H. (1994). Stomach NO synthesis. *Nature,* 368:502

Billecke, S.S., D'Alecy, L.G., Platel, R., Whitesall, S.E., Jamerson, K.A., Perlman, .L., & Gadegbeku, C.A. (2009). Blood content of asymmetric dimethylarginine: new insights into its dysregulation in renal disease. *Nephrol Dial Transplant,* 24(2):489-496

Blankenberg, S., Rupprecht, H.J., Bickel, C., Torzewski, M., Hafner, G., Tiret, L., Smieja, M., Cambien, F., Meyer, J., Lackner, K.J., & AtheroGene Investigators. (2003). Glutathione peroxidase 1 activity and cardiovascular events in patients with coronary artery disease. *N Engl J Med,* 349(17):1605–1613

Boyle, J.J., Weissberg, P.L., & Bennett, M.R. (2002). Human macrophage- induced vascular smooth muscle cell apoptosis requires NO enhancement of Fas/Fas–L interactions. *Arterioscler Thromb Vasc Biol,* 22:1624–1630

Busse, R., Luckhoff, A., & Bassenge, E. (1987). Endotheliumderived relaxant factor inhibits platelet activation. *Naunyn-Schmiedeberg's Arch Pharmacol,* 336:566–571

Castel, H., & Vaudry, H. (2001). Nitric oxide directly activates GABA (A) receptor function through a cGMP/protein kinase-independent pathway in frog pituitary melanotrophs. *J Neuroendocrinol,* 13:695–705

Chen, J., Kuhlencordt, P.J., Astern, J., Gyurko, R., & Huang, P.L. (2001). Hypertension does not account for the accelerated atherosclerosis and development of aneurysms in male apolipoprotein e/endothelial nitric oxide synthase double knockout mice. *Circulation,* 04(20):2391-2394

Clancy, R.M., Leszczynska, P., Piziak, J., & Abramson, S.B. (1992). Nitric oxide, an endothelial cell relaxation factor, inhibits neutrophil superoxide anion production via a direct action on NADPH oxidase. *J Clin Invest,* 90:1116–1121

Closs, EI., Scheld, J.S., Sharafi, M., & Förstermann, U. (2000). Substrate supply for nitric-oxide synthase in macrophages and endothelial ells: role of cationic amino acid transporters. *Mol Pharmacol,* 57:68–74

Cooke, J.P. (2004). Asymmetrical dimethylarginine: the Uber marker? *Circulation,* 109(15): 1813-1818

Crabtree, M.J., Smith, C..L, Lam, G., Goligorsky, M.S., & Gross, S.S. (2008). Ratio of 5,6,7,8-tetrahydrobiopterin to 7,8-dihydrobiopterin in endothelial cells determines glucose-elicited changes in NO vs. superoxide production by eNOS. *Am J Physiol Heart Circ Physiol,* 294:H1530-1540

de Nigris, F., Mancini, F.P., Balestrieri, M.L., Byrns, R., Fiorito, C., Wiiliams- Ignarro, S., Palagiano, A., Crimi, E., Ignarro, L.J., & Napoli, C. (2008). Therapeutic dose of nebivolol, a nitric oxide-releasing beta-blocker, reduces atherosclerosis in cholesterol-fed rabbits. *Nitric Oxide,* 19(1):57–63

d'Uscio, L.V., Milstien, S., Richardson, D., Smith, L., & Katusic, Z.S. (2003). Longterm vitamin C treatment increases vascular tetrahydrobiopterin levels and nitric oxide synthase activity. *Circ Res,* 92:88-95

d'Uscio, L.V., & Katusic, Z.S. (2006). Increased vascular biosynthesis of tetrahydrobiopterin in apolipoprotein E-deficient mice. *Am J Physiol Heart Circ Physiol,* 290:H2466-2471

Esper, R.J., Nordaby, R.A., Vilarino, J.O., Paragano, A., Cacharrón, J.L. & Machado, R.A. (2006). Endothelial dysfunction: a comprehensive appraisal. *Cardiovasc Diabetol,* 5:4 doi:10.1186/1475-2840-5-4

Fleming, I. & Busse, R. (2003). Molecular mechanisms involved in the regulation of the endothelial nitric oxide synthase. *Am J Physiol Regul Integr Comp Physiol,* 284:R1–12

Fleming, I. (2010). Molecular mechanisms underlying the activation of eNOS. *Pflügers Arch - Eur J Physiol,* 459:793-806

Förstermann, U., Closs, EI., Pollock, JS., Nakane, M., Schwarz, P., Gath, I., & Kleinert, H. (1994). Nitric oxide synthase isozymes. Characterization, purification, molecular cloning, and functions. *Hypertension,*.23(6, Part 2):1121-1131

Förstermann, U., & Münzel, T. (2006). Endothelial nitric oxide synthase in vascular disease: from marvel to menace. *Circulation,* 113:1708-1714

Förstermann, U. (2006). Janus-faced role of endothelial NO synthase in vascular disease: uncoupling of oxygen reduction from NO synthesis and its pharmacological reversal. *Biol Chem,* 387:1521–1533

Förstermann, U. (2008). Oxidative stress in vascular disease: causes, defense mechanisms and potential therapies. *Nat Clin Pract Cardiovasc Med,* 5:338-349

Förstermann, U. (2010). Nitric oxide and oxidative stress in vascular disease *Pflügers Arch - Eur J Physiol,* 459:923–939

Gao, Y.T., Roman, L.J., Martasek, P., Panda, S.P., Ishimura, Y., & Masters, B.S. (2007).Oxygen metabolism by endothelial nitric-oxide synthase. *J Biol Chem,* 282:28557- 28565

Gharavi, N.M., Baker, N.A., Mouillesseaux, K.P., Yeung, W., Honda, H.M., Hsieh, X., Yeh, M., Smart, E.J., & Berliner, J.A. (2006). Role of endothelial nitric oxide synthase in the regulation of SREBP activation by oxidized phospholipids. *Circ Res,* 98(6):768-776

Harrison, D., Griendling, K.K., Landmesser, U., Hornig, B., & Drexler, H. (2003). Role of oxidative stress in atherosclerosis. *Am J Cardiol,* 91:7A-11A

Heitzer, T., Krohn, K., Albers, S., & Meinertz, T. (2000). Tetrahydrobiopterin improves endothelium-dependent vasodilation by increasing nitric oxide activity in patients with Type II diabetes mellitus. *Diabetologia,* 43:1435-1438

Hemmens, B. & Mayer, B. (1998). Enzymology of nitric oxide synthases. *Methods Mol Biol,* 100:1–32

Herman, A. G., & Moncada, S. (2005). Therapeutic potential of nitric oxide donors in the prevention and treatment of atherosclerosis. *Eur Heart J,* 26(19):1945–1955

Hink, U., Li, H., Mollnau, H., Oelze, M., Matheis, E., Hartmann, M., Skatchkov, M., Thaiss, F., Stahl, R.A.K., Warnholtz, A., Meinertz, T., Griendling, K., Harrison, D.G., Förstermann, U., & Münzel, T. (2001). Mechanisms underlying endothelial dysfunction in diabetes mellitus. *Circ Res,* 88(2):E14-E22

Hodgin, J.B., Knowles, J.W., Kim, H.S., Smithies, O., & Maeda, N. (2002). Interactions between endothelial nitric oxide synthase and sex hormones in vascular protection in mice. *J Clin Invest,* 109:541-548

Horke, S., Witte, I., Wilgenbus, P., Kruger, M., Strand, D., & Förstermann, U. (2007). Paraoxonase-2 reduces oxidative stress in vascular cells and decreases endoplasmic reticulum stress-induced caspase activation. *Circulation,* 115:2055–2064

Hrabie, J.A., Klose, J.R., Wink, D.A., & Keefer, L.K. (1993). New nitric oxide- releasing zwitterions derived from polyamines. *J Org Chem,* 58:1472–1476

Ishikawa, K., Kanamasa, K., Ogawa, I., Takenaka, T., Naito, T., Kamata, N., Yamamoto, T., Nakai, S., Hama, J., Oyaizu, M., Kimura, A., Yamamoto, K., Aso, N., Arai, M., Yabushita, & H., Katori, Y. (1996). Long-term nitrate treatment increases cardiac events in patients with healed myocardial infarction. Secondary Prevention Group. *Jpn Circ J,* 60(10):779-788

Ishimaru, R.S., Leung, K., Hong, L., & LaPolt, P.S. (2001). Inhibitory effects of nitric oxide on estrogen production and cAMP levels in rat granulose cell cultures. *J Endocrinol,* 168:249–255 ISIS-4 (Fourth International Study of Infarct Survival) Collaborative Group. (1995). ISIS-4: arandomised factorial trial assessing early oral captopril, oral mononitrate, and intravenous magnesium sulphate in 58,050 patients with suspected acute myocardial infarction. *Lancet,* 345:669–685

Jiang, F., Roberts, S.J., Datla, S., & Dusting, G.J. (2006). NO modulates NADPH oxidasefunction via heme oxygenase-1 in human endothelial cells. *Hypertension* 48:950–957

John, S., Schlaich, M., Langenfeld, M., Weihprecht, H., Schmitz, G., Weidinger, G., &Schmieder, R.E.(1998). Increased bioavailability of nitric oxide after lipidlowering therapy in hypercholesterolemic patients: a randomized, placebo-controlled, double-blind study. *Circulation,*211–216

Jung, O., Marklund, S.L., Xia, N., Busse, R., & Brandes, R.P. (2007). Inactivation of extracellular superoxide dismutase contributes to the development of high-volume hypertension. *Arterioscler Thromb Vasc Biol,* 27:470–477

Kapil, V., Milsom, A.B., Okorie, M., Maleki-Toyserkani, S., Akram, F., Rehman, F.,Arghandawi, S., Pearl, V., Benjamin, N., Loukogeorgakis, S., Macallister, R., Hobbs, A.J., Webb, A.J., & Ahluwalia, A. (2010a). Inorganic nitrate supplementation lowers blood pressure in humans: role for nitrite-derived NO. *Hypertension,* 56(2):274-281

Kapil,V., Webb, A.J., & Ahluwalia, A. (2010b). Inorganic nitrate and the cardiovascularsystem. *Heart,* 96(21):1703-1709

Katusic, Z.S. (2001). Vascular endothelial dysfunction: does tetrahydrobiopterin play a role?*Am J Physiol Heart Circ Physiol,* 281: H981-986

Keefer, L.K., Nims, R.W., Davies, K.M., & Wink, D.A. (1996). 'NONOates' (1-substituteddiazen-1-ium-1,2-diolates) as nitric oxide donors: convenient nitric oxide dosage forms. *Meth Enzymol*, 268:281–293

Knowles, J.W., Reddick, R.L., Jennette, J.C., Shesely, E.G., Smithies, O., & Maeda N. (2000).Enhanced atherosclerosis and kidney dysfunction in eNOS(-/-)Apoe(-/-) mice are ameliorated by enalapril treatment. *J Clin Invest*, 105:451-845

Kockx, M.M., de Meyer, G.R., Muhring, J., Bult, H., Bultinck, J., & Herman, A.G. (1996).Distribution of cell replication and apoptosis in atherosclerotic plaques of cholesterol-fed rabbits. *Atherosclerosis*, 120:115–124

Kockx M.M. (1998). Apoptosis in the atherosclerotic plaque: quantitative and qualitativeaspects. *Arterioscler Thromb Vasc Biol*, 18:1519–1522

Kuhlencordt, P.J., Gyurko, R., Han, F., Scherrer-Crosbie, M., Aretz, T.H., Hajjar, R., Picard,M.H., & Huang, P.L. (2001). Accelerated atherosclerosis, aortic aneurysm formation, and ischemic heart disease in apolipoprotein E/endothelial nitric oxide synthase double-knockout mice. *Circulation*, 104(4):448-454

Kumar, V., Hong, S.Y., Maciag, A.E., Saavedra, J.E., Adamson, D.H., Prud' homme, R.K., Keefer, L.K., & Chakrapani, H. (2010). Stabilization of the nitric oxide (NO) prodrugs and anticancer leads, PABA/NO and double JS-K, through incorporation into PEG-protected nanoparticles. *Mol Pharm*, 7(1):291–298

Kureishi, Y., Luo, Z., Shiojima, I., Bialik, A., Fulton, D., Lefer, D.J., Sessa, W. C., & Walsh, K. (2000). The HMG-CoA reductase inhibitor simvastatin activates the protein kinase Akt and promotes angiogenesis in normocholesterolemic animals. *Nat Med*, 6:1004–1010

Landmesser, U., Dikalov, S., Price, S.R., McCann, L., Fukai, T., Holland, S.M., Mitch, W.E., &Harrison, D.G. (2003). Oxidation of tetrahydrobiopterin leads to uncoupling of endothelial cell nitric oxide synthase in hypertension. *J Clin Invest*, 111(8):1201-1209

Laufs, U., La Fata, V., Plutzky, J., & Liao, J.K. (1998). Upregulation of endothelial nitric oxidesynthase by HMG CoA reductase inhibitors. *Circulation*, 97:1129–1135

Laursen, J.B., Somers, M., Kurz, S., McCann, L., Warnholtz, A., Freeman, B.A., Tarpey, M., Fukai, T., & Harrison D.G. (2001). Endothelial regulation of vasomotion in apoE-deficient mice: implications for interactions between peroxynitrite and tetrahydrobiopterin. *Circulation*, 103(9):1282-1288

Lefer, D.J., & Lefer, A.M. (1988). Studies on the mechanism of the vasodilator action ofnicorandil. *Life Sci*, 42:1907–1914

Li, H., & Förstermann, U. (2000). Nitric oxide in the pathogenesis of vascular disease. *JPathol*, 190:244-254

Li, H., Wallerath, T., & Förstermann, U. (2002a). Physiological mechanisms regulating theexpression of endothelial-type NO synthase. *Nitric Oxide*, 7:132-147

Li, H., Wallerath, T., Münzel, T., & Förstermann, U. (2002b). Regulation of endothelial-typeNO synthase expression in pathophysiology and in response to drugs. *Nitric Oxide*, 7:149-164

Li, H., Witte, K., August, M., Brausch, I., Godtel-Armbrust, U., Habermeier, A., Closs, El.,Oelze, M., Münzel, T., & Förstermann, U. (2006). Reversal of endothelial nitric oxide synthase uncoupling and up-regulation of endothelial nitric oxide synthase expression lowers blood pressure in hypertensive rats. *J Am Coll Cardiol*, 47(12):2536-2544

Li, H., & Förstermann, U. (2009). Prevention of Atherosclerosis by Interference with theVascular Nitric Oxide System. *Curr Pharm Des*, 15(27):3133-3145

Lin, M.I., Fulton, D., Babbitt, R., Fleming, I., Busse, R., Pritchard, K.A. Jr., & Sessa, W.C. (2003). Phosphorylation of threonine 497 in endothelial nitric-oxide synthase coordinates the coupling of L-arginine metabolism to efficient nitric oxide production. *J Biol Chem*, 278: 44719–44726

Lloyd-Jones, IM., & Block, KD. (1996). The vascular biology of nitric oxide and its role inatherogenesis. *Annu Rev Med*,.47:365–375

Liu, VW., & Huang, PL. (2008). Cardiovascular roles of nitric oxide: a review of insightsfrom nitric oxide synthase gene disrupted mice. *Cardiovasc Res*,.77(1):19-29

Lundberg, J.O, Weitzberg, E., Lundberg, J.M., & Alving, K. (1994). Intragastric nitric oxideproduction in humans: measurements in expelled air. *Gut*. 35:1543–1546

Lundberg, J.O., & Weitzberg, E. (2005). NO Generation From Nitrite and Its Role in VascularControl. *Arterioscler Thromb Vasc Biol*, 25(5):915-922

Maas, R. (2005). Pharmacotherapies and their influence on asymmetric dimethylargine(ADMA). *Vasc Med*, 10(Suppl 1): S49-57

Mallis, R.J., Buss, J.E., & Thomas J.A. (2001). Oxidative modification of H-ras: S-thiolationand S-nitrosylation of reactive cysteines. *Biochem J*, 355:145–153

McNally, J.S., Davis, M.E., Giddens, D.P., Saha, A., Hwang, J., Dikalov, S., Jo, H., Harrison,D.G. (2003). Role of xanthine oxidoreductase and NAD(P)H oxidase in endothelial superoxide production in response to oscillatory shear stress. *Am J Physiol Heart Circ Physiol*, 285:H2290–H2297

Milkowski, A., Garg, H.K., Coughlin, J.R. & Bryan, N.S. (2010). Nutritional epidemiology inthe context of nitric oxide biology: A risk-benefit evaluation for dietary nitrite and nitrate. *Nitric Oxide*, 22(2):110-119

Moens, A.L., & Kass, D.A. (2006). Tetrahydrobiopterin and cardiovascular disease.*Arterioscler Thromb Vasc Biol*, 26:2439-2444

Moncada, S., Palmer, RM., & Higgs EA. (1991). Nitric oxide: physiology, pathophysiology,and pharmacology. *Pharmacol Rev*, 43(2):109–142

Mooradian, D.L., Hutsell, T.C., & Keefer, L.K. (1995). Nitric oxide (NO) donor molecules:effect of NO release rate on vascular smooth muscle cell proliferation in vitro. *J Cardiovasc Pharmacol*, 25:674–678

Morita, T. (2005). Heme oxygenase and atherosclerosis. *Arterioscler Thromb Vasc Biol*, 25: 1786–1795

Nakamura, Y., Moss, A.J., Brown, M.W., Kinoshita, M., & Kawai, C. (1999). Longterm nitrateuse may be deleterious in ischemic heart disease: A study using the databases from two large-scale postinfarction studies. Multicenter Myocardial Ischemia Research Group. *Am Heart J*, 138:577-585

Ohara, Y., Peterson, T.E., & Harrison, D.G. (1993). Hypercholesterolemia increasesendothelial superoxide anion production. *J Clin Invest*, 91:2546–2551

Ozaki, M., Kawashima, S., Yamashita, T., Hirase, T., Namiki, M., Inoue, N., Hirata, K., Yasui,H., Sakurai, H., Yoshida,Y., Masada, M., & Yokoyama, M. (2002). Overexpression of endothelial nitric oxide synthase accelerates atherosclerotic lesion formation in apoE-deficient mice. *J Clin Invest*, 110(3):331-340

Pritchard, K.A., Jr., Groszek, L., Smalley, D.M., Sessa, W.C., Wu, M., Villalon, P., Wolin,M.S., & Stemerman, M.B. (1995). Native low-density lipoprotein increases endothelial cell nitric oxide synthase generation of superoxide anion. *Circ Res*, 77(3):510-518

Psychogios, N., Hau, D.D., Peng, J., Guo, A.C., Mandal, R., Bouatra, S., Sinelnikov, I.,Krishnamurthy, R., Eisner, R., Gautam, B., Young, N., Xia, J., Knox, C., Dong, E., Huang, P., Hollander, Z., Pedersen, T.L., Smith, S.R., Bamforth, F., Greiner, R., McManus, B., Newman, J.W., Goodfriend, T., & Wishart, D.S. (2011). The human serum metabolome. *PLoS One*,16;6(2):e16957

Radomski, M.W., Palmer, R.M., & Moncada, S. (1987). The anti- aggregating properties ofvascular endothelium: interactions between prostacyclin and nitric oxide. *Br J Pharmacol,* 92:639–646

Ramachandran, A., Levonen, A.L., Brookes, P.S., Ceaser, E., Shiva, S., Barone, M.C., &Darley-Usmar, V. (2002). Mitochondria, nitric oxide, and cardiovascular dysfunction. *Free Radic Biol Med,* 33:1465–1474

Riccio, D.A., Dobmeier, K.P., Hetrick, E.M., Privett, B.J., Paul, H.S., & Schoenfisch, M.H. (2009). Nitric oxide-releasing S-nitrosothiol-modified xerogels. *Biomaterials,* 30:4494–502

Rosenson, R.S., & Tangney, C.C. (1998). Antiatherothrombotic properties of statins:implications for cardiovascular event reduction. *JAMA,* 279:1643–1650

Rozenberg, O., Shih, D.M., & Aviram, M. (2005). Paraoxonase 1 (PON1) attenuatesmacrophage oxidative status: studies in PON1 transfected cells and in PON1 transgenic mice. *Atherosclerosis,* 181:9–18

Ryoo, S., Lemmon, C.A., Soucy, K.G., Gupta, G., White, A.R., Nyhan, D., Shoukas, A.,Romer, L.H., & Berkowitz, D.E. (2006). Oxidized low-density lipoprotein-dependent endothelial arginase II activation contributes to impaired nitric oxide signaling. *Circ Res,* 99(9):951-960

Sarkar, R., Gordon, D., Stanley, J.C., & Webb, R.C. (1997). Cell cycle effects of nitric oxide onvascular smooth muscle cells. *Am J Physiol,* 272:H1810–1818

Schmidt, A., Geigenmüller, S., Völker, W., Seiler, P., & Buddecke, E. (2003). Exogenousnitric oxide causes overexpression of TGF-beta1 and overproduction of extracellular matrix in human coronary smooth muscle cells. *Cardiovasc Res,* 58: 671–678

Schmidt, A., Bilgasem, S., Lorkowski, S., Vischer, P., Völker, W., Breithardt, G., Siegel, G., &Buddecke, E. (2008). Exogenous nitric oxide regulates activity and synthesis of vascular endothelial nitric oxide synthase. *Eur J Clin Invest,* 38(7):476–485

Schmidt, T.S., & Alp, N.J. (2007). Mechanisms for the role of tetrahydrobiopterin inendothelial function and vascular disease. *Clin Sci (Lond),* 113:47-63

Schnabel, R., & Blankenberg, S. (2007). Oxidative stress in cardiovascular disease: successfultranslation from bench to bedside? *Circulation,* 116:1338-1340

Schulz, E., Anter, E., & Keaney, J.F. Jr. (2004).Oxidative stress, antioxidants, and endothelialfunction. *Curr Med Chem,* 11:1093–1104

Schulz, R., Kelm, M., & Heusch, G. (2004). Nitric oxide in myocardial ischemia/reperfusioninjury. *Cardiovasc Res,* 61(3):402- 413

Shinozaki, K., Kashiwagi, A., Nishio, Y., Okamura, T., Yoshida, Y., Masada, M., Toda, N., & Kikkawa, R. (1999). Abnormal biopterin metabolism is a major cause of impaired endothelium-dependent relaxation through nitric oxide/O2- imbalance in insulin-resistant rat aorta. *Diabetes,* 48(12):2437-2445

Sorescu, D., Weiss, D., Lassegue, B., Clempus, R.E., Szocs, K., Sorescu, G.P., Valppu, L.,Quinn, M.T., Lambeth, J.D., Vega, J.D., Taylor, W.R., & Griendling, K.K. (2002). Superoxide production and expression of nox family proteins in human atherosclerosis. *Circulation,* 105:1429–1435

Sowers, J.R. (2003). Effects of statins on the vasculature: implications for aggressive lipidmanagement in the cardiovascular metabolic syndrome. *Am J Cardiol,* 91:14B–22B

Stuehr, D., Pou, S., & Rosen, G.M. (2001). Oxygen reduction by nitric- oxide synthases. *J BiolChem,* 276:14533–14536

Sud, N., Wells, S.M., Sharma, S., Wiseman, D.A., Wilham, J., & Black, S.M. (2008).Asymmetric dimethylarginine inhibits HSP90 activity in pulmonary arterial endothelial cells: role of mitochondrial dysfunction. *Am J Physiol Cell Physiol,* 294:C1407-1418

Sullivan, J.C., Pollock, J.S. (2006). Coupled and uncoupled NOS: separate but equal?Uncoupled NOS in endothelial cells is a critical pathway for intracellular signaling. *Circ Res*, 98:717-719

Sun, J., Xin, C., Eu, J.P., Stamler, J.S., & Meissner, G. (2001). Cysteine-3635 is responsible forskeletal muscle ryanodine receptor modulation by NO. *Proc Natl Acad Sci USA*, 98:1158–1162

Tang, Y., Jiang, H., & Bryan, N.S. (2011). Nitrite and nitrate: cardiovascular risk-benefit andmetabolic effect. *Curr Opin Lipidol*, 22(1):11-15

Thomas, G.R., DiFabio, J.M., Gori, T., & Parker, J.D. (2007). Once daily Therapy WithIsosorbide-5-Mononitrate Causes Endothelial Dysfunction in Humans. *J Am Coll Cardiol*, 49:1289–1295

Torzewski, M., Ochsenhirt, V., Kleschyov, A.L., Oelze, M., Daiber, A., Li, H., Rossmann, H., Tsimikas, S., Reifenberg, K., Cheng, F., Lehr, H.A., Blankenberg, S., Förstermann, U., Münzel, T., & Lackner, K.J. (2007). Deficiency of glutathione peroxidase-1 accelerates the progression of atherosclerosis in apolipoprotein E-deficient mice. *Arterioscler Thromb Vasc Biol*, 27:850–857

Vasan, R.S. (2006). Biomarkers of Cardiovascular Disease: Molecular Basis and PracticalConsiderations. *Circulation*, 113:2335-23362

Vasquez-Vivar, J., Duquaine, D., Whitsett, J., Kalyanaraman, B. & Rajagopalan, S. (2002).Altered tetrahydrobiopterin metabolism in atherosclerosis: implications for use of oxidized tetrahydrobiopterin analogues and thiol antioxidants. *Arterioscler Thromb Vasc Biol*, 22:1655-1661

White, C.R., Darley-Usmar, V., Berrington, W.R., McAdams, M., Gore, J.Z., Thompson, J.A.,Parks, D.A., Tarpey, M.M., & Freeman, B.A. (1996). Circulating plasma xanthine oxidase contributes to vascular dysfunction in hypercholesterolemic rabbits. *Proc Natl Acad Sci USA*, 93:8745–8749

Xia, Y., Tsai, A.L., Berka, V., & Zweier, J.L. (1998). Superoxide Generation from endothelialnitric-oxide synthase. A a2+/calmodulin-dependent and tetrahydrobiopterin regulatory process. *J Biol Chem*, 273:25804-25808

Xue, H.M., He, G.W., Huang, J.H., & Yang, Q. (2010). New strategy of endothelial protectionin cardiac surgery: use of enhancer of endothelial nitric oxide synthase. *World J Surg*, 34:1461–1469

Yamawaki, H., Haendeler, J., & Berk, B.C. (2003). Thioredoxin: a key regulator ofcardiovascular homeostasis. *Circ Res*, 93:1029–1033

Yan, M.S., Matouk, C.C., & Marsden, P.A. (2010). Epigenetics of the vascular endothelium. *JAppl Physiol*, 109(3):916-926

Yang, H., Roberts, L.J., Shi, M.J., Zhou, L.C., Ballard, B.R., Richardson, A., & Guo, Z.M.(2004). Retardation of atherosclerosis by overexpression of catalase or both Cu/Zn-superoxide dismutase and catalase in mice lacking apolipoprotein E. *Circ Res*, 95:1075–1081

Young, D.V., Serebryanik, D., Janero, D.R., & Tam, S.W. (2000). Suppression of proliferationof human coronary artery smooth muscle cells by the nitric oxide donor, S-nitrosoglutathione, is cGMP-independent. *Mol Cell Biol Res Commun*, 4:32–36

Zhang, Y., Griendling, K.K., Dikalova, A., Owens, G.K., & Taylor, W.R. (2005). Vascularhypertrophy in angiotensin II-induced hypertension is mediated by vascular smooth muscle cell-derived H2O2. *Hypertension*. 46:732–737

Zou, M.H., Shi, C.,& Cohen, R.A. (2002). Oxidation of the zinc- thiolate complex anduncoupling of endothelial nitric oxide synthase by peroxynitrite. *J Clin Invest*, 109:817-826

13

An Anti-Inflammatory Approach in the Therapeutic Choices for the Prevention of Atherosclerotic Events

Aldo Pende and Andrea Denegri
Clinic of Internal Medicine 1, Department of Internal Medicine, University of Genoa School of Medicine, Genoa, Italy

1. Introduction

Atherosclerosis, with its dramatic events, represents a heavy burden in terms of morbidity and mortality throughout the entire world (Gibbons et al., 2008). Although the risk factors are very well known and addressed by every physician (genetic background, physical inactivity, hypertension, dyslipidemia, diabetes mellitus, obesity and metabolic syndrome, smoking), the precise mechanisms of the plaque formation and rupture are not completely clarified. These limitations are confirmed by the difficulties in obtaining better results in both primary and secondary prevention of cardiovascular events: recent results of completed clinical trials (such as NAVIGATOR, ACCORD, ROADMAP) suggest that we have reached a limit in terms of reducing events by simply addressing common risk factors appropriately (Zanchetti, 2009). As a matter of fact, at the present time we cannot prevent 70% of clinical events, also with administration of all well established anti-atherosclerotic therapeutics. In addition at least 10% of coronary events can occur in apparently healthy subjects in the absence of traditional risk factors (Baigent et al., 2005; Greenland et al., 2003).

The inflammatory paradigm has represented an important achievement in the understanding of the atherosclerotic process: abundant laboratory and clinical evidence accumulated over the last twenty years, also from our research group (Montecucco et al. 2010), confirming the hypothesis that inflammation exerts a major role through the different stages of atherosclerosis (Ross, 1999; Hansson, 2005; Hansson & Libby, 2006; Libby et al., 2009). Therefore it would be interesting to evaluate how the therapeutic choices exerted by physicians can modulate the inflammatory activation (the so called pleiotropic effects): in other terms do the drugs we use in the attempt of counteracting atherosclerosis (such as anti-hypertensive drugs, statins, fibrates, aspirin, anti-diabetic drugs) exert their protective effects through their main site of action (decrease of blood pressure, cholesterol, triglycerides, and glucose, anti-platelets actions) or can an additional anti-inflammatory effect be proposed, at least for some of them? This is the reason why recently Ridker proposed a clinical trial with low-dose methotrexate, a powerful anti-inflammatory drug extensively used in the treatment of auto-immune disease (suc as rheumatoid arthritis), in post-myocardial infarction (MI) patients (Ridker, 2009); another testable drug could be canakinumab, a human monoclonal antibody targeted against interleukin-1β (Libby et al., 2011).

In theory these approaches have a great appeal because their main target is represented by the basic mechanism of the atherosclerotic process, i.e. the inflammatory activation, but the risk of untoward effects can overcome the expected benefits: particularly in primary prevention the possible depression of the immune system and defense against cancer may be too dangerous in a substantially healthy population. In addition the involvement of the immune system, and consequently the inflammatory activation, is not completely elucidated because the entire network is particularly complex with many pathways, both redundant and with opposite effects, and many cells (Libby et al., 2011). Another reason for our difficulties is represented by the realization of the incomplete concordance between atherosclerosis in human vessels and the possible animal models (Bentzon & Falk, 2010): the hypotheses generated by the experimental research frequently do not find a confirmation in a clinical scenario.

The road of the anti-inflammatory approach in the treatment of atherosclerosis is paved by many defeats: table 1 tries to summarize the possible explanations.

Possible explanations	**Example**
Important side effects	NSAIDs, Corticosteroids, Torcetrapib
Activation of dangerous pathways	COX-2 inhibitors
Secondary target	Fibrates
Unfavourable effects on lipid profile	Rosiglitazone
Marked differences *in vitro* vs. *in vivo* conditions	Anti-oxidant agents
Too late and too shy treatment	All the possible options?

Table 1. Possible reasons of negative or partly successful trials for atherosclerosis

A new and theoretically safer way to modulate the inflammatory activation could involve new lipid anti-inflammatory mediators, such as lipoxins, resolvins, protectins, and maresins: these molecules derive from the transformation of both the ω-6 fatty acid arachidonic acid and the ω-3 fatty acids eicosapentaenoic acid and docosahexaenoic acid via actions of lipoxygenase, cyclooxygenase-2 and aspirin-acetylated COX-2 enzymes (Hersberger, 2010; Maskrey et al., 2011). These mediators exert significant effects favoring the resolution of the inflammatory process through the activation of a specific program, characterized by apoptosis and subsequent clearance of inflammatory cells. Again anti-inflammatory mediators are tightly linked, in terms of chemical structure and synthetic pathways, to pro-inflammatory molecules, such as leukotrienes. At the present time, among available drugs, aspirin and statins seem to be able to activate these pathways significantly (Spite & Serhan, 2010): the theoretical advantage would be represented by targeting inflammation without precipitating sustained immunosuppression.

Another important preliminary consideration is related to the ongoing debate about the appropriate timing of the beginning in anti-atherosclerotic treatments (Steinberg, 2010; Pletcher & Hulley, 2010). Although we need to never forget the fundamental role of healthy lifestyle choices, we know that some people are at potential high risk of vascular damage and consequently in this subset a more aggressive pharmacological approach can be advisable. The two opposite points of view are represented by physicians who support an aggressive therapy (at least with statins and antihypertensives, when indicated) at young age, i.e. at the beginning of the atherosclerotic process, and physicians who underline the risk of the creation of a "pseudodisease" (Lauer, 2011).

Directly linked to this topic is the role of biomarkers and vascular imaging in supporting treatment decisions: if we identify subclinical markers of atherosclerotic damage, we can use them in the prognostic stratification and consequently in rational therapeutic strategies. This consideration is an implicit criticism to the Framingham Risk Score (and other related risk calculators), a simple, relatively inexpensive, and useful way to predict cardiovascular events in the general population (Shah, 2010; Forrester, 2010). Limitations of the Framingham Risk Score include a substantial underestimation of lifetime risk and misclassification of some subgroups of subjects; in addition it does not incorporate family history and some components of the metabolic syndrome, important risk factors for coronary heart disease, and more importantly does not take into consideration the possible help of the noninvasive detection of subclinical atherosclerosis. Therefore we can reasonably affirm that Framingham Risk Score is very useful at the population level, but it remains suboptimal for individual subjects.

Subclinical atherosclerosis always begins with fatty streak lesions, which are already extensively diffuse by 30 years of age (Shah, 2010; Lauer, 2010): although we know that fatty streaks are reversible, we are also aware that this lesion is certainly the precursor of the stenotic plaque. Do we have validated imaging tools for subclinical atherosclerosis? Essentially, we can rely on coronary calcium score, obtained by computed tomography without contrast, and on carotid intima-media thickness, evaluated by B-mode ultrasonography (US). With some limitations (Shah, 2010; U.S. Preventive Services Task Force, 2009) they represent a useful aid in better classification of risk categories in human subjects: some years ago the SHAPE (Screening for Heart Attack Prevention and Education) Task Force recommended noninvasive atherosclerosis imaging of all asymptomatic men (age 45 - 75 years) and women (age 55 - 75 years), except those at very low risk, to augment conventional cardiovascular risk assessment algorithms (Naghavi et al., 2006): recently these guidelines were positively evaluated in the Dallas Heart Study, with significant bidirectional reclassification of eligibility for lipid-lowering therapy in the participants (See et al., 2008).

About serum biomarkers the role of high-sensitivity C-reactive protein (hsCRP) is well established and will be evaluated in depth for statins. Recently 30 biomarkers for atherosclerosis, or more in general cardiovascular diseases, were studied in two large cohorts totalling more than 9,000 subjects (Blankenberg et al., 2010): a consistent association with incident cardiovascular events was observed for hsCRP, B-type natriuretic peptide and cardiac troponin I. These observations allowed the development of a biomarker score which was positively validated in a cohort of male subjects.

The present article will present updated information about the anti-inflammatory effects of different classes of drugs and the possible therapeutic advantages obtained with this approach. Before starting the evaluation we need to never forget the fundamental protective role exerted by a healthy lifestyle: very recently we extensively reviewed these choices and their great social value (Pende & Dallegri, 2011). However we know that their implementation and long-term compliance is very low: a possible help is the potentiation of population-based strategies, such as smoking bans and food legislation against trans-fats and high amount of salt.

Table 2 gives some information about the clinical trials discussed in the review with full definition of the names.

Clinical trial acronym	Clinical trial name	Drugs tested
ACCORD-Lipid	Action to Control Cardiovascular Risk in Diabetes	Simvastatin, fenofibrate
AFCAPS/TexCAPS	Air Force/Texas Coronary Atherosclerosis Prevention Study	Statins
ARBITER 6-HALTS	Arterial Biology for the Investigation of the Treatment Effects of Reducing Cholesterol 6 - HDL and LDL Treatment Strategies in Atherosclerosis	Ezetimibe, niacin
ARIC	Atherosclerosis Risk in Communities	Multiple drugs
ARISE	Aggressive Reduction of Inflammation Stops Events	Succinobucol
A-to-Z	Aggrastat to Zocor	Simvastatin
CAMELOT	Comparison of Amlodipine vs Enalapril to Limit Occurrences of Thrombosis	Amlodipine, enalapril
CARE	Cholesterol and Recurrent Events	Pravastatin
DEFINE	Determining the Efficacy and Tolerability of CETP Inhibition with Anacetrapib.	Anacetrapib
HPS2-THRIVE	Treatment of High density lipoprotein to Reduce the Incidence of Vascular Events	Niacin/laropiprant
ILLUMINATE	Investigation of Lipid Level Management to Understand its Impact in Atherosclerotic Events	Torcetrapib
JUPITER	Justification for the Use of Statin in Prevention: an Intervention Trial Evaluating Rosuvastatin	Rosuvastatin
MIRACL	Myocardial Ischemia Reduction with Aggressive Cholesterol Lowering	Atorvastatin
NAVIGATOR	Nateglinide and Valsartan in Impaired Glucose Tolerance Outcomes Research	Nateglinide, valsartan
PLASMA	Phospholipase Levels And Serological Markers of Atherosclerosis	Varepladib
PROactive	Prospective Pioglitazone Clinical Trial in Macrovascular Events	Pioglitazone
PROVE IT-TIMI 22	Pravastatin or Atorvastatin Evaluation and Infection Therapy Thrombolysis in Myocardial Infarction 22	Pravastatin, atorvastatin
REVERSAL	Reversing Atherosclerosis with Aggressive Lipid Lowering	Pravastatin, atorvastatin
ROADMAP	Randomised Olmesartan and Diabetes Microalbuminuria Prevention	Olmesartan
SOLID-TIMI 52	Stabilization of Plaques Using Darapladib – Thrombolysis in Myocardial Infarction 52	Darapladib
STABILITY	Stabilization of Atherosclerotic Plaque by Initiation of Darapladib Therapy	Darapladib
VISTA-16	Vascular Inflammation Suppression to Treat Acute Coronary Syndrome for 16 Weeks	Varespladib

Table 2. Acronyms of clinical trials discussed in this review

2. HMG-CoA reductase inhibitors (statins)

Although the main mechanism of action of this class of drugs is the inhibition of the cholesterol synthesis, since the end of the last century a significant anti-inflammatory effect appeared to be present as additional explanation of the results in randomized controlled trials. The specific biomarker for inflammation was CRP and this molecule maintained its role in many different trials until present time.

Although the association between CRP and coronary artery disease was first observed more than two decades ago (Berk et al., 1990), researchers are still debating about the precise position of CRP in clinical and experimental atherosclerosis (Ridker, 2007; Schunkert & Samani, 2008; Casas et al., 2008; Nordestgaard, 2009; Anand & Yusuf, 2010; Boekholdt & Kastelein, 2010; Després, 2011; Keavney, 2011): some authors think that CRP exerts a fundamental role in the beginning of the vascular inflammatory process (for example through the activation of the classical complement pathway and enhancement of the innate immune response), instead a more conservative opinion regards CRP no more than a useful but unspecific biomarker of inflammation (an innocent bystander). In practical terms, its long half-life (about 19 h), its limited cost and possibility of replication of the assay in the follow-up without health issues for the patients represent good features. In addition CRP seems to meet most of the American Heart Association (AHA) statement criteria for use of a novel cardiovascular risk marker (proof of concept, prospective validation, incremental value beyond other risk factors, and clinical utility) (Hlatky et al., 2009). For these reasons Ridker et al. proposed and validated a new clinical risk algorithm, Reynolds risk score for both women (Ridker at al., 2007) and men (Ridker et al., 2008a), which incorporates information on both inflammation (hsCRP) and genetics (parental history of premature MI). The utility of hsCRP for risk reclassification was confirmed also in the Framingham Heart Study (Wilson et al., 2008).

Statins can exert their anti-inflammatory role through different effects: the combined actions are called pleiotropic effects and are abundantly reviewed in the literature (C.Y. Wang et al., 2007; Ludman et al., 2009). The main mechanism seems to be always related to the inhibition of HMG-CoA reductase enzyme, involved in the rate-limiting step in cholesterol biosynthesis, but also in the production of isoprenoid intermediates, such as farnesyl-pyrophosphate and geranyl-geranyl-pyrophosphate: these molecules are important for the post-translational modification of small GTP-binding proteins Ras, Rac, and Rho, which are known to modulate vascular smooth muscle cell proliferation, platelet aggregation, and plaque stability.

Returning to statin trials, CARE study of secondary prevention was able to demonstrate, in a post hoc analysis, that pravastatin decreased CRP levels significantly in comparison to placebo; this decrease did not correlate with the reduction in cholesterol levels (Ridker et al., 1999). Few years later similar results were obtained in a primary prevention study, the AFCAPS/TexCAPS trial (Ridker et al., 2001): an interesting observation was the absence of clinical benefits in subjects with low density lipoprotein (LDL)-cholesterol <150 mg/dl and hsCRP levels <2 mg/l, instead a significant benefit was found in those with LDL-cholesterol levels <150 mg/dl and hsCRP >2 mg/l. Further studies, such as MIRACL (Kinlay et al., 2003), REVERSAL (Nissen et al., 2005), A to Z (Morrow et al., 2006), and PROVE IT-TIMI 22(Ridker et al., 2005), demonstrated effects of statins on CRP. Again in all these studies the statin-induced reductions of CRP and LDL-cholesterol levels were only weakly correlated, whereas the decrease in CRP was correlated with slowed atherosclerosis progression, in an independent way with respect to LDL-cholesterol decrease. In PROVE IT-TIMI 22 and in A to Z trials the best outcomes were observed in individuals who reached both LDL-cholesterol levels <70 mg/dl and hsCRP <2.0 mg/l. Therefore the concept of a "dual target" for statin therapy (LDL-cholesterol and CRP) was introduced.

A step forward was represented by the JUPITER trial (Ridker et al., 2008b). JUPITER was a large, double-blind, placebo-controlled trial, multinational, primary prevention trial, which recruited 17,802 apparently healthy subjects with entry criteria of less than 130 mg/dl for LDL-cholesterol levels and hs-CRP levels of 2.0 mg/dl or higher. Subjects were randomly assigned to 20 mg/d of rosuvastatin or placebo and continued their usual standard care; the primary end point was a combination of MI, stroke, arterial revascularization, hospitalization for unstable angina, or death from cardiovascular causes.

The trial was terminated prematurely, after a mean of only 1.9 years of follow-up by an indipendent data and safety monitoring board. The absolute risk reduction was 1.2%, with the primary endpoint occurring in 2.8% of subjects in the placebo arm versus 1.6% of subjects in the rosuvastatin arm. The active treatment reduced the risk for first MI by 55%, the risk for venous thromboembolism by 52%, the need for coronary artery bypass grafting (CABG) or percutaneous coronary intervention (PCI) by 47%, and total mortality by 20%. On the basis of the Kaplan-Meier estimates and with a forward projection of the results, about 25 subjects would have to be treated for 5 years to prevent one primary endpoint. This estimate is very favourable, compared to trials evaluating statins in hyperlipidemic patients, where the 5-year number needed to treat patients was between 44 and 65; more strikingly in hypertension treatment the 5-year number needed to treat patients ranged between 86 and 140. The treatment with rosuvastatin was well tolerated even at very low attained levels of LDL-cholesterol (less than 50 mg/dl) with consequent lower risk of cardiovascular events (Hsia et al., 2011). Moreover the study demonstrated a 43% reduction in venous thrombosis. Another limited but important finding was the increase in the rate of diabetes mellitus as well as a small, significant increase in the median value of glycated hemoglobin: this observation was confirmed in a recent meta-analysis of 13 statin trials which showed a 9% increased risk of development of diabetes associated with statin therapy (Sattar et al., 2010).

The publication of the JUPITER trial spurred intense debate, sometimes with harsh criticisms to the authors (de Lorgeril et al., 2010; Kaul et al., 2010): the main points were the too early termination (with possible overestimation of the results), unprecise definitions of the endpoints (in particular about mortality), the undertreatment for the usual care of the involved patients, the increased health costs of this preventive approach, the excessive role of the pharmaceutical company. The trial however survived to the critics and convinced the United States Food and Drug Administration to approve the indication of rosuvastatin for reduction of acute MI, stroke, CABG, and PCI in men >50 years of age and women >60 years of age with hsCRP levels ≥2 mg/l who also have 1 additional cardiovascular risk factor. In addition in 2009 Canadian Cardiovascular Society guidelines included the results of the JUPITER trial recommending that also subjects at intermediate risk, defined as 10 - 20% risk at 10 years by Framingham criteria, should be treated with a statin when hsCRP is >2 mg/l.

JUPITER conclusions were similar to the results subsequently obtained in the ARIC study (Yang et al., 2009), again showing that, starting with individuals at highest risk, the relative cardiovascular event rates are high LDL-cholesterol + high CRP > high CRP + low LDL-cholesterol > high LDL-cholesterol + low CRP > low LDL-cholesterol + low CRP.

Another cholesterol-lowering drug, frequently administered with a statin, is ezetimibe, an inhibitor of the intestinal cholesterol transporter Niemann-Pick C1-like protein (NPC1L1): this drug can reduce LDL-cholesterol levels by almost 20% in individuals already taking a statin. However no clinical trial results have so far demonstrated that this combination will reduce cardiovascular events in comparison with statins only. In terms of anti-inflammatory effects ezetimibe per se did not reduce CRP levels, but it was able to help statin in decreasing CRP more deeply (Al Badarin et al., 2009).

3. High Density Lipoprotein (HDL)-modulating agents

Main focus of anti-atherosclerotic therapy is correctly the decrease in LDL-cholesterol levels. Although the success in terms of cardiovascular prevention was outstanding, we know that it is limited: as already stated, no more than 25-30% relative risk reduction was observed in statin monotherapy trials with a large amount of individuals in the active arm still suffering a cardiovascular event. This can be related to the different levels attained for LDL-cholesterol in the trials with progressive updates of the international guidelines for atherosclerosis with the motto "lower for LDL-cholesterol is always better" (Grundy, 2008), but undoubtedly a residual risk is still present: "lower LDL-cholesterol is better but it is not enough" (Superko & King III, 2008).

Another related observation, based on arteriographic findings, is the positive significant effect of statins on the decrease in the rate of atherosclerotic progression but the absent effect on any regression, something demonstrated on the contrary with a combined treatment (LDL-cholesterol reduction + HDL-cholesterol increase) (Superko & King III, 2008). This was confirmed recently by the conclusions of the ARBITER 6-Halts study which compared the effects of ezetimibe, an inhibitor of cholesterol absorption, and extended-release niacin in high risk patients already with statin therapy: the primary end point was the change in the intima-media thickness of common carotid artery (Taylor et al., 2009). Niacin was significantly superior to ezetimibe in the primary end point, suggesting again that the addition of a HDL-cholesterol raising drug to a statin is superior to a further LDL-cholesterol decreasing strategy.

Although a recent meta-analysis has suggested that increasing HDL-cholesterol does not reduce the risk of cardiovascular events in human subjects (Briel et al., 2009), animal studies have provided strong evidence that HDL-cholesterol is protective (Haas & Mooradian, 2011). HDL exerts a key role in the reverse cholesterol transport, whereby cholesterol is transported from peripheral cells to the liver and consequently fostering the removal of this molecule from the lipid-laden macrophages at the vascular level. In addition HDL particles have been shown to be involved in direct anti-oxidative, anti-apoptotic, anti-thrombotic, and also anti-inflammatory functions (Tabet & Rye, 2009), suggesting further protection against the atherosclerotic process. However we need to be aware that, during the inflammatory activation, HDL particles can shift to a "dysfunctional" setting, showing on the contrary pro-inflammatory properties (Säemann et al., 2010): therefore the functional properties of HDL reflect its role more appropriately than mere serum concentrations.

At the present time, among HDL-cholesterol-increasing drugs, niacin (nicotinic acid) is the most effective agent, raising HDL-cholesterol by 20-30% (Farmer, 2009) with an important side effect (flushing), which can be attenuated by both an extended-release formulation (Knopp et al., 1998) and a combination with a prostaglandin D2 receptor 1 antagonist, laropiprant (Perry, 2009). The results of the HPS2-THRIVE ongoing study will give us important information about the therapeutic role of this combination in the prevention of cardiovascular events. In the meantime we already know that niacin exerts direct anti-inflammatory effects, in particular an anti-oxidant and a CRP-decreasing activity (Sanyal et al., 2007; Thoenes et al., 2007).

The most effective way to increase HDL-cholesterol was thought to be the inhibition of the cholesteryl ester transfer protein (CETP), the enzyme responsible for the transfer of cholesteryl esters from HDL particles to very low-density lipoproteins and LDLs (Barter & Kastelein, 2006). The first developed CETP-inhibitor was torcetrapib, which was evaluated in the ILLUMINATE trial (Barter et al., 2007): in this study patients at high cardiovascular risk were randomly assigned to receive either torcetrapib + atorvastatin or placebo + atorvastatin. Despite the very favourable lipid changes obtained in the torcetrapib arm (a 72% increase in HDL-cholesterol and a 25% decrease in LDL-cholesterol), the rate of major cardiovascular events was increased by 25% and the deaths from cardiovascular causes by 40%; all-cause mortality was increased by 58% and an increase in blood pressure and aldosterone levels, therefore unrelated to CETP inhibition, was also observed in the active arm. Whereas the pressor and aldosterone-stimulating effects could explain the cardiovascular results, it was harder to understand the increased rate of deaths from noncardiovascular causes induced by torcetrapib: the increase was due to more deaths from cancers and infections. Since CETP inhibition alters the size and the composition of the HDL particles (Barter & Kastelein, 2006), these qualitative changes could predispose to an increased susceptibility to neoplasms and infections.

These negative results did not stop the development of other drugs of the same class: very recently the safety of anacetrapib was positively evaluated in the DEFINE study (Cannon et al., 2010) and the increased HDL particles exhibited a strong ability to suppress macrophage toll-like receptor 4-mediated inflammatory responses (Yvan-Charlet et al., 2010). A more direct way to stimulate the reverse cholesterol transport is the infusion of reconstituted HDL or Apo A-I mimetic peptides: with both therapeutic approaches a potent anti-inflammatory effect was observed (Natarajan et al., 2010).

4. Anti-platelet agents

Atherosclerotic thrombotic events are always characterized by an important inflammatory activation which is a consequence of the release of chemokines and cytokines from the platelets (Gurbel et al., 2009); however platelets are also involved in the initiation and the early progression of atherosclerosis mediating leukocyte recruitment and adhesion to the vascular wall (Antoniades et al., 2010). Many markers of platelet activation are currently investigated: in this context prospective studies and meta-analysis suggest a correlation between an increase in mean platelet volume and the risk of thrombosis (Gasparyan et al., 2011); in addition the soluble form of CD40 ligand has been studied in sera of human subjects and seems to have a prognostic role in atherothrombosis (Antoniades et al., 2010).

The most used anti-platelet drug, aspirin, is able to decrease serum CRP and patients with the highest baseline CRP levels derives the greatest benefit from this drug.

Trials of cardiovascular prevention with aspirin do not always confirm the positive effects of an anti-thrombotic approach, at least in the primary setting: also recently updated guidelines suggest judicious use of anti-platelet drug (Bell et al., 2011). The limited protective effects of aspirin have led to the concept of aspirin resistance (Gasparyan et al., 2008).

5. Phospholipase A_2 and ACAT inhibitors

In atherosclerosis the interactions between lipoprotein metabolism and inflammation are modulated by the complex phospholipase A_2 (PLA_2) superfamily. This family comprises five types of enzymes, of which the secretory PLA_2 ($sPLA_2$) and the lipoprotein-associated PLA_2 (Lp-PLA_2) have been associated with atherogenesis (Garcia-Garcia & Serruys, 2009). These enzymes catalyze the hydrolysis of the centre (sn-2) ester bond of phospholipids to produce non-esterified fatty acids (in particular arachidonic acid) and lysophospholipids (lysophosphatidylcholine): the atherogenic consequences are the formation of smaller and denser HDL and LDL particles, the formation of vascular LDL aggregates, the increased LDL oxidation, the synthesis of potent inflammatory lipid mediators such as prostaglandins and leukotrienes (Rosenson, 2009). Therefore inhibitors of the types of PLA_2 have been developed and have reached the phase III clinical evaluation, one for LpPLA2 (darapladib) and one for sPLA2 (varespladib).

In human studies darapladib induced a small but significant decrease in the inflammatory markers hsCRP and interleukin-6 with no changes in plasma lipid levels. In the IBIS-2 trial after 12 months the drug did not affect the primary end point, coronary plaque volume evaluated by intravascular ultrasound (IVUS); however necrotic core size remained unchanged in the active arm but increased in those treated with placebo (Boekholdt et al., 2008). Darapladib is now being evaluated in two large placebo-controlled cardiovascular outcome studies - STABILITY and SOLID-TIMI 52. As for varespladib, in the PLASMA Phase II the drug was demonstrated to induce a decrease in both oxidized LDL and CRP; an ongoing Phase III cardiovascular outcome study (VISTA-16) have recruited high risk patients.

Another important enzyme involved in the cellular cholesterol metabolism is acyl-coenzyme A:cholesterol acyltransferase (ACAT): this protein is able to catalyse cholesteryl ester formation by transfer of fatty acyl chain from acyl-coenzyme A to cholesterol. Two isozymes are present, one expressed in macrophages in atherosclerotic lesions (ACAT-1) and the other mainly expressed in small intestine (ACAT-2): therefore nonselective pharmacological inhibition of ACAT was expected to exert a double favourable effect, suppressing both foam cell formation in arterial walls and cholesterol intestinal absorption. Unfortunately results of the studies in human subjects were disappointing: avasimibe and pactimibe, the two nonselective ACAT inhibitors developed for clinical use, gave null or negative results (Fazio & Linton, 2006). Very recently a potent and selective ACAT-1 inhibitor, K-604, with significant anti-atherosclerotic effects *in vitro* and in experimental animals, entered a Phase II trial (Yoshinaka et al., 2010).

6. Leukotriene pathway inhibitors

Leukotrienes (LTs) belong to the family of eicosanoids and exert potent pro-inflammatory smooth muscle constrictive actions. It is well known their involvement in many inflammatory and allergic diseases, such as rheumatoid arthritis, inflammatory bowel disease, and bronchial asthma. Initially a leukotriene receptor blocker, i.e. montelukast, was administered to acute coronary syndrome patients to evaluate the endothelial function in brachial artery (clinicaltrials.gov NCT00351364, data unpublished). Subsequently inhibitors of both 5-lipoxygenase (5-LO) (atreleuton) and 5-lipoxygenase activating protein (FLAP) (veliflapon) were studied in human subjects. Atreleuton, a potent 5-LO inhibitor, was administered in acute coronary syndrome patients for 24 weeks and was able to reduce both the appearance of new coronary plaques and the volume of noncalcified plaques in comparison with placebo; these effects were paralleled by a 66% reduction of hsCRP (Tardif et al., 2010). Instead veliflapon, a weak FLAP inhibitor, induced a decrease in LTB4 production and myeloperoxidase activity with a nonsignificant reduction in CRP (Hakonarson et al., 2005).

7. CCR2 blockade

One of the main players in the inflammatory cascade induced by the atherosclerotic changes is chemokine CC motif ligand 2 (CCL2), also known as monocyte chemoattractant protein-1: this chemokine, through the interaction with its receptor chemokine receptor 2 (CCR2), efficiently induces the recruitment of circulating blood monocytes to become plaque macrophages. Very recently MLN1202, a highly specific humanized monoclonal antibody that recognizes CCR2 and inhibits CCL2 binding, was evaluated in a randomized, double-blind, placebo-controlled trial: the main aim was to measure possible decrease in hsCRP with the active treatment in cardiovascular high-risk patients (Gilbert et al., 2011). The results of this preliminary study confirmed a significant 26% reduction in the inflammatory marker, but obviously we need to perform outcome studies in order to establish a role of this new therapeutic approach in the treatment of atherosclerosis.

8. Peroxisome Proliferator-Activated Receptor (PPAR) agonists and Polyunsaturated Fatty Acids (PUFAs)

PPARs are ligand-activated transcription factors belonging to the nuclear receptor superfamily (Oyekan, 2011). Through cellular mechanisms called transactivation, binding of PPAR/nuclear retinoid receptor (RXR) heterodimers to PPAR response elements (PPREs) in the promoter region of target genes, and transrepression, interference with transcription factors such as nuclear factor-kB (NF-kB) and activator protein-1 (AP-1), these transcription factors exert multiple and complex effects involving the regulation of the vascular tone, inflammation and metabolism. The PPAR family consists of three isoforms, α, γ, and β/δ, which possess distinct functions, with corresponding agonists.

PPAR-α agonists (fibric acid derivatives = fibrates) have demonstrated potentially very favourable effects on serum lipids with a significant decrease in triglyceride levels and more modest effects on LDL-cholesterol (a decrease) and HDL-cholesterol (an increase); in addition LDL size is modified with a decrease of more atherogenic small dense particles. All these positive changes are theoretically complementary to those induced by statins

(Abourbih et al., 2009) and are paralleled by a significant anti-inflammatory modulation, as demonstrated both *in vitro* and *in vivo* (Adameova et al., 2009). Despite these considerations and the long time of clinical evaluation (more than 30 years in Europe), considerable controversy still remains about therapeutic efficacy, also after recent reevaluation (Jun et al., 2010; Goldfine et al., 2011).

The same negative results were observed in the ACCORD-Lipid substudy which compared a statin monotherapy with a combination therapy with a statin + a fibrate in type 2 diabetic patients, who are the population with the theoretical maximal advantage from the combination (Ginsberg et al., 2010). However a prespecified analysis showed a 31% reduction in the primary end point (nonfatal MI, nonfatal stroke, or death from cardiovascular causes) in the subgroup of patients with the most negative metabolic profile (baseline triglyceride levels >204 mg/dl and HDL-cholesterol levels <34 mg/dl).

PPAR-γ agonists (thiazolidinediones = glitazones) was known as anti-inflammatory agents for a long time (Duan et al., 2009): two molecules are available for administration in humans, pioglitazone and rosiglitazone. They have a specific therapeutic indication for type 2 diabetes mellitus due to their improvement in insulin sensitivity, supporting the interpretation of type 2 diabetes mellitus as an auto-inflammatory disease (Dinarello, 2010; N. Wang et al., 2011). *In vitro,* in human blood monocytes, pioglitazone reduces synthesis of IL-1β, tumor necrosis factor (TNF)-α, IL-6, MCP-1, Toll-like receptors (TLRs) (Dasu et al., 2009). Also *in vivo,* in human subjects, pioglitazone exerts potent anti-inflammatory effects with a significant decrease in hsCRP levels in both diabetic and nondiabetic individuals (Pfützner et al., 2010).

Like fibrates, cardiovascular end points evaluated in large randomized studies with glitazones gave disappointing results. The only published outcome trial with this group of drugs is the PROactive trial (Dormandy et al., 2005): in this study pioglitazone induced a nonsignificant reduction in the primary end point (a composite of death, nonfatal MI, stroke, major leg amputation, acute coronary syndrome, and coronary or leg revascularization); however the principal secondary end point (a composite of all-cause death, nonfatal MI, and stroke) was significantly reduced by 16%. On the contrary in different trials rosiglitazone gave some suspicions about detrimental effects on cardiovascular events: a large meta-analysis concluded that this drug may increase the risk of cardiovascular events (MI, death) (Nissen & Wolski, 2007), possibly through a more favourable effect of pioglitazone on the lipid profile (Goldberg et al., 2005). A possible step forward in the development of PPARs is the evaluation of a dual α/γ agonist: after the withdrawal of muraglitazar and tesaglitazar for important toxicities, aleglitazar is currently being investigated in type 2 diabetic patients (Paras et al., 2010).

Other drugs which are able to decrease triglyceride levels are omega-3 fatty acids: the attempt to copy Eskimo diet was successful in the secondary prevention of cardiovascular diseases with important complex anti-inflammatory effects, which probably involve the above mentioned mediators resolvins (De Caterina, 2011).

9. Succinobucol and fasudil

Another possible target for atherosclerosis treatment is represented by the blockade of the oxidative stress, and in particular of the oxidation of lipoproteins (Libby et al., 2011): this was the reason why anti-oxidant vitamins (vitamin C and E) were evaluated in randomized controlled trials, unfortunately with no success (Kris-Etherton et al., 2004). Two drugs exert similar potent *in vitro* anti-oxidant effects and have been studied in atherosclerotic patients: succinobucol and fasudil. Succinobucol is a derivative of probucol, previously withdrawn at Phase III evaluation for safety concerns, with well-demonstrated anti-inflammatory and anti-oxidant effects in endothelial and blood mononuclear cells (Kunsch et al., 2004). The ARISE trial recently examined the effects of succinobucol on cardiovascular events in patients with a recent acute coronary syndrome: there was no significant difference in the primary end point (cardiovascular death, resuscitated cardiac arrest, MI, stroke, unstable angina, or coronary revascularization); the composite secondary end point of cardiovascular death, MI, cardiac arrest and stroke was 19% lower in the succinobucol arm compared to placebo and reached statistical significance (Tardif et al., 2008). Another interesting observation of the study, tertiary end point, was the 63% relative reduction in the onset of new diabetes, related to a reduction in glycosilated haemoglobin in diabetic patients.

Fasudil is an inhibitor of Rho-kinase, an important downstream effector of the small GTP-binding protein RhoA (Satoh et al., 2011). It has been demonstrated that the RhoA/Rho-kinase pathway exerts a specific role in the pathogenesis of vasospasm, atherosclerosis, ischemia-reperfusion injury, hypertension, stroke, and heart failure. Fasudil is already marketed in Japan for the acute treatment of cerebral vasospasm but the possible additional indications in human subjects are not completely established (Zhou et al., 2011).

10. Anti-hypertensive drugs

Despite intensive research the pathogenesis of hypertension, the leading risk factor of death in the entire world (Ezzati et al., 2002), remains elusive. The hypothesis of a low-grade inflammatory activation could explain many aspects of the hypertensive process and therefore is actively investigated (Harrison et al., 2011; Leibowitz & Schiffrin, 2011; Montecucco et al., 2011). If we can translate these observation to the clinical ground, the therapeutic strategies should keep account of possible anti-inflammatory modulations of the hypotensive drugs adding more fuel to the controversy about the protective role exerted by the blood pressure reduction *per se* or the presence of additional pleiotropic actions of some classes of drugs with respect to others: "outcomes beyond blood pressure control?" (Sever et al., 2006; Staessen et al., 2010). In this context the renin-angiotensin system inhibitors (angiotensin-converting enzyme inhibitors, angiotensin II receptor blockers, renin inhibitors) could be the best choice since the fundamental role of this system in the activation of the vascular inflammation is widely demonstrated (Marchesi et al., 2008): this is confirmed by the *in vivo* demonstration of a significant decrease of various inflammatory markers induced by these drugs (reviewed in Montecucco et al., 2009).

However, the most comprehensive guidelines for the treatment of hypertension do not consider an inflammation-based approach: on the contrary the updated versions of the European Society of Hypertension/European Society of Cardiology guidelines did not confirm the role of CRP as a cardiovascular risk factor for the prognostic stratification, as proposed in the first edition (Mancia et al., 2007). All the hypertension guidelines emphasize the control of blood pressure levels as the main target for the therapeutic choices, without a classification of the different available drugs and suggesting that frequently we need to prefer a drug combination to improve effectiveness and limit side effects. In terms of the atherosclerotic process a partial confirmation of this approach comes from the IVUS substudy of the CAMELOT trial which demonstrated a significant slowing in the progression of the atheroma volume with a calcium-antagonist (amlodipine, a potent and possibly more effective hypotensive drug) compared to an angiotensin-converting enzyme inhibitor (enalapril) (Nissen et al., 2004).

11. Immunosuppressive agents

In this section we will discuss the anti-atherosclerotic effects of drugs developed for immunosuppression and therefore without a primary metabolic action. In terms of immunosuppression nothing is more powerful and studied than corticosteroids (Rhen & Cidlowski, 2005). 35 years ago corticosteroid administration was shown to exert deleterious effects in patients with MI (Roberts et al., 1976); however very recently oral prednisone was used successfully to prevent restenosis after PCI with bare metal stents in comparison with bare metal stents alone(better event-free survival) and drug-eluting stents (similar outcome) (Ribichini et al., 2011).

As discussed in the introduction, a proof-of-concept for the role of inflammation in the atherosclerotic process would be a clinical trial with well tolerated anti-inflammatory drugs, devoid of metabolic effects: methotrexate and canakinumab could be good choices and have been proposed recently.

For other drugs the tolerability in uncomplicated atherosclerotic subjects could be more problematic with a disadvantageous risk-benefit ratio, but their potentially positive cardiovascular effects in patients with a specific immunosuppressive indication can be carefully monitored in clinical trials for post hoc analysis (Westlake et al., 2010). Another possible application is the administration of these drugs for a limited period of time (e.g. for a few days after PCI).

TNF-α antagonists are extensively used in autoimmune diseases with a significant cardiovascular protection (Tracey et al., 2008), possibly related to the pivotal role of this cytokine in vascular dysfunction: recently, in a population of subjects who underwent carotid endarterectomy for a significant stenosis, we found an increase in TNF-α plasma levels in symptomatic patients for an ischemic cerebrovascular event with respect to asymptomatic patients (Montecucco et al., 2010). TNF-α antagonists have been evaluated in vascular disorders accompanying chronic disordes (Crohn' s disease and rheumatoid arthritis) with the demonstration of improvement in endothelial function (Schinzari et al., 2008; Hürlimann et al., 2002). In addition to the anti-inflammatory effects, these drugs also induce a favourable lipid profile with an increase in HDL-cholesterol and apolipoprotein A-I (van Eijk et al., 2009).

IL-1 seems to exert a central role in the intense inflammatory response which follows a MI. Using a recombinant form of the naturally occurring antagonist (anakinra), a pilot study was recently performed to test the safety and effects of this drug on post-MI left ventricular remodelling and CRP serum levels (Abbate et al., 2010). Anakinra was able to mitigate significantly left ventricular remodelling, evaluated with both cardiac magnetic resonance and echocardiography, and the changes in CRP levels correlated with the changes in cardiac anatomy.

Another new important inflammatory pathway involves p38 mitogen-activated protein kinase (MAPK). This phosphorylation cascade can be activated by a vascular injury, such as coronary stenting with subsequent neointimal proliferation and in-stent restenosis (Schieven, 2005), and represents an important intracellular switch for the production of key inflammatory cytokines (IL-1β, TNF-α, and IL-6), inflammatory enzyme cyclooxygenase-2 and matrix metalloproteases. Recently a p38 MAPK inhibitor (dilmapimod, SB-681323) has been shown to significantly attenuate the inflammatory activation induced by a PCI procedure with positive consequences in post-procedural outcomes (Sarov-Blat et al., 2010).

Interesting observations came from the administration of the immunosuppressive drug mycophenolate mofetil in atherosclerotic patients for a limited period of time: the drug, devoid of effects on both serum lipids and blood pressure, was able to attenuate cellular and biochemical inflammatory activation in the unstable carotid plaques of patients who subsequently underwent endarterectomy for advanced stenosis (van Leuven et al., 2006; Van Leuven et al., 2010). At the very beginning of the clinical evaluation are the inhibitors of Toll-like receptors, involved in the innate immune response (Hennessy et al., 2010; Cole & Monaco, 2010).

12. Conclusion

Recently the title of an editorial in Circulation was "Could direct inhibition of inflammation be the *next big thing* in treating atherosclerosis?" (Natarajan & Cannon, 2010). This is certainly a fascinating strategy because it tries to exert a fully pathogenetic approach, though we need not to forget the frustrations, caused by so many disappointing results. In this context we know that it is not always wise to found our evaluation on surrogate end points: only randomized controlled trials with cardiovascular hard end points can give the final answer.

Take-home messages

- Lifestyle choices are an essential part of the cardiovascular prevention and physicians must exert every effort to obtain a good compliance from patients
- In terms of therapeutic control of the different risk factors physicians must reach better results
- At the present time physicians have to focus at the single risk factors with the awareness that the inflammatory activation is important for the atherosclerotic process
- hsCRP represents a useful marker of inflammation and an excellent support for the prognostic stratification
- Additional help can derive from carotid US and coronary calcium score
- In the context of blockade of the inflammatory activation statins and RAS-inhibitors offer good choices in terms of safety and effectiveness
- Specific ant-inflammatory drugs need to be carefully evaluated with appropriate trials
- At the present time these drugs may be useful for a limited period of time (e.g.: after a PCI)
- Intense investigation on this topic will certainly suggest new therapeutic targets and strategies

In this review we tried to give an update of the experimental and clinical data with already marketed drugs or with Phase III therapeutic principles but we did not discuss the possible use of an immunomodulating (not immunosuppressive) approach: expansion of regulatory

T cells, a subset of T lymphocytes with a well demonstrated anti-inflammatory role, and atherosclerosis-specific immunization are thought as promising therapeutic opportunities and are actively investigated (Klingerberg & Hansson, 2009; van Puijvelde et al., 2008).

Although at the present time the physicians are confident with the use of drugs developed for particular aspects of the atherosclerotic spectrum (decrease of blood pressure, decrease in LDL-cholesterol, increase in HDL-cholesterol, decrease in glucose, etc.), the "unfinished business" of cardiovascular prevention (Libby, 2005) drives our efforts to find new targets and strategies against the pernicious activation of inflammation in atherosclerosis.

13. Acknowledgments

This work was supported by grant n. 2008.0812-132 from Fondazione Carige.

The authors declare that they have no conflicts of interest.

14. References

Abbate A., Kontos M., Grizzard J.D., Biondi-Zoccai G.G.L., Van Tassel B.W., Robati R., Roach L.M., Arena R.A., Roberts C.S., Varma A., Gelwix C.C., Salloum F.N., Hastillo A., Dinarello C.A., & Vetrovec G.W. (2010). Interleukin-1 blockade with anakinra to prevent adverse cardiac remodeling after acute myocardial infarction (Virginia Commonwealth University Anakinra Remodeling Trial [VCU-ART] Pilot Sudy). *American Journal of Cardiology,* Vol.105, No.10, (May 2010), pp. 1371-1377, ISSN 1879-1913

Abourbih S., Filion K.B., Joseph L., Schiffrin E.L., Rinfret S., Poirier P., Pilote L., Genest J., & Eisenberg M.J. (2009). Effect of fibrates on lipid profiles and cardiovascular outcomes: a systematic review. *American Journal of Medicine,* Vol.122, No.10, (August 2009), pp. 962e1-962e8, ISSN 1555-7162

Adameova A., Xu Y.J., Duhamel T.A., Tappia P.S., Shan L., & Dhalla N.S. (2009). Anti-atherosclerotic molecules targeting oxidative stress and inflammation. *Current Pharmaceutical Design,* Vol.15, No.27, (2009), pp. 3094-3107, ISSN 1381-6128

Al Badarin F.J., Kullo I.J., Kopecky S.L., & Thomas R.J. (2009). Impact of ezetimibe on atherosclerosis: is the jury still out? *Mayo Clinic Proceedings,* Vol.84, No.4, (April 2009), pp. 353-361, ISSN 1942-5546

Anand S.S., & Yusuf S. (2010). C-reactive protein is a bystander of cardiovascular disease. *European Heart Journal,* Vol.31, No.17, (July 2010), pp. 2092-2097, ISSN 1522-9645

Antoniades C., Bakogiannis C., Tousoulis D., Demosthenous M., Marinou K., & Stefanadis C. (2010). Platelet activation in atherogenesis associated with low-grade inflammation. Inflammation and Allergy Drug Targets, Vol.9, No.5, (December 2010), pp. 334-345, ISSN 1871-5281

Baigent C., Keech A., Kearney P.M., Blackwell L., Buck G., Pollicino C., Kirby A., Sourjina T., Peto R., Collins R., & Simes R. (2005). Efficacy and safety of cholesterol-lowering treatment: prospective meta-analysis of data from 90,056 participants in 14 randomised trials of statins. *Lancet,* Vol.366, No.9494, (June 2005), pp. 1267-1278, ISSN 1474-547X

Barter P.J., & Kastelein J.J.P. (2006). Targeting cholesteryl ester transfer protein for the prevention and management of cardiovascular disease. *Journal of the American College of Cardiology*, Vol.47, No.3, (February 2006), pp. 492-499, ISSN 1558-3597

Barter P.J., Caulfield M., Eriksson M., Grundy S.M., Kastelein J.J.P., Komajda M., Lopez-Sendon J., Mosca L., Tardif J.C., Waters D.D., Shear C.L., Revkin J.H., Buhr K.A., Fisher M., Tall A.R., & Brewer B. (2007). Effects of torcetrapib in patients at high risk for coronary events. *New England Journal of Medicine*, Vol.357, No.21, (November 2007), pp. 2109-2122, ISSN 1533-4406

Bell A.D., Roussin A., Cartier R., Chan W.S., Douketis J.D., Gupta A., Kraw M.E., Lindsay T.F., Love M.P., Pannu N., Rabasa-Lhoret R., Shuaib A., Teal P., Theroux P., Turpie A.G., Welsh R.C., & Tanguay J.F. (2011). The use of antiplatelet therapy in the outpatient setting: Canadian Cardiovascular Society guidelines executive summary. *Canadian Journal of Cardiology*, Vol.27, No.2, (March 2011), pp. 208-221, ISSN 1916-7075

Bentzon J.F., & Falk E. (2010). Atherosclerotic lesions in mouse and man: is it the same disease? *Current Opinion in Lipidology*, Vol.21, No.5, (October 2010), pp. 434-440, ISSN 1473-6535

Berk B.C., Weintraub, W.S., & Alexander R.W. (1990). Elevation of C-reactive protein in "active" coronary artery disease. *American Journal of Cardiology*, Vol.65, No.3, (January 1990), pp. 168-172, ISSN 1879-1913

Blankenberg S., Zeller T., Saarela O., Havulinna A.S., Kee F., Tunstall-Pedoe H., Kuulasmaa K., Yarnell J., Schnabel R.B., Wild P.S., Münzel T.F., Lackner K.J., Tiret L., Evans A., & Salomaa V. (2010). Contribution of 30 biomarkers to 10-year cardiovascular risk estimation in 2 population cohorts: the MONICA, risk, genetics, archiving, and monograph (MORGAM) biomarker project. *Circulation*, Vol.121, No.22, (June 2010), pp. 2388-2397, ISSN 1524-4539

Boekholdt S.M., de Winter R.J., & Kastelein J.J.P. (2008). Inhibition of lipoprotein-associated phospholipase activity by darapladib. Shifting gears in cardiovascular drug development: are anti-inflammatory drugs the next frontier? *Circulation*, Vol.118, No.11, (September 2008), pp. 1120-1122, ISSN 1524-4539

Boekholdt S.M., & Kastelein J.J.P. (2010). C-reactive protein and cardiovascular risk: more fuel to the fire. *Lancet*, Vol.375, No.9709, (January 2010), pp. 95-96, ISSN 1474-547X

Briel M., Ferreira-Gonzalez I., You J.J., Karanicolas P.J., Akl E.A., Wu P., Blechacz B., Bassler D., Wei X., Sharman A., Whitt I., Alves da Silva S., Khalid Z., Nordmann A.J., Zhou Q., Walter S.D., Vale N., Bhatnagar N., O'Regan C., Mills E.J., Bucher H.C., Montori V.M., & Guyatt G.H. (2009). Association between change in high density lipoprotein cholesterol and cardiovascular disease morbidity and mortality: systematic review and meta-regression analysis. *British Medical Journal*, Vol.338, No.92, (February 2009), doi:10.1136/bmj.b92, ISSN 1468-5833

Cannon C.P., Shah S., Dansky H.M., Davidson M., Brinton E.A., Gotto A.M., Stepanavage M., Liu S.X., Gibbons P., Ashraf T.B., Zafarino J., Mitchel Y., & Barter P. (2010). Safety of anacetrapib in patients with or at high risk of coronary heart disease. *New England Journal of Medicine*, Vol.363, No.25, (December 2010), pp. 2406-2415, ISSN 1533-4406

Casas J.P., Shah T., Hingorani A.D., Danesh J., & Pepys M.B. (2008). C-reactive protein and coronary heart disease: a critical review. *Journal of Internal Medicine*, Vol.264, No.4, (October 2008), pp. 295-314, ISSN 1365-2796

Cole J.E., & Monaco C. (2010). Treating atherosclerosis: the potential of Toll-like receptors as therapeutic target. *Expert Review of Cardiovascular Therapy*, Vol.8, No.11, (November 2010), pp. 1619-1635, ISSN 1477-9072

Dasu M., Park S., Devaraj S., & Jialal I. (2009). Pioglitazone inhibits Toll-like receptor expression and activity in human monocytes and db/db mice. *Endocrinology*, Vol.150, No.8, (August 2009), pp. 3457-3464, ISSN 1945-7170

De Caterina R. (2011). n-3 fatty acids in cardiovascular disease. *New England Journal of Medicine*, Vol.364, No.25, (June 2011), pp. 2439-2450, ISSN 1533-4406

de Lorgeril M., Salen P., Abramson J., Dodin S., Hamazaki T., Kostucki W., Okuyama H., Pavy B., & Rabacus M. (2010). Cholesterol lowering, cardiovascular diseases, and the rosuvastatin-jupiter controversy: a critical reappraisal. *Archives of Internal Medicine*, Vol.170, No.12, (June 2010), pp. 1032-1036, ISSN 1538-3679

Després J.P. (2011). CRP: star trekking the galaxy of risk markers. *Lancet*, Vol.377, No.9764, (February 2011), pp. 441-442, ISSN 1474-547X

Dinarello C.A. (2010). Anti-inflammatory agents: present and future. *Cell*, Vol.140, No.6, (March 2010), pp. 935-950, ISSN 1097-4172

Dormandy J.A., Charbonnel B., Eckland D.J.A., Erdmann E., Masi-Benedetti M., Moules I.K., Skene A.M., Tan, M.H., Lefebre P.J., Murray G.D., Standl E., Wilcox R.G., Mokan M., Norkus A., Pirags V., Podar T., Scheen A., Scherbaum W., Scherntaner G., Schmitz O., Skrha J., Smith U., & Taton J. (2005). Secondary prevention of macrovascular events in patients with type 2 diabetes in the PROactive Study (PROspective pioglitAzone Clinical Trial In macroVascular Events): a randomised controlled trial. *Lancet*, Vol.366, No.9493, (October 2005), pp. 1279-1289, ISSN 1474-547X

Duan S.Z., Usher M.G., & Mortensen R.M. (2009). PPARs: the vasculature, inflammation and hypertension. *Current Opinion in Nephrology and Hypertension*, Vol.18, No.2, (March 2009), pp. 128-133, ISSN 1473-6543

Ezzati M., Lopez A.D., Rodgers A., Vander Hoorn S., & Murray C.J.L. (2002). Selected major risk factors and global and regional burden of disease. *Lancet*, Vol.360, No.9343, (November 2002), pp. 1347-1360, ISSN 1474-547X

Farmer J.A. (2009). Nicotinic acid: a new look at an old drug. *Current Atherosclerosis Reports*, Vol.11, No.2, (March 2009), pp. 87-92, ISSN 1523-3804

Fazio S., & Linton M. (2006). Failure of ACAT inhibition to retard atherosclerosis. *New England Journal of Medicine*, Vol.354, No.12, (March 2006), pp. 1307-1309, ISSN 1533-4406

Forrester J.S. (2010). Redifining normal low-density lipoprotein cholesterol: a strategy to unseat coronary disease as the nation's leading killer. *Journal of the American College of Cardiology*, Vol.56, No.8, (August 2010), pp. 630-636, ISSN 1558-3597

Garcia-Garcia H.M., & Serruys P.W. (2009). Phospholipase A_2 inhibitors. *Current Opinion in Lipidology*, Vol.20, No.4, (August 2009), pp. 327-332, ISSN 1473-6535

Gasparyan A.Y., Watson T., & Lip G.Y. (2008). The role of aspirin in cardiovascular prevention: implications of aspirin resistance. *Journal of the American College of Cardiology*, Vol.51, No.19, (May 2008), pp. 1829-1843, ISSN 1558-3597

Gasparyan A.Y., Ayvazyan L., Mikhailidis D.P., & Kitas G.D. (2011). Mean platelet volume: a link between thrombosis and inflammation?. *Current Pharmaceutical Design*, Vol.17, No.1, (2011), pp. 47-58, ISSN 1873-4286

Gibbons R.J., Jones D.W., Gardner T.J., Goldstein L.B., Moller J.H., & Yancy C.W. (2008). The American Heart Association' s 2008 statement of principles for healthcare reform. *Circulation*, Vol.118, No.21, (November 2008), pp. 2209-2218, ISSN 1524-4539

Gilbert J., Lekstrom-Himes J., Donaldson D., Lee Y., Hu M., Xu J., Wyant T., & Davidson M. (2011). Effect of CC chemokine receptor 2 CCR2 blockade on serum C-reactive protein in individuals at atherosclerotic risk and with a single nucleotide polymorphism of the monocyte chemoattractant protein-1 promoter region. *American Journal of Cardiology*, Vol.107, No.6, (March 2011), pp. 906-911, ISSN 1879-1913

Ginsberg H.N., Elam M.B., Lovato L.C., Crouse III J.R., Leiter L.A., Linz P., Friedewald W.T., Buse J.B., Gerstein H.C., Probstfield J., Grimm R.H., Ismail-Beigi F., Bigger J.T., Goff Jr. D.C., Cushman W.C., Simons-Morton D.G., & Byington R.P. (2010). Effects of combination lipid therapy in type 2 diabetes mellitus: the ACCORD study group. *New England Journal of Medicine*, Vol.362, No.17, (April 2010), pp. 1563-1574, ISSN 1533-4406

Goldberg R.B., Kendall D.M., Deeg M.A., Buse J.B., Zagar A.J., Pinaire J.A., Tan M.H., Khan M.A., Perez A.T., & Jacober S.J. (2005). A comparison of lipid and glycemic effects of pioglitazone and rosiglitazone in patients with type 2 diabetes and dyslipidemia. *Diabetes Care*, Vol.28, No.7, (July 2005), pp. 1547-1554, ISSN 1935-5548

Goldfine A.B., Kaul S., & Hiatt W.R. (2011). Fibrates in the treatment of dyslipidemias - time for a reassessment. *New England Journal of Medicine*, Vol. 365, No.6, (August 2011), pp. 481-484, ISSN 1533-4406

Grundy S.M. (2008). Promise of low-density lipoprotein-lowering therapy for primary and secondary prevention. *Circulation*, Vol.117, No.4, (January 2008), pp. 569-573, ISSN 1524-4539

Greenland P., Knoll M.D., Stamler J., Neaton J.D., Dyer A.R., Garside D.B., & Wilson P.W. (2003). Major risk factors as antecedents of fatal and nonfatal coronary heart disease events. *Journal of the American Medical Association*, Vol.290, No.7, (August 2003), pp. 891-897, ISSN1538-3598

Gurbel P.A., Bliden K.P., Kreutz R.P., Dichiara J., Antonino M.J., & Tantry U.S. (2009). The link between heightened thrombogenicity and inflammation: pre-procedure characterization of the patient at high risk for recurrent events after stenting. *Platelets*, Vol.20, No.2, (March 2009), pp. 97-104, ISSN 1369-1635

Haas M.J., & Mooradian A.D. (2011). Inflammation, high-density lipoprotein and cardiovascular dysfunction. *Current Opinion in Infectious Diseases*, Vol.24, No.3, (June 2011), pp. 265-272, ISSN 1535-3877

Hakonarson H., Thorvaldsson S., Helgadottir A., Gudbjartsson D., Zink F., Andresdottir M., Manolescu A., Arnar D.O., Andersen K., Sigurdsson A., Thorgeirsson G., Jonsson A., Agnarsson U., Bjornsdottir H., Gottskalksson G., Einarsson A., Gudmundsdottir H., Adalsteinsdottir A.E., Gudmundsson K., Kristjansson K., Hardarson T., Kristinsson A., Topol E.J., Gulcher J., Kong A., Gurney M., Thorgeirsson G., & Stefansson K. (2005). Effects of a 5-lipoxygenase-activating protein inhibitor on biomarkers associated with risk of myocardial infarction: a randomized trial.

Journal of the American Medical Association, Vol.293, No.18, (May 2005), pp. 2245-2256, ISSN 1538-3598

Hansson G.K. (2005). Inflammation, atherosclerosis, and coronary artery disease. *New England Journal of Medicine*, Vol.352, No.16, (April 2005), pp. 1685-1695, ISSN 1533-4406

Hansson G.K., & Libby P. (2006). The immune response in atherosclerosis: a double-edged sword. *Nature Reviews Immunology*, Vol.6, No.7, (July 2006), pp. 508-519, ISSN 1474-1733

Harrison D.G., Guzik T.J., Lob H.E., Madhur M.S., Marvar P.J., Thabet S.R., Vinh A., & Weyand C.M. (2011). Inflammation, immunity, and hypertension. *Hypertension*, Vol.57, No.2, (February 2011), pp. 132-140, ISSN 1524-4563

Hennessy E.H., Parker A.E., & O'Neill L.A.J. (2010). Targeting Toll-like receptors: emerging therapeutics. *Nature Reviews Drug Discovery*, Vol.9, No.4, (April 2010), pp. 293-307, ISSN 1474-1784

Hersberger M. (2010). Potential role of the lipoxygenase derived lipid mediators in atherosclerosis: leukotrienes, lipoxins and resolvins. *Clinical Chemistry and Laboratory Medicine*, Vol.48, No.8, (August 2010), pp. 1063-1073, ISSN 1434-6621

Hlatky M.A., Greenland P., Arnett D.K., Ballantyne C.M., Criqui M.H., Elkind M.S.V., Go A.S., Harrell Jr. F.E., Hong Y., Howard B.V., Howard V.J., Hsue P.Y., Kramer C.M., McConnell J.P., Normand S.L.T., O'Donnell C.J., Smith S.C., & Wilson P.W.F. (2009). Criteria for evaluation of novel markers of cardiovascular risk: a scientific statement from the American Heart Association. *Circulation*, Vol.119, No.17, (May 2009), pp. 2408-2416, ISSN 1524-4539

Hsia J., MacFayden J.G., Monyak J., & Ridker P.M. (2011). Cardiovascular event reduction and adverse events among subjects attaining low-density lipoprotein cholesterol <50 mg/dl with rosuvastatin. The Jupiter Trial (Justification for the Use of Statins in Prevention: an Intervention Trial Evaluating Rosuvastatin). *Journal of the American College of Cardiology*, Vol.57, No.16, (April 2011), pp. 1666-1675, ISSN 1558-3597

Hürlimann D., Forster A., Noll G., Enseleit F., Chenevard R., Distler O., Béchir M., Spieker L.E., Neidhart M., Michel B.A., Gay R.E., Lüscher T.F., Gay S., & Ruschitzka F. (2004). Anti-tumor necrosis factor-α treatment improves endothelial function in patients with rheumatoid arthritis. *Circulation*, Vol.106, No.17, (October 2004), pp. 2184-2187, ISSN 1524-4539

Jun M., Foote C., Lv J., Neal B., Patel A., Nicholls S.J., Grobbee D.E., Cass A., Chalmers J., & Perkovic V. (2010). Effects of fibrates on cardiovascular outcomes: a systematic review and meta-analysis. *Lancet*, Vol.375, No.9729, (May 2010), pp. 1875-1884, ISSN 1474-547X

Kaul S., Morrissey R.P., & Diamond G.A. (2010). By Jove! What is a clinician to make of JUPITER? *Archives of Internal Medicine*, Vol.170, No.12, (June 2010), pp. 1073-1077, ISSN 1538-3679

Keavney B. (2011). C reactive protein and the risk of cardiovascular disease: are clearly linked but a causal associatiuon is unlikely. *British Medical Journal*, Vol.342, (February 2011), pp. 393-394, ISSN 1468-5833

Kinlay S., Schwartz G.G., Olsson A.G., Rifai N., Leslie S.J., Sasiela W.J., Szarek M., Libby P., & Ganz P. (2003). High-dose atorvastatin enhances the decline in inflammatory markers in patients with acute coronary syndromes in the MIRACL study. *Circulation*, Vol.108, No.13, (September 2003), pp. 1560-1566, ISSN 1524-4539

Klingenberg R., & Hansson G.K. (2009). Treating inflammation in atherosclerotic cardiovascular disease: emerging therapies. *European Heart Journal*, Vol.30, No.23, (December 2009), pp. 2838-2844, ISSN 1522-9645

Knopp R.H., Alagona P., Davidson M., Goldberg A.C., Kafonek S.D., Kashyap M., Sprecher D., Superko H.R., Jenkins S., & Marcovina S. (1998). Equivalent efficacy of a time-release form of niacin (Niaspan) given once-a-night versus plain niacin in the management of hyperlipidemia. *Metabolism*, Vol.47, No.9, (September 1998), pp. 1097-1104, ISSN 0026-0495

Kris-Etherton P.M., Lichtenstein A.H., Howard B.V., Steinberg D., & Witztum R. (2004). Antioxidant vitamin supplements and cardiovascular disease. *Circulation*, Vol.110, No.5, (August 2004), pp. 1726-1728, ISSN 1524-4539

Kunsch C., Luchoomun J., Grey J.Y., Olliff L.K., Saint L.B., Arrendale R.F., Wasserman M.A., Saxena U., & Medford R.M. (2004). Selective inhibition of endothelial and monocyte redox-sensitive genes by AGI-1067: a novel antioxidant and anti-inflammatory agent. *Journal of Pharmacology and Experimental Therapeutics*, Vol.308, No.3, (March 2004), pp. 820-829, ISSN 1521-0103

Lauer M.S. (2010). Screening asymptomatic subjects for subclinical atherosclerosis: not so obvious. *Journal of the American College of Cardiology*, Vol.56, No.2, (July 2010), pp. 106-108, ISSN 1558-3597

Lauer M.S. (2011). Pseudodisease, the next great epidemic in coronary atherosclerosis. *Archives of Internal Medicine*, Vol.171, No.14, (July 2011), pp. 1268-1269, ISSN 1538-3679

Leibowitz A, & Schiffrin E.L. (2011). Immune mechanisms in hypertension. *Current Hypertension Reports*, Epub. Ahead of Print, (August 2011), ISSN 1534-3111

Libby P. (2005). The forgotten majority: unfinished business in cardiovascular risk reduction. *Journal of the American College of Cardiology*, Vol.46, No.7, (October 2005), pp. 1225-1228, ISSN 1558-3597

Libby P., Ridker P.M., & Hansson G.K. (2009). Inflammation in atherosclerosis: from pathophysiology to practice. *Journal of the American College of Cardiology*, Vol.54, No.23, (December 2009), pp. 2129-2138, ISSN 1558-3597

Libby P., Ridker P.M., & Hansson G.K. (2011). Progress and challenges in translating the biology of atherosclerosis. *Nature*, Vol.473, No.7347, (May 2011), pp. 317-325, ISSN 1476-4687

Ludman A., Venugopal V., Yellon D.M., & Hausenloy D.J. (2009). Statins and cardioprotection - more than just lipid lowering ? *Pharmacology and Therapeutics*, Vol.122, No.1, (April 2009), pp. 30-43, ISSN 1879-016X

Mancia G., De Backer G., Dominiczak A., Cifkova R., Fagard R., Germanò G., Grassi G., Heagerty A.M., Kjeldsen S.E., Laurent S., Narkiewicz K., Ruilope L., Rynkiewicz A., Schmieder R.E., Struijker Boudier H.A.J., & Zanchetti A. (2007). 2007 guidelines for the management of arterial hypertension. *Journal of Hypertension*, Vol.25, No.9, pp. 1105-1187, ISSN 1473-5598

Marchesi C., Paradis P., & Schiffrin E.L. (2008). Role of the renin-angiotensin system in vascular inflammation. *Trends in Pharmacological Sciences*, Vol. 29, No.7, (July 2008), pp. 367-374, ISSN 0165-6147

Maskrey B.H., Megson I.L., Whitfield P.D., & Rossi A.G. (2011). Mechanisms of resolution of inflammation: a focus on cardiovascular disease. *Arteriosclerosis Thrombosis and Vascular Biology*, Vol.31, No.5, (May 2011), pp. 1001-1006, ISSN 1524-4636

Montecucco F., Pende A., & Mach F. (2009). The renin-angiotensin system modulates inflammatory processes in atherosclerosis: evidence from basic research and clinical studies. *Mediators of Inflammation*, Vol.2009, 752406, ISSN 1466-1861

Montecucco F., Lenglet S., Bertolotto M., Pelli G., Gayet-Ageron A., Palombo D., Pane B., Spinella G., Steffens S., Raffaghello L., Pistoia V., Ottonello L., Pende A., Dallegri F., & Mach F. (2010). Systemic and intraplaque mediators of inflammation are increased in patients symptomatic for ischemic stroke. *Stroke*, Vol.41, No.7, (July 2010), pp. 1394-1404, ISSN 1524-4628

Montecucco F., Pende A., Quercioli A., & Mach F. (2011). Inflammation in the pathophysiology of essential hypertension. *Journal of Nephrology*, Vol.24, No.1, (January-February 2011), pp. 23-34, ISSN 1724-6059

Morrow D.A., de Lemos J.A., Sabatine M.S., Wiviott S.D., Blazing M.A., Shui A., Rifai N., Califf R.M., & Braunwald E. (2006). Clinical relevance of C-reactive protein during follow-up of patients with acute coronary syndromes in the Aggrastat-to-Zocor Trial. *Circulation*, Vol.114, No.4, (July 2006), pp. 281-288, ISSN 1524-4539

Naghavi M., Falk E., Hecht H.S., & Shah P.K. (2006). The first SHAPE (Screening for Heart Attack Prevention and Education) guideline. *Critical Pathways in Cardiology*, Vol.5, No.4, (December 2006), pp. 187-190, ISSN 1535-2811

Natarajan P., & Cannon C.P. (2010). Could direct inhibition of inflammation be the "next big thing" in treating atherosclerosis. *Arteriosclerosis Thrombosis and Vascular Biology*, Vol.30, No.11, (November 2010), pp. 2081-2083, ISSN 1524-4636

Natarajan P., Ray K.K., & Cannon C.P. (2010). High-density lipoprotein and coronary heart disease: current and future therapies. *Journal of the American College of Cardiology*, Vol.55, No.13, (March 2010), pp. 1283-1299, ISSN 1558-3597

Nissen S.E., Tuczu E.M., Libby P., Thompson P.D., Ghali M., Garza D., Berman L., Shi H., Buebendorf E., & Topol E.J. (2004). Effect of antihypertensive agents on cardiovascular events in patients with coronary disease and normal blood pressure. The CAMELOT study: a randomized controlled trial. *Journal of the American Medical Association*, Vol.292, No.18, (November 2004), pp. 2217-2226, ISSN 1538-3598

Nissen S.E., Tuzcu E.M., Schoenhagen P., Crowe T., Sasiela W.J., Tsai J., Orazem J., Magorien R.D., O'Shaughnessy C., & Ganz P. (2005). Statin therapy, LDL cholesterol, C-reactive protein, and coronary artey disease. *New England Journal of Medicine*, Vol.352, No.1, (January 2005), pp. 29-38, ISSN 1533-4406

Nissen S.E., & Wolski K. (2010). Rosiglitazone revisited: an updated meta-analysis of risk for myocardial infarction and cardiovascular mortality. *Archives of Internal Medicine*, Vol.170, No.14, (July 2010), pp. 1191-1201, ISSN 1538-3679

Nordestgaard B.G. (2009). Does elevated C-reactive protein cause human atherothrombosis? Novel insights from genetics, intervention trials, and elsewhere. *Current Opinion in Lipidology*, Vol.20, No.5, (October 2009), pp. 393-401, ISSN 1473-6535

Oyekan A. (2011). PPARs and their effects on their cardiovascular system. *Clinical and Experimental Hypertension*, Vol.33, No.5, (August 2011), pp. 287-293, ISSN 1525-6006

Paras C., Hussain M.M., & Rosenson R.S. (2010). Emerging drugs for hyperlipidemia. *Expert Opinion on Emerging Drugs*, Vol.15, No.3, (September 2010), pp. 433-451, ISSN 1744-7623

Pende A., & Dallegri F. (2011). Anti-inflammatory approaches to reduce acute cardiovascular events: Not only benefits. *Current Pharmaceutical Biotechnology*, Epub. Ahead of Print, (April 2011), ISSN 1389-2010

Perry C.M. (2009). Extended-release niacin (nicotinic acid)/laropiprant. *Drugs*, Vol.69, No.12, (August 2009), pp. 1665-1679, ISSN 012-6667

Pfützner A., Schöndorf T., Hanefeld M., & Forst T. (2010). High-sensitivity C-reactive protein predicts cardiovascular risk in diabetic and nondiabetic patients: effects of insulin-sensitizing treatment with pioglitazone. *Journal of Diabetes Science and Technology*, Vol.4, No.3, (May 2010), pp. 706-716, ISSN 1932-2968

Pletcher M., & Hulley S.B. (2010). Statin therapy in young adults: ready for prime time? *Journal of the American College of Cardiology*, Vol.56, No.8, (August 2010), pp. 637-640, ISSN 1558-3597

Ribichini F., Tomai F., De Luca G., Boccuzzi G., Presbitero P., Pesarini G., Ferrero V., Ghini A.S., Abukaresh R., Aurigemma C., De Luca L., Zavalloni D., Soregaroli D., Marino P., Garbo R., Zanolla L., & Vassanelli C. (2011). Immunosuppressive therapy with oral prednisone to prevent restenosis after PCI. A multicenter randomized trial. *American Journal of Medicine*, Vol.124, No.5, (May 2011), pp. 434-443, ISSN 1555-7162

Ridker P.M., Rifai N., Pfeffer M.A., Sacks F.M., & Braunwald E. (1999). Long-term effects of pravastatin on plasma concentration of C-reactive protein. The Cholesterol and Recurrent Events (CARE) investigators. *Circulation*, Vol.100, Vol.3, (July 1999), pp. 230-235, ISSN 1524-4539

Ridker P.M., Rifai N., Clearfield M., Downs J.R., Weis S.E., Miles J.S., & Gotto Jr., A.M. (2001). Measurement of C-reactive protein for the targeting of statin therapy in the primary prevention of acute coronary events. *New England Journal of Medicine*, Vol.344, No.26, (June 2001), pp. 1959-1965, ISSN 1533-4406

Ridker P.M., Cannon C.P., Morrow D., Rifai N., Rose L.M., McCabe C.H., Pfeffer M.A., & Braunwald E. (2005). C-reactive protein levels and outcomes after statin therapy. *New England Journal of Medicine*, Vol.352, No.1, (January 2005), pp. 20-28, ISSN 1533-4406

Ridker P.M. (2007). C-reactive protein and the prediction of cardiovascular events among those at intermediate risk: moving an inflammatory hypothesis toward consensus. *Journal of the American College of Cardiology*, Vol.49, No.21, (May 2007), pp. 2129-2138, ISSN 1558-3597

Ridker P.M., Buring J.E., Rifai N., & Cook N.R. (2007). Development and validation of improved algorithms for the assessment of global cardiovascular risk in women: the Reynolds Risk Score. *Journal of the American Medical Association*, Vol.297, No.6, (February 2007), pp. 611-619, ISSN 1538-3598

Ridker P.M., Paynter N.P., Rifai N., Gaziano J.M., & Cook N.R. (2008a). C-reactive protein and parental history improve global cardiovascular risk prediction: the Reynolds Risk Score for Men. *Circulation*, Vol.118, No.22, (November 2008), pp. 2243-2251, ISSN 1524-4539

Ridker P.M., Danielson E., Fonseca F.A., Genest J., Gotto Jr., A.M., Kastelein J.J., Koenig W., Libby P., Lorenzatti A.J., MacFadyen J.G., Nordestgaard B.G., Shepherd J.,

Willerson J.T., & Glynn R.J. (2008b). Rosuvastatin to prevent vascular events in men and women with elevated C-reactive protein. *New England Journal of Medicine*, Vol.359, No.21, (November 2008), pp. 2195-2207, ISSN 1533-4406

Ridker P.M. (2009). Testing the inflammatory hypothesis of atherothrombosis: scientific rationale for the cardiovascular inflammation reduction trial (CIRT). *Journal of Thrombosis and Haemostasis*, Vol.7, No.Suppl.1, (July 2009), pp. 332-339, ISSN 1538-7836

Roberts R., DeMello V., Sobel B.E. (1976). Deleterious effects of methylprednisolone in patients with myocardial infarction. *Circulation*, Vol.53, No.Suppl. 3, (March 1976), pp. 1204-1206, ISSN 1524-4539

Rosenson R.S. (2009). Future role for selective phospholipase A_2 inhibitors in the prevention of atherosclerotic cardiovascular disease. *Cardiovascular Drugs and Therapy*, Vol.23, No.1, (February 2009), pp. 93-101, ISSN 1573-7241

Ross R. (1999). Atherosclerosis - an inflammatory disease. *New England Journal of Medicine*, Vol.340, No.2, (January 1999), pp. 115-126, ISSN 1533-4406

Säemann M.D., Poglitsch M., Kopecky C., Haidinger M., Hörl W.H., & Weichhart T. (2010). The versatility of HDL: a crucial anti-inflammatory regulator. *European Journal of Clinical Investigation*, Vol.40,No.12, (December 2010), pp. 1131-1143, ISSN 1365-2362

Sanyal S., Karas R.H., Kuvin J.T. (2007). Present-day uses of niacin: effects on lipid and non-lipid parameters. *Expert Opinion in Pharmacotherapy*, Vol.8, No.11, (August 2007), pp.1711-1717, ISSN 1744-7666

Sarov-Blat L., Morgan J.M., Fernandez P., James R., Fang Z., Hurle M.R., Baidoo C., Willette R.N., Lepore J.J., Jensen S.E., & Sprecher D.L. (2010). Inhibition of p38 mitogen-activated protein kinase reduces inflammation following coronary vascular injury in humans. *Arteriosclerosis Thrombosis and Vascular Biology*, Vol.30, No.11, (November 2010), pp. 2256-2263, ISSN 1524-4636

Satoh K., Fukumoto Y., & Shimokawa H. (2011). Rho-kinase: important new therapeutic target in cardiovascular diseases. *American Journal of Physiology Heart and Circulatory Physiology* , Vol.301, No.2, (August 2011), pp. H287-H296, ISSN 1522-1539

Sattar N., Preiss D., Murray H.M., Welsh P., Buckley B.M., de Craen A.J., Seshasai S.R., McMurray J.J., Freeman D.J., Jukema J.W., Macfarlane P.W., Packard C.J., Stott D.J., Westendorp R.G., Shepherd J., Davis B.R., Pressel S.L., Marchioli R., Marfisi R.M., Maggioni A.P., Tavazzi L., Tognoni G., Kjekshus J., Pedersen T.R., Cook T.J., Gotto A.M., Clearfield M.B., Downs J.R., Nakamura H., Ohashi Y., Mizuno K., Ray K.K., & Ford I. (2010). Statins and risk of incident diabetes: a collaborative meta-analysis of randomised statin trials. *Lancet*, Vol.375, No.9716, (February 2010), pp. 735-742, ISSN 1474-547X

Schieven G.L. (2005). The biology of p38 kinase: a central role in inflammation. *Current Topics in Medicinal Chemistry*, Vol.5, No.10, (September 2005), pp. 921-928, ISSN 1568-0266

Schinzari F., Armuzzi A., De Pascalis B., Mores N., Tesauro M., Melina D., & Cardillo C. (2008). Tumor necrosis factor-α antagonism improves endothelial dysfunction in patients with Crohn's disease. *Clinical Pharmacology and Therapeutics*, Vol.83, No.1, (January 2008), pp. 70-76, ISSN 1532-6535

Schunkert H., & Samani N.J. (2008). Elevated C-reactive protein in atherosclerosis – chicken or egg? *New England Journal of Medicine*, Vol.359, No.18, (October 2008), pp. 1953-1955, ISSN 1533-4406

See R., Lindsey J.B., Patel M.J., Ayers C.R., Khera A., McGuire D.K., Grundy S.M., & de Lemos J.A. (2008). Application of the Screening for Heart Attack Prevention and Education Task Force recommendations to an urban population: observations from the Dallas Heart Study. *Archives of Internal Medicine*, Vol.168, No.10, (May 2008), pp. 1055-1062, ISSN 1538-3679

Sever P.S., Poulter N.R., Elliott W.J., Jonsson M.C., & Black H.R. (2006). Management of hypertension: is it the pressure or the drug? *Circulation*, Vol.113, No.23, (June 2006), pp. 2754-2774, ISSN 1524-4539

Shah P.K. (2010). Screening asymptomatic subjects for subclinical atherosclerosis: can we, does it matter, and should we? *Journal of the American College of Cardiology*, Vol.56, No.2, (July 2010), pp. 98-105, ISSN 1558-3597

Spite M, & Serhan C.N. (2010). Novel lipid mediators promote resolution of acute inflammation: impact of aspirin and statins. *Circulation Research*, Vol.107, No.10, (November 2010), pp. 1170-1184, ISSN 1524-4571

Staessen J.A., Richart T., Wang Z., Thijs, L. (2010). Implications of recently published trials of blood pressure-lowering drugs in hypertensive or high-risk patients. *Hypertension*, Vol.55, No.4, (April 2010), pp. 819-831, ISSN 1524-4563

Steinberg D. (2010). Earlier intervention in the management of hypercholesterolemia: what are we waiting for? *Journal of the American College of Cardiology*, Vol.56, No.8, (August 2010), pp. 627-629, ISSN 1558-3597

Superko H.R., & King III S. (2008). Lipid management to reduce cardiovascular risk: a new strategy is required. *Circulation*, Vol.117, No.4, (January 2008), pp. 560-568, ISSN 1524-4539

Tabet F., & Rye K.A. (2009). High-density lipoproteins, inflammation and oxidative stress. *Clinical Science*, Vol.116, No.2, (January 2009), pp. 87-98, ISSN 1470-8736

Tardif J.C., McMurray J.J., Klug E., Small R., Schumi J., Choi J., Cooper J., Scott R., Lewis E.F., L'Allier P.L., & Pfeffer M.A. (2008). Effects of succinobucol (AGI-1067) after an acute coronary syndrome: a randomised, double-blind, placebo-controlled trial. *Lancet*, Vol.371, No.9626, (May 2008), pp. 1761-1768, ISSN 1474-547X

Tardif J.C., L'Allier P.L., Ibrahim R., Grégoire J.C., Nozza A., Cossette M., Kouz S., Lavoie M.A., Paquin J., Brotz T.M., Taub R., & Pressacco J. (2010). Treatment with 5-lipoxygenase inhibitor VIA-2291 (atreleuton) in patients with recent acute coronary syndrome. *Circulation Cardiovascular Imaging*, Vol.3, No.3, (May 2010), pp. 298-307, ISSN 1942-0080

Taylor A.J., Villines T.C., Stanek E.J., Devine P.J., Griffen L., Miller M., Weissman N.J., & Turco M. (2009). Extended-release niacin or ezetimibe and carotid intima-media thickness. *New England Journal of Medicine*, Vol.361, No.22, (November 2009), pp. 2113-2122, ISSN 1533-4406

Thoenes M., Oguchi A., Nagamia S., Vaccari C.S., Hammoud R., Umpierrez G.E., & Khan B.V. (2007). The effects of extended-release niacin on carotid intimal media thickness, endothelial function and inflammatory markers in patients with the metabolic syndrome. *International Journal of Clinical Practice*, Vol.61, No.11, (November 2007), pp. 1942-1948, ISSN 1368-5031

Tracey D., Klareskog L., Sasso E.H., Salfeld J.G., & Tak P.P. (2008). Tumor necrosis factor antagonist mechanisms of action: a comprehensive review. *Pharmacology and Therapeutics*, Vol.117, No.2, (February 2008), pp. 244-279, ISSN 0163-7258

U.S. Preventive Services Task Force (2009). Using nontraditional risk factors in coronary heart disease risk asessment: U.S. Preventive Services Task Force recommendation statement. *Annals of Internal Medicine*, Vol.151, No.7, (October 2009), pp. 474-482, ISSN 1539-3704

van Eijk I.C., de Vries M.K., Levels J.H., Peters M.J., Huizer E.E., Dijkmans B.A., van der Horst-Bruinsma I.E., Hazenberg B.P., van de Stadt R.J., Wolbink G.J., & Nurmohamed M.T. (2009). Improvement of lipid profile is accompanied by atheroprotective alterations in high-density lipoprotein composition upon tumor necrosis factor blockade: a prospective cohort study in ankylosing spondylitis. *Arthritis and Rheumatism*, Vol.60, No.5, (May 2009), pp. 1324-1330, ISSN 0004-3591

van Leuven S.I., Kastelein J.J., Allison A.C., Hayden M.R., & Stroes E.S. (2006). Mycophenolate mofetil (MMF): firing at the atherosclerotic plaque from different angles? *Cardiovascular Research*, Vol.69, No.2, (February 2006), pp. 341-347, ISSN 0008-6363

van Leuven S.I., van Wijk D.F., Volger O.L., de Vries J.P., van der Loos C.M., de Kleijn D.V., Horrevoets A.J., Tak P.P., van der Wal A.C., de Boer O.J., Pasterkamp G., Hayden M.R., Kastelein J.J., & Stroes E.S. (2010). Mycophenolate mofetil attenuates plaque inflammation in patients with symptomatic carotid artery stenosis. *Atherosclerosis*, Vol.211, No.1, (July 2010), pp. 231-236, ISSN 1879-1484

van Puijvelde G.H.M., van Es T., Habets K.L.L., Hauer A.D., van Berkel T.J.C., & Kuiper J. (2008). A vaccine against atherosclerosis: myth or reality? *Future Cardiology*, Vol.4, No.2, (March 2008), pp. 125-133, ISSN 1744-8298

Wang C.Y., Liu P.Y., & Liao J.K. (2008). Pleiotropic effects of statin therapy: molecular mechanisms and clinical results. *Trends in Molecular Medicine*, Vol.14, No.1, (January 2008), pp. 37-44, ISSN 1471-4914

Wang N., Yin R., Liu Y., Mao G., & Xi F. (2011). Role of peroxisome proliferator-activated receptor-γ in atherosclerosis: an update. *Circulation Journal*, Vol.75, No.3, (March 2011), pp. 528-535, ISSN 1346-9843

Westlake S.L., Colebatch A.N., Baird J., Kiely P., Quinn M., Choy E., Ostor A.J., & Edwards C.J. (2010). The effect of methotrexate on cardiovascular disease in patients with rheumatoid arthritis: a systematic literature review. *Rheumatology*, Vol.49, No.2, (February 2010), pp. 295-307, ISSN 1462-0332

Wilson P.W., Pencina M., Jacques P., Selhub J., D'Agostino Sr. R., & O'Donnell C.J. (2008). C-reactive protein and reclassification of cardiovascular risk in the Framingham Heart Study. *Circulation Cardiovascular Quality and Outcomes*, Vol.1, No.2, (November 2008), pp. 92-97, ISSN 1941-7705

Yang E.Y., Nambi V., Tang Z., Virani S.S., Boerwinkle E., Hoogeveen R.C., Astor B.C., Mosley T.H., Coresh J., Chambless L., & Ballantyne C.M. (2009). Clinical implications of JUPITER (Justification fo the Use of statins in Prevention: an Intervention Trial Evaluating Rosuvastatin) in a U.S. population. *Journal of the American College of Cardiology*, Vol.54, No.25, (December 2009), pp. 2388-2395, ISSN 1558-3597

Yoshinaka Y., Shibata H., Kobayashi H., Kuriyama H., Shibuya K., Tanabe S., Watanabe T., & Miyazaki A. (2010). *Atherosclerosis*, Vol.213, N.1, (November 2010), pp. 85-91, ISSN 1879-1484

Yvan-Charvet L., Kling J., Pagler T., Li H., Hubbard B., Fisher T., Sparrow C.P., Taggart A.K., & Tall A.R. (2010). Cholesterol efflux potential and antiinflammatory properties of high-density lipoprotein after treatment with niacin or anacetrapib. *Arteriosclerosis Thrombosis and Vascular Biology*, Vol.30, No.7, (July 2010), pp.1430-1438, ISSN 1524-4636

Zanchetti A. (2009). Bottom blood pressure or bottom cardiovascular risk? How far can cardiovascular risk be reduced? *Journal of Hypertension*, Vol.27, No.8, (August 2009), pp. 1509-1520, ISSN 1473-5598

Zhou Q., Gensch C., & Liao J.K. (2011). Rho-associated coiled-coil-forming kinases (ROCKs): potential targets for the treatment of atherosclerosis and vascular disease. *Trends in Pharmacological Sciences*, Vol.32, No.3, (March 2011), pp. 167-173, ISSN 1873-3735

14

Gender-Specific Aspects in the Clinical Presentation of Cardiovascular Disease

Chiara Leuzzi, Raffaella Marzullo,
Emma Tarabini Castellani and Maria Grazia Modena*
Department of Cardiovascular Disease, Women's Clinic
University of Modena and Reggio Emilia,
Italy

1. Introduction

In the industrialized countries, the cardiovascular disease (CVD) is the leading cause of mortality and morbidity in women after of 50 years. Genetic, hormonal and metabolic influences are involved in gender differences, including the epidemiology, symptoms, diagnosis, progression, prognosis and management of these pathologies.

Recent advances in the field of cardiovascular medicine have not led to significant drops in case fatality rates for women, compared to the dramatic reductions achieved for men. Such gender-specific difference in cardiovascular disease mortality are probably related to a knowledge gap about CVD in women. Thus, much of the evidence supporting contemporary recommendations for testing, prevention, and treatment of CVD in women is extrapolated from studies conducted predominantly on middle-aged men. For example pharmacological therapy is hampered by defective evidence.

Only recently, significant sex-related differences in prevalence, presentation, management and outcomes of CVD, have been evaluated and discovered.

The ability of knowing and recognizing gender differences in CVD may facilitate a rapid identification of cardiac signs and symptoms of warning and may avoid significant delays in diagnosis and treatment in women. This compendium will briefly summarize gender-related differences in several manifestations of CVD, with a special focus also on arrhythmias and heart failure.

2. Risk factors

Traditionally, guidelines classify women as being at high, intermediate or low risk on risk profile, based on Framingham risk scores. Despite major traditional risk factors are the same in both sexes, gender-specific differences are noted, and these differences are related to different outcome. For this reason, a new approach in evaluation of cardiovascular risk in

---

* Corresponding Author

women considers a multifactorial model that includes a complex interaction between sex hormones and traditional risk factors.

2.1 Traditional risk factors

There is also substantial gender-related differences in the prevalence and outcome in traditional risk factors. For example, overall rates of hypertension and smoking are higher in men, but their presence is associated with a worse outcome in women. The prevalence of hypertension is lower in pre-menopausal women than men, whereas in post-menopausal women it is higher than in men. In fact about 50% of post-menopausal women experience of moderate to severe hypertension or take antihypertensive therapy.

Several studies have clearly demonstrated a strong relationship between level of blood pressure and risk for cardiovascular events. In this setting, hypertension is one of the most risk factors for stroke, myocardial infarction, heart failure, aortic disease and chronic renal failure. Mechanisms responsible for the increase in blood pressure in post-menopausal women are complex and multifactorial, including loss of estrogen, oxidative stress, endothelial dysfunction, modification in renin-angiotensin system and sympathetic activation.

Hypertension may appears as an isolated disease, more typical of elderly women, or as part of the metabolic syndromes (MS), more frequently in early postmenopausal women. MS is a constellation of interrelated risk factors that promote the development of CVD. The presence of MS worsens the severity of hypertension and reduces the response to treatment. Than, MS is considered a unfavourable prognostic factor in hypertension post-menopausal women. On the other hand hypertension tends to associate with other metabolic risk factors and about one-half patients with essential hypertension are insulin resistant. In addition women with MS have chronic subclinical inflammation and systemic endothelial dysfunction. Endothelial dysfunction is common after the menopause and its detection may precede overt disease such as hypertension and diabetes.

Data derived from population studies demonstrate that total cholesterol measurements are higher in men until the fifth decade of life but, beyond this age, women have greater values. Examining the lipoprotein subclassis, women have less LDL particles than men and have about two-fold higher concentration of HDL particles then men. Particularly, HDL cholesterol inversely correlates with coronary artery disease (CAD) in young men and in women of all ages. Women typically experience a relatively mild decline in HDL cholesterol at the time of menopause.

Hypertriglyceridemia is also a more potent independent risk factor for CAD in women as compared with men. In fact, in presence of hypertriglyceridemia, the risk of CVD is twice in women.

Another strong risk factors in women is diabetes. Diabetic women have significantly higher cardiovascular mortality when compared with diabetic men, because diabetes eliminates the 'female advantage' of a lower CAD prevalence and outcome risk that exists for the female in general population. Furthermore diabetes is an independent predictor of 'atypical' presentation of acute myocardial infarction in women.

At the onset of diabetes-related cardiovascular complications, women have higher out-of-hospital mortality than men, and those who reach hospital are more likely to die from an initial cardiac event and are also at high risk of post-event complications.

2.2 Gender-specific risk factors

Other factors are unique to the female: menopause, which affects especially if early and hypothalamic-hypoestrogenism occurring in fertile women.

Menopause is a physiological condition associated with endothelial dysfunction, due to lack of estrogens. Than, the deficiency of female gonadal hormones may represent a major risk factor for menopausal hypertension, due to related modifications of blood vessel structure and the elicit response to a vasoactive substances.

Furthermore, dysfunction of the endotelium causes reduction or abolition of vasoprotective factors, inducing a proinflammatory, proliferative and procoagulatory milieu. These changes favour the development of cardiovascular risk factors, as hypertension.

Gender-specific opportunities for identifying women's risk (e.g., prior preeclampsia) also deserve further exploration.

Preeclampsia is a disorder of pregnancy diagnosed by gestational hypertension and proteinuria. Abnormal placentation resulting in preeclampsia and intrauterine growth restriction is a major cause of both maternal and perinatal morbidity and mortality.

Prior preeclampsia is associated with increased risk of CVD, including myocardial infarction, ischemic heart disease, stroke and endstage renal disease. Particularly, the increased risk for future vascular disease is more pronounced in women with early-onset preclampsia. Although the symptoms of preeclampsia resolve over a number of weeks after delivery, maternal vascular dysfunction may persist for years.

Endothelial dysfunction, however, is considered a central component of the pathophysiology of preeclampsia and known to contribute to the pathogenesis of hypertension and cardiovascular sequelae. Several factors contribute to the endothelial dysfunction in the post-partum state. Abnormal placenta, for example, release antiangiogenic factors, harmful to the vascular endothelium. Often, women with a history of peeclampsia or intrauterine growth restriction have high cholesterol levels, high blood pressure and insulin resistance.

Frequently, preeclamptic women are obese, and obesity associated with insulin resistance, may reduce endothelial dependent blood flow response.

Behavioral factors also, such as chronic stress, lack of social support, and family demands, as well as biological processes, including genetics, may contribute to the development of CVD in this setting.

Similarly, women with a history of polycystic ovary syndrome have a increased risk of CVD and have a greater frequency of multiple risk factors including central obesity, insulin resistance, and a greater prevalence of the metabolic syndrome and diabetes.

2.3 Inflammatory risk factors

Beside the traditional and female specific risk factors, novel risk markers such as inflammatory markers are being studied.

Women are at increased risk of inflammatory and autoimmune disease. The risk of mortality and morbidity from CVD is very high in autoimmune diseases, as systemic lupus erythematosus or rheumatoid arthritis. Various possible mechanisms have been proposed to explain the excess rate of cardiovascular mortality in patients with autoimmune disease.

A combination of traditional (dyslipidemia, hypertension, diabetes, and smoking) and nontraditional risk factors, including high inflammation, antiphospholipid antibodies and lipid oxidation, contribute to CVD in autoimmune diseases. Inflammation is a key component in the development of atherosclerosis in this setting. In fact, inflammation leads to the activation of endothelial cells, which, through an increase in the expression of leukocyte adhesion molecules, promotes a pro-atherosclerotic environment. Expression of proinflammatory cytokines and inflammatory mediators influences all stages of atherosclerosis development, from early atheroma formation to thrombus development responsible for events such as myocardial infarction. Proinflammatory cytokines may promote both traditional (e.g., dyslipidemia, insulin resistance) and nontraditional (e.g., oxidative stress) systemic cardiovascular risk factors.

Than in these patients, is commonly found a presence of endothelial dysfunction, a loss of arterial compliance and dysfunction in the microvascolature, resulting in myocardial flow heterogeneity.

Others factors contribute to poor prognosis: undertreatment of cardiovascular comorbidity may contribute to increased cardiovascular mortality in these patients. However, some drugs, largely used in this setting, may worsen cardiovascular profile: e.g. corticosteroids promote hypertension, dyslipidemia, and diabetes.

Then, novel risk stratification, including inflammatory markers and reproductive hormones, is developing to assess global cardiovascular risk in women.

3. Coronary heart disease

Coronary heart disease (CHD) is the most common cause of death amongst women, who experience more complications after acute myocardial infarction (AMI) than men.

It has been demonstrated that the epidemiology, the clinical manifestation and the progression of CHD are different in both sexes. The women developed CHD about 10-20 years later than men, in part by the influence of hormones and in part by the genetic sex.

Particularly, at the time of first experience of AMI, women are more likely to have diabetes mellitus or heart failure (HF) than men.

In addition, the prevalence of obstructive coronary disease is particularly low in premenopausal women, whilst increases dramatically for a woman after age 50.

The most common initial presentation of CHD is a AMI or sudden cardiac death and up to half of all women presenting with an acute myocardial infarction report no prior chest pain symptoms. There would appear to be an interaction effect of symptom presentation with age, in that older women often present in a similar way to men.

Several studies have indicated that women have "atypical" symptoms such as back pain, dyspnea, indigestion, nausea/vomiting and weakness. Frequently women reported pain in the jaw and neck and describe their symptoms as more anguished and frightening (emotional component) compared with men. Furthermore, prodromal symptoms are described up to 1 month before the onset of AMI such unusual fatigue (70.7%), sleep disturbance (47.8%) and shortness of breath (42.1%). The atypical presentation may explain the rate of under-diagnosed AMI, the under treatment of acute coronary syndromes and the worse outcomes characterized by increased hospital morbidity, higher mortality and fewer evidence-based therapies in women.

In the postmenopausal women, the plaque rupture is the main mechanism of acute coronary syndromes like as in the men. The higher mortality noted for younger women when compared with age-matched men is due the higher frequency of plaque erosion (Fig. 1). In an autopsy series, women also had a greater frequency of distal microvascular embolization in the setting of a fatal epicardial thrombosis when compared to men, independently of the type of thrombus or presence of necrosis. AMI and sudden death in women can occur also in spontaneous coronary artery dissection. This event is more frequent in the peri-partum period and can involve all coronary tree, but more frequently affects the left anterior descending artery. The dissection can involve every coronary, but in women frequently involves the left anterior descending coronary artery, whereas in man the right coronary artery is more frequently involved.

Many as 50% of patients undergoing coronary angiography for typical or atypical chest pain do not have obstructive CAD. An alternative mechanism of pain in women may be a coronary microvascular dysfunction, known as syndrome X. Most of these patients have an 'abnormal' exercise stress test, myocardial perfusion defects on gated Single-photon emission computed tomography or stress-induced wall motion abnormalities on echocardiography, but normal coronary angiography.

However, differentiation between these mechanisms of chest pain is important, because 'noncardiac' chest pain is not associated with cardiovascular sequelae and may require further medical evaluation and treatment. By contrast, syndrome X, which is thought to be caused by microvascular dysfunction, is associated with inducible metabolic ischaemia and can be treated by improving microvascular vasomotor tone with oral L-arginine, a precursor to vascular nitric oxide, and oestrogen.

Despite the absence of CAD and low risk for adverse cardiac events, a majority of those patients continue to have symptoms that contribute to a poor quality of life and consumption of large amounts of health care resources because of repeated evaluations and hospitalizations. Recently, Han et al. studied patients with obstructive CAD who underwent simultaneous intravascular ultrasound and coronary reactivity assessment and demonstrated that men have a greater atheroma burden and more diffuse epicardial endothelial dysfunction while women have more disease of the microcirculation. The coronary micro-vascular dysfunction, the smaller coronary artery lumens, the less collateral circulation than men and more prominent positive remodeling support the higher rate of angina, and acute coronary syndromes in the absence of obstructive CAD particularly during exertion or stress.

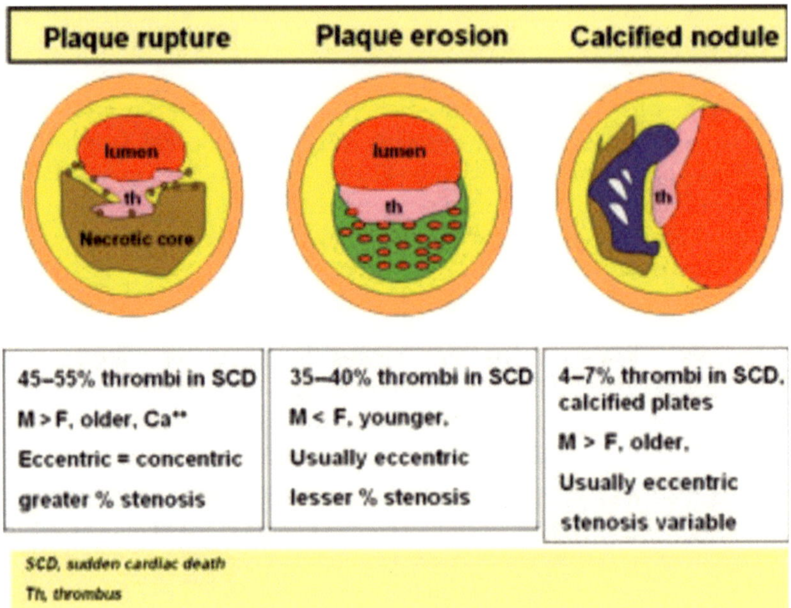

SCD, sudden cardiac death; Th, thrombus

Fig. 1. Gender differences in plaque morphologic features in an autoptic series of patients who died for sudden cardiac death, modified from reference 13.

4. Heart failure

The lifetime risk of developing HF is about 20% for both men and women. There are differences between men and women in clinical presentation, aetiology, treatment and outcome in HF, and these differences lead to different outcome.

The women are older than men and present more frequent hypertension and diabetes.

Diabetes mellitus is one of the strongest additional risk factors for the development of HF in women with CAD.

The systolic function is usually better preserved and the prevalence of ischemic etiology is lower respect to hypertension and valvular diseases. Another cause of HF includes cardiac toxicity from chemotherapeutic agents used to treat breast malignancy.

Mullens et al. show that the survival rate in women with non-ischemic cardiomyopathy was better than men, irrespective of baseline characteristics, while there was no advantage in presence of ischemic cause. The reason of different outcome remains unclear but might in part be related to sex differences in etiology.

The diagnosis of HF is a clinical diagnosis based on a constellation of symptoms and signs. Women with impaired systolic left ventricular function are more likely than men to have dependent edema, jugular venous distension, and an S3 gallop.

Furthermore, normal brain natriuretic peptide value, a biomarker used to identify patients with symptoms of HF, are higher in women versus men.

Current guidelines for HF therapy also are not sex specific due to under-representation of women and lack of sex-specific, prospective, randomized clinical trials. Indeed, women receive less life-prolonging treatment (ACE-I, beta-blockers and spironolactone) than men, in the presence of normal left ventricular function, while there no difference if etiology of HF is CAD.

Cardiac resynchronization therapy, an important therapy for HF, is beneficial for both women and men. Data suggest CRT is preferable to medical therapy alone in women for the combined end point of total mortality and hospital stay for major cardiovascular events.

A peculiar type of left ventricular dysfunction and HF typical in women is Takotsubo cardiomyopathy. This disease is typically observed in post-menopausal women and the highest frequency of occurrence is between the seventh and eighth decade of life.

The reason for the much more common occurrence in postmenopausal women is unclear.

It is characterized by a left ventricular dysfunction, electrocardiographic changes like an acute myocardial infarction and release of cardiac biomarkers, in the absence of obstructive coronary disease. The emotionally or physical stress are usually the triggers. The catecholamine-mediated cardio-toxicity, multi-vessels coronary vasospasm and abnormalities in coronary micro-vascular function have been postulated as pathophysiologic mechanisms.

The left ventricular dysfunction is reversible within weeks, despite a dramatic clinical presentation (similar to acute myocardial infarction but in the absence of obstructive coronary disease) and substantial risk of complications in the acute setting.

Another cause of left ventricular dysfunction and HF typical in women is peripartum cardiomyopathy (PPCM). This disease develops in the last month of pregnancy or within 5 months post-partum with no pre-existing cardiac disease or identifiable cause. The incidence is very low (<1%) and varies on the basis of the population studied. Risk factors include advanced maternal age, African descent, twin pregnancy, usage of tocolytics, and poverty.

The etiology remains unknown, but potential causes include abnormal immune response to pregnancy, increased myocyte apoptosis, genetic predisposition. Only 20% may worsen up to the death or transplantation, while one-half of PPCM patients recover normal systolic function within 6 months.

5. Arrhythmias

It is been demonstrated that women had a higher resting heart rate than did men (3 to 5 beats faster for minute). These finding may be explained by differences in exercise tolerance, autonomic modulation and intrinsic properties of the sinus node, influencing in part by hormonal influences. Burke et al. reported an higher average heart rate during the follicular or luteal phases of the menstrual cycle, although the response to double autonomic blockade was identical regardless of phase.

Several authors demonstrated differences in QT interval between men and women. Women have a longer corrected QT interval and the difference becomes more pronounced at lower heart rates. Rautaharju et al. reported that this difference was due to a drop in the corrected QT that occurred in males after puberty (when androgen levels are highest). Then, the interval in men gradually increased with age until 50 years, at which point it paralleled that of women. The actions of hormonal influences in QT differences was confirmed in families with genotipically characterized long QT syndrome. In addition, the torsades de pointes correlated to both congenital and acquired long QT Syndrome was more frequent in women.

There are many differences in incidence, prevalence, presentation and clinical course of many arrhythmias. Inappropriate sinus tachycardia is more common in women. Rodigruez et al. reported in patients undergoing invasive electrophysiologic testing for various tachycardias that the atrio-ventricular node reentrant tachycardia (AVNRT) was twice times more common in women, whereas atrial tachycardia affected both sexes equally. In addition, the atrio-ventricular reentrant (circus-movement) tachycardia (AVRT), atrial fibrillation (AF), and ventricular fibrillation (VF) occurred more often in men. These trends for supra-ventricular tachycardias (SVTs), AF, VF, were confirmed in the Framingham cohort. Myerburg and associates found that the inducing SVT during electrophysiologic testing was greatest at the onset of menses or during the premenstrual phase. Rossano et al. confirmed that the SVT prone state is hindered by estrogen and facilitated by progesterone.

The SVTs new- onset or exacerbation are most common arrhythmia during pregnancy and the postpartum period in absence o f structural heart disease. The mechanisms for increase in this situation may be related to progesteronerich gravid state, increased intravascular volume and autonomic tone.

The Atrial Fibrillation (AF) is the most prevalent in men, although its incidence increases with age both in men and women. Women with AF are more symptomatic, older and have lower quality of life and more co-morbidities than men. Also they present more likely a higher heart rate, longer episodes and increase incidence of embolic strokes compared to men. Data from the Euro Heart Survey on Atrial Fibrillation demonstrated that women are usually treated less aggressively, with fewer cardioversions and catheter ablations. In this study, albeit both genders received anticoagulation therapy, women experienced a significantly higher rate of stroke and major bleeding events.

6. References

[1] Leuzzi C, Sangiorgi GM and Modena MG (2010) Gender-specific aspects in the clinical presentation of cardiovascular disease Fundam Clin Pharmacol. N. 24(6):711-7

[2] Athyros VG, Ganotakis E, Kolovou GD et al (2011). Assessing The Treatment Effect in Metabolic Syndrome without Perceptible Diabetes (ATTEMPT): A Prospective-Randomized Study in Middle Aged Men and Women. Curr Vasc Pharmacol Apr 11. [Epub ahead of print].

[3] Leuzzi C, Modena MG (2011). Hypertension in postmenopausal women: pathophysiology and treatment. High Blood Press Cardiovasc Prev. N. 18;13-8.

[4] Shaw LJ, Bugiardini R, and Bairey Merz CN (2009) Women and Ischemic Heart Disease: Evolving Knowledge J. Am. Coll. Cardiol. N: 54;1561-1575

[5] Bairey Merz CN et al.(2006) Insights from the NHLBI-Sponsored Women's Ischemia Syndrome Evaluation (WISE) Study: Part II: gender differences in presentation,

diagnosis, and outcome with regard to gender-based pathophysiology of atherosclerosis and macrovascular and microvascular coronary disease. J. Am. Coll. Cardiol. N:47 S21–S29
[6] Vitale C, Miceli M, Rosano GM.(2007) Gender-specific characteristics of atherosclerosis in menopausal women: risk factors, clinical course and strategies for prevention. Climacteric. 2007 N.10; 16-20
[7] Association A.H.. Heart Disease and Stroke Statistics: 2004 Update. available at: http://americanheart.org/downloadable/heart/1072969766940HSStats2004Update.pdf
[8] Yinon Y, Kingdom JCP, Odutayo A (2010). Vascular Risk Vascular Dysfunction in Women With a History of Preeclampsia and Intrauterine Growth Restriction : Insights Into Future. Circulation N. 122, 1846-1853
[9] Bairey Merz N et al.(2004) Women's Ischemic Syndrome Evaluation: current status and future research directions: report of the National Heart, Lung and Blood Institute workshop: October 2–4, 2002: executive summary. Circulation N:109, 805–807
[10] Bugiardini R, Estrada JL, Nikus K et al. (2010) Gender bias in acute coronary sindromes. Curr Vasc Pharmacol. N.8;276-84
[11] Vaccarino V et al.(1999) Sex-based differences in early mortality after myocardial infarction. National Registry of Myocardial Infarction 2 Participants. N. Engl. J. Med. N:341 217–225
[12] Nabel EG et al.(2002) Women's Ischemic Syndrome Evaluation: current status and future research directions: report of the National Heart, Lung and Blood Institute workshop: October 2–4, 2002: Section 3: diagnosis and treatment of acute cardiac ischemia: gender issues. Circulation N: 109 e50–e52. 25
[13] Kolodgie FD et al. (2004) Pathologic assessment of the vulnerable human coronary plaque. Heart N: 90 1385–1391. 26
[14] Farb A et al. (2003) Pathological mechanisms of fatal late coronary stent thrombosis in humans. Circulation N:108, 1701–1706
[15] Shaver PJ, Carrig TF and Baker WP (1978)Postpartum coronary artery dissection. Br. Heart J. N: 40 83–86
[16] Basso C, Morgagni G.L., Thiene G.(1996) Spontaneous coronary artery dissection: a neglected cause of acute myocardial ischaemia and sudden death. Heart N: 75, 451–454
[17] Han SH et al.(2008)Sex differences in atheroma burden and endothelial function in patients with early coronary atherosclerosis. Eur Heart J N: 29, 1359–69
[18] Lloyd-Jones DM.(2001) The risk of congestive heart failure: sobering lessons from the Framingham Heart Study. Curr. Cardiol. Rep. N:3, 184–190
[19] O'Meara E et al.(2007) Sex differences in clinical characteristics and prognosis in a broad spectrum of patients with heart failure: results of the Candesartan in Heart failure: Assessment of Reduction in Mortality and morbidity (CHARM) program. Circulation N: 115 3111- 3120
[20] Hsich EM and Pina IL. (2009) Heart failure in women: a need for prospective data. J. Am. Coll. Cardiol. N: 54 491–498
[21] Mullens W et al. (2008) Gender differences in patients admitted with advanced decompensated heart failure. Am. J. Cardiol. N:102, 454–458
[22] Komajda M et al. (2003) The EuroHeart Failure Survey programme – a survey on the quality of care among patients with heart failure in Europe. Part 2: treatment. Eur.Heart J. N:24, 464–474

[23] Koeth O et al.(2008) Clinical, angiographic and cardiovascular magnetic resonance findings in consecutive patients with Takotsubo cardiomyopathy. Clin. Res. Cardiol. N:97, 623–627

[24] Gianni M et al.(2006) Apical ballooning syndrome or takotsubo cardiomyopathy: a systematic review. Eur. Heart J. N: 27, 1523–1529

[25] Hsich EM and Piña IL. (2009). Heart Failure in Women: A Need for Prospective Data. J Am Coll Cardiol N.54; 491-498

[26] Liu K et al. (1989) Ethnic differences in blood pressure, pulse rate, and related characteristics in young adults. The CARDIA study. Hypertension N:14:218-26

[27] Linde C.(2000) Women and arrhythmias. Pacing Clin Electrophysiol N: 23:1550-60

[28] Kadish AH. (1995) The effects of gender on cardiac electrophysiology and arrhythmias. In: Zipes DP, Jalife J, editors. Cardiac electrophysiology: from cell to bedside. 2nd ed. Philadelphia: WB Saunders; p. 1268-75

[29] Huikuri HV et al. (1996) Sex-related differences in autonomic modulation of heart rate in middle-aged subjects. Circulation N:94,122-5

[30] Burke JH et al.(1997) Gender-specific differences in the QT interval and the effect of autonomic tone and menstrual cycle in healthy adults. Am J Cardiol N:79,178-81

[31] Stramba-Badiale M et al.(1997) Gender and the relationship between ventricular repolarization and cardiac cycle length during 24-h Holter recordings. Eur Heart J N:18:1000-6

[32] Lehmann MH et al. (1997) Age-gender influence on the rate-corrected QT interval and the QT-heart rate relation in families with genotypically characterized long QT syndrome. J Am Coll Cardiol N:29, 93-9

[33] Locati EH et al.(1998) Age- and sex-related differences in clinical manifestations in patients with congenital long-QT syndrome: findings from the International LQTS Registry. Circulation N: 97, 2237-44

[34] Yarnoz MJ and Curtis AB.(2008) More reasons why men and women are not the same (gender differences in electrophysiology and arrhythmias). Am. J. Cardiol. N: 101 1291–1296

[35] Rollo P et al.(2001) Gender and Cardiac Arrhythmias Tex Heart Inst J 28, 265-75

[36] Lee RJ, Shinbane JS.(1997) Inappropriate sinus tachycardia. Diagnosis and treatment. Cardiol Clin N:15,599-605

[37] Morillo CA, Klein GJ, Thakur RK, Li H, Zardini M, Yee R.(1994) Mechanism of 'inappropriate' sinus tachycardia. Role of sympathovagal balance. Circulation N:90,873-7

[38] Rodriguez LM et al. (1992) Age at onset and gender of patients with different types of supraventricular tachycardias.Am J Cardiol N:70:1213-5

[39] Benjamin EJ et al.(1994) Independent risk factors for atrial fibrillation in a population-based cohort. The Framingham Heart Study. JAMA N:271,840-4

[40] Myerburg RJ et al. (1999) Cycling of inducibility of paroxysmal supraventricular tachycardia in women and its implications for timing of electrophysiologic procedures. Am J Cardiol N:83:1049-54

[41] Rosano GM et al.(1996) Cyclical variation in paroxysmal supraventricular tachycardia in women. Lancet N:347, 786–788

[42] Yarnoz MJ, Curtis AB.(2008) More reasons why men and women are not the same (gender differences in electrophysiology and arrhythmias. Am. J. Cardiol. N:101, 1291–1296

[43] Dagres N et al. (2007) Gender-related differences in presentation, treatment, and outcome of patients with atrial fibrillation in Europe: a report from the Euro Heart Survey on Atrial Fibrillation. J Am Coll Cardiol N: 49, 572–577

15

The Role of Stress in a Pathogenesis of CHD

Taina Hintsa[1], Mirka Hintsanen[1,2],
Tom Rosenström[1] and Liisa Keltikangas-Järvinen[1]
[1]*IBS, Unit of Personality Work and Health Psychology, University of Helsinki*
[2]*Helsinki Collegium for Advanced Studies, University of Helsinki*
Finland

1. Introduction

Stress has been commonly seen as a risk factor of diseases of major public health relevance including Type 2 diabetes and coronary heart disease (CHD). An influence of stress in their development has been considered a "well-known fact" even to the extent that a pathogenesis of those diseases has been widely attributed to stress. Empirical evidence is, however, somewhat conflicting. Even though studies showing an association between work stress and CHD are great in number, negative findings also exist. Thus, there is no consensus on the clinical importance of work stress in a development of CHD. Consequently, work stress is currently not included in the list of established risk factors of CHD (www.americanheart.org).

There are, however, several reasons explaining the conflicting findings, and several aspects have been omitted in stress research. Even an assessment of stress is far from unambiquity. The present paper was taken with a purpose to highlight complicated associations between different kind of stress reactions and risk factors of CHD.

This review will capitalize on the longitudinal population based birth cohort study of the *Young Finns Study*. Here, the representative, population based sample of 3596 healthy subjects from six age cohorts have been followed for 30 years and monitored in 9 study phases in order to discover the lifelong development of risk factors of coronary heart disease. From the great multidisciplinary reservoir of risk factors available in the Young Finns settings, stress is the focus of the current paper.

In this chapter we focus on different types of stress, e.g. psychological, psychosocial, physiological stress and work stress. Special issues to be highlighted here are as follows: Do the origins of stress proneness lie in childhood? Is stress vulnerability inherited?, Which is worse in regard to health: chronic or acute stress?, Does stress really have health consequences? Do genetic predispositions explain an association between stress and its health outcomes? What are the problems with statistical analyses in epidemiological studies?

2. Coronary heart disease

Coronary artery disease (CAD) which gradually progresses to coronary heart disease (CHD) is still the leading cause of death in industrialized countries. According to World Health

Organization cardiovascular diseases are the number one cause of death globally. In 2004, cardiovascular diseases were globally the cause of death of 29% of all deaths. Of those deaths, approximately 7.2 million were due to CHD (www.who.int/mediacentre/factsheets/fs317/en/index.html). In Finland, among the working aged population, in men there were 1218 and in women 231 deaths due to CHD in 2008 (http://www3.ktl.fi/stat/).

Atherosclerosis is the pathogenic process that underlies most cardiovascular diseases including CHD. Recently, a non-invasive technique such as an ultrasound measure of intima-media thickness has been developed to assess early stages of atherosclerosis. Carotid artery intima-media thickness (IMT) is a marker of subclinical atherosclerosis and increased IMT has been shown to predict CHD (O'Leary & Polak 2002).

Although the inherited, even a genetic disposition to CHD has been documented, CHD is seen as a lifestyle disease. Certain lifestyle factors may contribute to the manifestation of genetic disposition, and eventually have an effect on the onset of CHD. American Heart Association lists traditional risk factors for CHD: increasing age, male sex and heredity; smoking, high blood cholesterol, high blood pressure, physical inactivity and obesity (modifiable risk factors), and stress, alcohol and diet/nutrition as other risk factors of CHD.The traditional behavioural risk factors of CHD include smoking, alcohol consumption and physical inactivity. Behavioural and personality characteristics may be seen as lifestyle factors too, because they contribute to significant choices and decisions that individuals make during their lives. A systematic review of the epidemiological literature of prospective cohort studies, that is articles between 1966-1997 identify four psychosocial or behavioural risk factors of CHD: Type A behaviour,/hostility, depression, psychosocial work characteristics, and social support (Hemingway & Marmot 1999). According to a prognosis of World Health Organization stressful life events and psychosocial stress will the most detrimental risk factors for the development of cardiovascular diseases in the near future (http://www.who.int/en/).

In this chapter we introduce some recent findings about childhood and adolescent origins of stress, stress-health associations, e.g. temperament and early atherosclerosis (Hintsanen et. al., 2009a), the association between chronic stress and preclinical atherosclerosis (Chumaeva et. al., 2009a), and long-lasting chronic stress strengthening the physiological stress reactions in acute stress (Chumaeva et. al., 2010a). Furthermore, the topic whether stress has implications for CHD risk and what are the potential mechanisms are discussed.

3. The Young Finns study

In the literature, The Bogalusa Heart Study and the Young Finns Study are the only population-based prospective follow-up studies that have examined cardiovascular disease and CHD risks since childhood that have collected psychological information. The collection of psychological information in the Bogalusa Heart Study continued until the end of 1980s, and since then the Young Finns Study has been collecting psychological data. Thus, the Young Finns data is worldwide quite unique and it makes possible to study psychological risk factors of CHD from childhood on.

The Young Finns Study is a multi-centre study which was carried out in five university cities in Finland which have medical schools (Helsinki, Kuopio, Oulu, Tampere and Turku), and in rural municipalities nearby (Fig. 1). The areas of Helsinki, Tampere and Turku represented the west of the country, and the Kuopio and Oulu areas represented eastern Finland. The rural municipalities were chosen using the criteria of correspondence of industrial structure with average municipalities in the province, the age cohort being sufficiently large. The sample included an equal number of urban and rural populations in the area (Åkerblom et. al., 1991).To ensure equal and sufficiently large samples from east and west, and to include some communities in the extreme east, the sample size in Kuopio was twice that in other cities, with four instead of two rural municipalities included in the study (Åkerblom et al 1991). Two of the easternmost rural municipalities studied in the Kuopio area belonged to the province of North Karelia, where CHD morbidity and mortality among adults have been especially high (Menotti et. al., 1989). In 1980 the baseline study sample consisted of 4326 invited participants of which over 3500 children and adolescents aged from 3 to 18 participated (83.1%). The study included medical examinations and questionnaires (both self- and parent reports). These participants have had medical examinations and have filled questionnaires including demographic, socioeconomic/social and psychological information in the follow-up studies conducted in 1983, 1986, 1989, 1992, 1997, 2001, 2007 and 2011. The study design and the number of participants and the response rates at each data collection phases are outlined in Figure 2.

The participants have reported several aspects of their lives during 31 years, at several time points. These aspects include a wide range of CHD risk factors such as socioeconomic conditions, social life, health behaviour, dietary habits, environmental factors and personality.

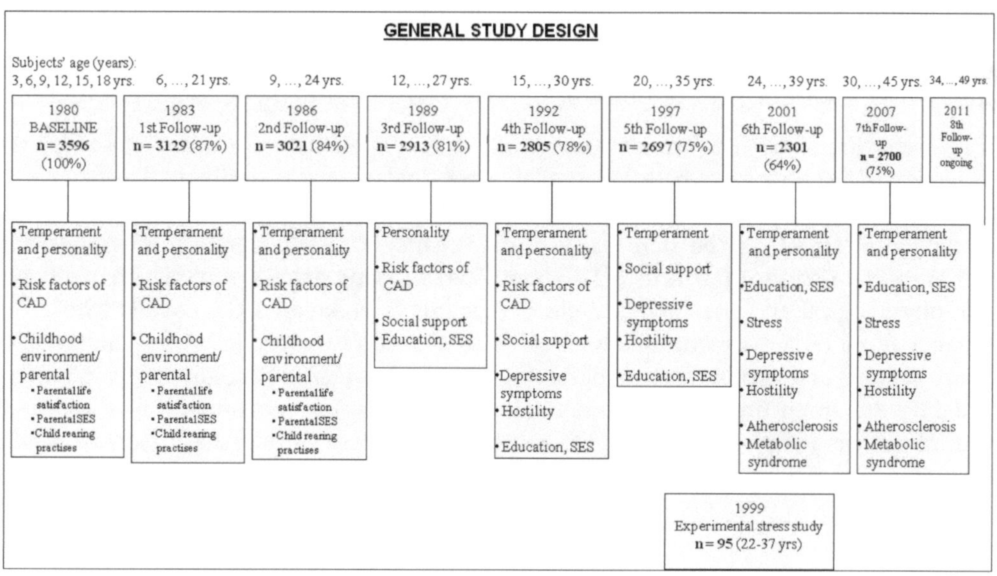

Fig. 1. The general study desing of the Young Finns Study.

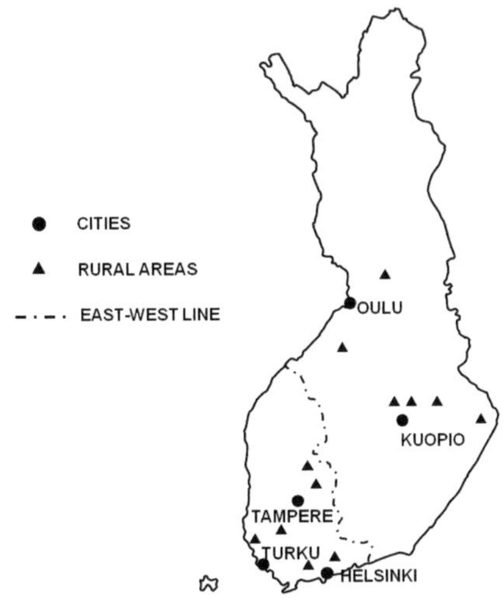

Fig. 2. The Young Finns Study: participating universities in Finland.

4. Stress

The purpose of this chapter is to highlight complicated associations between different kind of stress reactions and risk factors of CHD. Generally the term stress refers to experiences of endangering one's physical or psychological wellbeing. Physiological stress refers to bodily adaptation processes and the maintenance of body's balance (McEwen 1998; Selye 1973). Selye (1973) defined stress as a function of elevated corticosteroid levels and used the term stress to refer to the effects of any agent that threatens the homeostasis of the organism. McEwen and Stellar introduced (1993) the term allostasis which refers to the body's ability to achieve stability. The allostatic load is assumed to be caused by frequent stress, lack of adaptation to repeated stress, and inability to shut down the allostatic response when the stress is over and inadequate response or dysfunction of the stress systems (McEwen 1998).

In the behavioural sciences, stress refers to a mental experience of distress caused by the evaluation of the imbalance between available personal resources (individual appraisals of stressful encounters) and environmental demands (e.g. stressful life events). Thus, psychological stress can be defined as a discrepancy between personal capacities and environmental demands (Lazarus & Folkman 1984). Somatic stress symptoms are related to both physiological and psychological stress (Lazarus & Folkman 1984; Lovallo 1997). The different types of stressors are likely to elicit divergent stress reactions. The multifaceted nature of stress and various sources of stress must also be taken into account. It is important to define the stress precisely in epidemiological studies. Consequently, stress has been determined here in terms of stressful life events, experience of chronic stress, experimentally induced mental and physiological stress reactions and work stress.

4.1 Work stress

European Foundation for the improvement of living and working conditions (2007) reports that work stress is affecting more than 40 million individuals across the European Union, and is among the most often reported cause of illness by employees. Work stress has been suggested to increase the CHD risk via several different pathways and mechanisms. Therefore it is important to focus also on psychosocial characteristics at work in regard to cardiovascular health. The work stress models that are presented here have been used extensively in studies of occupational and cardiovascular health (Belkic et. al., 2004; van Vegchel et. al., 2005).

Theories of work stress focus on various aspects in the work environment. Contemporary models on work stress include factors that are long-term harmful stressors at work. There are several work stress models, but the scientifically most tested concepts include The Job Demands-Job control Model (Karasek & Theorell 1990) and the Effort-Reward Imbalance (ERI) model (Siegrist et. al., 2004). More recently organisational justice has been hypothesized to form an important source of stress at work (Elovainio et. al., 2010; Kivimäki et. al., 2005).

The two-dimensional Job Demands-Job Control model involves work-related aspects of job demands and job control. Job demands refer to time pressures and an excessive work load, and job control involves employees' decision latitude and opportunities to use social, organisational and personal resources in their work. The model proposes that employees who have high job demands together with low job control are suffering from job strain, and if prolonged, have increased risk of stress-related diseases. The ERI model of work stress is based on social exchange theory and it has broadened the view from proximal work aspects into descriptive and evaluative information on job demands, i.e. efforts, and more distant aspects of work, i.e. rewards. Efforts denote quantative and qualitative load, and increase in total load at work. Rewards refer to financial reward, esteem reward, reward related to promotion aspects and job security (Siegrist et al 2004).

Research on the psychosocial health determinants has recently extended the focus also to organizational justice, that is, social relations, decision making and managerial procedures at work (Colquitt 2001; Kivimäkii et. al., 2005). Organizational justice can be defined as "the extent to which employees are treated with justice at their workplace" (Colquitt 2001; Moorman 1991). Organisational justice includes four components: 1) procedural justice, 2) interpersonal justice, 3) informational justice and (4) distributive justice. Procedural justice refers to being able to express your views and feelings during organisational procedures, perceiving that they have been consistently applied. Interpersonal justice denotes aspects of supervisors' behaviour, i.e. have they treated the person with respect and dignity. Informational justice consists of communicating and giving details about the decisions. Distributive justice refers to the perception of whether outcomes at work reflect the effort one has put into work and whether the outcome is appropriate.

5. Do the origins of stress-proneness lie in childhood?

It may be suggested that origins of one's stress proneness lie in childhood. This has not been studied a lot in humans, but rationale for this suggestion has been derived from animal studies. Several studies conducted on rats and nonhuman primates have shown that lack of nurturing behavior does affect the stress systems of the pups so that pups that have received less nurturing develop altered physiological stress responsiveness and show increased behavioral stress reactivity in adulthood (Caldji et. al., 1998; Coplan et. al., 1996; Ladd et. al., 1996; Liu et. al., 1997).

The effect of maternal care to the development of offspring stress responsiveness has been examined with various research designs. For example, by handling the pups it is possible to increase the nurturing behaviors performed by the mother such as licking and grooming, and this makes it possible to compare pups that have received high nurturing by the mother and pups who have received normal care (Liu et al 1997). Studies have also used maternal separation for instant by comparing the physiological stress responsiveness of pups that have not been separated and pups that have been separated from their mother for varying periods of time (Stanton et. al., 1988). However, this kind of design might be suspected to reflect effects of food deprivation rather than deprivation of maternal nurturing. To examine whether this is the case, a study by Stanton, Gutierrez and Levine (1988) specifically examined whether increased stress responsiveness is related to lack of maternal nurturing or to lack of nutrition offered by the lactating mother. Their results showed that the association was partly dependent on the age of the examined rat pups so that in younger ages (12 and 16 days of age), lack of maternal nurturing increased stress reactivity, whereas when the pups grew somewhat older (20 days of age), the lack of maternal nurturing as well as the lack of nutrition increased stress reactivity assessed as elevated corticoid levels in response to novelty situation (Stanton et al 1988). Based on these results, it seems that maternal nurturing has an independent effect that cannot be explained by food deprivation.

Still other design was used by Coplan and colleagues (1996) who compared offspring of mother monkeys (bonnet macaques) who had differing conditions in which they foraged for food. One group of mothers foraged in uncertain conditions (the amount of needed foraging varied) whereas the other group foraged in predictable conditions (the amount of needed foraging was either constantly low or constantly high) (Coplan et al 1996). As it has been shown that unpredictable need for foraging lowers the amount of grooming the mother directs towards the monkey infants (Rosenblum & Paully 1984), comparing different foraging groups allows to compare the effects of higher and lower maternal nurturing behaviors.

In general, the studies conducted on animals that have examined effects of maternal nurturing to the stress responsiveness of the infants in their adulthood, have shown that those infants who have received less nurturing from their mothers show various alterations in their hypothalamic-pituitary-adrenal (HPA) -axis functioning later in life (Caldji et al 1998; Coplan et al 1996; Liu et al 1997). For instance, in response to acute stressors, offspring have shown changed physiological stress reactivity measured with plasma levels of adrenocorticotrophin hormone (ACTH), levels of corticosterone, glucocorticoid feedback sensitivity, and levels of hypothalamic corticotrophin-releasing hormone messenger RNA (Liu et al 1997). Furthermore, stable increases in corticotrophin releasing factor (CRF) in the cerebrospinal fluid have been found in grown up offspring of less nurturing mothers (Coplan et al 1996). Also changes in behaviour are observable, and offspring of less nurturing mothers show higher rates of behaviours reflecting stress (e.g. fearfulness) (Caldji et al 1998).

There are also several other findings that show that changes in stress reactivity in response to lower maternal nurturing can be found also in humans. For instance, Repetti, Taylor and Seeman (2002) have reviewed the literature and concluded that childhood unsupportive family relations (e.g. high rate of conflicts in the family and low nurturing) affect physiological stress responsiveness of HPA-axis functioning and sympathetic-adrenomedullary (SAM) functioning as well as emotion regulation and coping with stress. However, long-term prospective studies are rare.

6. Is stress vulnerability inherited?

Temperament refers to biologically rooted, partly inherited, relatively stable individual differences in reactivity to stimuli (Cloninger et. al., 1993; Gray 1991; Lewis & Haviland 1993; Strelau 1998). The inheritance of stress refers here to an innate temperament. Rationale is as follows: temperament a) has a biological basis, b) is highly inherited, and c) explains what one experiences as a stress and partly determines what the health consequences are. The common assumption in several temperament theories is that temperament plays important role in moderating stress (Strelau 1998). Temperament traits are closely related to emotions that have been suggested to be a possible source of stress-related individual differences (Lovallo 1997). Temperament is considered to be an important determinant in what one indentifies as a stressor, a state of stress, in how one copes with stress and therefore also the physiological consequences of stress (Strelau 1998). Temperament may explain a perception of stress and may predispose to negative emotional stress reactions.

7. Acute stress vs. chronic stress

Acute stress refers to a very short-time stress that can both be positive (eustress) and more distressing experience such as daily hassles or stressful encounters in day-to-day life. Chronic stress is the type of stress that is ongoing for a longer period of time and often feels unmanageable. Both acute and chronic stress may be detrimental to health (Lovallo 1997). It is not clear which is more detrimental to health, acute or chronic stress. What is likely that they may have different effects on health.

Acute stress is a normal adaptive reaction to threat of the sympathetic-adrenal-medullary axis (SAM) releasing catecholamines and the hypothalamic-pituitary-adrenal (HPA) axis secretion of glucocorticoids (Sapolsky et. al., 2000). Even though acute stress reaction is adaptive and necessary, it may have detrimental influences on cardiac health. Acute stress may trigger cardiac events or lead to sudden death (Culic 2007; Hemingway et. al., 2001).

Chronic stress is likely to influence the autonomic nervous system function, and may alter the endocrine system and the immune system function. If a person is exposed to chronic stress, the SAM and HPA axis are continuously over-activated or in imbalance, and overcompensation or collapse of these systems may leave the individual susceptible to stress-related diseases (Korte et. al., 2005). Prolonged secretion of epinephrine, norepinephrine and cortisol, i.e. primary stress mediators, may affect the stress system so that their ability to protect the organism is compromised and instead starting to damage the brain and the body (McEwen 2008). The secondary outcomes of the wear and tear condition processes are the metabolic parameters such as insulin, cholesterol, triglycerides which may reach sub-clinical level at this stage of stress. The final stage of stress may include the wear and tear of the body, i.e. allostatic exhaustion (McEwen 1998; 2008).

8. Work stress

Several epidemiological studies have shown the association between work stress and CHD risk (Belkic et al 2004; Kivimäki et. al., 2006; van Vegchel et al 2005). Job strain has been suggested to be a risk factor for CHD and cardiac events (Belkic et al 2004; Kivimäki et. al., 2002; Kivimäkii et. al., 2006). A review of 45 empirical studies on effort-reward imbalance between 1986-2003 reports that the extrinsic effort-reward hypothesis (high effort combined with low rewards increase disease risk) has shown a good explanatory power for the incidence of CHD (van Vegchel et al 2005).

Previous studies report lower levels of organisational justice to be associated with lower wellbeing, higher self reported morbidity, higher medically certified absence from work, and increased mental health problems (Elovainio et. al., 2000; Elovainio et. al., 2001; Kivimäki et. al., 2003; Kivimäki et. al., 2005). Injustice at work has been related to impaired cardiovascular regulation among women (Elovainio et. al., 2006b), and cardiovascular mortality (Elovainio et al 2006b). Low organizational justice has been reported to be a risk to the health of employees (Elovainio et. al., 2006a). Furthermore, it has been reported that employees who experience high organisational justice at work had lower risk of incident CHD than those with low or an intermediate level of justice (Kivimäki et. al., 2005).

When studying work stress-CHD risk associations, it is important to examine the role of third variables such as pre-employment origins of work stress. We have examined the childhood origins of work stress which is a novel perspective in work stress research. Furthermore, it is also important to extend work stress research towards taking individual differences and genetic influences into account.

9. Does stress have implications for CHD risk and what are the potential mechanisms?

Showing the causal link between stress and the outcome requires evidence and knowledge about the potential mechanisms. The research of the Young Finns Study provides epidemiological and experimental evidence on the importance of stress in early atherosclerosis and in the pathogenesis of CHD, and also shows that the associations between stress and cardiovascular risk are complicated.

Stress may influence health via several different pathways, i.e. alterations in autonomic nervous system, neuroendocrine activity, immune system functions, behavioral and cognitive functions (Lovallo 1997). Prolonged stress may alter the function of autonomic nervous system, neuroendocrine functions and inflammation systems (McEwen 1998; Sapolsky 1996; Sapolsky et al 2000), and it may affect individuals' health-behaviour in terms of increased smoking and alcohol consumption, and decreased physical activity, and may increase anxiety, depression and psychological distress and include alterations in memory functions and attention (Hemingway & Marmot 1999; Lovallo 1997). Being exposed to chronic stress may lead to different types of health problems such as mental disorders, vital exhaustion, burnout and increase of CHD disease risk via several different pathways (Lovallo 1997).

9.1 Epidemiological evidence

The findings presented in this chapter are mainly from the Young Finns study (YFS) and they focus on early atherosclerosis. The results of a smaller sample of men describe the associations between psychological factors and hormonal variables and Insulin resistance syndrome risk factors.

In the YFS, an association between job strain and IMT has been documented among men aged 32.3 years on average (Hintsanen et. al., 2005). This implies that among men job strain may be linked to atherosclerosis in its early non-symptomatic stages. A recent longitudinal study on the association between job strain and IMT reports that large decreases in job strain from 2001 to 2007 in men was associated with slower progression of IMT and decreases in both job control and demands (a change towards passive jobs) were associated with greater IMT progression (Rosenström et. al., 2011). These results imply that temporal changes in job demands and control are linked with IMT.

Our research has focused in three temperament theories: Gray's neurobiological model of temperament, Cloninger's psychobiological theory of temperament, and the EAS theory of temperament by Buss and Plomin. Gray's temperamental model assumes three fundamental systems with independent neurobiological mechanisms in the mammalian central nervous system (CNS): the behavioral inhibition system (BIS), the behavioral approach system (BAS) and the fight/flight system (FFS). The BIS is activated by aversive stimuli and is assumed to cause behavioral inhibition, and increase in attention levels and negative affects. The BAS is primarily activated by appetitive stimuli causing approach behavior and positive affects. There are individual differences in the sensitivity or functioning strength of these systems. Thus, some individuals are more prone to react to incentives and to experience positive affects, that is BAS sensitive, while some are fixed to threats in the environment and more likely to experience negative affects than others (Corr 2008; Gray 1991).

Cloninger's psychobiological theory of temperament, measured by temperament and character inventory (TCI) includes three genetically independent dimensions of temperament: novelty seeking (NS), harm avoidance (HA) and reward dependence (RD) (Cloninger et al 1993). Persistence (P) was added to the model a little bit later (Cloninger et al 1993). Novelty seeking, linked with dopaminergic activity, refers to tendency to respond strongly to novelty. High novelty seeking is characterized by exploratory behaviors, impulsivity, excitability and disorderliness. Harm avoidance, related to serotonergic activity, denotes that high harm avoidant persons are cautious, fearful, inhibited and prone to anxiety and fatigue. Reward dependence, associated with noradrenalin activity, refers to sensitivity to social cues, empathy and sentimentality. Persistence is a tendency to act persistently regardless of weariness and frustration, and high persistence is characterized by perseverance.

The emotionality-activity-sociability (EAS) theory of temperament focuses on broad temperament traits that are likely to be present in majority of situations (Buss & Plomin 1984). The temperament traits are negative emotionality, sociability and activity. Negative emotionality is characterized by tendency to get upset easily and equals to stress sensitivity. Sociability is a preference to be in a company of other people. Activity refers to the tempo of physical actions and vigor referring to the strength with which these actions are performed.

Temperament and early atherosclerosis. Temperament traits in terms of Cloninger's temperament theory explain between-individual variation in atherosclerosis (Hintsanen et al 2009a). Higher NS and RD, and lower HA were associated with preclinical atherosclerosis. The effect sizes of the associations found were comparable to those of traditional risk factors of CHD, which is an important finding. Novelty seekers are likely to seek for novel situations and environments, and via that encounter stressful situations continuously, i.e. be exposed to stress frequently. High RD persons seek for approval and have desire to please others, potentially even at the expense of their own wellbeing. Harm avoidant persons are characterised by stress-proneness and therefore a positive relation between high HA and higher IMT would have been expected. Stress reactions of highly harm avoidant persons increase in experimental settings, but in real life, however, they may have successfully learned to avoid stressful situations and thus be less exposed to stress.

In women, childhood hyperactivity has been shown to predict IMT in adulthood (Keltikangas-Järvinen et. al., 2006). It was concluded that childhood temperament may directly contribute to the development on IMT in women. This association might partly be explained by different environmental expectations for boys and girls. The same temperament plays a different roles in boys and girls (Kerr et. al., 1997). The association between childhood hyperactivity and adulthood IMT among women might be due to that high hyperactivity in girls may enhance the misfit with the environment which, in turn, may be related to chronic stress (Keltikangas-Järvinen et. al., 2006).

We have found an association between active temperament and early atherosclerosis among men. The results of a study on emotionality-activity-sociability temperament and preclinical atherosclerosis showed that a highly active temperament may contribute to early atherosclerosis in men, and that body mass may mediate this association (Pulkki-Råback et. al., 2011).

Chronic stress and cardiac responsiveness. Endothelial dysfunction is a marker of atherosclerotic risk (Bonetti et. al., 2003), and arterial elasticity indicated by carotid arterial compliance (CAC) may be an additional indicator of early atherosclerosis (Anderson 2006). We studied the role of chronic stress, endothelial dysfunction and arterial elasticity in regard to IMT. Chronic stress was indexed by vital exhaustion which is a state of unusual fatigue, a loss of mental and physical energy and increased irritability (Appels et. al., 1987), and has been referred as an indicator of long-term mental stress (Ingles et. al., 1999). Endothelial dysfunction was indexed by brachial flow-mediated dilation (FMD), and carotid elasticity by CAC. A significant VE and FMD, and VE and CAC interactions on IMT were found in participants with the very lowest FMD and CAC. It was concluded that chronic stress may especially harmful if the endothelium is not working properly (Chumaeva et al 2009a). Chronic stress was negatively related to FMD, which may imply that chronic stress may contribute to endothelial dysfunction. A study on the possible sex differences in the combined effect of chronic stress with impaired vascular endothelium functioning and the development of early atherosclerosis showed a significant VE x CAC interaction on IMT among men. High VE level was related to higher IMT among those men with low CAC (Chumaeva et. al., 2010b). These results imply that vital exhaustion is a risk only if it has resulted in ineffective cardiac stress reactivity. Chronic stress may induce imbalance of the autonomic function which may be the mechanism linking vital exhaustion and cardiac responsiveness to an increased risk of atherosclerosis.

Chronic stress in terms of major stressful life events and vital exhaustion has been related to arrhythmic events (Hintsa et. al., 2010c). A history of stressful life events and prolonged mental stress have been associated with arrhythmic events among subjects who are genetically predisposed to cardiac vulnerability (a sample of molecularly defined patients with long QT syndrome). In this group of patients the interaction of a gene defect and the environmental loading may contribute to the manifestation of arrhythmic events.

Psychological factors and IRS. Stress may be a trigger for the neuroendocrine and metabolic abnormalities characteristic to the metabolic syndrome. It has been shown that chronic stress may exert effects on waist-hip -ratio (WHR) and on subsequent metabolic alterations.

Chronic stress is suggested to exert a pathophysiological effect on WHR, on alterations in insulin and lipid metabolism, in fibrinolysis and in blood pressure. Perceived stress modifies an association between neuroendocrine mechanisms and metabolic syndrome. The associations may be explained by HPA-axis dysfunction, that is, a failure to adrenal hypoactivity to prevent overshooting of reactions to stress (Räikkönen et. al., 1997).

Psychological factors may explain a proportion of HPA-axis responses that are related to Insulin resistance syndrome (IRS). Type A behavior was related to a high level of mean basal ACTH and a low level of cortisol response to ACTH stimulation after dexamethasone suppression. Hostility was linked to a high level of mean basal cortisol and a high cortisol in cortisol/ACTH –ratio. Vital exhaustion that indexes chronic stress was related to a low level of mean basal ACTH and a decreased ACTH in relation to cortisol (Keltikangas-Järvinen et. al., 1997; Keltikangas-Järvinen et. al., 1996b). Stress modulated adrenal responsiveness may partly explain the IRS risk, and the risk of atherosclerosis, too. Chronic stress and stressful life-style have been related to the IRS (Räikkönen et. al., 1996b). Chronic stress in terms of vital exhaustion, and a stressful life-style (Type A behavior, hostility and anger) were associated with hyperinsulinemia, hyperglycemia, dyslipidemia, hypertension, and increased abdominal obesity. The secondary outcomes of allostatic load include metabolic, cardiovascular and immune parameters' alterations and potential to reach sub-clinical levels of these (McEwen 1998; 2008; McEwen & Stellar 1993). Therefore it is important to further investigate the role of stress-related personality and behavioral factors in regard to metabolic alterations.

Psychological factors and HPA-axis responses. The studies presented in this paragraph have been conducted among middle-aged male managers who responded questionnaires, participated in laboratory analyses, and were clinically examined in Helsinki University Central hospital (n=64-90). Results of a study on the relationships between the pituitary adrenal hormones, insulin and glucose in regard to chronic stress showed that basal ACTH level during oral glucose tolerance test was positively related to the cortisol response to ACTH at 60 minutes, the fasting insulin level, and the insulin to glucose ratio among chronically stressed men (Keltikangas-Järvinen et. al., 1998).

A neuroendocrine pattern characterized by an elevation in cortisol response to ACTH stimulation and dominance of cortisol in the ratio of mean basal cortisol level to mean basal ACTH level denoting a defeat type of reaction to stress differentiated borderline hypertensive men from normotensive men (Räikkönen et. al., 1996a). The results may imply that the variance shared by chronic stress, emotional distress and pituitary-adrenocortical hormones could be the mechanism by which stress influences and increased risk for hypertension.

Author, year	**Study focus**	**Main findings**
Hintsanen et. al., 2005	IMT: job strain and social support	In men, job strain was related to higher IMT.
Rosenström et al., 2010	IMT and job strain (2001 and 2007)	An association between job strain and IMT in 2001 among men. In men with large decreases in job strain-slower progression of IMT.
Hintsanen et. al., 2009a	IMT and Cloninger temperament	Higher NS and RD, and lower HA was associated with IMT.
Keltikangas-Jarvinen et. al., 2006	IMT and childhood temperament	In women, childhood hyperactivity predicted adulthood IMT.

Author, year	Study focus	Main findings
Pulkki-Råback et. al., 2011	IMT and EAS temperament	A highly active temperament may contribute to early atherosclerosis in men, and that body mass may mediated this association.
Chumaeva et. al., 2009a	IMT and chronic stress (VE) and endothelial dysfunction (FMD)	Significant VE and FMD, and VE and CAC interactions on IMT were found in participants with the very lowest FMD and CAC.
Chumaeva et. al., 2010b	IMT and chronic stress (VE), flow-mediated dilation (FMD), Carotid elasticity (CAC)	In men, a significant VE x CAC interaction on IMT. High VE level was related to higher IMT among those men with low CAC.
Hintsa et. al., 2010c	Arrhythmic events and chronic stress	A history of stressful life events and prolonged mental stress are associated with arrhythmic events in LQTS patients. The association between stressful life events and arrhythmic events was independent of age, sex, specifically focused drugs and LQTS subtype.
Räikkönen et. al., 1997	IRS and chronic stress (VE)	Chronic stress excerted effects on WHR and on subsequent metabolic alterations which denote a chance of adrenal steroid biosynthesis.
Keltikangas-Järvinen et. al., 1996b	IRS and psychological factors	A link between VE-anger out and net-increment of cortisol and the IRS.
Räikkönen et. al., 1996b	IRS and stress inducing life style (Type A behaviour, hostility and anger)	Chronic stress in terms of vital exhaustion, and a stressful life-style (Type A behavior, hostility and anger) were associated with hyperinsulinemia, hyperglycemia, dyslipidemia, hypertension, and increased abdominal obesity.
Keltikangas-Järvinen et. al., 1998	HPA-axis and chronic stress	Basal ACTH level during OGTT was positively related to the cortisol response to ACTH at 60 minutes, the fasting insulin level, and the insulin to glucose ratio among exhausted men.
Keltikangas-Järvinen et. al., 1997	HPA-axis responses and Type A behaviour (TABP), hostility, chronic stress (VE)	TABP was related to a high level of mean basal ACTH and a low level of cortisol response to ACTH stimulation after dexamethasone suppression; Hostility was related to a high level of mean basal cortisol and a high cortisol in cortisol/ACTH ratio, and VE was related to a low level of mean basal ACTH and a decreased ACTH in relation to cortisol.
*Räikkönen et.al., 1996a	HPA-axis and Chronic stress (VE), anger	A neuroendocrine pattern characterized by an elevation in cortisol response to ACTH stimulation and dominance of cortisol in the ratio of mean basal cortisol level to mean basal ACTH level denoting a defeat type of reaction to stress differentiated borderline hypertensive men from normotensive men.

Table 1. Summary of results of the epidemiological studies.

9.2 Experimental studies

In the series of our studies on experimental stress we have found that psychological factors are related to experimentally induced stress. The typical psychological stressors in the laboratory are an acoustic startle probe, a mental arithmetic task, and a public speaking task. The experimental stressors in the laboratory in our studies were a mental arithmetic (the three best participants would be awarded a prize of $40, appetitive task), and a startle and a reaction time tasks (aversive tasks). Exaggerated heart rate reactivity to stress may imply disease proneness. It has been suggested that heightened heart rate responses to stress may be a risk for development of atherosclerosis and coronary heart disease (Matthews, 1986, Krantz & Manuck, 1984). Temperament may also be important in regard to stress-related cardiac reactivity and may even predispose the individual to elevated risk profile of the metabolic parameters. Temperament refers to individual differences in arousability of behavioural and physiological systems. There are prominent individual differences in the mode of autonomic response to stress (Cacioppo 1994).

The self-reported emotions have been measured according to the Larsen and Diener (1992) circumplex model of affects (Larsen & Diener 1992). Emotions can be defined as action tendencies or action dispositions (Lewis & Haviland 1993). Two general dimensions of affects are valence (pleasant/unpleasant) and activation or arousal (Larsen & Diener 1992). The two-dimensional circumplex model of affect consists of eight sections which are: high/low activation, unpleasant/pleasant, activated/ unactivated unpleasant, and activated/unactivated pleasant. We have also used the Watson's and Tellegen's model of positive affectivity (PA) and negative affectivity (NA) to measure the general affective orientation during laboratory tasks (Watson et. al., 1988) in our studies.

Temperament may predispose the person to stress and negatively biased environmental and personal interpretations. In an experimental study it has been reported that temperament in terms of Gray's concept explains emotional reactions during laboratory stress (Heponiemi et. al., 2003). This model was used to structure the self-reported affects in our study. The experimental stressors in the laboratory were a mental arithmetic, a startle and a reaction time tasks. The main finding was that BIS sensitivity was related to activated unpleasant affects (e.g. anxious, fearful, tense) during reaction time and startle tasks whereas BAS sensitivity was associated with activated pleasant affects (e.g. vigorous, lively) during mental arithmetic task. BIS sensitivity is, thus, likely to predispose a person to emotional distress in stressful situation regardless of the nature of the stressor, and also probably to a higher stress proneness. Thus, BIS sensitivity may increase one's stress vulnerability by predisposing the person to poor and inactive coping. BIS has been previously related to negative affectivity (Heponiemi et al 2003). BIS sensitivity may also influence person's focus of attention and predispose to bias towards negative cues of the environment because it has been suggested that high BIS-persons would be negatively biased in environmental interpretations.

We have found that temperament trait persistency (in terms of Cloninger's concept) interacted with chronic stress predisposing to a high physiological stress reactivity (Keltikangas-Järvinen & Heponiemi 2004). Chronic stress was indexed by vital exhaustion. Vital exhaustion was associated with parasympathetic withdrawal, i.e. low RSA magnitude, during stressful tasks in laboratory. Temperament trait persistence was likely to strengthen cardiac stress reactivity of exhausted women. Findings suggest that background stress may decrease one's capacity to cope with acute stress and be related to continuous physiological stress.

According to Gray's theory, BAS sensitivity refers to strong reaction to incentives and thus BAS is assumed to primarily be activated by appetitive stimuli such as reward and termination of punishment (Gray 1991). We found that BAS sensitivity was related to heart rate reactivity and parasympathetic withdrawal during the tasks (Heponiemi et. al., 2004). The relationship between BAS temperament and cardiac reactivity might be mediated by the parasympathetic nervous system. HR expresses the balance between the parasympathetic and sympathetic nervous system. Normal parasympathetic control of heart is suggested to promote good health, may protect the heart and dampen the sympathetic reactions to stress (Porges 1992) whereas low parasympathetic control of HR has been associated with cardiovascular diseases (Tsuji et. al., 1996).

Temperament in terms of Cloninger's concept, that is HA, has been related to chronic stress, and when associated with vital exhaustion, likely to predispose negative affects when accompanied by exhaustion (Heponiemi et. al., 2005). The level of vital exhaustion among healthy persons was related to unpleasant affects such as sadness, fear, anxiety and anger. In other words, the participants with high level of vital exhaustion felt more tense, fearful, anxious, sad, depressed, angry and irritated during stress, and less lively than participants with low levels of vital exhaustion. Furthermore, inherited temperament may increase proneness to exhaustion and predispose to negative affects when feeling exhausted. The results imply that temperamental tendency to perseverance combined with stressful environmental loading may predispose to exhaustion. Temperament may predispose an exhausted person to negative affects and lead to individual differences in stress vulnerability.

Cloninger's psychobiological model of temperament and character postulates that each of the temperament dimensions is associated with a specific emotional experience. We tested this assumption and found that NS was associated with dullness during monotonous and aversive situations and with a higher level of pleasantness during the initial baseline period and the appetitive situation. HA was associated with higher levels of fear and unpleasant emotions and lower levels of positive emotions, depending on the situational cues. The study provides support for the validity of Cloninger's temperament dimensions as predictors of emotional responses during different challenges. Especially, novelty seeking and harm avoidance appear to have a significant influence on emotional experience (Puttonen et. al., 2005).

Temperament in terms of Cloninger's concept is related to a perception of stress during experimentally induced stress (Ravaja et. al., 2006). HA was consistently associated with high anticipated threat prior to stressors and high perceived stress after the stressors. In addition, the interaction of HA and NS predicted threat appraisals prior the task. Low HA and high NS was associated with higher threat before the social task (public speech). Individual differences in perceived threat may be important because it is assumed that the primary appraisal of threat affects psychological and physiological responses to stressors (Lazarus & Folkman 1984).

Novelty seeking temperament has been associated with higher IMT (Hintsanen et. al., 2009b). Cardiac stress reactivity and recovery was studied among extremely high and extremely low scorers of novelty seeking. We examined whether novelty seeking is associated with cardiac reactions to a laboratory challenge. The results suggest that, that high novelty seekers may be more stress resilient because they might have faster cardiac recovery after stress (Hintsanen et. al., 2009b).

A study of hemodynamic and other autonomically mediated responses to mental stress in laboratory and the parameters of IRS among adolescent boys showed that a high level and an increasing trend of heart rate (HR) and finger blood volume (FBV)were related during challenging tasks (Keltikangas-Järvinen et. al., 1996a). Automatically mediated physiological responses (HR, HRV, FBV and skin conductance level, SCL) to experimentally induced stress are related to serum insulin level and other parameters of IRS in adolescent boys. The finding suggests that trends of psychophysiological responses to task-induced stress implicate important individual differences in stress modulation. In addition, results imply a relationship between stress-induced sympathetically mediated physiological responses and the metabolic and anthropometric parameters constituting IRS in healthy adolescent boys.

Individuals differ widely in the extent to which they are prone to experience normal daily challenges as positive or negative. Watson's and Tellegen's model of positive affectivity (PA) and negative affectivity (NA) was used to measure the general affective orientation during laboratory tasks (Watson et al 1988). PA included emotions such as active, enthusiastic and energetic, and NA refers to being distressed, fearful and nervous. A study examining the relationship between PA and NA to autonomic cardiac reactivity during laboratory tasks reports that participants with high levels of PA during varying laboratory tasks exhibited high parasympathetic reactivity and heart rate reactivity (Heponiemi et. al., 2006). However, against expectations, high levels of NA were not related to sympathetic arousal. It was concluded that cardiac reactivity may be associated with positive involvement and enthusiasm, and thus, should not be automatically considered as pathological.

Acute mental stress may contribute to the cardiovascular disease progression via autonomic nervous system controlled negative effects on the endothelium. We examined the interactive effect of acute mental stress-induced cardiac reactivity/recovery and endothelial function on the prevalence of carotid atherosclerosis. The results showed a significant interaction of FMD and cardiac RSA recovery for IMT, and a significant interaction of FMD and pre-ejection period (PEP). P recovery for IMT. Among participants with low FMD, slower PEP recovery was related to higher IMT. Among individuals with high FMD, slow RSA recovery predicted higher IMT. It seems that the development of endothelial dysfunction may be one possible mechanism linking slow cardiac recovery and atherosclerosis via autonomic nervous system mediated effect. Cardiac recovery plays a role in progression of atherosclerosis in persons with high and low FMD. The role of sympathetically mediated cardiac activity seems to be more important in those with impaired FMD, and parasympathetically mediated in those with relatively high FMD (Chumaeva et al 2010a; Chumaeva et. al., 2009b).

High parasympathetic reactivity during stress is considered as appropriate stress response whereas an inability to suppress parasympathetic tone is related to experienced stress and stress vulnerability (Porges 1992). When considering the potential mechanisms (summary over all our findings including the temperament-related experiments) between stress and CHD risk slow cardiac recovery is of high importance. It seems that the important role of stress in CHD risk is played rather by parasympathetic underactivity than sympathetic overactivity.

Author, year	Study focus	Main findings
Heponiemi et. al., 2003	Self-rated affects and BIS-BAS temperament (n= 95)	BAS was related to pleasant affects with an especially great increase of activated pleasant affect (vigorous, peppy, lively) during an appetitive task. BIS was related to unpleasant affects with a great increase of activated unpleasant affects (anxious, fearful, tense) during an aversive task.
Keltikangas-Järvinen et. al., 1996	Cardiac reactivity, chronic stress (VE) and temperament (n=76)	Chronic stress was related to parasympathetic withdrawal. Chronically stressed women expressed the highest level of physiological reactivity. Among the chronically stressed the initial parasympathetic tone had no effect whereas in the non-chronically stressed parasympathetic reactivity was greatest when initial parasympathetic tone was high.
Heponiemi et. al., 2004	Cardiac autonomic stress profiles and BIS-BAS temperament (n=65)	BAS was related to HR reactivity and parasympathetic withdrawal during the tasks.
Heponiemi et. al., 2005	Affects, chronic stress and temperament (n=76)	Chronic stress was related to unpleasant state affects other than state fatigue. Temperament modified the relationship between chronic stress and affects. Chronic stress was related to harm avoidance.
Puttonen et. el., 2005	Affective responses during challenge and temperament	NS was associated with dullness during monotonous and aversive situations and with a higher level of pleasantness during the initial baseline period and the appetitive situation. HA was associated with higher levels of fear and unpleasant emotions and lower levels of positive emotions.
Ravaja et. al., 2006	Threat, stress and performance appraisalsand temperament (n= 97)	Temperament traits are related to threat, stress and performance appraisals. HA was related to high anticipated threat prior to the stressors.
Hintsanen et. al., 2009b	Cardiac stress reactivity and recovery and temperament (n= 29)	High novelty seekers may be more stress resilient because they had faster cardiac recovery than others.
Keltikangas-Järvinen et. al., 1996a	IRS parameters (insulin, HDL, TG, SBP, SSF, STR) and mental stress (n=48)	Automatically mediated physiological responses (HR, HRV, FBV and SCL) to experimentally induced stress are related to serum insulin level and other parameters of IRS in adolescent boys.
Heponiemi et. al., 2006	Cardiac reactivity, facial muscle movements and positive and negative affects (n=77)	Experiencing positive affects was related to more pronounced parasympathetic, heart rate, and orbicularis oculi reactivity.
Chumaeva et. al., 2009b	IMT and chronic stress (VE), cardiac stress reactivity and recovery (n=69)	Among the highly exhausted men aged 28-37, lower HR reactivity was related to greater IMT.
Chumaeva et. al., 2010a	IMT and chronic stress (VE), cardiac stress reactivity and recovery, flow-mediated dilation (FMD) (n= 81)	A FMD and cardiac RSA interaction, and FMD and PEP recovery for IMT. Among participants with low FMD, slower PEP recovery was related to higher IMT. Among individuals with high FMD, slow RSA recovery predicted thicker IMT.

Table 2. Summary of the results of experimental studies.

9.3 Work stress

Several epidemiological studies have shown the association between work stress and CHD risk but there are also non-significant findings (Belkic et al 2004; Lange et al 2003; van Vegchel et al 2005). To explain conflicting findings, it is important to study whether the excess CHD risk among employees with high job strain is confounded by the pre-employment, personality and genetic effects. Therefore, we have focused on a novel perspective of examining effects of biological, psychological and socioeconomic factors in early life and adolescence, i.e. the period before entering work life, on perceptions of work stress and early atherosclerosis.

Pre-employment factors and work stress. We have examined whether pre-employment factors influence perceptions of work stress in adulthood. The socioeconomic conditions in childhood and adolescence may also contribute to perceptions of work stress in adulthood. Lower parental socioeconomic position (SEP), that is low paternal and maternal education and low family income, has been shown to predict increased job strain of the offspring in adulthood (Hintsa et. al., 2006). Part of the effect of low parental SEP on job strain and job control was mediated by participants' education. In addition, high parental SEP in the childhood family predicted higher rewards at work in adulthood among women (Hintsa et. al., 2007). We also found a strong positive relationship between parental SEP and the participants' educational attainment. A potential explanation for the predictive relationship between parental SEP and participants' education is that highly educated parents may offer good educational resources and through that enhance the educational attainment of their offspring. These findings indicate that pre-employment factors should be taken into account as potential confounders in future research on job strain-CHD risk associations.

Stressful childhood environments are suggested to contribute to later stress vulnerability. It has been shown that deficient nurturing attitudes in childhood predict offspring's work stress and low job control in adulthood (Hintsanen et. al., 2010). Deficient nurturing attitudes were indicated by intolerance of the mother towards the normal activity of the child, and low emotional warmth by the mother towards to the child. Deficient nurturance may also have indirect stress-inducing effects: the development of social skills has previously been related to child-rearing styles (Steelman et. al., 2002). Social skills are very important in the contemporary work as team work and personal networks have become increasingly important. Furthermore, inadequate social skills are likely to be sources of stress.

Temperament and personality in perceptions of work stress. Temperament traits may predispose the individual to experience work stress. Temperament in terms of Cloninger's concept is related to work stress, also to the components that are expected to reflect environmental loading by characteristics at work (Hintsa et. al., 2010a). Low NS and high HA predicted higher job strain. High NS, low HA and high P predicted higher long-term job control. Partly inherited, quite stable temperamental tendencies seem to contribute to job strain and its components. High NS seems to protect from job strain whereas high HA may predispose the individual to long-term work stress. HA may increase the number of stressful encounters at work because the individual predisposition to experience stress more easily. HA has previously been related to inefficient coping strategies such as rumination, resignation and escaping from stressful situations. Therefore, HA may lead to the selection of less efficient coping strategies and subsequently influence the time it takes to recover from stress.

Furthermore, it has been documented that temperament traits negative emotionality and sociability predict work stress. Negative emotionality refers to tendency to easily react with anger or fear and sociability a tendency to enjoy being in the company of others and to search for others company (Buss & Plomin 1984). The results have shown that higher negative emotionality and lower sociability systematically predict higher perceived job strain and effort-reward imbalance (ERI) (Hintsanen et. al., 2011).

Type A behaviour – work stress. Personality may also predispose a person to experience work stress. Type A behaviour is a stress—related personality type originally found by Friedman and Rosenman, and it has been related to risk of CHD. Type behaviour is characterized by aggressiveness, feelings of time urgency, competitiveness, easily aroused anger/hostility, and hard-driving elements. Ambition and competitiveness are very relevant traits in regard to work context. Type A persons have high need for control, and demanding and challenging situations are likely to elicit Type A behaviour. Of the components of Type A behaviour, high leadership was found to predict low long-term work stress while high hard-driving (taking things seriously, high responsibility and competitiveness,) predicted higher long-term work stress (Hintsa et. al., 2010b). Furthermore, high aggression and eagerness-energy may predispose the employee to unfavourable effort-reward condition. Thus, it seems that different Type A behaviour components may have divergent influence on long-term work stress. These results suggest that more attention should be paid to individual factors and stress vulnerability in work stress research. Our findings strongly suggest that stress sensitivity may have childhood roots.

Do pre-employment factors explain work stress-CHD risk association? We have also aimed at examining the possible explanation for conflicting findings in work stress - CHD risk research. Therefore a series of studies examining the role of confounding factors in the work stress - CHD risk associations have been conducted. A prospective study on the contribution of biological, familial and socioeconomic risk factors in adolescence to the association between adulthood job strain and IMT reported that these pre-employment factors did not confound the relationship between job strain and early atherosclerosis in men (Kivimäki et. al., 2007). The findings of this study support the role of job strain as a risk factor for increased CHD risk.

In a study among Finnish men, it was found that personality trait leadership (willingness to always win, being selected as a leader in group activities, being socially active and having many hobbies), which is a component of Type A behaviour, attenuated the association between job strain and IMT (Hintsa et. al., 2008). Low leadership in adolescence predicted higher job strain 15 years later, and this personality characteristic attenuated the association between job strain and IMT by 17% to nonsignificant. It was concluded that leadership component of Type A behaviour may represent a non-risk component of Type A behaviour, and that personality characteristics might also be important to include in work stress-CHD risk studies.

A study among British male civil servants showed that selected pre-employment factors such as family history of CHD, height, paternal education and social class, and number of siblings were related to increased risk for CHD. The significant hazard ratios (HR) for CHD found were 1.33 for family history of CHD, 1.18 for each quartile decrease in height, and 1.16 for each category increase in number of siblings. Psychosocial factors at work also predicted CHD: the significant HR was 1.72 both for low job control and low organisational justice (Hintsa et. al., 2010d). However, the association between psychosocial factors at work and CHD incidence was largely independent of selected pre-employment factors.

Author, year	**Study focus**	**Main findings**
Hintsa et. al., 2006	Job strain and pre-employment factors	Lower parental SEP and higher parental life dissatisfaction independently of the number of siblings and educational level predicted job strain in adulthood 18 years later. The effects were partly mediated by participants' education.
Hintsa et. al., 2007	ERI and pre-employment factors	High rewards were predicted by high parental life satisfaction in men and by high parental SEP in women.
Hintsanen et. al., 2010	Job strain, ERI and maternal nurturing attitudes	Deficient emotional warmth in childhood predicted lower adulthood job control and higher job strain.
Kivimäki et. al., 2007	Job strain-IMT association and early risk factors	Pre-employment influences did not confound the association between job strain and IMT.
Hintsa et. al., 2008	Job strain-IMT association and pre-employment factors	Type A personality leadership component attenuated the association between job strain and IMT by 17% to non-significant. Pre-employment family factors had only modest effect on this association.
Hintsanen et. al., 2007	Job strain-IMT association and NRG-1	Job strain was associated with increased IMT among men with T/T genotype of NRG-1. A direct association between NRG-1 and IMT was found in women.
Hintsanen et. al., 2008	Job strain-IMT association and COMT	In men, job strain was associated with increased IMT in Val/Val carriers.
Hintsa et. al., 2010d	Psychosocial factors at work and CHD, and pre-employment factors	The association between psychosocial factors at work (low job control and organisational justice) and CHD was largely independent of the selected pre-employment factors. Increase in number of siblings, quartile decrease in height and family history of CHD predicted development of CHD.
Hintsanen et. al., 2010	Job strain, ERI and maternal nurturing attitudes	Deficient emotional warmth in childhood predicted lower job control and higher job strain in adulthood independently of age, sex, SES in childhood, maternal mental problems, and participants' hostility and depressive symptoms.
Hintsa et. al., 2010a	Long-term job strain, job control and job demands (6 years) and temperament	Low NS and high HA predicted higher long-term job strain. Higher NS, lower HA and higher P predicted higher long-term job control. Higher HA and higher P predicted higher long-term job demands.
Hintsanen et. al., 2011	Job strain, ERI and temperament	Higher negative emotionality and lower sociability systematically predicted higher perceived job strain and ERI. Activity predicted higher perceived ERI.
Hintsa et. al., 2010b	Job strain, ERI and personality (Type A behaviour)	High leadership (Type A dimension) predicted lower long-term job strain and higher long-term job control. High hard-driving predicted higher long-term job strain. High aggression, hard-driving and eagerness-energy predicted ERI.

Table 3. Summary of results of the work stress studies.

Do genetic factors contribute to the association between work stress and IMT? We have extended our research to clarify whether genetic predispositions explain an association between stress and its health outcomes. When trying to indentify groups at risk, examining whether an interaction between genotype and job strain may predispose to increased atherosclerotic processes is important. Another study reports that the association between job strain and greater IMT was found only among men with the T/T genotype of NRG-1 gene (Hintsanen et. al., 2007). Thus, the T/T genotype may be a marker of genetic susceptibility to the negative health effects of job strain on early atherosclerosis in men. Job strain has been related to higher IMT among men with Val/Val genotype of the catechol-O-methyltranferase (COMT) gene (Hintsanen et. al., 2008). This implies that Val/Val carriers may be at higher risk for negative health effects of job strain. It seems that the new study strategy of taking the genetic influences into account in identifying groups at risk for negative effects of work stress on cardiovascular risk may be worthwhile.

In sum, all the findings described here imply that although work stress seems to increase the CHD risk, there are some pre-employment factors that should be taken into account in work stress-CHD risk studies. In addition, this evidence should motivate the development of systematic intervention strategies for large-scale studies testing whether reducing work stress, giving employees a stronger say in decisions about their work and enhancing a righteous manner of treating employees at work would reduce CHD.

9.4 Statistical problems

In this section we discuss shortly three general problems in statistical modelling of population data that we think are particularly central for behavioural epidemiology. If objective of science is to go beyond what can be seen with naked eyes, implication is that our observations depend on the instruments we use. One such instrument is the statistical model. Careful scrutiny of instrument limitations is every bit as important as the results they provide.

Linear models between behavioural variables are most frequently used in epidemiological studies, while psychological theories rarely assume independency or linearity, and also many of the above cited studies demonstrated some interaction effects. Questionnaire-based measures are typically thought to contain measurement error. Measurement error makes the estimation of nonlinear and interactive effects between variables notoriously hard (Carroll et. al., 2006; Griliches & Ringstad 1970). A lot of methodological development is warranted regarding modelling of general nonlinearities in this context, and either more precise measurements or more precise models of measurement error may be the prerequisite. Also, exponentially increasing amounts of data are required for the data-driven exploration of increasingly high dimensional interactions (Wasserman 2006). In below, we turn to problems that are present even when linear approximation is reasonable.

Often questionnaire-based measurement instruments entertain floor/ceiling-effect (inadequate sampling of true variation) and/*or* measurement error. Using a variable suffering from either one as a covariate in ordinary (and generalized) linear regression model can results in bias and false findings if the covariate is correlated with another 'independent' (predictor) variable (Austin & Brunner 2003; Brunner & Austin 2009; Carroll et al 2006). These problems could be addressed, along with those arising from more familiar overfitting problem (Babyak 2004), from the point of view of combined cross-validation and partial least squares regression (Abdi 2010; Rosipal & Kramer 2006).

In this young field of science, often little is known about precise type of measurement error, and model assumptions rarely are firmly established. Partial least squares regression handles well a range of error types (Reis & Saraiva 2004) and cross-validation is able to control for errors in assumptions (Arlot & Celisse 2010). For these (and other) reasons this combination holds promise beyond many more commonly encountered choices of explorative data analysis.

Finally, both linear and nonlinear models typically assume that model holds over entire study population, whereas often only a part of the study population displays an effect. Genetic vulnerability and gene-environment interactions are clear examples of interacting variables that may not always be available in the data (Caspi et. al., 2010; Keltikangas-Järvinen & Jokela 2010). A statistical null finding can thus result from an inappropriate combination of heterogeneous groups instead of the lack of association. Such grouping of data according to latent (unobserved) variable can be modelled with mixture (weighted sum) of statistical models (McLahlan & Peel 2000).

Although mixture models are frequently referred as readily available and their utility is apparent, they are not a similarly well-researched topic as many other familiar statistical models. Their estimation actually involves technical difficulties known as singularities of parameter space (Watanabe 2009). This is a way of saying that more than one set of model parameters can result in the exact same model and that miniscule chances in parameters may cause drastic changes in the resulting model. This is undesirable phenomenon because one often interprets the data in terms of model parameters (e.g. regression slope). Mathematical theories that are most frequently used to analyze statistical models cannot cope with these difficulties, and new developments seem important (Watanabe 2009).

Above we discussed of some pertinent difficulties that still hinder most statistical modelling attempts in the field, from linear to nonlinear and mixture models. We feel that scientists applying these methods are not always sufficiently informed about involved difficulties. Current section attempted to fill this gap to a small degree and point some important methodological research topics, not to discourage researchers from doing their best possible work.

10. Conclusions

The findings of the Young Finns Study imply that stress is related to an increase of CHD risk through several pathways. The results also imply that more attention should be paid to pre-employment factors and individual differences in work stress research.

Stress affects people differently, that is, there are differences in individuals in stress proneness and what is considered as a stressor. These individual differences in stress experience stem from inherited characteristics and life experiences from childhood on. The influence of stress on cardiovascular health may be mediated through several different mechanisms. Based on our research it seems that the important role of stress in CHD risk is played rather by parasympathetic underactivity than sympathetic overactivity. Stress has to be measured appropriately and accurately keeping several different aspects of stress in mind: source of stress, the duration of stress, and individual vulnerability to stress have to be kept in mind when studying the role of stress in pathogenesis of CHD.

However, the research also shows that studying stress-health associations and the etiological role of stress in CHD is complicated and needs accurate measuring, appropriate statistical methods and population-based longitudinal study designs.

11. References

Abdi H. 2010. Partial least squares regression and projection on latent structure regression (PLS-regression) *Wiley Interdisciplinary Reviews: Computational Statistics* 2:97-106.

Anderson TJ. 2006. Arterial stiffness or endothelial dysfunction as a surrogate marker of vascular risk. *Canadian Journal of Cardiology* 22 Suppl B:72B-80B.

Appels A, Hoppener P & Mulder P. 1987. A questionnaire to assess premonitory symptoms of myocardial infarction. *International Journal of Cardiology* 17:15-24.

Arlot S & Celisse A. 2010. A survey of cross-validation procedures for model selection. *Statistics Surveys* 4 40-79.

Austin PC & Brunner LJ. 2003. Type I error inflation in the presence of a ceiling effect *The American Statistician* 57:97-104.

Babyak MA. 2004. What you see may not be what you get: a brief, nontechnical introduction to overfitting in regression-type models. *Psychosomatic Medicine* 66:411-21.

Belkic KL, Landsbergis PA, Schnall PL & Baker D. 2004. Is job strain a major source of cardiovascular disease risk? *Scandinavian Journal of Work, Environment & Health* 30:85-128.

Bonetti PO, Lerman LO & Lerman A. 2003. Endothelial dysfunction: a marker of atherosclerotic risk. *Arteriosclerosis, Thrombosis and Vascular Biology* 23:168-75.

Brunner J & Austin PC. 2009. Inflation of type I error rate in multiple regression when independent variables are measured with error. *Canadian Journal of Statistics* 37:33-46.

Buss AH & Plomin R. 1984. *Temperament: Early developing personality traits.* Hillsdale, NJ: Lawrence Erlbaum Associates Inc.

Cacioppo JT. 1994. Social neuroscience: autonomic, neuroendocrine, and immune responses to stress. *Psychophysiology* 31:113-28.

Caldji C, Tannenbaum B, Sharma S, Francis D, Plotsky PM & Meaney MJ. 1998. Maternal care during infancy regulates the development of neural systems mediating the expression of fearfulness in the rat. *Proceedings of the National Academy of Sciences of the United States of America* 95:5335-40.

Carroll RJ, Ruppert D, Stefanski LA & Crainiceanu CM. 2006. *Measurement error in nonlinear models: A modern perspective* Boca Raton, USA: Chapman & Hall/CRC.

Caspi A, Hariri AR, Holmes A, Uher R & Moffitt TE. 2010. Genetic sensitivity to the environment: the case of the serotonin transporter gene and its implications for studying complex diseases and traits. *American Journal of Psychiatry* 167:509-27.

Chumaeva N, Hintsanen M, Hintsa T, Ravaja N, Juonala M, Raitakari OT & Keltikangas-JärvinenL. 2010a. Early atherosclerosis and cardiac autonomic responses to mental stress: a population-based study of the moderating influence of impaired endothelial function. *BMC Cardiovascular Disorders* 10:16.

Chumaeva N, Hintsanen M, Juonala M, Raitakari OT & Keltikangas-Järvinen L. 2010b. Sex differences in the combined effect of chronic stress with impaired vascular endothelium functioning and the development of early atherosclerosis: the Cardiovascular Risk in Young Finns study. *BMC Cardiovascular Disorders* 10:34.

Chumaeva N, Hintsanen M, Ravaja N, Juonala M, Raitakari OT & Keltikangas-Järvinen L. 2009a. Chronic stress and the development of early atherosclerosis: moderating effect of endothelial dysfunction and impaired arterial elasticity. *International Journal of Environmental Research and Public Health* 6:2934-49.

Chumaeva N, Hintsanen M, Ravaja N, Puttonen S, Heponiemi T, Pulkki-Råback L, Juonala M, Raitakari OT, Viikari JS & Keltikangas-Järvinen L. 2009b. Interactive effect of long-term mental stress and cardiac stress reactivity on carotid intima-media thickness: The Cardiovascular Risk in Young Finns study. *Stress* 12:1.

Cloninger CR, Svrakic DM & Przybeck TR. 1993. A psychobiological model of temperament and character. *Archives of General Psychiatry* 50:975-90.

Colquitt JA. 2001. On the dimensionality of organizational justice: a construct validation of a measure. *Journal of Applied Psychology* 86:386-400.

Coplan JD, Andrews MW, Rosenblum LA, Owens MJ, Friedman S, Gorman JM & Nemeroff CB. 1996. Persistent elevations of cerebrospinal fluid concentrations of corticotrophin-releasing factor in adult nonhuman primates exposed to early-life stressors: Implications for the pathophysiology of mood and anxiety disorders. *Proceedings of the National Academy of Sciences of the United States of America* 93:1619-23.

Corr PJ. 2008. Reinforcement sensitivity theory: introduction. In *The reinforcement sensitivity theory of personality*, ed. PJ Corr. Cambridge: Cambridge University Press.

Culic V. 2007. Acute risk factors for myocardial infarction. *International Journal of Cardiol* 117:260-9.

Elovainio M, Heponiemi T, Kuusio H, Sinervo T, Hintsa T & Aalto AM. 2010. Developing a short measure of organizational justice: a multisample health professionals study. *J Occupational and Environmental Medicine* 52:1068-74.

Elovainio M, Kivimäki M, Puttonen S, Lindholm H, Pohjonen T & Sinervo T. 2006a. Organisational injustice and impaired cardiovascular regulation among female employees. *Occupational and Environmental Medicine* 63:141-4.

Elovainio M, Kivimäki M, Steen N & Kalliomaki-Levanto T. 2000. Organizational and individual factors affecting mental health and job satisfaction: a multilevel analysis of job control and personality. *Journal of Occupational Health Psychology* 5:269-77.

Elovainio M, Kivimäki M & Helkama K. 2001. Organizational justice evaluations, job control and occupational strain. *Journal of Applied Psychology* 86:418-24.

Elovainio M, Leino-Arjas P, Vahtera J & Kivimäki M. 2006b. Justice at work and cardiovascular mortality: a prospective cohort study. *Journal of Psychosomatic Research* 61:271-4.

Gray JA. 1991. The neuropsychology of temperament. In *Explorations in temperament: International perspectives on theory and measurement. Perspectives on individual differences.*, ed. J Strelau, A Angleitner, pp. 105-28.

Griliches Z & Ringstad V. 1970. Error-in-the-variables bias in nonlinear contexts. . *Econometrica: Journal of the Econometric Society*, 38:368-70.

Hemingway H, Malik M & Marmot M. 2001. Social and psychosocial influences on sudden cardiac death, ventricular arrhythmia and cardiac autonomic function. *European Heart Journal* 22:1082-101.

Hemingway H & Marmot MG. 1999. Psychosocial factors in the aetiology and prognosis of coronary heart disease: systematic review of prospective cohort studies. *British Medical Journal* 318:1460-7.

Heponiemi T, Keltikangas-Järvinen L, Kettunen J, Puttonen S & Ravaja N. 2004. BIS-BAS sensitivity and cardiac autonomic stress profiles. *Psychophysiology* 41:37-45.

Heponiemi T, Keltikangas-Järvinen L, Puttonen S & Ravaja N. 2003. BIS/BAS sensitivity and self-rated affects during experimentally induced stress. *Personality and Individual Differences* 34:943-57.

Heponiemi T, Keltikangas-Järvinen L, Puttonen S & Ravaja N. 2005. Vital exhaustion, temperament, and the circumplex model of affect during laboratory-induced stress. *Cognition & Emotion* 19:879-97.

Heponiemi T, Ravaja N, Elovainio M, Näätänen P & Keltikangas-Järvinen L. 2006. Experiencing positive affect and negative affect during stress: relationships to cardiac reactivity and to facial expressions. *Scandinavian Journal of Psychology* 47:327-37.

Hintsa T, Hintsanen M, Jokela M, Elovainio M, Raitakari OT & Keltikangas-Järvinen L. 2010a. The influence of temperament on long-term job strain and its components: The Cardiovascular Risk in Young Finns Study. *Personality and Individual Differences* 49:700-5.

Hintsa T, Hintsanen M, Jokela M, Pulkki-Råback L & Keltikangas-Järvinen L. 2010b. Divergent influence of different type a dimensions on job strain and effort-reward imbalance. *Journal of Occupational and Environmental Medicine* 52:1-7.

Hintsa T, Kivimäki M, Elovainio M, Hintsanen M, Pulkki-Råback L & Keltikangas-JärvinenL. 2007. Pre-employment family factors as predictors of effort/reward imbalance in adulthood: a prospective 18-year follow-up in the Cardiovascular Risk in Young Finns study. *Journal of Occupational and Environmental Medicine* 49:659-66.

Hintsa T, Kivimäki M, Elovainio M, Keskivaara P, Hintsanen M, Pulkki-Råback L & Keltikangas-Järvinen L. 2006. Parental socioeconomic position and parental life satisfaction as predictors of job strain in adulthood: 18-year follow-up of the Cardiovascular Risk in Young Finns Study. *Journal of Psychosomatic Research* 61:243-9.

Hintsa T, Kivimäki M, Elovainio M, Vahtera J, Hintsanen M, Viikari JS, Raitakari OT & Keltikangas-Järvinen L. 2008. Is the association between job strain and carotid intima-media thickness attributable to pre-employment environmental and dispositional factors? The Cardiovascular Risk in Young Finns Study. *Occupational and Environmental Medicine* 65:676-82.

Hintsa T, Puttonen S, Toivonen L, Kontula K, Swan H & Keltikangas-Järvinen L. 2010c. A history of stressful life events, prolonged mental stress and arrhythmic events in inherited long QT syndrome. *Heart* 96:1281-6.

Hintsa T, Shipley M, Gimeno D, Elovainio M, Chandola T, Jokela M, Keltikangas-Järvinen L, Vahtera J, Marmot MG & Kivimäki M. 2010d. Do pre-employment influences explain the association between psychosocial factors at work and coronary heart disease? The Whitehall II study. *Occupational and Environmental Medicine* 67:330-4.

Hintsanen M, Elovainio M, Puttonen S, Kivimäki M, Lehtimaki T, Kahonen M, Juonala M, Rontu R, Viikari JS, Raitakari OT & Keltikangas-Järvinen L. 2008. Val/Met polymorphism of the COMT gene moderates the association between job strain and early atherosclerosis in young men. *Journal of Occupational and Environmental Medicine* 50:649-57.

Hintsanen M, Elovainio M, Puttonen S, Kivimäki M, Raitakari OT, Lehtimäki T , Rontu R, Juonala M, Kahonen M, Viikari J & Keltikangas-Järvinen L. 2007. Neuregulin-1 genotype moderates the association between job strain and early atherosclerosis in young men. *Annals of Behavioral Medicine* 33:148-55.

Hintsanen M, Hintsa T, Widell A, Kivimäki M, Raitakari OT & Keltikangas-Järvinen L. 2011. Negative emotionality, activity, and sociability temperaments predicting long-term job strain and effort-reward imbalance: A 15-year prospective follow-up study. *Journal of Psychosomatic Research* 71:90-6.

Hintsanen M, Kivimäki M, Elovainio M, Pulkki-Råback L, Keskivaara P, Juonala M, Raitakari OT & Keltikangas-Järvinenn L. 2005. Job strain and early atherosclerosis: the Cardiovascular Risk in Young Finns study. *Psychosomatic Medicine* 67:740-7.

Hintsanen M, Kivimäki M, Hintsa T, Theorell T, Elovainio M, Raitakari OT, Viikari JSA & Keltikangas-Järvinen L. 2010. A prospective cohort study of deficient maternal nurturing attitudes predicting adulthood work stress independent of adulthood hostility and depressive symptoms. *Stress*:1-10.

Hintsanen M, Pulkki-Råback L, Juonala M, Viikari JS, Raitakari OT & Keltikangas-Järvinen L. 2009a. Cloninger's temperament traits and preclinical atherosclerosis: the Cardiovascular Risk in Young Finns Study. *Journal of Psychosomatic Research* 67:77-84.

Hintsanen M, Puttonen S, Järvinen P, Pulkki-Råback L, Elovainio M, Merjonen P & Keltikangas-Järvinen L. 2009b. Cardiac Stress Reactivity and Recovery of Novelty Seekers. *International Journal of Behavioral Medicine*:16:236-40.

Ingles JL, Eskes GA & Phillips SJ. 1999. Fatigue after stroke. *Archives of Physical Medical Rehabilitation* 80:173-8.

Karasek RA & Theorell T. 1990. *Healthy work: Stress, productivity and the reconstruction of working life.* New York: Basic Books.

Keltikangas-Järvinen L & Jokela M. 2010. Nature and nurture in personality *Focus* 8:180-6.

Keltikangas-Järvinen L & Heponiemi T. 2004. Vital exhaustion, temperament, and cardiac reactivity in task-induced stress. *Biological Psychology* 65:121-35.

Keltikangas-Järvinen L, Pulkki-Råback L, Puttonen S, Viikari J & Raitakari OT. 2006. Childhood hyperactivity as a predictor of carotid artery intima media thickness over a period of 21 years: the cardiovascular risk in young Finns study. *Psychosomatic Medicine* 68:509-16.

Keltikangas-Järvinen L, Ravaja N, Räikkönen K, Hautanen A & Adlercreutz H. 1998. Relationships between the pituitary-adrenal hormones, insulin, and glucose in middle-aged men: moderating influence of psychosocial stress. *Metabolism* 47:1440-9.

Keltikangas-Järvinen L, Ravaja N, Räikkönen K & Lyytinen H. 1996a. Insulin resistance syndrome and autonomically mediated physiological responses to experimentally induced mental stress in adolescent boys. *Metabolism* 45:614-21.

Keltikangas-Järvinen L, Räikkönen K & Adlerkreutz H. 1997. Response of the pituitary-adrenal axis in terms of Type A behavior, hostility and vital exhaustion in healthy middle aged men. *Psychology and Health* 12:533-42.

Keltikangas-Järvinen L, Räikkönen K, Hautanen A & Adlercreutz H. 1996b. Vital exhaustion, anger expression, and pituitary and adrenocortical hormones. Implications for the insulin resistance syndrome. *Arteriosclerosis, Thrombosis and Vascular Biology* 16:275-80.

Kerr M, Tremblay RE, Pagani L & Vitaro F. 1997. Boys' behavioral inhibition and the risk of later delinquency. *Archives of General Psychiatry* 54:809-16.

Kivimäki M, Elovainio M, Vahtera J & Ferrie JE. 2003. Organisational justice and health of employees: prospective cohort study. *Occupational & Environmental Medicine* 60:27-34.

Kivimäki M, Ferrie JE, Brunner E, Head J, Shipley MJ, Vahtera J & Marmot MG. 2005. Justice at work and reduced risk of coronary heart disease among employees: the Whitehall II Study. *Archives of Internal Medicine* 165:2245-51.

Kivimäki M, Hintsanen M, Keltikangas-Järvinen L, Elovainio M, Pulkki-Råback L, Vahtera J, Viikari JSA & Raitakari OT. 2007. Early risk factors, job strain, and atherosclerosis among men in their 30s: the Cardiovascular Risk in Young Finns Study. *American Journal of Public Health* 97:450-2.

Kivimäki M, Leino-Arjas P, Luukkonen R, Riihimäki H, Vahtera J & Kirjonen J. 2002. Work stress and risk of cardiovascular mortality: prospective cohort study of industrial employees. *British Medical Journal* 325:857-61.

Kivimäki M, Virtanen M, Elovainio M, Kouvonen A, Väänänen A & Vahtera J. 2006. Work stress in the etiology of coronary heart disease--a meta-analysis. *Scandinavian Journal of Work, Environment and Health* 32:431-42.

Korte SM, Koolhaas JM, Wingfield JC & McEwen BS. 2005. The Darwinian concept of stress: benefits of allostasis and costs of allostatic load and the trade-offs in health and disease. *Neuroscience and Biobehavioral Reviews* 29:3-38.

Ladd CO, Owens MJ & Nemeroff CB. 1996. Persistent changes in corticotrophin-releasing factor neuronal systems induced by maternal deprivation. *Endocrinology* 137:1212-8.

Larsen RJ & Diener E. 1992. Promises and problems with the circumplex model of emotion. In *Review of personality and social psychology: Emotion*, ed. MS Clark. Newbury Park, CA: Sage.

Lazarus RS & Folkman S. 1984. *Stress, appraisal and coping*. New York: Springer Publishing Company

Lewis M & Haviland JM. 1993. *Handbook of emotions*. New York, NY: Guilford Press

Liu D, Diorio J, Tannenbaum B, Caldji C, Francis D, Freedman A, Sharma S, Pearson D, Plotsky PM & Meaney MJ. 1997. Maternal care, hippocampal glucocorticoid receptors, and hypothalamic-pituitary-adrenal responses to stress. *Science* 277:1659-62.

Lovallo WR. 1997. *Stress & Health. Biological and Psychological interactions.* Thousand Oaks: SAGE publications, Inc.

McEwen BS. 1998. Protective and damaging effects of stress mediators. *New England Journal of Medicine* 338:171-9.

McEwen BS. 2008. Central effects of stress hormones in health and disease: Understanding the protective and damaging effects of stress and stress mediators. *European Journal of Pharmacology* 583:174-85.

McEwen BS & Stellar E. 1993. Stress and the individual. Mechanisms leading to disease. *Arch Intern Med* 153:2093-101.

McLahlan G & Peel D. 2000. *Finite mixture models.* . New York, USA John Wiley & Sons, Inc.

Menotti A, Keys A, Aravanis C, Blackburn H, Dontas A, Fidanza F, Karvonen MJ, Kromhout D, Nedeljkovic S, Nissinen A & et al. 1989. Seven Countries Study. First 20-year mortality data in 12 cohorts of six countries. *Annals of Medicine* 21:175-9.

Moorman RH. 1991. Relationship between organizational justice and organizational citizenship behaviors: do fairness perception influence employee citizenship? *Journal of Applied Psychology* 76:845-55.

O'Leary DH & Polak JF. 2002. Intima-media thickness: a tool for atherosclerosis imaging and event prediction. *American Journal of Cardiology* 90:18L-21L.

Porges SW. 1992. Vagal tone: a physiologic marker of stress vulnerability. *Pediatrics* 90:498-504.

Pulkki-Råback L, Puttonen S, Elovainio M, Raitakari OT, Juonala M & Keltikangas-Järvinen L. 2011. Adulthood EAS-temperament and carotid artery intima-media thickness: the Cardiovascular Risk in Young Finns study *Psychological Health* 26:61-75.

Puttonen S, Ravaja N & Keltikangas-Järvinen L. 2005. Cloninger's temperament dimensions and affective responses to different challenges. *Comprehensive Psychiatry* 46:128-34.

Räikkönen K, Hautanen A & Keltikangas-Järvinen L. 1996a. Feelings of exhaustion, emotional distress, and pituitary and adrenocortical hormones in borderline hypertension. *Journal of Hypertension* 14:713-8.

Räikkönen K, Keltikangas-Järvinen L, Adlercreutz H & Hautanen A. 1996b. Psychosocial stress and the insulin resistance syndrome. *Metabolism* 45:1533-8.

Räikkönen K, Keltikangas-Järvinen L, Hautanen A & Adlerkreutz H. 1997. Neuroendocrine mechanisms in chronic perceived stress: associations with the metabolic syndrome. *Endocrinology and Metabolism* 4:247-54.

Ravaja N, Keltikangas-Järvinen & Kettunen J. 2006. Cloninger's temperament dimensions and threat, stress, and performance appraisals during different challenges among young adults. *Journal of Personality* 74:287-310.

Reis MS & Saraiva PM. 2004. A comparative study of linear regression methods in noisy environments. *Journal of Chemometrics,* 18:526-36.

Repetti RL, Taylor SE & Seeman TE. 2002. Risky families: family social environments and the mental and physical health of offspring. *Psychological Bulletin* 128:330-66.

Rosenblum LA & Paully GS. 1984. The effects of varying environmental demands on maternal and infant behavior. *Child Development* 55:305-14.

Rosenström T, Hintsanen M, Kivimäki M, Jokela M, Juonala M, Viikari JS, Raitakari OT & Keltikangas-Järvinen L. 2011. Change in job strain and progression of atherosclerosis: The Cardiovascular Risk in Young Finns study. *Journal of Occupational Health Psychology* 16:139-50.

Rosipal R & Kramer N. 2006. Overview and recent advances in partial least squares. . *Lecture Notes in Computer Science* 3940:34-51.

Sapolsky RM. 1996. Stress, Glucocorticoids, and Damage to the Nervous System: The Current State of Confusion. *Stress* 1:1-19.

Sapolsky RM, Romero LM & Munck AU. 2000. How do glucocorticoids influence stress responses? Integrating permissive, suppressive, stimulatory, and preparative actions. *Endocrine Reviews* 21:55-89.

Selye H. 1973. The evolution of the stress concept. *American Scientist* 61:692-9.

Siegrist J, Starke D, Chandola T, Godin I, Marmot M, Niedhammer I & Peter R. 2004. The measurement of effort-reward imbalance at work: European comparisons. *Social Science & Medicine* 58:1483-99.

Stanton ME, Gutierrez YR & Levine S. 1988. Maternal deprivation potentiates pituitary-adrenal stress responses in infant rats. *Behavioral Neuroscience* 102:692-700.

Steelman LM, Assel MA, Swank PR, Smith KE & Landry SH. 2002. Early maternal warmth responsiveness as a predictor of child social skills: direct and indirect paths of influence over time. *Applied Developmental Psychology* 23:135-56.

Strelau J. 1998. *Temperament. A Psychological Perspective*. New York: Plenum Press

Tsuji H, Larson MG, Venditti FJ, Jr., Manders ES, Evans JC, Feldman CL & Levy D. 1996. Impact of reduced heart rate variability on risk for cardiac events. The Framingham Heart Study. *Circulation* 94:2850-5.

van Vegchel N, de Jonge J, Bosma H & Schaufeli W. 2005. Reviewing the effort-reward imbalance model: drawing up the balance of 45 empirical studies. *Social Science & Medicine* 60:1117-31.

Wasserman L. 2006. *All of nonparametric statistics.* . New York, USA: Springer-Verlag

Watanabe S. 2009. *Algebraic geometry and statistical learning theory*. New York, USA: Cambridge University Press

Watson D, Clark LA & Tellegen A. 1988. Development and validation of brief measures of positive and negative affect: the PANAS scales. *Journal of Personality and Social Psychology* 54:1063-70.

Åkerblom HK, Uhari M, Pesonen E, Dahl M, Kaprio EA & Nuutinen E. 1991. Cardiovascular risk in young Finns. *Annals of Medicine* 23:35-40.

16

Pulse Pressure and Target Organ Damage

Adel Berbari and Abdo Jurjus
American University of Beirut,
Lebanon

1. Introduction

Hypertension remains the major risk for cardiovascular disease, stroke and end-stage nephropathy. Hypertension is traditionally defined in terms of elevated systolic and or diastolic blood pressure (BP). Recently, however, there has been increased recognition of the importance of high brachial pulse pressure (PP) as an important and independent predictor of increased cardiovascular morbidity and mortality, especially in senior subjects (Franklin et al., 2001). This paradigm shift is attributed to the aging of the population. The aging process is associated with an increased incidence of systolic hypertension, and in particular isolated systolic hypertension (ISH) (Franklin et al., 1999; Franklin et al. 2001; National High Blood Pressure Education Program Working Group, 1994). Both systolic and isolated systolic hypertension are characterized by wide (high) PP (Franklin et al. 2001 & National High Blood Pressure Education Program Working Group, 1994).

Increased pulse pressure (PP) defined as the difference between inappropriately elevated systolic blood pressure (SBP) and reduced diastolic blood pressure (DBP) at any value of mean arterial pressure (MAP) is a surrogate measure of increased arterial stiffness of central elastic arteries (aorta and its major branches) (Figure 1) (Dart & Kingwell, 2001; Safar et al., 2003). Arterial stiffness has emerged as an important independent predictor of adverse cardiorenal outcome in the general population (Figure 2) (Boutouyrie et al., 2002). Central PP is considered an accurate indicator of arterial stiffness (Boutouyrie et al., 2002). However, brachial PP is a widely accepted marker of arterial stiffness in the elderly and in some middle-aged individuals because central PP equalizes brachial PP during aging due to PP augmentation by early wave reflection (Dart & Kingwell, 2001).

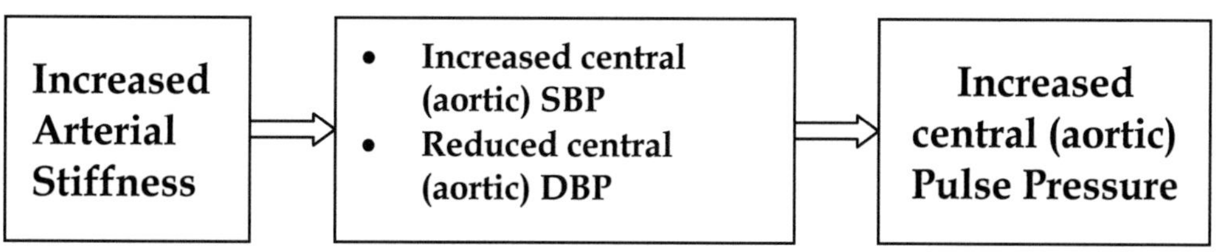

SBP= Systolic blood pressure, DBP= Diastolic blood pressure

Fig. 1. Determinants of Central Pulse Pressure

The relationship between PP and age is reported to be J-shaped, negative in subjects younger than 50 years and becoming positive after the age of 50 years. These findings suggest different pathophysiologic implications in younger versus older subjects. In subjects younger than 50 years of age, with preserved left ventricular dynamics, PP is related to a hyperdynamic cardiovascular state whereas, after the age of 60 years, arterial stiffening becomes a major determinant (Wilkinson et al., 2001). In fact, after the age of 60 years, the increase in PP results both from continuous elevation in SBP and a decrease in DBP (Franklin et al., 2001).

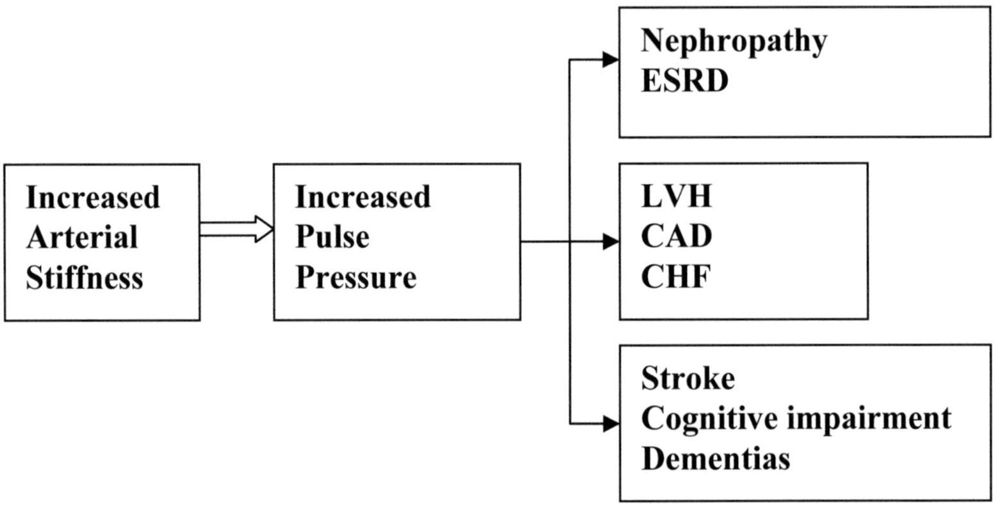

LVH= Left ventricular hypertrophy, CAD= Coronary artery disease, CHF= Congestive heart failure, ESRD= Endstage renal disease

Fig. 2. Relationship between increased arterial stiffness, increased pulse pressure and target organ disease

Several observational and clinical studies have indicated that, in both normotensive and hypertensive middle-aged and older subjects, wide PP is a better predictor of cardiovascular events and target organ disease than increased SBP and MAP adjusted for age, sex and other cardiovascular risk factors (Franklin et al., 2001). Further, a level of PP that predicts cardiovascular events in hypertensive patients appears to be equal or greater than 60-63mmHg (De Simone et al., 2005).

An increased brachial PP is an independent predictor of cardiovascular mortality not only in hypertensive men but also in normotensive men aged 40-69 years (Benetos et al., 1998). Thus, normotensive men with PP > 55mmHg were shown to have a 40% increased cardiovascular risk compared to normotensive men with same age but PP< 45mmHg (Benetos et al., 1998). Further, the predictive value of PP was observed even in well controlled hypertensive subjects (Benetos et al., 1998). Finally, the predictive power of PP has been demonstrated in subjects with evidence of other target organ involvement such as left ventricular dysfunction, endstage renal failure and in those with diabetes mellitus (Schram et al., 2002).

In contrast, in subjects younger than 50 years, brachial PP is not associated with a poor prognostic implication. In these subjects, the central arteries are more distensible and velocity of reflected pulse wave is low (Kotsis et al., 2011). As a result, SBP and PP increase significantly by about 12-14mmHg from central to peripheral arteries. This is known as the amplification phenomenon (Franklin et al., 2001 & Karamanoglu et al., 1993). Central and peripheral MAP and DBP, however, are not significantly different. Consequently, the peripheral (brachial) SBP and PP overestimate central (aortic) values (Franklin et al., 2001 & Karamanoglu et al., 1993). After the age of 55-60 years, as a result of arterial aging, central SBP and PP may increase even more than peripheral pressures. As a result, central SBP and PP become equal to or higher than peripheral (brachial) SBP and PP (Figure 3) (Franklin et al., 2001; Karamanoglu et al., 1993; Kotsis et al., 2011).

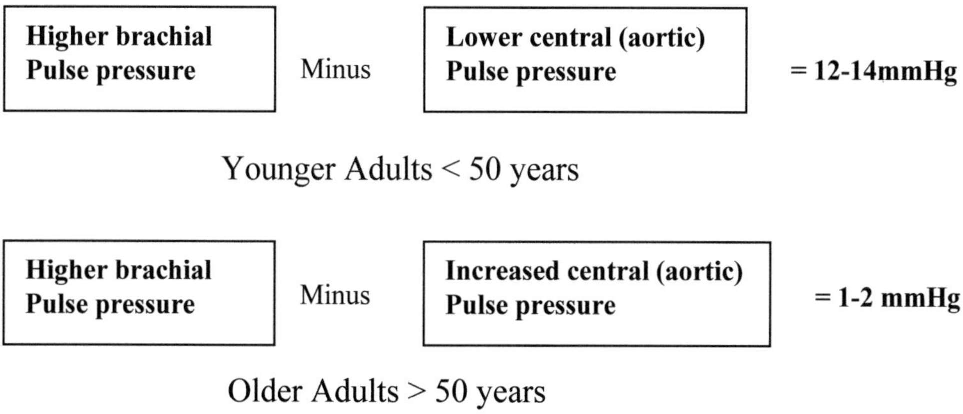

Fig. 3. Amplification phenomenon in younger and older adults

2. Genesis of the pulse pressure

The various BP components in the systemic circulation are the resultant of an interaction between left ventricular outflow (ejection) and properties of the large arterial system (aorta and its proximal major branches) (Benetos et al., 2010 & Van Bortel et al., 2001).

Ejection of blood from the left ventricle (LV) generates flow and pressure waves (Safar et al., 2003 & Wilkinson et al., 2001). The pressure wave generated by the LV travels down the arterial tree and is reflected back at any discontinuity of the arterial wall, namely at the multiple resistance arterioles and their bifurcation (Safar et al., 2003). The pressure waveform recorded at any site of the arterial tree is the sum of a forward traveling waveform, the incident pulse wave generated by left ventricular ejection and a back travelling wave, the reflected pulse wave (Safar et al., 2003 & Wilkinson et al., 2001).

2.1 Youth and early adulthood

In youth and early adulthood, the peak pressure recorded in the proximal aorta during LV ejection represents the SBP. Due to high distensibility of the system, the pressure wave form travels at low velocity (low pulse wave velocity- PWV) to the periphery and the reflected wave returns to the heart after closure of the aortic valve, so that it does not create an additional pressure load to the contracting LV (Safar et al., 2003). It does, however, increase the pressure during early diastole thereby enhancing DBP and improving coronary perfusion (Safar et al., 2003).

PP which represents pressure fluctuations resulting from episodic cardiac contraction is approximately 25mmHg in the aorta and is amplified to 40mmHg in the brachial and radial arteries.

2.2 Aging

In humans, the aging process is associated with structural and functional changes in the aorta and proximal elastic arteries. These vessels dilate and stiffen.

With increased arterial stiffness, the pulse wave travels faster, and reflected pulse wave merges earlier with the incident wave, augmenting aortic systolic blood pressure, rather than diastolic blood pressure (Safar et al., 2003 & Wilkinson et al., 2001). As a result, left ventricular load is increased and coronary perfusion is compromised (Safar et al., 2003 & Wilkinson et al., 2001).

3. Amplification phenomenon

BP amplification is defined as the elevation of PP from the central aorta towards the periphery and is mainly attributed to an increase in SBP (Benetos et al., 2011; McEniery et al., 2005). Pressure wave amplification can be explained by the reflection phenomenon of the oscillating BP wave (Benetos et al., 2011; McEniery et al., 2005). In the presence of compliant (i.e. low stiffness) central elastic arterial system as in young adults, PWV is low, the reflected pulse wave will attain the peripheral arteries (i.e. radial arteries) during systole due to their proximity to the reflecting sites, and the central arteries during the diastolic period (Benetos et al., 2011). This mechanism explains PP phenomenon namely why the peripheral (brachial, radial) is higher than the central (aortic) PP. The ratio of brachial / central PP varies from 70% in subjects younger than 20 years to 20% in those older than 80 years (McEniery et al., 2005). When expressed in absolute change in mmHg, the difference between brachial and central PP varies from 20 to 7 mmHg (Benetos et al., 2011; McEniery et al., 2005). Loss of PP amplification, associated with an increase in central PP and PWV have been shown to be significant predictors of all cause and cardiovascular mortality (Benetos et al., 2010).

3.1 Determinants of PP amplification

Several factors have been postulated to alter PP amplification including aging, gender, and traditional risk factors (McEniery et al., 2005).

In youth and early adulthood, PP increases significantly from central (aorta / proximal elastic arteries) to peripheral (brachial) arteries, leading to PP amplification. This phenomenon is attributed to higher SBP and slightly lower DBP in peripheral (brachial, radial) arteries. In contrast, MAP gradient between central and peripheral arteries is only 1-2mmHg.

In middle-aged and elderly subjects, the increasing stiffness of central elastic arterial system is associated with elevation of central SBP, reduction in DBP, widening of central PP and loss of PP amplification.

Females have a lower PP amplification than males of similar age which is attributed to:

i. i) shorter arterial tree;
ii. ii) additional gender related factors.

Subjects with hypertension, diabetes, dyslipidemia or established CV disease tend to have a low PP amplification independent of age, height or gender.

Age and gender remain the major determinants of PP amplification.

4. Kidney damage and pulse pressure

It is well established that hypertension and chronic kidney disease (CKD) are closely linked. Hypertension is the second most common primary diagnosis in patients with incident or prevalent endstage renal disease (ESRD). Further, most forms of CKD are etiologically related to hypertension (Udani et al., 2011). In addition, coexistent or superimposed hypertension is the major risk for progression of CKD (Hsu et al., 2005; Perry et al., 1995; Udani et al., 2011). The rates of CKD and ESRD in the USA attributed to hypertension have been steadily increasing partly attributed to the aging process (Udani et al., 2011).

Epidemiologic data and several clinical studies have documented a graded relationship between degree of BP elevation and renal functional impairment. Malignant hypertension, characterized by marked BP elevations (SBP/DBP ≥ 220/120mmHg) leads, if untreated, to severe renal damage and irreversible renal failure which is attributed to occlusive intra-renal arterial and arteriolar lesions (Bidani and Griffin, 2004). Conversely, data from several cohort studies provide strong support for nonmalignant hypertension as a causal risk for development of CKD and endstage renal failure (ESRD). In 12000 hypertensive patients from multiple Veterans Administration Centers followed up for 15 years, Perry et al. reported that uncontrolled hypertension was associated with a risk for development of CKD/ESRD(Perry et al., 1995). Specifically, the risk ratio for CKD was 2.8 for a pre-treatment SBP= 166-180mmHg, and 7.6 for a pre-treatment SBP>180mmHg (Perry et al., 1995).

Even modest BP elevation in the non-hypertensive range appears to confer increased risk of CKD. Compared to BP< 120/80mmHg, the adjusted risk ratio for developing ESRD was 1.62 for BP=120-129/80-84 mmHg and 1.98 for BP=130-139/84-89 mmHg in a cohort of 316675 adult members of the Kaiser Permanente of Northern California (Hsu et al., 2005).

4.1 Hypertensive nephropathy

4.1.1 Histopathologic patterns

Hypertension-induced kidney damage can be classified into two clinical and histopathologic patterns: 1) vascular, 2) glomerular.

The vascular pattern, often referred as nephrosclerosis can be further subdivided into two forms - namely benign and malignant nephrosclerosis (Bidani and Griffin, 2004). Benign nephrosclerosis, the most frequent form which occurs in the majority of patients with essential hypertension, is characterized by hyaline arteriosclerosis which is slowly progressive but does not compromise the vascular lumen (Bidani and Griffin, 2004). Accordingly, significant loss of nephrons and compromise of renal function are infrequent (Bidani and Griffin, 2004). In contrast, malignant hypertension is characterized by marked

BP elevation (SBP/DBP ≥ 220/120 mmHg) and occlusive arterial and arteriolar preglomerular lesions with prominent fibrinoid necrosis leading to ischemic glomerular injury (Bidani and Griffin, 2004). Rapid deterioration of renal function and irreversible renal failure can develop in the absence of adequate BP reduction (Bidani and Griffin, 2004). However, with the availability of effective modern antihypertensive therapy, malignant hypertension has become an uncommon cause of ESRD.

The glomerular pattern, characterized by an accelerated segmental or global glomerulosclerosis, is an increasingly recognized lesion of hypertension-induced kidney damage (Bidani and Griffin, 2002 & Bidani et al., 2009). It is often superimposed on the underlying primary nephropathy and occurs even with mild to moderate BP elevations. Further, these histopathologic renal changes are independent of presence of nephrosclerosis (Bidani and Griffin, 2002 & Bidani et al., 2009). In fact, vascular lesions are not prominent.

4.1.2 Mechanisms of hypertension-induced nephropathy (CKD)

The mechanisms of hypertension-induced renal injury and appearance of hypertensive nephropathy have not been completely elucidated. A growing body of evidence suggests a link between aortic stiffness and renal function (Mimran, 2006). Aortic stiffness causes increased SBP and wide (increased) PP, both factors associated with increased rates of decline in renal function and progression to renal impairment (Mimran, 2006).

4.2 Renal autoregulation

Disturbances in the mechanisms of renal autoregulation appear to play important roles in the appearance and progression of hypertensive nephropathy (Loutzenhiser et al., 2006).

One of most striking features of the renal circulation is the phenomenon of autoregulation by which the kidney maintains constant renal blood flow (RBF) and glomerular filtration rate (GFR) in the face of wide fluctuations of systemic BP (Loutzenhiser et al, 2002). This dual regulation of both RBF and GFR is achieved by proportionate changes in the tone of the preglomerular and postglomerular resistances (Loutzenhiser et al, 2002). This process is initiated by combination and integration of two mechanisms, the faster renal myogenic response and the slower tubuloglomerular feedback (TGF) system (Loutzenhiser et al, 2002). TGF involves a flow-dependent signal that is sensed at the macula densa and alters the tone of the adjacent preglomerular and postglomerular resistances (Loutzenhiser et al, 2002). The renal myogenic response involves a direct vasoconstriction of the afferent arteriole when this vessel is exposed to an increase in transmural pressure (Loutzenhiser et al, 2002, 2006).

By using the hydronephrotic rat kidney preparation, Loutzenhiser et al reported that the myogenic response is influenced only by the SBP, even when MAP is kept constant (Loutzenhiser et al, 2002, 2006).

Normally, increases in systemic BP, whether sustained or intermittent are prevented from fully reaching the renal microcirculation by proportionate vasoconstriction of the preglomerular afferent arterioles (Loutzenhiser et al, 2002, 2006). Systolic BP and PP appear to be the major determinants of the tone of the afferent arterioles, independent of MAP and DBP (Loutzenhiser et al, 2002, 2006). In fact, recent clinical studies indicate that hypertensive renal injury correlates most strongly with SBP and PP (Ford et al., 2010; Mimran, 2006; Safar, 2004; Verhave et al., 2005).

In contrast to the microcirculation of other organs, the renal microcirculation presents two special features. First, glomerular MAP and pulsatile pressures are high, representing about 60% of the aortic pressures (Mitchell, 2004). Second, because the resistance is higher in the efferent arteriole than in the afferent arteriole, the pressure drop across the afferent arteriole is low (Mitchell, 2004). These hemodynamic characteristics allow the maintenance of glomerular filtration but expose the glomerular microcirculation to high pressure injury and biotrauma (Mitchell, 2010). Under normal conditions, the renal myogenic response prevents transmission of the elevated MAP and pulsatile pressure from reaching the glomerular capillaries (Loutzenhiser et al, 2002).

Renal autoregulation mediates hypertension-induced nephropathy (CKD) by 2 mechanisms: i) intact renal autoregulation associated with elevated systemic BP levels within or beyond the autoregulatory threshold; ii) impaired renal autoregulatory process.

4.2.1 Intact renal autoregulation

4.2.1.1 Elevated systemic BP levels within the autoregulatory threshold

In mild to moderate uncomplicated essential hypertension, the renal autoregulatory mechanisms are intact and BP levels remain within the autoregulatory threshold (Bidani & Griffin, 2002, 2004). The elevated systemic BP enhances the myogenic tone of the afferent arteriole, preserving the relative constancy of the glomerular capillary hydrostatic pressures and insulating the renal microcirculation from biotrauma (Bidani & Griffin, 2002, 2004). Renal functional impairment is minimal and development of CKD and ESRD is infrequent (Bidani & Griffin, 2002, 2004). However, prolonged exposure of the renal circulation to elevated systemic BP levels may initiate the pattern of benign nephrosclerosis in the afferent arterioles which is characterized by vascular lesions of nonspecific hyaline arteriosclerosis (Bidani & Griffin, 2002, 2004).

4.2.1.2 Elevated systemic BP beyond the autoregulatory threshold

In contrast, in malignant hypertension, although the autoregulatory process is still preserved, the markedly elevated MAP levels, which exceed the upper threshold of the process, may cause severe renal vascular and glomerular disruptive lesions, resulting in severe renal functional impairment (Bidani & Griffin, 2002, 2004). However, with the advent of renal vascular disease, renal autoregulatory responses may become secondarily impaired leading to amplification of the renal damage.

A sudden severe BP elevation is much more likely to exceed the autoregulatory threshold than a progressive rise in BP to the same levels. This is due to the protection afforded by the rightward shift of the upper and lower limits of autoregulation, a characteristic feature in chronic hypertension (Bidani & Griffin, 2004).

4.2.2 Impaired renal autoregulation

Impaired renal autoregulation is frequently reported in states such as diabetes and CKD (Bidani & Griffin, 2004). This hemodynamic alteration tends to be manifested as dilatation of the afferent arteriole, glomerular hypertrophy, hyperfiltration injury and subsequent extracellular matrix production and glomerulosclerosis with irreversible reduction in GFR (Bidani & Griffin, 2004). In addition, increased aortic stiffness may contribute directly to renal injury by favoring increased transmission of PP to the renal microcirculation (Bidani & Griffin, 2004). Unlike benign and malignant nephrosclerosis, the histological lesions are glomerular, being characterized by glomerulosclerosis (Bidani & Griffin, 2004).

4.3 Clinical studies – Relation between SBP/PP and renal vascular nephropathy

Several longitudinal and cross-sectional studies indicate a relation between an increase in arterial stiffness and its corollaries, increased SBP/PP, and injury to the renal microcirculation.

4.3.1 Essential hypertension

4.3.1.1 Systolic blood pressure (SBP)

In the Systolic Hypertension in the Elderly Program (SHEP) conducted in subjects older than 65 years with ISH, SBP emerged as the best predictor of an increase in serum creatinine within a 5-year period (Young et al., 2002). Similarly in a cohort of 722 subjects with treated essential hypertension, the decrease in GFR, within a 7-year observation period, was preferentially associated with baseline SBP (Vupputuri et al., 2003).

4.3.1.2 Pulse pressure (PP)

Other clinical investigations revealed an association between PP and decline in renal function in older subjects. Fesler et al reported that in 132 never treated essential hypertension patients at baseline followed on treatment for 6.5 years, the yearly change in GFR was strongly and inversely correlated with PP independent of baseline GFR, age, MAP, body mass index, and microalbuminuria (Fesler et al., 2007). Gosse et al reported similar findings (Gosse et al., 2009). Measured either on clinic examination or by ambulatory BP monitoring in 375 patients with uncomplicated essential hypertension without proteinuria over a mean follow-up period of 14 years, initial baseline PP was an independent determinant of decline in renal function, pointing to the role of BP pulsatility as a glomerular biotrauma (Gosse et al., 2009).

4.3.2 Chronic Kidney Disease (CKD)

Aortic stiffening has been shown to predict loss of renal function also in CKD. Ford et al evaluated the relation between arterial stiffness and changes in renal function in 120 patients with CKD stage 3 and 4 enrolled in the prospective ACADEMIC (Arterial Compliance and Oxidant Stress as Predictors of Loss of Renal Function, Morbidity and Mortality in Chronic Kidney Disease (CKD) study) cohort (Ford et al., 2010). These investigators noted that, compared to those with lower PWV (12.3 m/sec), patients with higher PWV (13.9 m/s) experienced a greater progression of CKD, as determined by a greater decrease in the reciprocal of serum creatinine and greater than 25% decline in estimated glomerular filtration rate during 1 year follow-up (Ford et al., 2010).

Conversely, decreasing renal function may promote risk of accelerated rate of aortic stiffening. In 1290 untreated normotensive and hypertensive subjects with a serum creatinine < 130 μmol/L (< 1.47 mg/dl), Mourad et al reported an inverse association between aortic PWV and creatinine clearance calculated by the Cockcroft-Gault formula (Mourad et al., 2001). However the aortic PWV was significantly enhanced only in subjects exhibiting a reduced creatinine clearance in the lower tertile of normal values particularly in younger than 55 years of age. Baseline serum creatinine was the only predictor of the changes in arterial function (Mourad et al., 2001).

Similar associations between reduction in GFR and an acceleration of PWV were reported in the CRIC study in which unadjusted analysis indicated that each $10ml/min/1.73m^2$ decrease in estimated GFR was associated cross-sectionally with a 0.5 m/s increase in aortic PWV (Townsend et al., 2010).

In patients with ESRD (stage V) , increased aortic stiffening, as measured by PWV may be a contributor to further deterioration in renal structure and function. Several uremia related factors have been postulated to account for the disease of the large arterial system (Udani et al., 2011).

4.4 Aging

The aging process is often associated with reduced renal function (Mimran, 2006). In the Multiple Risk Factor Intervention Trial (MRFIT), a high risk of ESRD was reported in patients with isolated systolic hypertension (ISH) (Klag et al., 1996). In a cohort of 212 patients with ISH, an inverse relationship between PP and GFR and effective renal plasma flow (ERPF) was documented in subjects 60 years of age and older independent of age, MAP and known cardiovascular factors (Verhave et al., 2005). This inverse relationship, however, was observed in elderly subjects exhibiting the highest tertile of PP (Verhave et al., 2005).

4.5 Microalbuminuria and pulse pressure

Increased urinary albumin excretion (UAE) is a well recognized risk for cardiovascular morbidity and mortality and a predictor of renal involvement (Sarnak et al., 2003).

The pathophysiologic mechanisms causing increased UAE have not been fully elucidated. However a link between BP and UAE is well recognized. Although earlier studies emphasized an association between DBP/MAP and UAE, more recent studies report stronger relations between SBP/PP and UAE (Farasat et al., 2010). In a cross-sectional study that included 211 untreated controls, patients with essential hypertension or clinically stable cardiovascular disease, Pedrinelli et al found that PP was the best predictor of UAE, defined as UAE≥15 μg/min (Pedrinelli et al., 2000). Similarly in a longitudinal study of 450 normotensive and untreated hypertensive subjects drawn from the Baltimore Study of Aging, only longitudinal levels of SBP and PP, pulsatile BP components, were independent predictors of UAE in men (Pedrinelli et al., 2000).

4.6 Renal transplantation and pulse pressure

Increased PP, a sign of arterial stiffness, is frequently recorded in renal transplant recipients (Fernandez-Fresnedo et al., 2005).

Several studies have demonstrated a relationship between PP and renal allograft function and survival. In a cohort of 493 renal transplant recipients with a median follow-up of 6.3

years, increased PP, recorded 3 months post-transplant emerged as an early and strong marker of poor allograft outcome (Bahous et al., 2006; Vetromile et al., 2009).Further, recent data suggest that immunosuppressive regimens which include Calcineurin inhibitors may also mediate both an increased risk of arterial stiffness and allograft dysfunction (Seckinger et al., 2008). Adequate BP control and immunosuppressive therapy free of Calcineurin inhibitors have been recommended to improve allograft outcome and prevent nephrotoxicity (Seckinger et al., 2008 & Vetromile et al., 2009).

5. Cardiovascular disease and pulse pressure

Epidemiologic surveys and clinical observations have established a strong association between indices of arterial stiffness (peripheral PP, central PP, aortic PWV, pressure wave amplification) and cardiovascular events in hypertensive and older subjects.

5.1 Structural and functional changes in the cardiovascular system

Arterial stiffness is associated with structural and functional changes in the central elastic arteries (aorta and proximal elastic branches). These vessels dilate and stiffen (Lakatta, 2003). The primary cause of the stiffening is marked disorganization of the normal elastic pattern, increased deposition of less extensible collagen fibers, fibrosis, inflammation, medial smooth muscle necrosis, calcification and diffusion of macromolecules into the arterial wall (Lakatta, 2003). The repetitive cycles of distension of the arterial wall which occur with each heart beat lead to fatigue, fraying and fracture of the elastic fibers and subsequent extensive impairment of the medical elastin fiber network (Lakatta, 2003).

With increasing stiffness of the central elastic arteries, pulse wave velocity is faster, leading to summation of reflected and incident pulse waves in systole, enhancing central SBP, reducing DBP and widening central PP (Benetos et al., 2010). The elevation in central SBP increases myocardial oxygen demand, enhances left ventricular load, generates a heightened LV systolic pressure to sustain a constant blood flow and impairs ventricular ejection. Moreover, the contemporary reduction in DBP, the latter being a determinant of coronary blood supply, compromises coronary perfusion, predisposes to subendocardial ischemia, myocardial infarction and arrhythmias (Mosley et al., 2007). Both an elevated SBP and wide PP promote hypertrophy of the left ventricle, with impaired left ventricular relaxation and diastolic heart failure (Mosley et al., 2007). Finally, PP, an index of oscillatory hemodynamic forces, is a significant modulator of formation and rupture of atherosclerotic plaques (Mosley et al., 2007).

Endothelial dysfunction and reduced bioavailability of nitric oxide, frequently associated with arterial stiffness, impair and limit the vasoactive and antiatherosclerotic properties of the vascular endothelium (Mosley et al., 2007).

A cross-talk has been recently documented between the central elastic arterial system and microcirculation of target organ damage (O'Rourke and Safar, 2005). Arterial stiffness and PP have a negative impact on the microcirculation of the kidney and brain, predisposing to renal impairment and deterioration in neurocognitive function (O'Rourke and Safar, 2005).

5.2 Clinical studies

Recent prospective and retrospective epidemiologic and clinical studies have demonstrated that an elevated PP is independently related, in both middle aged and older subjects, to an increased risk of cardiovascular events. In two independent French untreated male cohorts, the IPC (Investigations Preventives et Cliniques) composed of 15561 men aged 20 to 82 years who had 2 visits spaced 4 to 10 years apart, and the Paris Prospective Study including 6246 men aged 42 to 53 years examined over a period of 4 years, Benetos et al reported that an increase in SBP combined with a reduction in DBP, a hemodynamic pattern characteristic of wide PP, was associated with a highest risk of cardiovascular mortality, independent of age, initial BP levels and other risk factors (Benetos et al., 2000). In a different study, these same investigators noted that in untreated subjects, a spontaneous evolution towards a pattern of combined increase in SBP and reduced DBP over an extended period was associated with a 2 fold increase in cardiovascular mortality compared to those without changes in SBP and DBP (Benetos et al., 2000).

The relationship between pulsatile BP components and risk of cardiovascular events was also explored in 1109 patients with coronary artery disease. Intra-aortic BP indices were recorded during coronary angiography in these patients (Jankowski et al., 2008). After a 4.5 year follow-up, the ascertained primary endpoints (cardiovascular death, myocardial infarction, stroke, cardiac arrest, cardiac transplantation or myocardial revascularization) occurred in 22% of the patients (Jankowski et al., 2008). Central pulsatility (defined as PP/MAP) and central PP emerged as the primary endpoints with ratios of 1.3 and 1.25 respectively suggesting that central pulsatile BP indices were more important determinants of risk of cardiovascular events than steady BP components in patients with coronary artery disease (Chirinos et al. & Jankowski et al., 2008).

Premature stiffening of the arterial tree is frequently reported in insulin resistance and diabetes (Kengne et al., 2009 & Stehouwer et al., 2008). In the recent ADVANCE (Action in Diabetes and Vascular Disease: Preterax and Diamicron- Modified Release Controlled Evaluation Study) a clinical trial which enrolled 1140 subjects with type 2 diabetes, older than 55 years and one additional cardiovascular risk factor, the hazard ratio for cardiovascular events was 1.17 for SBP, 1.20 for PP, 1.12 for MAP and 1.04 for DBP. The investigators concluded that SBP and PP were the two best and DBP the least effective determinants of risk of major cardiovascular outcomes in relatively older diabetic patients (Kengne et al., 2009).

PP has been shown to be a predictor of heart failure especially in the elderly. In a sample of 2512 subjects aged ≥ 65 years, participants in the Established Population for Epidemiologic Study for the Elderly Program free of cardiovascular heart disease (CHD) and congestive heart failure (CHF) at baseline, a 10mmHg increment in PP was associated with an increased risk of CHD, CHF and overall mortality of 12%, 14% and 6% respectively both in normotensive subjects and in those with ISH (Vaccarino et al., 2000).

6. Cerebrovascular disease, stroke, neurocognitive dysfunction and pulse pressure

Several studies, in both population and patient-based cohorts have demonstrated a strong association between increased brachial PP and excess risk of stroke and neurocognitive dysfunction in both elderly and middle aged subjects (Hanon et al, 2005; Paultre & Mosca, 2005).

6.1 Mechanisms of cerebrovascular events

An increased arterial stiffness can enhance the risk of stroke through several mechanisms. An elevation in central PP enhances arterial remodeling both at the site of the extracranial and intracranial arteries, increasing carotid wall thickness, and predisposing to carotid stenosis, formation of atherosclerotic plaques and the likelihood of their rupture (Laurent et al., 2009). Central PP has been associated with increased prevalence and severity of cerebral white matter lesions (Kim et al., 2011 & Scuteri et al., 2011). A second mechanism relates to the specific features of the cerebral circulation. The torrential cerebral blood flow and low cerebrovascular resistance expose the cerebral microcirculation to high pressure fluctuations in the carotid and vertebral arteries which tend to increase three-to fourfold with age (O'Rourke & Safar, 2005). Finally, coronary heart disease and heart failure, often associated with arterial stiffness and high central PP, are also risk factors for stroke (Selvetella et al., 2003).

6.2 Clinical studies

Several epidemiologic surveys and clinical studies have documented that, in the elderly, high brachial PP was more predictive for stroke incidence and mortality than elevated SBP (>140mmHg). In the Boston Veterans Administration Study, PP was a stronger predictor for fatal cardiovascular outcome than were SBP and DBP among elderly subjects aged 60-85 years (Waldstein et al., 2008). Similar observations were reported in a prospective study of 5092 Chinese subjects. In this study, the incidence of total stroke, either ischemic or hemorrhagic, was related to PP (Zhang et al., 2004). In contrast, several other prospective studies identified SBP as a stronger predictor for incidence and mortality of stroke than PP (Miura et al., 2009).

Further, there is growing evidence that response of PP to antihypertensive therapy may also be relevant to outcome. In a post-hoc analysis of Systolic Hypertension in the Elderly Program (SHEP) trial data, an increase in PP (>10mmHg) on active drug treatment was associated with an increased risk of stroke (Vaccarino et al., 2001).. Another analysis of the same study revealed the enhanced risk of stroke resulted from excessive reduction in DBP with a threshold at about 60mmHg (Somes et al., 1999).

Elderly patients often have multiple comorbid conditions. These subjects are at increased postoperative complications when undergoing major surgical procedures. In a recent prospective study, a high brachial PP (>72mmHg) was reported to be associated with an increased risk of stroke during the postoperative period (Benjo et al., 2007).

In contrast to the well established relationship between brachial PP and risk of stroke in the elderly, data in middle aged subjects are controversial. A meta-analysis of prospective cohort studies reported that PP was not an independent risk factor for stroke. However, in a recent large cohort Japanese study which included 33372 participants free of cardiovascular disease at baseline and followed for 12 years, the JPHC study, PP was an independent stroke predictor among middle aged subjects with SBP<140mmHg, but not among those with higher SBP (Okada et al., 2011). Among persons of SBP<140mmHg, a 10mmHg higher PP at baseline was associated with 8.31mmHg higher SBP and 1.69mmHg lower DBP at baseline (Okada et al., 2011). These data suggest that, in middle aged subjects with SBP<140mmHg, it is the low DBP rather than the non hypertensive SBP which impacts the excess stroke risk (Okada et al., 2011).

Increased brachial PP is also a risk predictor for neurocognitive dysfunction in healthy elderly and middle aged normotensive and hypertensive individuals (Robbins et al., 2005). Impairment of cognitive function and memory loss are frequent in the aging population, especially among the elderly subjects (Henskens et al., 2008). Alzheimer's disease and vascular dementia are the most devastating manifestations of these neurocognitive disorders. Several longitudinal studies have emphasized an association between these dementias with increased PWV and a wide brachial PP, both indices of increased arterial stiffness (Qiu et al., 2003). In a community based cohort of 1270 elderly subjects (mean age ≥ 75 years) free of dementia at baseline, higher brachial PP (> 84 versus 70-84mmHg) was associated with increased risks of both Alzheimer's disease and vascular dementia (adjusted relative risks of 1.9 and 1.7 respectively) (Qiu et al., 2003). The association was particularly pronounced among women.

7. Therapeutic approaches

It is well established that reduction in BP and or improvement in arterial stiffness are associated with a reduction in risk of cardiovascular events (Dart & Kingwell, 2001). However it is often difficult to separate the effects of antihypertensive therapy on BP reduction alone from their direct effects on vascular wall properties. In fact, interventions that reduce BP and improve cardiovascular outcome are often associated with improvement in indices of arterial stiffness (PWV, PP) (Laurent et al., 2006; Laurent & Boutouyrie, 2007; Van Bortel et al., 2001).

Therapeutic mechanisms include both lifestyle issues and pharmacologic treatment.

7.1 Lifestyle measures

A large number of lifestyle measures have been postulated to reduce both BP and arterial stiffening. These include body weight reduction, exercise, lowering salt intake, smoking cessation and moderation of alcohol consumption.

7.1.1 Weight reduction

Intentional weight reduction in obese hypertensive subjects is associated with significant fall in BP. Several clinical studies have shown that obese subjects whether normotensive or hypertensive exhibit increased arterial stiffness with its associated hemodynamic indices (increased PWV and PP) (Orr et al., 2008). In these subjects, weight loss with a hypocaloric diet improved arterial stiffness and reduced PWV and PP (Dengo et al., 2010). In some studies, an improvement in endothelial function was also reported (Miyaki et al., 2009).

7.1.2 Dietary supplement

Several dietary supplements appear to improve functional characteristics of the elastic arterial system. Supplementation with n-3 polyunsaturated fatty acids reduces arterial stiffness in dyslipidemic subjects, probably by decreasing serum triglycerides (Nestel et al., 2002). A high dietary intake of isoflavones, the non-steroidal plant derived compounds rich in soy beans, and administration of red clover isoflavones reduce PWV (Van Der Schouw et al., 2002). These effects have been attributed to the affinity of isoflavones to human estrogen receptors.

Recent reports have demonstrated that cocoa use ameliorated endothelial function, as evidenced by improved endothelial flow mediated vasorelaxation (Ferri, 2006). Changes were more striking in older subjects. The amelioration in endothelial function has been attributed to the flavanols, a subclass of flavanoids, present in large quantities in cocoa beans (Ferri, 2006). Controlled experiments conducted with beverages rich in flavanoids (wine, fruit, vegetable, tea, purple grape juice) have documented similar endothelial benefits (Ferri, 2006).

The cocoa related improved endothelial functions have been linked to increased bioavailability of nitric oxide (Ferri, 2006). In clinical trials, cocoa supplementation has been associated with BP reduction in subjects with grade I hypertension, with ISH and in younger soccer players (Ferri, 2006; Taubert et al., 2003).

7.1.3 Salt intake

Salt is the most potent modulator of arterial stiffness (Zieman et al., 2005). High salt intake enhances the age-related changes in the vascular system (Zieman et al., 2005). High salt intake increases MAP and triggers structural and functional pressure-independent changes in the vascular wall. In experimental animals, exposure to high salt diet has been associated with alterations in the composition of the vascular wall that precede BP elevations by several weeks (Limas et al., 1980). In the human, short- and long-term salt restriction causes an improvement in arterial distensibility independent from the effect on BP levels (Aviolo et al., 1986). In a group of elderly subjects (mean age 64 ± 2 years) with isolated systolic hypertension, dietary salt restriction for 4 weeks was associated with fall in both supine resting SBP (≈ 6mmHg), ambulatory SBP (≈ 3mmHg) and enhanced carotid artery compliance by 46% (Gates et al., 2004).

7.1.4 Alcohol consumption

An association between alcohol consumption and increased arterial stiffness has been reported in several studies (Sierksma et al., 2004; Zieman et al., 2005). Conversely, moderation of alcohol intake appears to reduce significantly PWV in both genders, independently of changes in BP levels (Sierksma et al., 2004; Zieman et al., 2005).

7.1.5 Physical exercise

The age related increase in arterial stiffness can be partly reversed by a program of physical training. In middle aged sedentary men, 3 months of aerobic training (walking or jogging 40 minutes daily at 70-75% of maximum heart rate) enhanced arterial compliance to levels observed in similarly aged endurance trained subjects (Tanaka et al., 2000). However, moderate exercise does not appear to improve arterial stiffening in elderly subjects with isolated systolic hypertension (Miyachi et al., 2003; Tanaka et al., 2000; Zieman et al., 2005).

In contrast, resistance training (weight lifting) has been reported to increase arterial stiffness and is associated with more severe increase in left ventricular mass compared to sedentary controls (Bertovic et al., 1999).

7.2 Pharmacologic approach

Although antihypertensive therapy has targeted brachial (peripheral) BP parameters, recent studies suggest that control of central hemodynamic indices (central SBP, PP, PWV) afford better cardiorenal protection (The CAFÉ Investigators, for the Anglo-Scandinavian Cardiac Outcomes Trial (ASCOT) Investigators, 2006).

The therapeutic benefits of antihypertensive drugs are influenced by two major effects: i) the effect due to BP reduction; ii) the direct effect of the drug on the vessel wall (Weber et al., 2005). Drug therapy that favorably influences blood vessel function appears to directly enhance the mechanical properties of arterial wall, independent of BP changes. In a therapeutic trial on patients with endstage renal failure, a population at very high cardiovascular risk, longer survival was strongly related to the drug-induced reversibility of aortic stiffness measured by PWV independently of BP evaluation (Guerin et al., 2001).

Although all classes of antihypertensive drugs reduce BP effectively, they do not exert similar benefits on arterial structure and function (Van Bortel et al., 2001). Antihypertensive therapy should focus on modulating high PP, the latter parameter contributing to major risk of cardiorenal events in older hypertensive subjects (Van Bortel et al., 2001). In these subjects who frequently exhibit ISH or a disproportionate increase in SBP over DBP, causing a selective widening in PP, the goal of treatment should aim at decreasing SBP with maintenance or even enhancing DBP. These targets may be attained by an active improvement in arterial stiffness, change in wave reflection and reduction in left ventricular ejection (Van Bortel et al., 2001).

Inhibitors of the renin-angiotensin-aldosterone system (RAAS), calcium channel antagonists, nitrosovasodialtors, diuretics and 3-methylglutaryl-coenzyme A inhibitors (statins) appear to modulate arterial stiffness (Staessen and Birkenhager, 2005).

The RAAS inhibitors reduce arterial stiffness by inhibition of the vasoconstrictive action of angiotensin II and improvement in endothelial function (Van Bortel et al., 2001). In a substudy of the RENAAL clinical trial, administration of Losartan to diabetic patients with baseline PP≥90mmHg led to 53.5% risk reduction for ESRD alone and 35.5% risk reduction for ESRD or death (Bakris et al., 2003). A similar mode of action has been postulated for the aldosterone antagonists (Van Bortel et al., 2001). Calcium channel blockers, by exerting direct relaxing effects on vascular smooth muscle cells, appear to also achieve a reduction in arterial stiffness and wave reflection. Nitrosovasodialtors effectively reduce central SBP and PP, especially in patients with stiff arteries and enhanced wave reflections. The benefits provided by nitrates and phosphodiesterase type-5 inhibitors have been attributed to the increase in cyclic guanosine monophosphate in vascular smooth muscles (Weber et al., 2005). Diuretics reduce arterial stiffness by decreasing systemic BP (Cushman et al., 2001 & Weber et al., 2005).

In contrast, in clinical trials, atenolol or pure beta-blockade based-therapy did not provide cardiovascular protection compared to that afforded by newer classes of BP lowering agent, despite similar brachial BP levels (Conduit Artery Function Evaluation [CAFÉ] Study – Anglo Scandinavian Cardiac Outcomes Trial [ASCOT], 2006).

Administration of statins to overweight and obese subjects was associated with an improvement in arterial stiffness as evidenced by a significant reduction in PWV, independent of baseline cardiometabolic risk factors (Orr et al., 2009).

8. Conclusion

Increased PP, defined as the difference between inappropriately elevated SBP and reduced DBP at any value of MAP has recently emerged as an important and independent predictor of enhanced cardiovascular morbidity and mortality, especially in senior subjects. Central PP represents a surrogate measure of increased arterial stiffness of the central elastic arteries. However, brachial PP is a widely accepted marker of arterial stiffness in older subjects due to loss of amplification phenomenon and equalization with central PP.

In the general population, PP and age are positively correlated after the age of 50 years, whereas a negative correlation between these 2 parameters is found in adults younger than 50 years.

Interaction between left ventricular outflow and elastic properties of the central arteries creates incident forward propagating and reflected backward traveling pulse waves which summate either in diastole or systole. In young adults, due to high arterial distensibility, both pulse waves summate in diastole boosting central DBP, whereas in older subjects, due to increased arterial stiffness, summation occurs in late systole, generating a high SBP and loss of peripheral amplification.

Epidemiologic surveys and clinical studies have demonstrated, in the elderly, a close relationship between increased brachial PP and cardiovascular events, stroke, impairment in neurocognitive function and dementia, and vascular nephropathy and progression of CKD.

Therapeutic regimens include lifestyle modifications and pharmacologic medications. Therapeutic benefits have been reported when BP reduction has been associated with improved arterial function and reduced arterial stiffness.

9. References

Aviolo, AP., Clyde, KM., Beard, TC., Cooke, HM., Ho, KK., O'Rourke, MF. (1986). Improved Arterial Distensibility in Normotensive Subjects on a Low Salt Diet. *Arteriosclerosis*, Vol.6, pp. 166-169

Bahous, SA., Stephan, A., Blacher, J. & Safar, ME. (2006). Aortic Stiffness, Living Donors and Renal Transplantation. *Hypertension*, Vol. 47, pp. 216-221

Bakris, GL., Weir, MR., Shanifar, S., Zhang, Z., Douglas, J., Van Dijk, DJ., Brenner, BM., for the RENAAL Study Group. (2003). Effects of Blood Pressure level on Progression of Diabetic Nephropathy: Results from the RENAAL Study. *Archives of Internal Medicine*, Vol. 163, pp. 1555-1565

Benetos, A., Rudnichi, A., Safar, M. & Guize, L., (1998). Pulse Pressure and Cardiovascular Mortality in Normotensive and Hypertensive Subjects. *Hypertension*, Vol. 32, pp. 560-564

Benetos, A., Zureik, M., Morcet, J., Thomas, F., Bean, K., Safar, M., Ducimetiere, P., & Guize, L. (2000). A Decrease in Diastolic Blood Pressure Combined with an Increase in Systolic Blood Pressure Is Associated with a Higher Cardiovascular Mortality in Men *Journal of the American College of Cardiology*, Vol. 35, pp. 673-680

Benetos, A., Thomas, F., Joly, L., Blacher, J., Pannier, B., Labat, C., Salvi, P., Smulyan, H. & Safar, ME. (2010). Pulse Pressure Amplification: a Mechanical Biomarker of Cardiovascular Risk. *Journal of the American College of Cardiology*, Vol. 55, pp. 1032-1037

Benetos, A., Salvi, P. & Lacolley, P. (2011). Blood Pressure Regulation during the Aging Process: the End of the "Hypertension Era"? *Journal of Hypertension*, Vol. 29, pp. 646-652

Benjo, A., Thompson, RE., Fine, D., Hogue, CH., Alejo, D., Kaw, A., Gerstenblith, G., Shah, A., Berkowitz, DE. & Nyhan, D. (2007). Pulse Pressure is an Independent Predictor of Stroke Development after Cardiac Surgery. *Hypertension*, Vol. 50, pp. 630-635

Bertovic, DA., Waddell, TK., Gatzka, CD., Cameron, JD., Dart, AM. & Kingwell, BA. (1999). Muscular Strength Training is Associated with Low Arterial Compliance and High Pulse Pressure. *Hypertension*, Vol. 33, pp. 1385-1391

Bidani, AK. & Griffin, KA. (2002). Long-Term Renal Consequences of Hypertension for Normal and Diseased Kidneys. *Current Opinion in Nephrology and Hypertension*, Vol. 11, pp. 73-80

Bidani, AK. & Griffin, KA. (2004). Pathophysiology of Hypertensive Renal Damage-Implications for Therapy. *Hypertension*, Vol. 44, pp. 595-601

Bidani, AK., Griffin, AK., Williamson, G., Wang, X. & Loutzenhiser, R. (2009). Protective Importance of the Myogenic Response in the Renal Circulation. *Hypertension*, Vol. 54, pp. 393-398

Boutouyrie, P., Tropeano, AI., Asmar, R., Gautier, I., Benetos, A., Lacolley, P. & Laurent, S. (2002). Aortic Stiffness is an Independent Predictor of Primary Coronary Events in Hypertensive Patients - A Longitudinal Study. *Hypertension*, Vol. 39, pp. 10-15

Chirinos, JA., Zambrano, JP., Chakko, S., Veerani, A., Schob, A., Willens, HJ., Perez, G. & Mendez, AJ. (2005). Aortic Pressure Augmentation Predicts Adverse Cardiovascular Events in Patients with Established Coronary Artery Disease. *Hypertension*, Vol.45, pp. 980-985

CAFÉ Investigators for the Anglo-Scandinavian Cardiac Outcomes Trial (ASCOT) Investigators, CAFÉ Steering Committee and Writing Committee, Williams, B., Lacy, PS., Thom, SM., Cruickshank, K., Stanton, A., Collier, D., Hughes, AD., Thurston, H. & O'Rourke, M. (2006). Differential Impact of Blood Pressure-Lowering Drugs on Central Aortic Pressure and Clinical Outcomes: Principal Results of the Conduit Artery Function Evaluation (CAFÉ) Study. *Circulation*, Vol. 113, pp. 1213-1225

Cushman, WC., Materson, BJ., Williams, DW., Reda, DJ & for the Veterans Affairs Cooperative Study Group on Antihypertensive Agents. (2001). Pulse Pressure Changes with Six Classes of Antihypertensive Agents in a Randomized Controlled Trial. *Hypertension*,Vol. 38, pp. 953-957

Dart, AM. & Kingwell, BA. (2001). Pulse Pressure - A Review of Mechanisms and Clinical Relevance. *Journal of the American College of Cardiology*, Vol. 37, pp. 975-984

Dengo, AL., Dennis, EA., Orr JS., Marinik, EL., Ehrlich, E., Davy, B. & Davy KJ. (2010). Arterial Destiffening with Weight Loss in Overweight and Obese Middle-Aged and Older Subjects. *Hypertension*, Vol. 55, pp. 855-861

De Simone, G., Roman MJ., Alderman, MH., Galderisi, M., De Divitiis, O. & Devereux, RB. (2005). Is High Pulse Pressure a Marker of Preclinical Cardiovascular Disease. *Hypertension,* Vol. 45, pp. 575-579

Farasat, SM., Valdes, C., Shetty, V., Muller, DC., Egan, JM., Metter, EJ., Ferrucci, L. & Najjar, SS. (2010). Is Longitudinal Pulse Pressure a Better Predictor of 24-Hour Urinary Albumin Excretion than Other Indices of Blood Pressure. *Hypertension,* Vol. 55, pp. 415-421

Fernandez-Fresnedo, G., Escallada, R., Martin de Francisco, AL., Ruiz, JC., Sanz de Castro, S., Gonzalez Cotorruelo, J. & Arias, M. (2005). Association between Pulse Pressure and Cardiovascular Disease in Renal Transplant Patients. *American Journal of Transplantation,* Vol. 5, pp. 394-398

Ferri, C., Grassi, D. & Grassi, G. (2006). Cocoa Beans, Endothelial Function and Aging: an Unexpected Friendship. *Journal of Hypertension,* Vol. 24, pp. 1471-1474

Fesler, P., Safar, ME., Du Cailar, G., Ribstein, J. & Mimran, A. (2007). Pulse Pressure is an Independent Determinant of Renal Function During Treatment of Essential Hypertension. *Journal of Hypertension,* Vol. 25, pp. 1915-1920

Ford, ML., Tomlinson, LA., Chapman, TP., Rajkumar, C. & Holt, SG. (2010). Aortic Stiffness is Independently Associated with Rate of Renal Function Decline in Chronic Kidney Disease Stages 3 and 4. *Hypertension,* Vol. 55, pp. 1110-1115

Franklin, SS., Khan SA., Wong ND., Larson, MG. & Levy, D. (1999). Is Pulse Pressure Useful in Predicting Risk for Coronary Heart Disease? The Framingham Heart Study. *Circulation,* Vol. 100, pp. 354-360

Franklin, SS., Jacobs, MJ., Wong, ND., L'Italien, GJ. & Lapuerta, P. (2001). Predominance of Isolated Systolic Hypertension among Middle-Aged and Elderly US Hypertensives: Analysis Based on National Health and Nutrition Survey (NHANES) III. *Hypertension,* Vol. 37, pp. 869-874

Franklin, SS., Larson, MG., Khan, AS., Wong, ND., Leip EP., Kannel, WK. & Levy, D. (2001). Does the Relation of Blood Pressure to Coronary Heart Disease Risk Change with Aging? The Framingham Heart Study. *Circulation,* Vol. 103, pp. 1245-1249

Gates, PE., Tanaka, H., Hiatt, WR. & Seals, DR. (2004). Dietary Sodium Restriction Rapidly Improves Large Artery Elastic Compliance in Older Adults with Systolic Hypertension. *Hypertension,* Vol. 44, pp. 35-41

Guerin, AP., Blacher, J., Pannier, B., Marchais, SJ., Safar, ME. & London, GM. (2001). Impact of Aortic Stiffness Attenuation on Survival of Patients in End-Stage Renal Failure. *Circulation,* Vol. 103, pp. 987-992

Gosse, P., Coulon, P., Papaioannou, G., Litalien, J. & Lemetayer, P. (2009). Long-Term Decline in Renal Function is Linked to Initial Pulse Pressure in the Essential Hypertensive. *Journal of Hypertension,* Vol. 27, pp. 1303-1308

Hanon, O., Haulton, S., Lenoir, H., Seux, ML., Rigaud, AS., Safar, M., Girerd, X. & Forette, F. (2005). Relationship Between Arterial Stiffness and Cognitive Function in Elderly Subjects with Complaints of Memory Loss. *Stroke,* Vol. 36, pp. 2193-2197

Henskens, LHG., Kroon, AA., Van Oostenbrugge, RJ., Gronenschild, EHBM., Fuss-Lejeune, MMJJ., Hofman, PAM., Lodder, J. & De Leeuw, PW. (2008). Increased Pulse Wave Velocity is Associated With Silent Cerebral Small-Vessel Disease in Hypertensive Patients. *Hypertension,* Vol. 52, pp. 1120-1126

Hsu, C-Y., McCulloch, CE., Darbinian, J., Go, AS. & Iribarren, C. (2005). Elevated Blood Pressure and Risk of End-Stage Renal Disease in Subjects Without Baseline Kidney Disease. *Archives of Internal Medicine,* Vol. 165, pp. 923-928

Jankowski, P., Kawecka-Jaszcz, K., Czarnecka, D., Brzozowska-Kiszka, M., Styczkiewicz, K., Loster, M., Kloch-Badelek, M., Wilinski, J., Curylo, AM. & Dudek, D. on behalf of the Aortic Blood Pressure and Survival Study Group. (2008). Pulsatile but Not Steady Component of Blood Pressure Predicts Cardiovascular Events in Coronary Patients. *Hypertension*, Vol. 51, pp. 1-8

Karamanoglu, M., O'Rourke, MF., Avolio, AP. & Kelly, RP. (1993). An Analysis of the Relationship Between Central Aortic and Peripheral Upper Limb Pressure Waves in Man. *European Heart Journal*, Vol. 14, pp. 160-167

Kengne, AP., Czernichow, S., Huxley, R., Grobbee, D., Woodward, M., Neal, B., Zoungas, S., Cooper, M., Glasziou, P., Hamet, P., Harrap, SB., Mancia, G., Poulter, N., Williams, B. & Chalmers, J. on behalf of the ADVANCE Collaborative Group. (2009). Blood Pressure Variables and Cardiovascular Risk: New Findings from ADVANCE. *Hypertension*, Vol. 54, pp. 399-404

Kim, CK., Lee, SH., Kim, BJ., Ryu, WS. & Yoon, BW. (2011). Age-Independent Association of Pulse Pressure with Cerebral White Matter Lesions in Asymptomatic Elderly Individuals. *Journal of Hypertension*, Vol. 29, pp. 325-329

Klag, MJ., Whelton, PK., Randall, BL., Neaton, JD., Brancati, FL., Ford, CE., Shulman, NB. & Stamler, J. (1996). Blood Pressure and End-Stage Renal Disease in Men. *New England Journal of Medicine*, Vol. 334, pp. 13-18

Kotsis, V., Stabouli, S., Karafillis, I. & Nilsson, P. (2011). Early Vascular Aging and the Role of Central Blood Pressure. *Journal of Hypertension*, Vol., 29, pp. 1847-1853

Lakatta, EG. (2003). Arterial and Cardiac Aging: Major Shareholders in Cardiovascular Disease Enterprises. Part III: Cellular and Molecular Clues to Heart and Arterial Aging. *Circulation*, Vol. 107, pp. 490-497

Laurent, S., Tropeano, A-I. & Boutouyrie, P. (2006). Pulse Pressure Reduction and Cardiovascular Protection. *Journal of Hypertension*, Vol. 24 (Suppl 3), pp. S13-S18

Laurent, S. & Boutouyrie, P. (2007). Recent Advances in Arterial Stiffness and Wave reflection in Human Hypertension. *Hypertension*, Vol. 49, pp. 1202-1206

Laurent, S., Briet, M. & Boutouyrie, P. (2009). Large and Small Artery Cross-Talk and Recent Morbidity-Mortality Trials in Hypertension. *Hypertension*, Vol. 54, pp. 388-392

Limas, C., Westrum, B., Limas, CJ. & Cohn, JN. (1980). Effect of Salt on the Vascular Lesions of Spontaneously Hypertensive Rats. *Hypertension*, Vol.2, pp. 477-489

Loutzenhiser, R., Bidani, A. & Chilton, L. (2002). Renal Myogenic Response-Kinetic Attributes and Physiologic Role. *Circulation Research*, Vol. 90, pp. 1316-1324

Loutzenhiser, R., Griffin, K., Williamson, G. & Bidani, A. (2006). Renal Autoregulation: New Perspectives Regarding the Protective and Regulatory Roles of the Underlying Mechanisms. *American Journal of Physiology-Regulatory, Integrative and Comparative Physiology*, Vol. 290, pp. R1153-R1167

McEniery, CM., Yasmin., Hall, IR., Qasem, A., Wilkinson, IB. & Cockroft, JR. on behalf of the ACCT Investigators. (2005). Normal Vascular Aging: Differential Effects on Wave Reflection and Aortic Pulse Wave Velocity: the Anglo-Cardiff Collaborative Trial (ACCT). *Journal of the American College of Cardiology*, Vol. 46, pp. 1753-1760

Mimran, A. (2006). Consequence of Elevated Pulse Pressure on Renal Function. *Journal of Hypertension*, Vol. 24 (Suppl.3), pp. S3-S7

Mitchell, G. (2004). Increased Aortic Stiffness: an Unfavorable Cardiorenal Connection. *Hypertension*, Vol. 43, pp. 151-153

Mitchell, GF., Hwang, S-J., Vasan, RS., Larson, MG., Pencina, MJ., Hamburg, NM., Vita, JA., Levy, D. & Benjamin, EJ. (2010). Arterial Stiffness and Cardiovascular Events. The Framingham Heart Study. *Circulation,* Vol. 121, pp. 505-511

Miura, K., Nakagawa, H., Ohashi, Y., Harada, A., Taguri, M., Kushiro, T., Takahashi, A., Nishinaga, M., Soejima, H. & Ueshima, H. for the Japan Arteriosclerosis Longitudinal Study (JALS) Group. (2009).Four Blood Pressure Indexes and the Risk of Stroke and Myocardial Infarction in Japanese Men and Women: A Meta-Analysis of 16 Cohort Studies. Circulation, Vol. 119, pp. 1892-1898

Miyachi, M., Donato, AJ., Yamamoto, K., Takahashi, K., Gates, PE., Moreau, KL. & Tanaka, H. (2003). Greater Age-Related Reductions in Central Arterial Compliance in Resistance-Trained Men. *Hypertension,* Vol. 41, pp. 130-135

Miyaki, A., Maeda, S., Yoshizawa, M., Misono, M., Saito, Y., Sasai, H., Endo, T., Nakata, Y., Tanaka, K. & Ajisaka, R. (2009). Effect of Weight Reduction with Dietary Intervention on Arterial Distensibility and Endothelial Function in Obese Men. *Angiology,* Vol. 60, pp. 351-357

Mosley II, WJ., Greenland, P., Garside, DB. & Lloyd, Jones. (2007). Predicitve Utility of Pulse Pressure and Other Blood Pressure Measures for Cardiovascular Outcomes. *Hypertension,* Vol. 49, pp. 1256-1264

Mourad, JJ., Pannier, B., Blacher, J., Rudnichi, A., Benetos, A., London, GM. & Safar, ME. (2001). Creatinine Clearance, Pulse Wave Velocity, Carotid Compliance and Essential Hypertension. *Kidney International,* Vol. 59, pp. 1834-1841

National High Blood Pressure Program Working Group. (1994). National High Blood Pressure Program Working Group Report on Hypertension in the Elderly. Hypertension, Vol. 23, pp. 275-285

Nestel, P., Shige, H., Pomeroy, S., Cehun, M., Abbey, M., & Raederstorff D., (2002). The n-3 Fatty Acids Eicosapentaenoic and Docosahexaenoic Acid Increase Systemic Arterial Compliance in Humans. *The American Journal of Clinical Nutrition.* Vol. 76, pp.326-330

Okada, K., Iso, H., Cui, R., Inove, M. & Tsugane, S. (2011). Pulse Pressure is an Independent Risk Factor for Stroke among Middle-Aged Japanese with Normal Systolic Blood Pressure: the JPHC Study. *Journal of Hypertension,* Vol. 29, pp. 319-324

O'Rourke, MF. & Safar, ME. (2005). Relationship between Aortic Stiffening and Microvascular Disease in Brain and Kidney: Cause and Logic of Therapy. *Hypertension,* Vol. 46, pp. 200-204

Orr, JS., Gentile, CL., Davy, BM. & Davy, KP. (2008). Large Artery Stiffening with Weight Gain in Humans: Roll of Visceral fat Accumulation. *Hypertension,* Vol. 51, pp. 1519-1524

Orr, JS., Dengo, L., Rivero, JM., & Davy, KP. (2009). Arterial Destiffening with Atorvastatin in Overweight and Obese Middle-Aged and Older Adults. *Hypertension,* Vol. 54, pp. 763-768

Paultre, F. & Mosca, L. (2005). Association of Blood Pressure Indices and Stroke Mortality in Isolated Systolic Hypertension. *Stroke,* Vol. 36, pp. 1288-1290

Pedrinelli, R., Dell'omo, G., Penno, G., Bandinelli, S., Bertini, A., Di Bello, V. and Mariani, M. (2000). Microalbuminuria and Pulse Pressure in Hypertensive and Atherosclerotic Men. *Hypertension,* Vol. 35, pp. 48-54

Perry, HMJr., Miller, JP., Fornoff, JR., Baty, JD., Sambhi, MP., Rutan, G., Moskowitz, DW. & Carmody, SE. (1995). Early Predictors of 15-Year End Stage Renal Disease in Hypertensive Patients. *Hypertension,* Vol. 25, pp. 587-594

Qiu, C., Winblad, B., Viitanen, M. & Fratiglioni, L. (2003). Pulse Pressure and Risk of Alzheimer Disease in Persons Aged 75 Years and Older: A Community-Based, Longitudinal Study. *Stroke*, Vol. 34, pp. 594-599

Robbins, MA., Elias, MF., Elias, PK. & Buoge, MM. (2005). Blood Pressure and Cognitive Function in an African-American and Caucasian-American Sample: the Maine-Syracuse Study. *Psychosomatic Medicine*, Vol. 67, pp. 707-714

Safar, ME., Levy, BI. & Struitjker-Boudier, H. (2003). Current Perspectives on Arterial Stiffness and Pulse Pressure in Hypertension and Cardiovascular Diseases. *Circulation*, Vol. 107, pp. 2864-2869

Safar, ME. (2004). Peripheral Pulse Pressure, Large Arteries and Microvessels. *Hypertension*, Vol. 44, pp. 121-122

Sarnak, MJ., Levey, AS., School Werth, AC., Coresh, J., Culleton, B., Hamm, LL., McCullough, PA., Kasike, BL., Kelepouris, E., Klag, MJ., Parfrey, P., Pfeffer, M., Raij, L., Spinosa, DJ. & Wilson PW. (2003). Kidney Disease as a Risk Factor for Development of Cardiovascular Diseases: a Statement from the American Heart Association Councils on Kidney in Cardiovascular Disease, High Blood Pressure Research, Clinical Cardiology, and Epidemiology and Prevention. *Circulation*, Vol. 108, pp. 2154-2169

Schram, MT., Kostense, PJ., Van Dijk, R.A.J.M., Dekker, JM., Nijpels, G., Bouter, LM., Heine RJ. & Stehouwer, C.D.A. (2002). Diabetes, Pulse Pressure and Cardiovascular Mortality: the Hoorn Study. *Journal of Hypertension*, Vol. 20, pp. 1743-1751

Scuteri, A., Nilsson, PM., Tzourio, C., Redon, J. & Laurent, S. (2011). Microvascular Brain Damage with Aging and Hypertension: Pathophysiological Consideration and Clinical Implications. *Journal of Hypertension*, Vol. 29, pp. 1469-1477

Seckinger, J., Sommerer, C., Hinkel, U-P., Hoffmann, O., Zeier, M., Schwenger, V. (2008). Switch of Immunosuppression from Cyclosporine A to Everolimus: Impact on Pulse Wave Velocity in Stable De Novo Renal Allograft Recipients. *Journal of Hypertension*, Vol. 26, pp. 2213-2219

Selvetella, G., Notte, A., Maffei, A., Calistri, V., Scamardella, V., Frati, G., Trimarco, B.,Colonnese, C. & Lembo, G. (2003). Left Ventricular Hypertrophy is Associated with Asymptomatic Cerebral Damage in Hypertensive Patients. *Stroke*, Vol. 34, pp. 1766-1770

Sierksma, A., Muller, M., Van Der Schouw, YT., Grobbee, DE., Hendriks, HF. & Bots, ML. (2004). Alcohol Consumption and Arterial Stiffeness in Men. *Journal of Hypertension*, Vol. 22, pp. 357-362

Somes, GW., Pahor, M., Shorr, RI., Cushman, WC. & Applegate, WB. (1999). The Role of Diastolic Blood Pressure When Treating Isolated Systolic Hypertension. *Annals of Internal Medicine*, Vol. 159, pp. 2004-2009

Staessen, JA. & Birkenhäger, WH. (2005). Evidence that New Antihypertensives are Superior to Older Drugs. *Lancet*, Vol. 366, issue 9489, pp. 869-871

Stehouwer, CD., Henry, RM. & Ferreira, I. (2008). Arterial Stiffness in Diabetes and the Metabolic Syndrome: a Pathway to Cardiovascular Disease. *Diabetologia*, Vol. 51, pp. 527-539

Tanaka, H., Dinenno, FA., Monahan, KD., Clevenger, CM., Desouza, CA. & Seals, DR. (2000). Aging Habitual Exercise and Dynamic Arterial Compliance. *Circulation*, Vol. 102, pp. 1270-1275

Taubert, D., Berkels, R., Roesen, R. & Klaus, W. (2003). Chocolate and Blood Pressure in Elderly Individuals with Isolated Systolic Hypertension. *Journal of the American Medical Association*, Vol. 290, pp. 1029-1030

Townsend, RR., Wimmer, NJ. & Chirinos, JA. (2010). Aortic PWV in Chronic Kidney Disease: a CRIC Ancillary Study. *American Journal of Hypertension,* Vol. 23, pp. 282-289

Udani, S., Lazich, I. & Bakris, GL. (2011). Epidemiology of Hypertensive Kidney Disease. *Nature Reviews of Nephrology,* Vol. 7, pp. 11-21

Vaccarino, V., Holford, TR. & Krumholz, HM. (2000). Pulse Pressure and Risk for Myocardial Infarction and Heart Failure in the Elderly. *Journal of the American College of Cardiology,* Vol. 36, pp. 130-138

Vaccarino, V., Berger, AK., Abramson, J., Black, HR., Setaro, JF., Davey, JA. & Krumholz, HM. (2001). Pulse Pressure and Risk of Cardiovascular Events in the Systolic Hypertension in the Elderly Program. *American Journal of Cardiology,* Vol. 88, pp. 980-986

Van Bortel, LMAB., Struitjker-Boudier, HAJ. & Safar, ME. (2001). Pulse Pressure, Arterial Stiffness and Drug Treatment of Hypertension. *Hypertension,* Vol. 38, pp. 914-921

Van Der Schouw, YT., Pijpe, A., Lebrun, CEI., Bots, ML., Peeters, PHM., Van Staveren, WA., Lamberts, SWJ. & Grobbee, DE. (2002). Higher Usual Dietary Intake of Phytoestrogens Is Associated with Lower Aortic Stiffness in Postmenopausal Women. *Arteriosclerosis, Thrombosis and Vascular Biology,* Vol. 22, pp. 1316-1322

Verhave, JC., Fesler, P., Du Cailar, G., Ribstein, J., Safar, ME. & Mimran, A.(2005). Elevated Pulse Pressure Is Associated with Low Renal Function in Elderly Patients with Isolated Systolic Hypertension. *Hypertension,* Vol. 45, pp. 586-591

Vetromile, F., Szwarc, I., Garrigue, V., Delmas, S., Fesler, P., Mimran, A., Ribstein, J. & Mourad, G. (2009). Early High Pulse Pressure is Associated with Graft Dysfunction and Predicts Poor Kidney Allograft Survival. *Transplantation,* Vol. 88, pp. 1088-1094

Vupputuri, S., Batuman V., Muntner, P., Bazzano, LA., Lefante, JJ., Whelton, PK. & He, J. (2003). Effect of Blood Pressure on Early Decline in Kidney Function among Hypertensive Men. *Hypertension,* Vol. 42, pp. 1144-1149

Waldstein, SR., Rice, SC., Thayer, JF., Najjar, SS., Scuteri, A. & Zonderman, AB. (2008). Pulse Pressure and Pulse Wave Velocity are Related to Cognitive Decline in the Baltimore Longitudinal Study of Aging. *Hypertension,* Vol. 51, pp. 99-104

Weber, T., Auer, J., O'Rourke, MF., Kvas, E., Lassnig, E., Lamm, G., Stark, N., Rammer, M. & Eber, B. (2005). Increased Arterial Wave Reflections Predict Severe Cardiovascular Events in Patients Undergoing Percutaneous Coronary Interventions. *European Heart Journal,* Vol. 26, pp. 2657-2663

Wilkinson, IB., Franklin, SS., Hall, IR., Tyrrell, S. & Cockroft, JR. (2001). Pressure Amplification Explains why Pulse Pressure is Unrelated to Risk in Young Subjects. *Hypertension,* Vol. 38, pp. 1461-1466

Young, JH., Klag, MJ., Muntner, P., Whyte, JL., Pahor, M. & Coresh, J. (2002). Blood Pressure and Decline in Kidney Function: Findings from the Systolic Hypertension in the Elderly Program (SHEP). *Journal of the American Society of Nephrology,* Vol. 13, pp. 2776-2782

Zhang, XF., Attia, J., D'Este, C. & Yu, XH. (2004). Prevalence and Magnitude of Classical Risk Factors for Stroke in a Cohort of 5092 Chinese Steelworkers over 13.5 Years of Follow-Up. *Stroke,* Vol. 35, pp. 1052-1056

Zieman, SJ., Melenovsky, V., & Kass, DA. (2005). Mechanisms, Pathophysiology and Therapy of Arterial Stiffness. *Arteriosclerosis, Thrombosis, Vascular Biology,* Vol. 25, pp. 932-934

17

Low-Level Exposure to Lead as a Cardiovascular Risk Factor

Anna Skoczynska and Marta Skoczynska
Wroclaw Medical University, Poland

1. Introduction

Cardiovascular diseases are the main cause of death in many developed and developing countries around the world. Cardiovascular end points (myocardial infarction, stroke or sudden death) are strictly connected with prevalence of classic cardiovascular risk factors, such as smoking, sedimentary lifestyle, obesity, atherosclerotic lipid pattern and arterial hypertension. Also, many 'new' factors have been identified, e.g. hyperhomocysteinemia, increased fraction of small, dense LDL or lipoprotein (a), increased C-reactive protein, increased apo-B/apo-A ratio or some enzymes' increased activities (Skoczynska, 2006). However, traditional risk factors alone (nonmodifiable and modifiable alike) do not fully explain high incidence and mortality from these diseases. The effectiveness of different strategies concentrating on reducing known risk factors does not translate to a satisfactory reduction of incidence and mortality from myocardial infarction or stroke. It is essential to introduce strategies concerning 'new' risk-factors, as well as to identify those that remain unknown.

Heavy metals, such as lead, cadmium and mercury, are the most abundant xenobiotics in human environment. These metals are present in the air, house dust, soil, water, consumer products and some herbal remedies. Main toxicological problems result from these metals' accumulation in soil, water, plants and animals, which is responsible for human exposure to toxic metals many years after the cessation of the emission. The intrauterine exposure, which is especially dangerous, as metals pass the placental barrier (Bellinger et al., 1987), as well as lead exposure in early childhood (Roy et al., 2009), affects strongly immature tissues, mainly the central nervous system. Lead exposure during pregnancy has a clear impact on mental and behavioral development (Hu et al., 2006; Nie et al., 2011). It has been documented that there is no safe lead blood level and that its toxic action is present at levels much lower than previously suspected. Another problem is the existence of combined exposure to heavy metals, toxic and essential alike, in human natural environment. The disturbance in the homeostasis of trace metals (zinc, copper, calcium, iron, selenium) affects lead toxicity in the cardiovascular system (Faure et al., 1991; Kuliczkowski et al., 2004; Skoczynska et al., 1994).

Although the knowledge on low lead exposure effects on the heart and blood vessels is incomplete, it seems justified to put forward a thesis that environmental exposure to lead is a risk factor for developing a cardiovascular event. In case of this thesis' positive verification, conducted studies, aside from contributing new facts to the knowledge on lead toxicity, may become a set-point for solving practical issues, i.e. means for identification and reduction of lead exposure sources, diagnosis and monitoring of lead toxicity, prophylaxis and treatment of individuals with an increased body lead burden. This would allow to achieve long-term social benefits, such as a decrease in incidence and mortality from cardiovascular diseases.

2. The global decrease in exposure to lead

Together with industrialization and motorization, the world lead production had been rising till 1980s, when it reached over 3.8 million tons per year (Kelly & Matos, 2005). However, since the 1990s, in general, the exposure to lead around the world has declined. It has been caused by the elimination of leaded petrol, the decrease in sales of lead containing water pipes and canned foods, and the recall from production of lead containing paints.

In 1991, US Centers for Disease Control and Prevention (CDC) adopted the blood lead level of 10 µg/dL as a threshold for lead toxicity. In 1995, the same value was assumed by the World Health Organization. The United States National Health and Nutrition Examination Surveys (NHANES) have documented a dramatic decline in blood lead concentrations in US adults and children (Muntner et al., 2005). A decline in blood lead level has been found also in Australia (Rossi, 2008).

Despite legislative changes, in some developing countries the exposure to lead persists on an unchanged level. Only in 2000, in about 100 countries there was an exposure to leaded petrol. Lead is also used in the production of paints that are employed in maritime industry or to paint external building parts (Tong et al., 2000). In industrialized Asian, South and Latin American regions, also lead mining, smelting, battery factories, cottage industries, crystal glass foundries and glazed ceramics manufacturing are important antropogenic lead sources. In the nineties, in some industrial areas of China, the proportion of children with blood lead level exceeding 10 µg/dL reached 99% but in non-industrial regions was about 50% (Shen et al. 1996). Among children older than 18 months, living in the area of Mexico City, 44% had blood lead level higher than 10 µg/dL (Romieu et al., 1995). Similarly, in populations of children living in industrial regions of India, these proportions were disturbingly high and ranged from 40% to 62% (Conference on Lead Poisoning, Bangalore, 1999).

Still, the worst situation concerns Africa and is caused by lack of legislative regulations, low number of epidemiologic studies and little toxicological information (Mathee et al., 2006).

In many developed European countries, i.e. Belgium, Germany, Sweden and the United Kingdom, there was a decline in blood lead level between 1978 and 1988 (Tong et al., 2000). The research project entitled Public Health Impact of long-term, low-level Mixed Element exposure (PHIME) in a susceptible population revealed that the European population has been subjected to a dramatically lower exposure to lead since the abolition of lead from petrol. In spite of this fact, at PHIME Seminar 'Effects of exposure to metals; no margin of safety in Europe' at the European Environment Agency on 10th of February 2011, it was emphasized that 'lead pollution sources must continually be hunted down and stopped'. This recommendation is based on the observation that the level of exposure to lead associated with a reduced IQ in children seems to be much lower than previously known (Report of PHIME, 2011).

The exposure to lead in populations of Central-Eastern European countries is still dangerously high (Bogunia et al., 2007; Pawlas et al., 2008; Trzcinka-Ochocka et al., 2005). It is a consequence of political and economical neglect in the last decades. One of the main problems is lack of information on the factual level of environmental lead exposure.

3. The dependence of circulatory system changes on body lead burden

Lead does not fulfill any physiological function in the body and can be toxic even at a small blood concentration. At present, it is well documented that some neurological and cardiovascular effects of lead emerge at a blood lead level lower than adopted as a threshold, i.e. below 10 μg/dL. It has been estimated that blood lead level in a natural, non-contaminated environment amounts to 0.016 μg/dL, i.e. about 600 times lower than the standard adopted for children by the CDC (Flegal & Smith, 1992). In the 1980s-90s, it was shown that lead-induced hypertension develops as a result of the environmental exposure associated with the blood lead concentration of 10-40 μg/dL (Cheng et al., 2001; Harlan et al., 1985; Pirkle et al., 1985). Simultaneously, lead-induced changes in blood pressure were not large. Results of 31 meta-analyses showed only a slight increase in blood pressure at a doubled blood lead level; on average 1 mmHg for systolic and 0.6 mmHg for diastolic pressure (Nawrot & Staessen, 2002).

Also other studies performed in the 1980s-90s showed a toxic action of lead at a relatively low exposure, i.e. corresponding to the blood lead concentration of less than 25 μg/dL (Tong et al., 1998). In 2006, in *Circulation,* Menke et al. published data from NHANES analysis showing the association between blood lead level and mortality from both myocardial infarction and stroke. This association was significant at the lead level lower than 10 μg/dL (Menke et al., 2006).

The dependence of changes in the circulatory system on blood lead level is not clear. On the basis of literature, it seems likely that there is an inverse relationship, i.e. a lower exposure is associated with greater cardiovascular changes, similarly to the case of neurotoxic effects of lead in children (Lanphear et al., 2005).

In population studies of people exposed to lead, lead is determined in blood, urine and bone. The most frequently measured indicator of exposure is the blood concentration. Due to a relatively short half-life of lead in the blood (approximately 30 days), this biomarker does not reflect the body lead burden but rather a recent exposure to external or intrinsic sources (e.g. lead released into the blood from storage sites, in conditions such as acidosis, fever or infection). Therefore, a more reliable indicator of quantities of lead accumulated in the body is the bone concentration. Lead is measured in the skeletal system (in the tibia or in the patella) using the method of K-shell x-ray fluorescence (KXRF) (Arora et al., 2009).

The positive correlation between blood lead level and arterial pressure has been well documented. However, lead concentration in the patella better correlates with the occurrence of coronary heart disease than arterial hypertension. Also, it has been suggested that blood lead level is a better predictor of cardiovascular diseases in young people, and lead concentration in the skeleton in elderly (Weisskopf et al., 2009).

4. The lead effect on the cardiovascular system

4.1 Lead and arterial blood pressure

On the basis of numerous population studies in different settings, including prospective studies, it has been well documented that lead induces arterial hypertension. The majority of cross-sectional and prospective studies showed a significant association between blood lead level and systolic or diastolic blood pressure (Apostoli et al., 1992; Ding et al., 1998; Hu et al., 1996; Malvezzi et al., 2001; Micciolo et al., 1994; Schwartz, 1991; Takebayashi et al., 2011; Tsao et al., 2000; Weiss et al., 1988). These associations have been found in populations with different geographic, ethnic, and socioeconomic backgrounds (Martin et al., 2006). A positive correlation was also established between umbilical blood lead level and the occurence of arterial hypertension in pregnancy (Rabinowitz et al., 1987). The development of hypertension in workers chronically exposed to high lead levels has been interpreted as a consequence of lead-induced nephropathy (Agency for Toxic Substances and Disease Registry, 1999; U.S. Environmental Protection Agency, 2006). However, in workers occupationally exposed to lower than nephrotoxic lead levels, low blood lead concentration was found as a predictor of an increased systolic blood pressure (Sirivarasai et al., 2004; Telisman et al., 2001). Similarly, prospective studies showed a correlation between lead bone concentration and systolic blood pressure (Cheng et al. 2001; Glenn et al., 2003).

The impact of confounding factors on the relationship between body lead burden and arterial blood pressure can be reduced in experimental studies. Results of many studies performed on numerous experimental models, on various experimental animals (rats, rabbits, calf), have confirmed the hypertensive effect of small doses of lead and explained various mechanisms of this action. These mechanisms result from lead action on the central and peripheral nervous system (Hoffer et al., 1987; Nehru & Sidhu 2001; Silbergeld 1992; Reckziegel et al., 2011), the vessel wall (Ding et al., 1998; Dursun et al., 2005), the renin-angiotensin system (Rodriguez-Iturbe et al., 2005; Sharifi et al., 2004), the kallikrein system (Carmignani et al., 1999), metabolic processes (Skoczynska et al., 1993; Skoczynska et al., 2004), the generation of free radicals (Stohs & Bagchi 1995; Vaziri et al. 2001; Vaziri & Sica 2004), and intracellular signalling pathways (Carmignani et al., 2000), leading to an increase in the vascular tone, and the peripheral vascular resistance (Fig. 1).

It has been concluded that the evidence is sufficient to infer a causal relationship between lead exposure and arterial hypertension (Brown et al., 2011; Navas-Acien et al., 2007; Weisskopf et al., 2009). However, the most important mechanisms explaining the hypertensive effect of chronic low exposure to environmental lead still need an explanation. Hypertension induced by high doses of lead can be partially explained by the nephrotoxic action of this metal (Batuman, 1993; Navas-Acien et al., 2009). It is possible that also in low-lead exposed individuals an impaired renal function is responsible for a persistent increase in blood pressure, as an inverse association between the glomerular filtration rate and blood lead has been observed in people with blood lead levels as low as 10 µg/dL (Fadrowski et al., 2010), or even 5 µg/dL (Ekong et al., 2006). One of the problems to examine in the future is the exploration of dose - response relationship and the determination of the latency period for lead - induced hypertension.

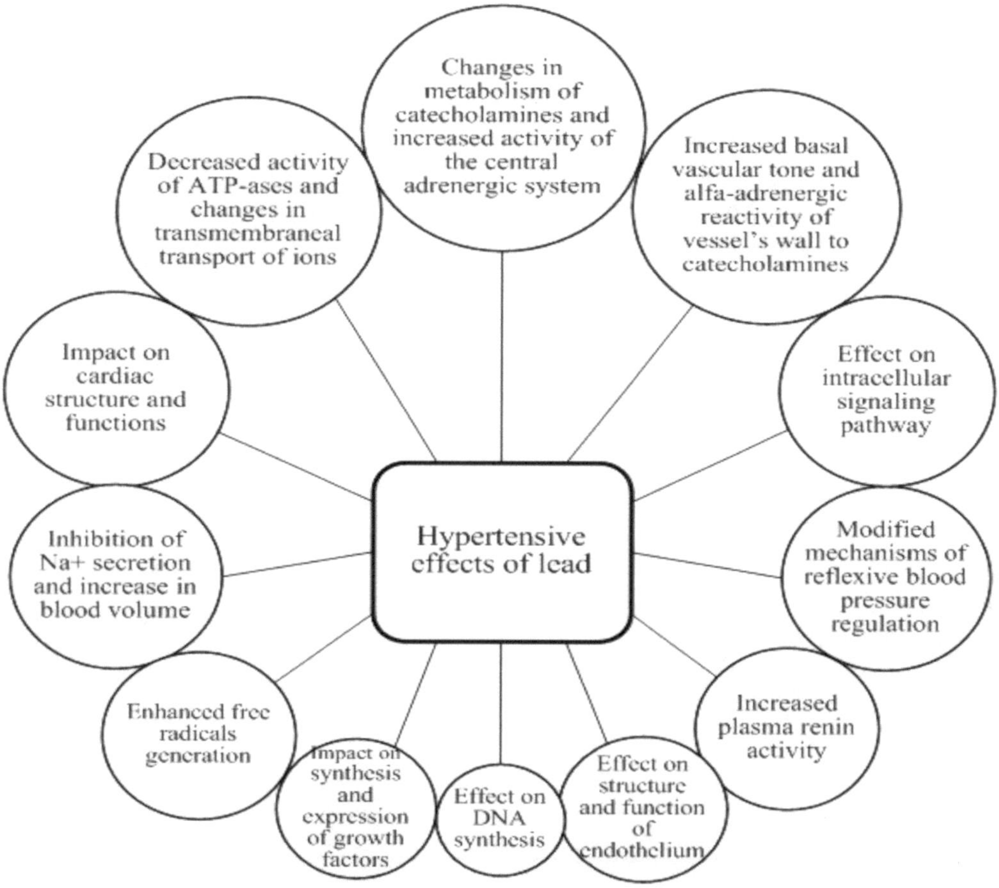

Fig. 1. Cardiovascular mechanisms of the hypertensive effect of low doses of lead (Skoczynska, 2006)

4.2 Lead and atherosclerosis

Aside from arterial hypertension, small amounts of lead cause also metabolic, functional and structural changes in the vessel wall. Some of these changes can accelerate the process of atherosclerosis. In the 1980s, in animal models, low-lead doses induced atherosclerosis was obtained (Revis et al., 1980,1981). Long-term lead exposure, measured by body lead store, was identified as a potential risk of intracranial carotid atherosclerosis in human (Lee et al., 2009). Some of the documented pro-atherosclerotic changes include: changes in lipid metabolism (Gatagonova, 1994; Kasperczyk et al., 2005a), endothelial dysfunctions (Ding et al., 1998; Vaziri et al., 2001), disturbances in essential metals' homeostasis (De Castro et al., 2010; Othman and Missiry, 1998; Wang et al., 2011), as well as an increase in free radicals' generation (Stohs and Bagchi 1995; Vaziri et al. 2001), a procoagulant state (Fujiwara et al., 2000; Kaji et al., 1991) and an inflammatory response (Heo et al., 1998) (Fig. 2).

In our previous studies performed on experimental animals exposed to small doses of lead, we have shown that an increased vessel wall reactivity to the catecholamines vasoconstricting action (Skoczynska et al., 1986; Skoczynska et al., 1987; Skoczynska et al.,

2001), an impaired vasodilatatory effect of acetylcholine (Skoczynska et al., 2005) and changes in vasoactive mediators blood levels (Skoczynska et al., 2003) are preceded by atherogenic dyslipidemia (Skoczynska et al., 1993), an increased lipid peroxidation, especially in the brain (Skoczynska et al.,1994), changes in the renin-angiotensin system (Wrobel & Skoczynska, 2002), and copper and zinc homeostasis (Skoczynska et al., 1994). In copper foundry workers exposed to lead, we have observed changes in vasoactive mediators blood levels (Skoczynska et al., 2002), hypertriglyceridemia (Skoczynska et al., 2007), an increased serum lipid peroxidation (Turczyn et al., 2010) and changes in copper and zinc homeostasis (Skoczynska et al., 2001).

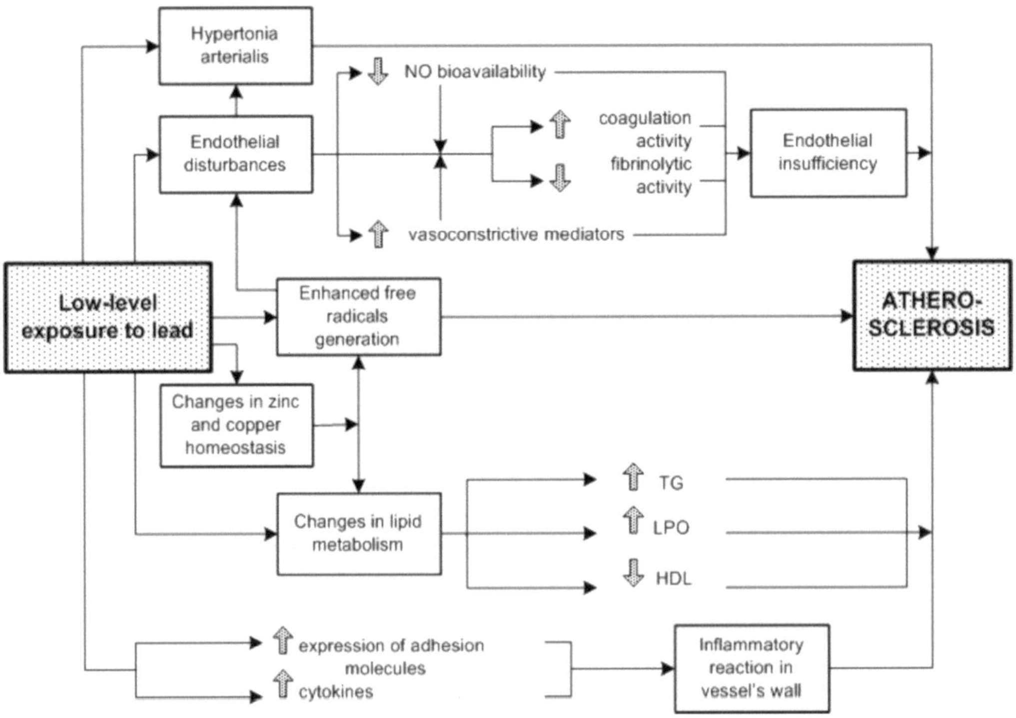

Fig. 2. Possible mechanisms of the pro-atherosclerotic action of lead (Skoczynska, 2006)

4.3 Lead and intermediate or immediate cardiovascular end points

Lead-induced changes in the circulatory system affect the occurrence of cardiovascular end points in lead exposed populations. Intermediate indicators of these events are functional and structural changes in the heart, such as changes in the left ventricular mass, heart rate, heart rate variability or electrocardiographic abnormalities. The 24-hour electrocardiographic evaluation performed in our centre in groups of men occupationally exposed to lead (copper foundry workers) showed that various heart rhythm disorders were more frequent as compared to the controls. A more frequent incidence of tachycardia (Gajek et al., 2004; Poręba et al., 2010a), a decreased heart rate variability (Poręba et al., 2011), and abnormal parameters of heart rate turbulence (Poręba et al., 2010a) were observed. In another group of men with arterial hypertension, occupationally exposed to lead, the study has demonstrated a significantly more frequent manifestation of left ventricular diastolic dysfunction and an increase in local arterial stiffness (Poręba et al., 2010b). However, lead exposed workers without hypertension also had an impaired diastolic function, compared with nonexposed controls (Beck & Steinmetz-Beck, 2005). In our earlier study, it was estimated that a ten-year risk of fatal cardiovascular disease (SCORE) in crystal glassworks' employees exposed to lead was higher in comparison to other workers (Doroszko et al., 2008). Also lipid disturbances were associated with the occupational exposure to lead (Skoczynska et al., 2007). All these changes were related to a relatively high blood lead level (above 40 μg/dL). Our newest experimental studies, using nuclear magnetic resonance, seem to confirm an increased incidence of left ventricular diastolic dysfunction in rats poisoned with small doses of lead (data in press).

In other studies, steel workers (Kasperczyk et al.,2005b) or battery workers (Tepper et al., 2001) exposed to lead displayed a higher left ventricular mass and/or a lower ejection fraction, compared to administrative workers from the same factories. On the other hand, in other studies, the interventricular septum and the left ventricular wall thickness determined in refinery workers with high blood lead level were similar to those determined in workers with lower blood lead concentration. Simultaneously, the decrease of diastolic cardiac function was more significant in the lead poisoned group (Zou et al., 1995). It may be concluded that results of studies performed on populations occupationally exposed to lead are inconsistent and the data on how lead affects the heart is insufficient. It remains unknown, for example, if lead, regardless of its hypertensive effect, leads to left ventricular diastolic dysfunction or changes heart rate variability.

There is no conclusion regarding the exact nature of lead influence on ECG. Since the 1970s, it has been known that lead increases heart sensitivity to noradrenaline arrhythmogenic action and causes bradycardia. Lead negative chronotropic action was associated with the blocking of heart beta adrenoreceptors activity (Bertel et al., 1978; Tsao et al. 2000). In various electrocardiographic studies, a significantly higher prevalence of heart ventricles repolarization disorders and heart rhythm disturbances was observed in groups of workers exposed to lead, in comparison to controls (Gatagonova 1995; Sroczynski et al., 1990). Among 775 men who participated in the Normative Aging Study, bone lead levels were found to be positively associated with heart rate, corrected QT and QRS intervals, especially in younger men. Additionally, a risk of intraventricular or atrioventricular block increased in men with elevated bone lead levels, whereas blood lead level was not associated with any of the electrocardiographic disturbances (Cheng et al., 1998; Eum et al., 2011). Authors of these studies suggest that the cumulative exposure to low lead levels causes electrocardiographic conduction disturbances. These disorders may be associated with the occurrence of different variants of genes involved in iron metabolism, such as hemochromatosis or heme oxygenase-1 genes. Park et al. found evidence that these genes' variants increase the impact of low-level lead exposure on the prolonged QT interval (Park et al., 2009). However, intermediate cardiovascular outcome varied across studies, and findings were incoherent.

Similarly, results of epidemiologic studies on the association between environmental low-lead exposure and immediate cardiovascular disease end points (coronary heart disease, stroke and cardiovascular disease other than arterial hypertension) are inconsistent. One of the first studies that analyzed a correlation between blood lead level and the incidence of coronary heart disease or stroke was The British Regional Heart Study. In this study, 7371 men aged 40 to 59 from 24 British towns were followed-up for 6 years. After allowing confounding effects of cigarette smoking and a town of residence, there was no evidence that blood lead level is a risk factor for major ischemic heart disease or stroke (Pocock et al., 1988). Also the study performed among 1052 inhabitants of Copenhagen County, who had the mean blood lead concentration of about 7 µg/dL in women and 18 µg/dL in men, and were observed for over 14 years, demonstrated a significant ($p<0.03$) risk for total mortality associated with blood lead but the risk for fatal and nonfatal cardiovascular disease or coronary complications was not significant (Møller & Kristensen, 1992).

On the contrary, studies published during 2002-2006 showed an increased cardiovascular mortality in the general population environmentally exposed to lead among individuals with blood lead levels from 20 µg/dL to 5 µg/dL.

The Second National Health and Nutrition Examination Survey (NHANES II), a national cross-sectional survey of the general US population conducted from 1976 to 1980, showed that individuals with blood lead levels of 20 to 29 µg/dL between 1976 and 1980 (15% of the US population at the time) experienced significantly increased all-cause, circulatory, and cardiovascular mortality from 1976 through 1992. After including the role of potential confounders, individuals with baseline blood lead levels of 20 to 29 µg/dL had a 46% increase in all-cause mortality (rate ratio (RR), 1.46; 95% confidence interval (CI), 1.14-1.86) and a 39% increase in circulatory mortality (RR, 1.39; 95% CI, 1.01-1.91), when compared to those with blood lead levels of less than 10 µg/dL (<0.5 µmol/L). All-cause mortality for those with blood lead levels of 10 to 19 µg/dL (0.5-0.9 µmol/L) was intermediately increased and statistically insignificant (Lustberg & Silbergeld, 2002).

The association between blood lead levels and increased all-cause and cardiovascular mortality was observed also at blood lead levels substantially lower than 20 µg/dL. In the Third National Health and Nutrition Examination Survey, which from 1988 to 1994 recruited 13,946 adult participants who were followed-up for up to 12 years for all-cause and cause-specific mortality, the geometric mean blood lead level in study participants was 2.58 µg/dL. After the multivariate adjustment, hazard ratios (95% CI) of participants in the highest tertile of blood lead (≥ 3.62 µg/dL) and those in the lowest tertile (< 1.94 µg/dL) were 1.25 (1.04 to 1.51; P(trend) across tertiles = 0.002) for all cause mortality and 1.55 (1.08 to 2.24; P(trend) across tertiles = 0.003) for cardiovascular mortality. Blood lead level was significantly related to both myocardial infarction and stroke mortality, and the association was evident at levels ≥ 2 µg/dL) (Menke et al., 2006).

The second study based on the Third NHANES US community concerned 9,757 participants ≥ 40 years old put in three categories, depending on blood lead level: <5 µg/dL (the reference category), 5 to <10 and ≥10 µg/dL. The relative risk of mortality from all causes was 1.24 (95% confidence interval (CI), 1.05-1.48) for those with blood levels of 5 to <10 µg/dL and 1.59 (95% CI, 1.28-1.98) for those with blood levels ≥ 10 µg/dL (p for trend < 0.001) (Schober et al., 2006). To conclude, both studies based on the Third NHANES have documented an association between blood lead below 10 µg/dL and mortality among U.S. adults.

Also occupational exposure seems to be associated with an increased risk of cardiovascular diseases. In 1963, Dingwall-Fordyce and Lane published results of an analysis of the causes of death among workers who had been exposed to lead. There were 425 pensioners, 184 of whom had died; additionally, 153 deaths occurred among an unknown number of employees who had not yet reached the retirement age. This analysis provided evidence that heavy exposure to lead was associated with an increased incidence of deaths from cerebrovascular catastrophes (Dingwall-Fordyce & Lane, 1963). The study of 1261 typesetters exposed to low lead doses, started in 1961 and followed until the end of 1984, confirmed the increased cerebral mortality in workers subjected to prolonged exposure. The all-cause standardized mortality ratio was 0.74, the cardiac mortality ratio was 0.63, whereas the ratio for cerebrovascular disease was 1.35 (at the edge of statistical significance). For printers employed for 30 years or more, the cardiovascular mortality ratio was 1.68 (95% CI: 1.18-2.31; $p = 0.002$) (Michaels et al., 1991). In turn, in the prospective study described by Robinson in 1974, over 20 years (1947-67) the risk of mortality in a group of 592 tetraethyl lead workers and in a group of 660 non-exposed workers was similar. No difference between the two groups in either total mortality or mortality from specific diseases was found (Robinson, 1974). Other retrospective observation which covered 4.556 workers occupationally exposed to lead, diagnosed during 1970-1992, revealed increased total mortality (670 deaths; SMR = 108; 95% CI: 100-116) in comparison to the general population. However, the risk of cardiovascular mortality was significantly increased only in the subcohort with high exposure (153 deaths; SMR = 129; 95% CI: 109-151) (Wilczynska et al., 1998).

In analyses of results obtained from 13,043 South Korean lead workers with mean geometrical blood lead level of 6.01 μg/dL, the impact fractions for cardiac disease among lead workers would be estimated as about 5-13 times higher than those of the general population. Manufacture of accumulators, manufacture of other electronic valves, tubes, and components, and manufacture of accessories for motor vehicles were identified as a relatively important industry. Other industrial processes of relative importance included battery assembly, acid treatment and other soldering (Kim et al., 2008). Also in population of 420 male bus drivers in Thailand, with blood lead level ranging from 2.5 to 16.2 μg/dL (the mean of 6.3 ± 2.2 μg/dL), using the second derivative finger photoplethysmogram (SDPTG) as a marker of the cardiovascular risk, and allowing age, body mass index and lifestyle factors, a significant correlation between blood lead and SDPTG-AI was found (Kaewboonchoo et al., 2010).

4.4 Lead and peripheral artery disease

There have been no prospective studies on the association of blood lead with peripheral arterial disease (PAD). However, the relative risk for PAD, comparing blood lead levels $\geq$ 2.47 μg/dL versus $<$ 1.03 μg/dL, in a cross-sectional analysis of NHANES 1999–2002, was 1.92. Data was obtained from 1999 to 2000, from 2125 participants who were $\geq$ 40 years of age. Peripheral arterial disease was defined as a condition with an ankle brachial index lower than 0.9 in at least one leg (Muntner et al., 2005). After adjustment for demographic and cardiovascular risk factors, the odds ratios of peripheral arterial disease, comparing the second, third and fourth quartile of blood lead level with the lowest quartile, were 1.63, 1.92 and 2.88, respectively. It was concluded that blood lead (as well as cadmium) is associated with an increased prevalence of peripheral arterial disease in the general U.S. population (Navas-Acien et al., 2004). Simultaneously, lead levels in urine (contrary to cadmium) were not associated with PAD at the levels found in this population (Navas-Acien et al., 2005). In turn, the observed association of homocysteine level and PAD can be completely explained by confounding due to smoking, increased blood lead and cadmium levels and impaired renal function (Guallar et al., 2006). The disturbances in homocysteine metabolism (Poręba et al., 2005) and the negative linear correlation between blood lead levels and the ankle-brachial index (Doroszko et al., 2008) were found also in workers occupationally exposed to lead; however, the latter relationship was discovered only in a subgroup of workers with a normal lipid pattern. Results obtained by Schafer et al. showed that hyperhomocysteinemia could be a mechanism that underlies lead effects on the cardiovascular and central nervous systems, possibly offering new targets for prevention of long-term consequences of lead exposure (Schafer et al., 2005).

In 2009, Weisskopf et al. published results of the analysis of all observational studies from database searches and citations regarding lead, intermediate and immediate cardiovascular end points. Studies in general populations have identified a positive association between lead exposure and coronary heart disease, cardiac mortality, cerebral mortality and peripheral arterial disease. Estimates of the relative risk of cardiovascular mortality in workers exposed to lead varied widely across occupational studies; with positive, inverse or null correlations. The positive association between lead levels and cardiovascular mortality occurred in workers with the heaviest exposure. Authors concluded that the evidence is suggestive but not sufficient to infer a causal relationship of lead exposure and clinical cardiovascular outcomes. There is also a suggestive but insufficient evidence to infer a causal relationship of lead exposure and heart rate variability (Weisskopf et al., 2009).

5. Genetic polymorphisms and lead toxicity

Human sensitivity to toxic effect of heavy metals differs depending on age, sex, general health status, quantitative and qualitative alimental deficiency, diet, smoking, lifestyle, place of inhabitancy and socioeconomical status, hygienic habituation, total occupational and environmental exposure to xenobiotics. Some of the critical effects of lead result from lead interference with enzymatic processes responsible for the synthesis of heme. These include the inhibition of delta-aminolevulinic acid dehydratase (ALAD), changes in the concentration of delta-aminolevulinic acid in urine (ALA-U), blood (ALA-B) or plasma (ALA-P), changes in the concentration of coproporhyrin in urine and zinc protoporphyrin (ZP) in blood. As a result of exposure to lead, there is a decrease in activity of blood pyrimidine nucleotidase (P5'N) and nicotinamide adenine dinucleotide synthetase (NADS), as well as changes in nucleotides' blood content. All these effects have been used as biomarkers of lead toxicity (Skoczynska, 2006). Genetic polymorphisms that affect lead toxicokinetics and toxicodynamics may be important factors modifying the risk of harmful effects of lead in vulnerable populations.

Differences in lead effect on the heme synthesis pathway, observed between different representatives of the same population exposed to lead, may be determined by different types of the ALAD gene. In turn, the differences between heme precursors levels in different ALAD genotypes can be related to a varied lead affinity to different ALAD isozymes. Thus, ALAD1 homozygotes (a genotype more frequent than ALAD 1-2) might be more susceptible to disturbances in heme metabolism caused by lead exposure than ALAD2 carriers (Sakai et al., 2000; Suzen et al., 2003). ALAD 1-1 subjects might be also more susceptible to the cytogenetic effect of lead than ALAD 1-2 subjects (Alexander et al., 1998; Dyudu & Suzen 2003). ALAD polymorphisms may be also involved in the emergence of lead-induced arterial hypertension. In terms of exposure to large doses of lead, ALAD polymorphisms are associated with lead-induced renal hyperfiltration (Weaver et al., 2003). It has been shown, that ALAD 1-2 variants affect the presence of the association between renal function and bone (the tibia or the patella) lead level. Similarly, variant B of the vitamin D receptor gene modifies renal sufficency, although only in young population exposed to high doses of lead (Weaver et al., 2006). Also the impact of endothelial nitric oxide synthase (eNOS) gene polymorphisms on kidney function has been demonstrated in employees exposed chronically to lead: the presence of the Asp allele was associated with higher serum creatinine than the genotype Glu/Glu (Weaver et al., 2003). Lead and selected genes, i.e. vitamin D receptor (VDR) and ALAD genes, may influence blood pressure and risk of hypertension. In a group of workers, 798 exposed to lead and 135 non-exposed, VDR genotypes (BB and Bb vs. Bb), lead concentration in the blood and in the tibia, and the amount of lead bound by dimercapto-succinic acid were all positive predictors of systolic blood pressure. Lead exposed individuals with the VDR B allele, mainly heterozygotes, had systolic blood pressures that were 2.7-3.7 mm Hg higher than in workers with the bb genotype. VDR genotype was also associated with diastolic blood pressure; lead workers with the VDR B allele had diastolic blood pressures that were 1.9-2.5 mm Hg higher than in lead workers with the VDR bb genotype (p = 0.04). In addition, compared to lead workers with the VDR bb genotype, workers with the VDR B allele had a higher prevalence of hypertension (adjusted odds ratio (95% confidence interval) = 2.1 (1.0, 4.4), p = 0.05) and a larger increase in blood pressure with age (Lee et al., 2001).

In the analysis described by Scinicariello et al., on the basis of data obtained from adults who participated in the Third NHANES, whose DNA was available (n=6,016), multivariable logistic and linear regressions stratified by race/ethnicity were used to examine whether blood pressure was associated with the ALAD gene and blood lead levels. Blood lead level was associated with systolic pressure in non-Hispanic whites and with hypertension, systolic and diastolic pressures in non-Hispanic blacks, but not in Mexican Americans. Non-Hispanic white ALAD2 carriers of the highest blood lead level quartile had a significantly higher adjusted prevalence odds ratio for hypertension compared with ALAD1 homozygous individuals. In addition, a significant interaction between lead concentration and the ALAD2 allele, in relation to systolic blood pressure, was shown in non-Hispanic whites and non-Hispanic blacks (Scinicariello et al., 2010).

Also a mutation of the hemochromatosis gene (HFE H63D) has been associated with changes in blood pressure, examined as the pulse pressure (the difference between systolic and diastolic blood pressure) within the Normative Aging Study between 1991-2001. Baseline bone lead levels, markers of the cumulative lead exposure, are associated with steeper increases in pulse pressure in men with at least one H63D allele (p-interaction = 0.03 for tibia and 0.02 for patella), compared with men with only wild types or C282Y variant (Zhang et al., 2010). HFE variants are associated also with increased blood lead levels in young children (Hopkins et al., 2008).

Lead induces arterial hypertension in the consequence of low exposure, which may be not manifested by a toxic effect on the marrow, kidneys or other organs. The existence of lead hypertensive effect, in the range of blood concentration lower than 40 µg/dL, has been supported by numerous experimental and population studies. However, the presence of a significant correlation between blood lead level and systolic and/or diastolic blood pressure has not been confirmed by all of performed epidemiologic tests. These discrepancies can be explained by the fact that lead-induced hypertension results rather from the past than from the current exposure, and hence arterial pressure values should be rather related to bone than to blood lead level. The occurrence of polymorphisms of genes involved in lead toxic effect may stand for another explanation. Interactions between lead toxicity and ALAD or HFE genes polymorphisms were observed in occupational and epidemiologic studies. These polymorphisms, occurring singularly or in an association with other polymorphisms (e.g. the vitamin D receptor gene), seem to be involved in lead-induced hypertension. Results of experimental studies indicate that the correlation between lead exposure, arterial blood pressure and the presence of polymorphisms of angiotensin converting enzyme and beta(2)adrenergic receptor genes should be analyzed in the general population. It is likely that studies of these polymorphisms, gene-to-gene interactions and interactions between genes and environmental factors may provide the identification of causes of so called spontaneous hypertension (Skoczynska, 2008).

6. Problems related to lead toxicity

It has been established that low level exposure to lead induces arterial hypertension. However, the data of many studies is suggestive but insufficient to infer that low level exposure to lead increases the occurrence of cardiovascular end points. The causal interference between lead exposure and immediate as well as some of intermediate end points needs a further explanation. The dose-effect relationship in the cardiovascular action of lead also remains unclear. It is possible that only low and recent exposure to lead is associated with arterial hypertension. Perhaps, there is an inverse relationship between blood lead levels and blood pressure values, similarly as in neurotoxic effects of lead in young organisms. It is also possible that cardiac end points are associated with long-term exposure to lead, which would be implied by the existent relationship between the patella lead and the occurrence of coronary heart disease.

Subsequently, blood lead level, most often determined spectrophotometrically, is variable and depends not only on external but also internal exposure. Factors such as fever, alcohol and acidosis cause a mobilization of lead from organs and from the skeleton. A single measurement of blood lead should be therefore verified, which is frequently practiced in occupationally exposed but would be difficult to apply to the general population. In turn, bone (the tibia or the patella) lead concentration, an established marker of accumulated lead, is determined using the method of K-shell x-ray fluorescence. This marker is more stable in comparison to blood lead but more difficult and expensive to measure.

In the population analysis of data on lead cardiovascular effects, it is indispensable to determine the role of confounding factors. The presence of a greater number of these factors cause incoherence in studies' results. Factors such as race, education, income, urban versus rural location and socioeconomic status should be considered. There are especially great difficulties in establishing how hypertension impacts relations between low exposure to lead and other than hypertension lead effects. Hypertension may result from lead action or occur independently but in each case constitutes a factor that confounds relations between lead and e.g. coronary heart disease or stroke. Similarly, disturbances in lipid and homocysteine metabolism or trace metals homeostasis may be simultaneously confounding factors and results of lead action.

7. Chelation treatment for lead poisoning

The chelation treatment has historically been used to reduce body lead burden in patients with severe symptoms of poisoning with lead. Chelating agents are organic compounds capable of linking together metal ions to form complex ring-like structures, which are subsequently excreted with urine. Effectiveness of chelation depends on whether the chelating agent is able to reach the intracellular site where the heavy metal is firmly bound. This intracellular availability is conditioned by many factors, e.g. ionic diameter, intra/extracellular compartmentalization and excretion pathway. Hydrophilic chelators are most effective in metals' excretion with urine, but they weaken complex intracellular metal deposits, whereas lipophilic chelators can redistribute toxic metals to lipid-rich organs, e.g. the brain (Andersen & Aaseth, 2002).

The chelation is usually performed using calcium disodium ethylenediamine tetra acetic acid ($CaNa_2EDTA$) and a preceeded administration of calcium. A contraindication to chelation is hypocalcemia or renal insufficiency. Also D-penicillamine and British anti-lewisite (BAL) have been used as antidotes for acute and chronic poisoning. 2, 3-dimercaprol (BAL) has long been the mainstay of chelation therapy for lead or arsenic poisoning. A thiol chelating agent, meso-2,3,-dimercaptosuccinic acid (DMSA), an analogue of BAL, has been tried successfully in animals as well as in a few cases of human lead and arsenic intoxication. DMSA could be a safe and effective method of treatment, but one of the major disadvantages of chelation with DMSA is its inability to remove lead from the intracellular sites because of its lipophobic nature (Kalia & Flora, 2005).

Even after many years of chelation, an effective treatment of patient poisoned with lead is difficult to obtain. New trends in chelation therapy including combined treatment are promising. This includes the use of structurally different chelators or a combination of an adjuvant and a chelator to provide better clinical and biochemical recovery, in addition to lead mobilization. Kalia et al. compared the therapeutic efficacy of captopril and DMSA, either individually, or in combination, against arsenite induced oxidative stress and metal mobilization in rats. Interestingly, combined administration of captopril and DMSA had a remarkable effect in depleting total arsenic concentration from blood and soft tissues. In addition, captopril administration during chelation treatment had beneficial effects particularly on the protection of inhibited blood ALAD activity (Kalia et al., 2007).

The therapeutic efficacy of melatonin or N-acetylcysteine (NAC) in reducing lead concentration in blood and other soft tissues was studied individually and in combination with DMSA. Administration of melatonin and NAC individually provided protection to the antioxidant defense, which disturbed by lead may significantly compromise a normal cellular function. Administration of melatonin and NAC (a thiol containing antioxidant) provided an increase in tiobarbituric acid levels, reduced glutathione and oxidized glutathione contents in tissues, which suggests these drugs' ability to act as free radical scavengers and to protect cells against toxic insult. In turn, a combined treatment of DMSA and NAC provided more pronounced efficacy in restoring altered biochemical variables and in reducing body lead burden than monotherapy with DMSA. The results suggest the involvement of ROS in lead toxicity and a pronounced beneficial role of NAC in therapeutic implications of lead poisoning, when co-administered with a thiol chelator (DMSA). They also support the hypothesis that cellular redox status may be significantly reversed by utilizing a thiol containing an antioxidant compound. Authors concluded that combined therapy with an antioxidant moiety and a thiol-chelating agent may be a better choice for treating plumbism (Flora et al., 2004a).

It has been suggested that a concomitant administration of an antioxidant could play a significant and important role in abating a number of toxic effects of lead, when administered with thiol chelators. Flora et al. also investigated the effect of taurine, an amino acid and a known antioxidant, either alone or in combination with DMSA, in the treatment of subchronic lead intoxication in male rats. DMSA was able to increase the activity of ALAD, while both taurine and DMSA were able to significantly increase GSH level and bring them towards normal. In animals treated with taurine, there has been a reduction of changes of biochemical parameters indicative of oxidative stress, especially in the brain. The data also implied a promising role of taurine during chelation of lead, as a possible potentiator of the depletion of blood, liver and brain lead, compared to DMSA alone (Flora et al., 2004b).

Chelation is a beneficial therapy in case of chronic intoxication with heavy metals. This therapy is of smaller significance in case of acute poisoning, which is a result of a complex clinical situation. Acute metal intoxication usually proceeds with multiorgan distress syndrome, determining contraindications to treatment with chelators. Symptoms of kidney or liver dysfunction limit credibility of indicators monitoring chelator's effectiveness. As a rule, patients need the intensive care and symptomatic treatment. However, the moment chelators are allowed to include, the chelation therapy can determine the prognosis. In workers occupationally exposed to heavy metals, chelation can serve as a prognostic procedure, useful in occupational risk estimation. It also enables to undertake appropriate actions. Temporary or lasting discontinuation of work in exposition to lead, before clinical symptoms appear, results in a significant decrease in the occupational lead poisoning.

However, due to metal accumulation in tissues, chelation is not a fully effective therapy and needs repeated doses of drugs, usually administered through the parenteral way. A combined therapy, an antioxidant plus chelator, does not seem to be the best choice for all of the patients poisoned with metals. This therapy can be beneficial only if an antioxidant is simultaneously a chelator, as it is in case of N-acetylcysteine. Then, the additive impact of both chelators is expected. The effectiveness of the therapy with an antioxidant is significantly dependent on patient's oxidative status at the beginning of the treatment. This effect, due to the antioxidant potential, can be beneficial as well as aggravating. It concerns especially metals which do not undergo Fenton's reaction: cadmium, lead, mercury. Additionally, the use of antioxidants without chelators, i.e. in the prevention of cardiovascular diseases, showed only equivocal benefits resulting from the antioxidant supplementation. Moreover, some of patients showed an increased number of cardiovascular end points and incidence of neoplasms. New long-term chelators, consisting of structurally different components (including N-acetylcysteine), are needed.

To summarize, chelation is a common therapy in case of poisoning with toxic metals but it is only partially satisfactory because of metal accumulation in tissues. A combined therapy with long term, structurally different chelators could become a viable alternative in the future.

In developed countries, workers occupationally exposed to lead at high concentrations (i.e. copper founders) are subjected to biological monitoring. Chelation, which is practised as a part of the monitoring, decreases body burden with toxic metals. In the nearest future, it is essential to began a study on the effect of chelation on arterial blood pressure and cardiovascular end points in workers exposed to lead.

8. Plan for the future

Current investigations, which will continue after previous clinical, epidemiologic and experimental studies, are to explain whether environmental exposure to lead is a risk factor for development of vascular changes in the heart, brain and legs. They are also designed to explain the role of homocysteine and lead-iron interactions in cardiac and vascular effects of lead. The final purpose of project is the assessment of environmental exposure to lead as a lowering average life expectation factor.

Further cross-sectional and prospective studies, combined epidemiological and toxicological, on the presence of the relationship between blood lead concentrations and prevalence of coronary heart disease, stroke and peripheral artery disease are needed. Confounding factors' (male sex, age over 65, smoking, hypertension, diabetes and abnormal lipid pattern) influence on studied relations should be considered. DNA isolation should be conducted in order to determine the frequency of genetic polymorphisms that may influence the presence of a relationship between blood lead levels and ischemic heart disease or stroke. It should also be researched whether polymorphisms of determined genes (e.g. beta receptor and vitamin D receptor genes, or PPAR alpha and lipoprotein lipase genes) affect lead-induced hypertension or lead-induced changes in the lipid pattern. Moreover, the determination of iron and homocysteine role in lead toxic effects is needed.

Obtained results may confirm the thesis that environmental exposure to lead is a risk factor for developing a cardiovascular event. In case of a positive verification, conducted studies may become a set-point for solving practical issues, i.e. providing means of reducing sources of lead exposure and/or lead toxicity (chelators, antioxidants). Probably, current environmental safety standards for blood lead level ought to be lowered. A criterion for elevated lead exposure screening needs to be verified not only in children but also in adults. The risk assessment of lead exposure impact should include lead cardiovascular effects. The risk assessment of cardiovascular end points should include the information on lead exposure.

9. References

Alexander B.H., Checkoway H., Costa-Mallen P., Faustman E.M., Woodes J.S., Kelsey K.T., VanNetten C., Costa L.G. Interaction of blood lead and delta-aminolevulinic acid dehydratase genotype on markers of heme synthesis and sperm production in lead smelter workers. Environ Health Perspect. 1998; 106(4):213-6.

Andersen O., Aaseth J. Molecular mechanisms of in vivo metal chelation: implications for clinical treatment of metal intoxications. Environ Health Perspect. 2002; 5:887-90.

Apostoli P., Maranelli G., Micciolo R. Is hypertension a confounding factor in the assessment of blood lead reference values? Sci Total Environ. 1992; 120: 127-134.

Arora M., Weuve J., Weisskopf M.G., Sparrow D., Nie H., Garcia R.I., Hu H. Cumulative lead exposure and tooth loss in men: the normative aging study. Environ Health Perspect. 2009 Oct;117(10):1531-4. Epub 2009 Jun 15.

Batuman V. Lead nephropathy, gout and hypertension. Am J Med Sci. 1993; 305: 241–247.

Beck B., Steinmetz-Beck A. Echocardiographic evaluation of left ventricular function in persons with chronic professional exposure to lead. Adv Clin Exp Med. 2005; 14(5):905-916

Bellinger D., Leviton A., Waternaux C., Needleman H., Rabinowitz M. Longitudinal analyses of prenatal and postnatal lead exposure and early cognitive development. N Engl J Med. 1987 Apr 23;316(17):1037-43.

Bertel O., Bühler F.R., Ott J. Lead-induced hypertension: blunted beta-adrenoceptor-mediated functions. Br Med J. 1978 Mar 4;1(6112):551

Bogunia M., Kwapuliński J., Bogunia E., Brodziak B., Ahnert B., Nogaj E., Kowol J., Rzepka J., Winiarska H., Wojtanowska M. Lead content in blood of children living near zinc smelter plant exposure on environmental tobacco smoking (ETS). Przegl. Lek. 2007;64(10):723-8.

Brown M.J., Raymond J., Homa D., Kennedy C., Sinks T. Association between children's blood lead levels, lead service lines, and water disinfection, Washington, DC, 1998-2006. Environ Res. 2011 Jan;111(1):67-74. Epub 2010 Nov 26.

Carmignani M., Boscolo P., Poma A., Volpe A.R. Kininergic system and arterial hypertension following chronic exposure to inorganic lead. Immunopharmacology, 1999, 44(1-2), 105-10.

Carmignani M., Volpe A.R., Boscolo P., Qiao N., Di Gioacchino M., Grilli A. Catcholamine and nitric oxide systems as targets of chronic lead exposure in inducing selective functional impairment.Life Sci. 2000; 68(4): 401-15.

Cheng Y., Schwartz J., Sparrow D., Aro A., Weiss S.T., Hu H. Bone lead and blood lead levels in relation to baseline blood pressure and the prospective development of hypertension: the Normative Aging Study. Am J Epidemiol. 2001 15;153(2):164-71.

Cheng Y., Schwartz J., Vokonas P.S., Weiss S.T., Aro A., Hu H. Electrocardiographic conduction disturbances in association with low-level lead exposure (the Normative Aging Study). Am J Cardiol. 1998 Sep 1;82(5):594-9.

De Castro C.S., Arruda A.F., Da Cunha L.R., SouzaDe J.R., Braga J.W., Dórea J.G. Toxic metals (Pb and Cd) and their respective antagonists (Ca and Zn) in infant formulas and milk marketed in Brasilia, Brazil. Int J Environ Res Public Health. 2010 Nov;7(11):4062-77.

Ding Y., Vaziri N.D., Gonick H.C.: Lead - induced hypertension. II. Response to sequential infusions of L-arginine, superoxide dismutase, and nitroprusside. Environ Res. 1998; 76:107-113.

Dingwall-Fordyce I., Lane R.E. A follow-up study of lead workers. Br J Ind Med. 1963 Oct;20:313-5.

Doroszko A., Skoczynska A., Drożdż K., Kreczyńska B. Cardiovascular risk in workers ocupationally exposed to lead. Part II. The impact of lead on the cardiovascular function on the basis of ECG, ABI and intima media thickness evaluation. Med.Pracy 2008; 59(5): 355-363. 29.

Dursun N., Arifoglu C., Süer C., Keskinol L. Blood pressure relationship to nitric oxide, lipid peroxidation, renal function, and renal blood flow in rats exposed to low lead levels. Biol Trace Elem Res. 2005 May; 104(2):141-9.

Duydu Y., Suzen H.S. Influence of delta-aminolevulinic acid dehydratase (ALAD) polymorphism on the frequency of sister chromatid exchange (SCE) and the number of high-frequency cells (HFCs) in lymphocytes from lead-exposed workers. Mutat Res. 2003; 540(1):79-88.

Eum K.D., Nie L.H., Schwartz J., Vokonas P.S., Sparrow D., Hu H., Weisskopf M.G. Prospective cohort study of lead exposure and electrocardiographic conduction disturbances in the Department of Veterans Affairs Normative Aging Study. Environ Health Perspect. 2011 Jul; 119(7):940-4. Epub 2011 Mar 16.

Fadrowski J., Navas-Acien A., Tellez-Plaza M., Guallar E., Weaver V.M., Furth S.L. Blood lead level and kidney function in US adolescents: The Third National Health and Nutrition Examination Survey. Arch Intern Med. 2010; 170(1):75-82.

Faure P., Roussel A.M., Richard M.J., Foulon T., Groslambert P., Hadjian A., Favier A. Effect of an acute zinc depletion on rat lipoprotein distribution and peroxidation. Biol Trace Elem Res. 1991 Feb; 28(2):135-46.

Flegal A.R., Smith D.R. Current needs for increased accuracy and precision in measurements of low levels of lead in blood. Environ Res. 1992 Aug; 58(2):125-33.

Flora S.J., Pande M., Bhadauria S., Kannan G.M. Combined administration of taurine and meso 2,3-dimercaptosuccinic acid in the treatment of chronic lead intoxication in rats. Hum Exp Toxicol. 2004; 23:157-66 (a).

Flora S.J., Pande M., Kannan G.M., Mehta A. Lead induced oxidative stress and its recovery following co-administration of melatonin or N-acetylcysteine during chelation with succimer in male rats. Cell Mol Biol (Noisy-le-grand). 2004; 50 Online Pub:OL543-51 (b).

Fujiwara Y., Yamamoto C., Kaji T. Proteoglycans synthesized by cultured bovine aortic smooth muscle cells after exposure to lead: lead selectively inhibits the synthesis of versican, a large chondroitin sulfate proteoglycan. Toxicology, 2000; 154: 9-19.

Gajek J., Zyśko D., Chlebda E. Heart rate variability in workers chronically exposed to lead. Kardiol Pol. 2004; 61(7):21-30.

Gatagonova T.M. Bioelectrical activity of the myocardium and cardiac pump function in workers engaged in lead production. Gig Sanit. 1995 May-Jun; (3):16-9.

Gatagonova T.M. Characteristics of the serum lipids in workers of lead industry. Med Tr Prom Ekol. 1994; (12):17-21.

George Foundation. Project lead-free: a study of lead poisoning in major Indian cities. In: Proceedings of the International Conference on Lead Poisoning, Bangalore, India, 8-10 February 1999. Bangalore, The George Foundation, 1999: 79-86.

Glenn B.S., Stewart W.F., Links J.M., Todd A.C., Schwartz B.S. The longitudinal association of lead with blood pressure. Epidemiology 2003; 14(1):30-6.

Guallar E., Silbergeld E.K., Navas-Acien A., Malhotra S., Astor B.C., Sharrett A.R., Schwartz B.S. Confounding of the relation between homocysteine and peripheral arterial disease by lead, cadmium, and renal function. Am J Epidemiol. 2006 Apr 15; 163(8):700-8. Epub 2006 Feb 16.

Harlan W.R., Landis J.R., Schmouder R.L., Goldstien N.G., Harlan L.C. Blood lead and blood pressure. JAMA. 1985; 253: 530–534.

Heo Y., Lee W.T.: Lawrence D.A.: Differential effects of lead and cAMP on development and activities of Th1- and Th2-lymphocytes. Toxicol. Sci., 1998, 43, 172-178.

Hoffer B.J., Olson L., Palmer M.R. Toxic effects of lead in the developing nervous system: in oculo experimental models. Environ Health Perspect. 1987; 74:169-75.

Hopkins M.R., Ettinger A.S., Hernández-Avila M., Schwartz J., Téllez-Rojo M.M., Lamadrid-Figueroa H., Bellinger D., Hu H., Wright R.O. Variants in iron metabolism genes predict higher blood lead levels in young children. Environ Health Perspect. 2008 Sep; 116(9):1261-6.

Hu H., Hashimoto D., Besser M. Levels of lead in blood and bone of women giving birth in a Boston hospital.Arch Environ Health. 1996; 51(1): 52-8.

Hu H., Téllez-Rojo M.M., Bellinger D., Smith D., Ettinger A.S., Lamadrid-Figueroa H., Schwartz J., Schnaas L., Mercado-García A., Hernández-Avila M. Fetal lead exposure at each stage of pregnancy as a predictor of infant mental development. Environ Health Perspect. 2006 Nov; 114(11):1730-5.

Kaewboonchoo O., Morioka I., Saleekul S., Miyai N., Chaikittiporn C., Kawai T. Blood lead level and cardiovascular risk factors among bus drivers in Bangkok, Thailand. Ind Health. 2010; 48(1):61-5.

Kaji T., Sakamoto M. Stimulation of heparan sulphate release from cultured endothelial cells by plasmin. Blood Coagul Fibrinolysis. 1991; 2(3): 419-23.

Kalia K., Flora S.J. Strategies for safe and effective therapeutic measures for chronic arsenic and lead poisoning. J Occup Health. 2005; 47:1-21.

Kalia K., Narula G.D., Kannan G.M., Flora S.J. Effects of combined administration of captopril and DMSA on arsenite induced oxidative stress and blood and tissue arsenic concentration in rats. Comp Biochem Physiol C Toxicol Pharmacol. 2007; 144:372-9.

Kasperczyk J. Lipids, lipid peroxidation and 7-ketocholesterol in workers exposed to lead. Hum Exp Toxicol. 2005 Jun; 24(6):287-95.

Kasperczyk S., Przywara-Chowaniec B., Kasperczyk A., Rykaczewska-Czerwińska M., Wodniecki J., Birkner E., Dziwisz M., Krauze-Wielicka M. Function of heart muscle in people chronically exposed to lead. Ann Agric Environ Med. 2005; 12(2):207-10.(b)

Kelly T.D. & Matos G.R. Historical statistics for mineral and material commodities in the United States. In: U.S. Geological Survey, 140, 2005, Lead: 20.08.2011, at http://pubs.usgs.gov/ds/2005/140/.

Kim K.R., Lee S.W., Paik N.W., Choi K. Low-level lead exposure among South Korean lead workers, and estimates of associated risk of cardiovascular diseases. J Occup Environ Hyg. 2008 Jun; 5(6):399-416.

Kuliczkowski W., Jołda-Mydłowska B., Kobusiak-Prokopowicz M., Antonowicz-Juchniewicz J., Kosmala W. Effect of heavy metal ions on function of vascular endothelium in patients with ischemic heart disease. Pol Arch Med Wewn. 2004 Jun; 111(6):679-85.

Lanphear B.P., Hornung R., Khoury J., Yolton K., Baghurst P., Bellinger D.C., Canfield R.L., Dietrich K.N., Bornschein R., Greene T., Rothenberg S.J., Needleman H.L., Schnaas L., Wasserman G., Graziano J., Roberts R. Low-level environmental lead exposure and children's intellectual function: an international pooled analysis. Environ Health Perspect. 2005 Jul; 113(7):894-9.

Lead-related nephrotoxicity: a review of the epidemiologic evidence. Ekong E.B., Jaar B.G., Weaver V.M. Lead-related nephrotoxicity: a review of the epidemiologic evidence. Kidney Int. 2006 Dec; 70(12):2074-84.

Lee B.K., Lee G.S., Stewart W.F., Ahn K.D., Simon D., Kelsey K.T., Todd A.C., Schwartz B.S. Associations of blood pressure and hypertension with lead dose measures and polymorphisms in the vitamin D receptor and delta-aminolevulinic acid dehydratase genes. Environ Health Perspect. 2001: 109(4):383-9.

Lee T.H., Tseng M.C., Chen C.J., Lin J.L. Association of high body lead store with severe intracranial carotid atherosclerosis. Neurotoxicology. 2009 Nov; 30(6):876-80. Epub 2009 Jul 16.

Lustberg M. & Silbergeld E. Blood lead levels and mortality. Arch Intern Med. 2002; 162:2443-2449.

Malvezzi C.K., Moreira E.G., Vassilieff I, Vassilieff V.S., Cordellini S.: Effect of L-arginine, DMSA and the association of L-arginine and DMSA on tissue lead mobilization and blood pressure level in plumbism. Brazilian J of Medical and Biological Research. 2001; 34: 1341-1346.

Martin D., Glass T.A., Bandeen-Roche K., Todd A.C., Shi W., Schwartz B.S. Association of blood lead and tibia lead with blood pressure and hypertension in a community sample of older adults. Am J Epidemiol. 2006 Mar 1; 163(5):467-78. Epub 2006 Jan 18.

Mathee A., Röllin H., von Schirnding Y., Levin J., Naik I. Reductions in blood lead levels among school children following the introduction of unleaded petrol in South Africa. Reductions in blood lead levels among school children following the introduction of unleaded petrol in South Africa

Menke A., Muntner P., Batuman V., Silbergeld E.K., Guallar E. Blood lead below 0.48 µmol/L (10 µg/dL) and mortality among US adults. Circulation. 2006; 114: 1388–1394.

Micciolo R., Canal L., Maranelli G., Apostoli P. Non-occupational lead exposure and hypertension in northern Italy. Int J Epidemiol. 1994; 23: 312-320.

Michaels D., Zoloth S.R., Stern F.B. Does low-level lead exposure increase risk of death? A mortality study of newspaper printers. Int J Epidemiol. 1991 Dec;20(4):978-83.

Møller L. & Kristensen T.S. Blood lead as a cardiovascular risk factor. Am J Epidemiol. 1992; 136: 1091–1100.

Muntner P., Menke A., DeSalvo K.B., Rabito F.A., Batuman V. Continued decline in blood lead levels among adults in the United States: the National Health and Nutrition Examination Surveys. Arch Intern Med. 2005 Oct; 10;165(18):2155-61.

Navas-Acien A., Guallar E., Silbergeld E.K., Rothenberg S.J. Lead exposure and cardiovascular disease--a systematic review. Environ Health Perspect. 2007 Mar; 115(3):472-82.

Navas-Acien A., Selvin E., Sharrett A.R., Calderon-Aranda E., Silbergeld E., Guallar E. Lead, cadmium, smoking, and increased risk of peripheral arterial disease. Circulation. 2004; 109: 3196–3201.

Navas-Acien A., Silbergeld E.K., Sharrett R., Calderon-Aranda E., Selvin E., Guallar E. Metals in urine and peripheral arterial disease. Environ Health Perspect. 2005 Feb; 113(2):164-9.

Navas-Acien A., Tellez-Plaza M., Guallar E., Muntner P., Silbergeld E., Jaar B., Weaver V. Blood cadmium and lead and chronic kidney disease in US adults: a joint analysis. Am J Epidemiol. 2009 Nov 1; 170(9):1156-64. Epub 2009 Aug 21.

Nawrot T.S., Thijs L., Den Hond E.M., Roels H.A., Staessen J.A. An epidemiological re-appraisal of the association between blood pressure and blood lead: a meta-analysis. J Hum Hypertens. 2002 Feb;16(2):123-31.

Nehru B., Sidhu P. Behavior and neurotoxic consequences of lead on rat brain followed by recovery. Biol Trace Elem Res. 2001; 84(1-3):113-21.

Nie L.H., Wright R.O., Bellinger D.C., Hussain J., Amarasiriwardena C., Chettle D.R., Pejović-Milić A., Woolf A., Shannon M. Blood lead levels and cumulative blood lead index (CBLI) as predictors of late neurodevelopment in lead poisoned children. Biomarkers. 2011 Sep; 16(6):517-24. Epub 2011 Aug 9.

Othman A.I., El Missiry M.A. Role of selenium against lead toxicity in male rats. j Biochem Mol Toxicol. 1998; 12(6):345-9.

Park S.K., Hu H., Wright R.O., Schwartz J., Cheng Y., Sparrow D., Vokonas P.S., Weisskopf M.G. Iron metabolism genes, low-level lead exposure, and QT interval. Environ Health Perspect. 2009 Jan; 117(1):80-5. Epub 2008 Aug 22.

Pawlas K., Pawlas N., Kmiecik-Malecka E., Malecki A. The relationship between children's blood lead level and postural stability. J Human Kinetics; 2008, 20:71-80.

Pirkle J.L., Schwartz J., Landis J.R., Harlan W.R. The relationship between blood lead levels and blood pressure and its cardiovascular risk implications. Am J Epidemiol. 1985; 121: 246–258.

Pocock S.J., Shaper A.G., Ashby D., Delves H.T., Clayton B.E. The relationship between blood lead, blood pressure, stroke, and heart attacks in middle-aged British men. Environ Health Perspect. 1988 Jun; 78:23-30.

Poręba R., Gać P., Poręba M., Andrzejak R. The relationship between occupational exposure to lead and manifestation of cardiovascular complications in persons with arterial hypertension. Toxicol Appl Pharmacol. 2010 Nov 15; 249(1):41-6. (b)

Poręba R., Gać P., Poręba M., Derkacz A., Andrzejak R. Tachycardia as an independent risk factor in chronic lead poisoning. In: Sobieszczańska M, Jagielski J, Macfarlane PW (Eds.). Electrocardiology 2009. JAKS Publishing Company, Wroclaw 2010, pp. 251-261. (a)

Poręba R., Poręba M., Gać P., Steinmetz-Beck A., Beck B., Pilecki W., Andrzejak R., Sobieszczańska M. Electrocardiographic changes in workers occupationally exposed to lead. Ann Noninvasive Electrocardiol. 2011; 16(1):33-40.

Poręba R., Skoczyńska A., Derkacz A., Szymańska-Chabowska A., Andrzejak R. Serum homocysteine level in person occupationaly exposed to lead. Adv.Clin.Exp.Med. 2005 Vol.14 no.3; s.537-543.

Rabinowitz M., Bellinger D., Leviton A., Needleman H., Schoenbaum S. Pregnancy hypertension, blood pressure during labor, and blood lead levels. Hypertension. 1987; 10(4):447-51.

Reckziegel P., Dias V.T., Benvegnú D., Boufleur N., Silva Barcelos R.C., Segat H.J., Pase C.S., Dos Santos C.M., Flores E.M., Bürger M.E. Locomotor damage and brain oxidative stress induced by lead exposure are attenuated by gallic acid treatment. Toxicol Lett. 2011; 203(1):74-81. Epub 2011 Mar 22.

Report of the PHIME Seminar at European Environment Agency "*Effects of exposure to metals; no margin of safety in Europe*" on 10th of February 2011.

Revis N.W., Major T.C., Horton C.Y. The effects of calcium, magnesium, lead, or cadmium on lipoprotein metabolism and atherosclerosis in the pigeon. J Environ Pathol Toxicol. 1980 Sep; 4(2-3):293-303.

Revis N.W., Zinsmeister A.R., Bull R. Atherosclerosis and hypertension induction by lead and cadmium ions: an effect prevented by calcium ion. Proc Natl Acad Sci U S A. 1981 Oct; 78(10):6494-8.

Robinson T.R. 20-year mortality of tetraethyl lead workers. J Occup Med. 1974 Sep;16(9):601-5.

Rodríguez-Iturbe B., Sindhu R.K., Quiroz Y., Vaziri N.D. Chronic exposure to low doses of lead results in renal infiltration of immune cells, NF-kappaB activation, and overexpression of tubulointerstitial angiotensin II. Antioxid Redox Signal. 2005 Sep-Oct; 7(9-10):1269-74.

Romieu I., Carreon T., Lopez L., Palazuelos E., Rios C., Manuel Y., Hernandez-Avila M. Environmental urban lead exposure and blood lead levels in children of Mexico City. Environ Health Perspect. 1995 Nov; 103(11):1036-40.

Rossi E. Low level environmental lead exposure--a continuing challenge. Clin Biochem Rev. 2008 May; 29(2):63-70.

Roy A., Bellinger D., Hu H., Schwartz J., Ettinger A.S., Wright R.O., Bouchard M., Palaniappan K., Balakrishnan K. Lead exposure and behavior among young children in Chennai, India Environ Health Perspect. 2009 Oct; 117(10):1607-11. Epub 2009 Jun 26.

Sakai T., Morita Y., Araki T., Kano M., Yoshida T. Relationship between delta-aminolevulinic acid dehydratase genotypes and heme precursors in lead workers. Am J Ind Med. 2000; 38(3):355-60.

Schafer J.H., Glass T.A., Bressler J., Todd A.C., Schwartz B.S. Blood lead is a predictor of homocysteine levels in a population-based study of older adults. Environ Health Perspect. 2005 Jan; 113(1):31-5. 25.

Schober S.E., Mirel L.B., Graubard B.I., Brody D.J., Flegal K.M. Blood lead levels and death from all causes, cardiovascular disease, and cancer: results from the NHANES III mortality study. Environ Health Perspect. 2006; 114(10):1538-41

Schwartz J. Lead, blood pressure, and cardiovascular disease in men and women. Environ Health Perspect. 1991, 91:71-5.

Scinicariello F., Yesupriya A., Chang M.H., Fowler B.A. Modification by ALAD of the association between blood lead and blood pressure in the U.S. population: results from the Third National Health and Nutrition Examination Survey. Environ Health Perspect. 2010 Feb; 118(2):259-64.

Sharifi A.M., Darabi R., Akbarloo N., Larijani B., Khoshbaten A. Investigation of circulatory and tissue ACE activity during development of lead-induced hypertension. Toxicol Lett. 2004 Nov 2; 153(2):233-8.

Shen X., Rosen J.F., Guo D., Wu S. Childhood lead poisoning in China. Sci Total Environ. 1996 Mar 15; 181(2):101-9.

Silbergeld EK. Mechanisms of lead neurotoxicity, or looking beyond the lamppost. FASEB J. 1992 Oct; 6(13):3201-6.

Sirivarasai J., Kaojarern S., Wananukul W., Deechakwan W., Srisomerarn P.. Non-occupational lead and cadmium exposure and blood pressure in Thai men. Asia Pac J Public Health. 2004; 16:133-137.

Skoczynska A. Genetic aspects of hypertensive effects of lead. Med Pr. 2008; 59(4):325-32.

Skoczynska A. In: Lead as cardiovascular risk factor. Ed: W.Górnicki Wyd. Med. 2006

Skoczynska A., Gruber K., Belowska-Bień K., Mlynek V. Risk of cardiovascular diseases in lead-exposed workers of crystal glassworks. Part I. Effect of lead on blood pressure and lipid metabolism. Med Pr. 2007;58(6):475-83.

Skoczynska A., Juzwa W., Smolik R., Szechiński J., Behal F.J. Response of the cardiovascular system to catecholamines in rats given small doses of lead.Toxicology. 1986; 39(3):275-89.

Skoczynska A., Martynowicz H., Poręba R., Antonowicz-Juchniewicz J., Sieradzki A., Andrzejak R. Trehalase concentration in urine as a marker of renal dysfuncton in workers occupationally exposed to lead. Med Pr. 2001; 52: 247-252.

Skoczynska A., Martynowicz H., Rupnik A., Turczyn B., Wojakowska A., Górecka H. Glycosaminoglycans content in the organs of rats chronically treated with lead. Metal Ions Biol Med. 2004, 8, 364-367.

Skoczynska A., Poręba R., Derkacz A. Endothelial dysfunction in workers exposed to lead. In: Atherosclerosis: risk factors, diagnosis and treatment. Monduzzi Editore, International Proceedings Division, Salzburg. 2002; July 7-10: 77-81.

Skoczynska A., Smolik R. The effect of combined exposure to lead and cadmium on serum lipids and lipid peroxides level in rats. Int J Occup Med Environ Health, 1994, 7, 263-271

Skoczynska A., Smolik R., Jeleń M. Lipid abnormalities in rats given small doses of lead. Arch Toxicol 1993, 67, 200-4.

Skoczynska A., Smolik R., Milian A. The effect of combined exposure to lead and cadmium on the concentration of zinc and copper in rat tissues. Int J Occup Med Environ Health. 1994; 7(1):41-9.

Skoczynska A., Stojek E. The impact of subchronic lead poisoning on the vascular effect of nitric oxide in rats. Environ Toxicol Pharmacol. 2005; 19: 99-106.

Skoczynska A., Stojek E., Górecka H., Wojakowska A. The serum vasoactive agents in lead-treated rats. Int J Occup Med Environ Health. 2003; 16: 169-177.

Skoczynska A., Szechiński J., Juzwa W., Smolik R., Běhal F. Carotid sinus reflexes in rats given small doses of lead. Toxicology 1987, 43, 161-171.

Skoczynska A., Wróbel J., Andrzejak R. Lead-cadmium interaction effect on the responsiveness of rat mesenteric vessels to norepinephrine and angiotensin II. Toxicology, 2001; 162: 157-170.

Sroczyński J., Biskupek K., Piotrowski J., Rudzki H. Effect of occupational exposure to lead, zinc and cadmium on various indicators of the circulatory system of metallurgical workers. Med Pr. 1990; 41(3):152-8.

Stohs S.J., Bagchi D. Oxidative mechanisms in the toxicity of metal ions. Free Rad Biol Med. 1995; 18: 321-336.

Suzen H.S., Duydu Y., Avdin A., Isimer A., Vural N. Influence of the delta-aminolewulinic acid dehydratase (ALAD) polymorphism on biomarkers of lead exposure in Turkish storage battery manufacturing workers. Am J Ind Med. 2003; 43(2):165-71.

Takebayashi T. Epidemiologic review of long-term, low-level exposure to environmental chemicals and cardiovascular disease: an exposure-response relationship. Nippon Eiseigaku Zasshi. 2011; 66(1):13-21.

Telisman S., Jurasović J., Pizent A., Cvitković P. Blood pressure in relation to biomarkers of lead, cadmium, copper, zinc, and selenium in men without occupational exposure to metals. Environ Res. 2001; 87(2):57-68.

Tepper A., Mueller C., Singal M., Sagar K. Blood pressure, left ventricular mass, and lead exposure in battery manufacturing workers. Am J Ind Med. 2001 Jul; 40(1):63-72.

Tong S., Baghurst P.A., Sawyer M.G., Burns J., McMichael A.J. Declining blood lead levels and changes in cognitive function during childhood: the Port Pirie Cohort Study. JAMA. 1998 Dec 9; 280(22):1915-9.

Tong S., von Schirnding Y.E., Prapamontol T. Environmental lead exposure: a public health problem of global dimensions. Bull World Health Organ. 2000; 78(9):1068-77.

Trzcinka-Ochocka M., Jakubowski M., Raźniewska G. Asessment of occupational exposure to lead in Poland. Med Pr. 2005; 56(5):395-404.

Tsao D.A., Yu H.S., Cheng J.T., Ho C.K., Chang H.R. The change of beta-adrenergic system in lead-induced hypertension. Toxicol Appl Pharmacol. 2000; 164(2):127-33.

Turczyn B., Skoczynska A., Wojakowska A. Serum and urinary glycosaminoglycans in workers chronically exposed to lead. Med. Pr. 2010; 61(5):553-60.

Vaziri N.D., Ding Y., Ni Z.: Compensatory up-regulation of nitric oxide synthase isoforms in lead-induced hypertension; reversal by a superoxide dismutase-mimetic drug. J Pharm Exp Ther. 2001; 298(2): 679-685.

Vaziri N.D., Sica D.A. Lead-induced hypertension: role of oxidative stress. Curr Hypertens Rep. 2004 Aug; 6(4):314-20.

Wang L., Zhou X., Yang D., Wang Z. Effects of lead and/or cadmium on the distribution patterns of some essential trace elements in immature female rats. Hum Exp Toxicol. 2011 Apr 18. (Epub ahead of print).

Weaver V.M., Lee B.K., Todd A.C., Ahn K.D., Shi W., Jaar B.G., Kelsey K.T., Lustberg M.E., Silbergeld E.K., Parsons P.J., Wen J., Schwartz B.S. Effect modification by dela-aminolevulinic acid dehydratase, vitamin D receptor, and nitric oxide synthase gene polymorphisms on associations between patella lead and renal function in lead workers. Environ. Res. 2006, 102(1):61-9.

Weaver V.M., Schwartz B.S., Ahn K.D., Stewart W.F., Kelsey K.T., Todd A.C., Wen J., Simon D.J., Lustberg M.E., Parsons P.J., Silbergeld E.K., Lee B.K. Associations of renal function with polymorphisms in the delta-aminolevulinic acid dehydratase, vitamin D receptor, and nitric oxide synthase genes in Korean lead workers. Environ Health Perspect. 2003; 111(13):1613-9.

Weiss S.T., Munoz A., Stein A., Sparrow D., Speizer F.E. The relationship of blood lead to systolic blood pressure in a longitudinal study of policemen. Environ Health Perspect. 1988; 78: 53-6.

Weisskopf M.G., Jain N., Nie H., Sparrow D., Vokonas P., Schwartz J., Hu H. A prospective study of bone lead concentration and death from all causes, cardiovascular diseases, and cancer in the Department of Veterans Affairs Normative Aging Study. Circulation. 2009 Sep; 22;120(12):1056-64. Epub 2009 Sep 8.

Wilczyńska U., Szeszenia-Dabrowska N., Sobala W. Mortality of men with occupational lead poisoning in Poland. Med Pr. 1998; 49(2):113-28.

Wrobel J., Skoczynska A. The activity of angiotensin converting enzyme in vascular mesenteric bed of rats poisoned with lead and cadmium. Med Pr. 2002; 53(2):131-6.

Zhang A., Park S.K., Wright R.O., Weisskopf M.G., Mukherjee B., Nie H., Sparrow D., Hu H. HFE H63D polymorphism as a modifier of the effect of cumulative lead exposure on pulse pressure: the Normative Aging Study. Environ Health Perspect. 2010 Sep; 118(9):1261-6. Epub 2010 May 14.

Zou H.J., Ding Y., Huang K.L., Xu M.L., Tang G.F., Wu M.H., Wang S.Y. Effects of lead on systolic and diastolic cardiac functions. Biomed Environ Sci. 1995 Dec;8(4):281-8.

18

Obstructive Sleep Apnoea Syndrome as a Systemic Low-Grade Inflammatory Disorder

Carlos Zamarrón[1], Emilio Morete[1] and Felix del Campo Matias[2]
[1]*Servicio de Neumología, Hospital Clínico Universitario, Santiago,*
[2]*Hospital Universitario Rio Hortega, Valladolid,*
Spain

1. Introduction

Obstructive sleep apnea syndrome (OSAS) is a common disorder characterized by recurrent upper airway collapse during sleep. A reduction or complete cessation of airflow occurs despite ongoing inspiratory efforts and leads to arousals, sleep fragmentation, and oxyhemoglobin desaturation (Remmers et al., 1978; Young et al., 1993).

Though clinically recognized for more than four decades (Gastaut et al., 1965), general awareness of OSAS has been slow to develop. OSAS has been associated with cardiovascular disease (Marin et al., 2005; Duran-Cantolla et al., 2010; Barbe et al., 2010), automobile accidents (Teran-Santos et al., 1999), chronic obstructive pulmonary disease (Chaouat et al., 1995), heart failure (Oldenburg et al., 2007) and health related quality of life deterioration (Pichel et al., 2004). OSAS often coexists with obesity and has been related to insulin resistance and metabolic syndrome (Choi et al., 2008).

Patients with OSAS experience repetitive episodes of hypoxia and reoxygenation during transient cessation of breathing that may have systemic effects. These patients also present increased levels of biomarkers linked to endocrine-metabolic and cardiovascular alterations (Zamarron et al., 2008). Moreover, OSAS may involve sleep fragmentation, tonic elevation of sympathetic neural activity, oxidative stress, inflammation, hypercoagulability and endothelial dysfunction (Bradley & Floras, 2009; Fava et al., 2011). All of this indicates that OSAS should be considered a systemic disease rather than a local abnormality.

The present review analyses the pathophysiology related to the systemic consequences of OSAS and the mechanisms involved in the association between OSAS and systemic diseases (Figure 1).

2. Sleep fragmentation

Extreme sleep habits can affect health and have been associated with increased inflammation. Significant changes in habitual sleep duration can lead to chronic low-grade systemic inflammation (Meisinger et al., 2005; Patel et al., 2009). Activation of pro-inflammatory pathways may represent a mechanism. In a recent study in pediatric OSAS patients, increased TNF-α levels were primarily driven by sleep fragmentation and body mass index. These levels were closely associated with the degree of sleepiness, as measured by the Multiple Sleep Latency Test. Surgical treatment of OSAS resulted in significant reductions in TNF-α levels with reciprocal prolongations in sleep latency (Gozal et al., 2010).

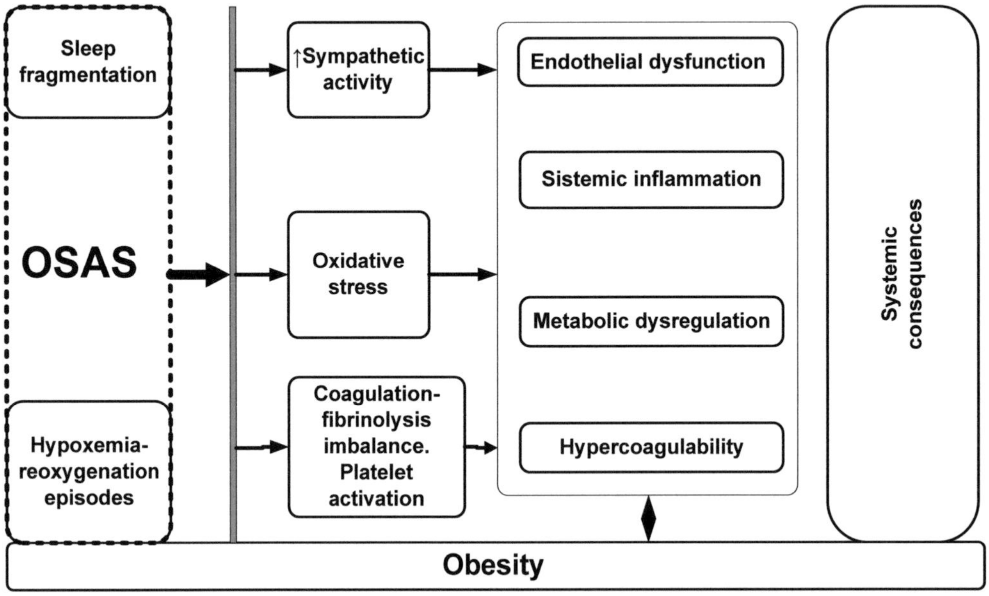

Fig. 1. A schematic summary of the proponed sequence of events in OSAS starting from episodic hypoxia and ending with systemic consequences.

Sleep fragmentation increases sympathetic nervous activity, which, in turn, results in a higher metabolic rate and elevated catecholamine secretion. Furthermore, severe sleep fragmentation can disturb nocturnal renin and aldosterone secretion profiles, and increase nighttime urine excretion. Moller et al. found that long-term CPAP reduced blood pressure, which was correlated with reductions in plasma renin and angiotensin II levels (Moller et al., 2003).

Although the mechanism of this altered inflammatory status in humans undergoing experimental sleep loss is unknown, it is likely that autonomic activation and metabolic changes play key roles (Mullington et al., 2010).

3. Enhanced sympathetic traffic

In OSAS patients, tonic activation of chemoreflex activity produces enhanced sympathetic traffic (Somers et al., 1988). Cyclic intermittent hypoxia (IH) and hypercapnia provides the causal link between upper airway obstruction during sleep and sympathetic activation during awakening. In a recent study in healthy humans, IH significantly increased sympathetic activity and daytime blood pressure after a single night of exposure. The baroreflex control of sympathetic outflow declined (Tamisier et al., 2011). Surges in sympathetic nervous system activity associated with apneic events have also been related to antifibrinolytic activity reflected by elevations in PAI-1 (von & Dimsdale, 2003). During apneic events, there is an up-regulation of the renin-angiotensin system and down-regulation of nitric oxide synthases (Fletcher et al., 1999; Prabhakar et al., 2001).

The increased sympathetic activity and IH associated with apneic episodes has been proposed as a possible mechanism behind the association between OSAS, systemic inflammation and cardiovascular disease. CPAP reduces sympathetic nerve activity (Maser et al., 2008), increases arterial baroreflex sensitivity (Marrone et al., 2011) and decreases vascular risk (Kohler et al., 2008).

4. Oxidative stress

There is an emerging consensus that OSAS is an oxidative stress disorder. In a recent study involving children with OSAS, Malakasioti found an increase of hydrogen peroxide levels in exhaled breath condensate, which is an indirect index of altered redox status in the respiratory tract (Malakasioti et al., 2011).

Apnea produces a decline in oxygen levels followed by reoxygenation when breathing resumes. The cyclical episodes of hypoxia-reoxygenation, analogous to cardiac ischemia/reoxygenation injury causing ATP depletion and xanthine oxidase activation, and increases the generation of oxygen-derived free radicals. CPAP therapy decreases the levels of oxidative stress in OSAS patients (Chin et al., 2000; Alonso-Fernandez et al., 2009).

Oxidative stress can profoundly regulate the cellular transcriptome through activation of transcription factors, including specificity protein-1, hypoxia-inducible factor-1, c-jun, and possibly nuclear factor-kappaB. Activation of redox-sensitive gene expression is suggested by the increase in some protein products of these genes, including VEGF (Teramoto et al., 2003), EPO (Marrone et al., 2008), endothelin-1 (Belaidi et al., 2009), inflammatory cytokines and adhesion molecules (Ohga et al., 1999; Dyugovskaya et al., 2002; Ohga et al., 2003).

Increased oxidative stress has been associated with development of cardiovascular diseases and can be promoted by the chronic intermittent hypoxia characteristic of OSAS (Park et al., 2007). A variety of studies suggest that oxidative stress is present in OSAS at levels relevant to tissues such as the arterial wall (Grebe et al., 2006; Barcelo et al., 2006). This process enhances lipid uptake into human macrophages and may contribute to atherosclerosis in OSAS patients (Lattimore et al., 2005). Furthermore, OSAS decreases blood antioxidant status in high BMI subjects and may change the relationship between oxidative stress markers (Wysocka et al., 2008). After CPAP, expression of eNOS and phosphorylated eNOS was found to be significantly increased whereas expression of nitrotyrosine and nuclear factor-kappaB significantly decreased (Jelic et al., 2010) but some studies shown that CPAP may not affect antioxidant defense (Alzoghaibi & Bahammam, 2011).

Recently, Nair reported that oxidative stress is mediated, at least in part, by excessive NADPH oxidase activity. This author suggests that pharmacological agents targeting NADPH oxidase may provide a therapeutic strategy in OSAS (Nair et al., 2011).

5. Systemic inflammation

Local and systemic inflammation is present in OSAS. Insofar as local inflammation, bronchial and nasal changes are especially relevant (Devouassoux et al., 2007). In a recent study, patients showed a significant increase in IL-8 and ICAM concentrations in both plasma and exhaled condensate. In addition, they showed a higher neutrophil percentage in induced sputum. These findings were significantly and positively correlated to AHI (Carpagnano et al., 2010), however, CPAP-therapy did have a significant effect (Lacedonia et al., 2011).

Several studies have reported changes in circulating levels of adhesion molecules in OSAS patients (El-Solh et al., 2002; Zamarron-Sanz et al., 2006). Dyugovskaya analysed polymorphonuclear apoptosis and expression of adhesion molecules in vitro in patients with moderate to severe OSAS. Decreased apoptosis and increased expression of adhesion molecules were observed. Although adhesion molecules may facilitate increased polymorphonuclear-endothelium interactions, decreased apoptosis may further augment these interactions and facilitate free radical and proteolytic enzymes (Dyugovskaya et al., 2008).

OSAS patients present increased levels of inflammatory mediators such as TNFα and IL-6 (Imagawa et al., 2004; Bravo et al., 2007) that decrease with CPAP treatment (Arias et al., 2008; Steiropoulos et al., 2009).

Systemic inflammation is increasingly being recognized as a risk factor for a number of complications including atherosclerosis (Ross, 1999) and is a well-established factor in the pathogenesis of cardiovascular disease (Hansson, 2005). Certain acute-phase proteins that have been associated in humans with cardiovascular disease, such as serum amyloid (Svatikova et al., 2003), C-reactive protein (Taheri et al., 2007; Punjabi & Beamer, 2007) which have been associated in humans with cardiovascular disease are elevated in OSAS patients and improve with CPAP treatment (Yokoe et al., 2003; Kuramoto et al., 2009).

The mechanisms by which inflammation contributes to OSAS-induced vascular dysfunction are not known. Reoxygenation after a brief period of hypoxia as experienced repetitively and systematically by OSAS patients may predispose to cell stress. It has been suggested that such events favor the activation of a proinflammatory response as mediated through the nuclear transcription factor nuclear factor-kappaB, a master regulator of inflammatory gene expression.

Inflammation may be an important link between increased sympathetic nervous system activity and vascular dysfunction in OSAS. Chronically elevated sympathetic activity produced an inflammatory response in several organs and vascular beds (Yu et al., 2005).

Some authors point to the role of the T-lymphocyte. This cell is known to play an important role in ANG II-induced hypertension and endothelial dysfunction via NADPH oxidase-induced superoxide production (Guzik et al., 2007).

Increased expression of inflammatory cytokines may contribute to endothelial dysfunction and subsequent cardiovascular complications (Ryan et al., 2005; Foster et al., 2007). Currently, some studies suggest that pentraxin 3, an acute phase response protein, is rapidly produced and released by several cell types, in particular by mononuclear phagocytes, and endothelial cells in response to primary inflammatory signals, may play a significant role in OSAS-associated vascular damage (Kasai et al., 2011). Arnaud report that some inhibition of molecules such as RANTES/CCL5, a cytokine that is a a selective attractant for memory T lymphocytes and monocytes may play a significant role in athesroscletoric remodeling OSAS-associated vascular damage (Arnaud et al., 2011)

However, mesenchymal stem cells triggered an early anti-inflammatory response in rats subjected to recurrent obstructive apneas, suggesting that these stem cells could play a role in the physiological response to counterbalance inflammation in OSAS (Carreras et al., 2010).

In a recent study on healthy human males, Querido et al. analysed the effect over 10 days of nightly IH in the following systemic inflammatory markers: serum granulocyte macrophage colony-stimulating factor, interferon-gamma, interleukin-1 β, interleukin-6, interleukin-8, leptin, monocyte chemotactic protein-1, vascular endothelial growth factor, intracellular adhesion molecule-1, and vascular cell adhesion molecule-1. There was no significant change in any of the markers. These findings suggest that a more substantial or a different pattern of hypoxemia might be necessary to activate systemic inflammation, that the system may need to be primed before hypoxic exposure, or that increases in inflammatory markers OSAS patients may be more related to other factors such as obesity or nocturnal arousal (Querido et al., 2011).

6. Hypercoagulability

Hypercoagulability resulting from increased coagulation or inhibited fibrinolysis is associated with an increased risk for cardiovascular disease (Zouaoui et al., 2006). This is another factor implicated in the association between this disease and OSAS (Peled et al., 2008).

A variety of findings support the existence of a relation between hypercoagulability, OSAS and cardiovascular disease. Firstly, patients with OSAS present higher plasma levels of several procoagulant factors such as fibrinogen (Reinhart et al., 2002; Tkacova et al., 2008), activated clotting factor FVII, FXIIa and thrombin/antithrombin III complexes (von et al., 2005) and the fibrinolysis-inhibiting enzyme plasminogen activator inihibitor (PAI-1) (von et al., 2006; Zamarron et al., 2008). Secondly, increased D-dimer levels in untreated OSAS have been correlated with severity of nocturnal hypoxemia, characteristic of OSAS (Shitrit et al., 2005). Thirdly, sleep fragmentation and sleep efficiency data have been associated with increased levels of von Willebrand factor and soluble tissue factor, two markers of a prothrombotic state (von et al., 2007).

OSAS is associated with platelet activation (Akinnusi et al., 2009). Platelet activation is a link in the pathophysiology of diseases prone to thrombosis and inflammation (Gasparyan et al., 2011). In these patients, platelet activation is associated with greater levels of oxygen desaturation (Oga et al., 2009;Rahangdale et al., 2011) that decreases after CPAP treatment (Varol et al., 2011).

In a current article, thromboelastography, a simple test of hemostasis, has been proposed for evaluating the risk of future cardiovascular disease in patients with OSAS (Othman et al., 2010).

7. Endothelial dysfunction

Endothelial dysfunction is an early marker of vascular abnormality preceding clinically overt cardiovascular disease (Giannotti & Landmesser, 2007; Halcox et al., 2009).

The intact endothelium regulates vascular tone and repair capacity, maintaining proinflammatory, anti-inflammatory, and coagulation homeostasis. Alteration of these homeostatic pathways results in endothelial dysfunction before structural changes in the vasculature. The hypoxia, hypercapnia, and pressor surges accompanying obstructive apneic events may serve as potent stimuli for the release of vasoactive substances and for impairment of endothelial function.

In OSAS, endothelial dysfunction could be caused by both hypoxia-reoxygenation cycles and chronic sleep fragmentation produced by repetitive arousals. A causal relationship between OSAS and endothelial dysfunction was demonstrated by a study in which flow-mediated dilation in the forearm was improved by CPAP treatment (Ip et al., 2004; Trzepizur et al., 2009). Levels of nitric oxide, a major vasodilator substance released by the endothelium, have been found to be decreased in OSAS patients, and these levels normalize with CPAP therapy (Haight & Djupesland, 2003).

A number of studies with OSAS patients indicate an associated endothelial dysfunction (Nieto et al., 2004). In patients with OSAS, increased production of superoxide by neutrophils (Schulz et al., 2000), increased biomarkers of lipid peroxidation (Lavie et al., 2004), and increased levels of 8-isoprostanes (Alonso Fernandez 2009; Carpagnano et al., 2003) have been observed.

Among the most important vasoconstrictive substances is endothelin-1, a peptide hormone secreted under the influence of hypoxia (Kanagy et al., 2001). Several studies have reported higher endothelin-1 levels in OSAS patients (Phillips et al 1999; Saarelainen & Hasan, 2000) however, Grimpen reports conflicting findings (Grimpen et al., 2000). This divergence might be explained by differences in study design. The groups studied by Phillips (Phillips et al., 1999) and Saarelainen (Saarelainen & Hasan, 2000) had more severe disease and, thus, underwent more severe oxygen desaturations that acted as a trigger for endothelin-1 secretion. Gjorup showed that hypertensive OSAS patients had greater nocturnal and diurnal endothelin-1 plasma levels than healthy controls, suggesting that OSAS does not affect plasma endothelin-1 levels in the absence of coexistent cardiovascular diseases (Gjorup et al., 2007).

The inconsistency of the above endothelin-1 levels likely reflects the predominantly abluminal release of endothelin. Using rat models of arterial hypertension, several authors have reported elevated vascular production of endothelin-1, while circulating levels remained similar to controls (Pohl & Busse, 1989; Rossi & Pitter, 2006). This demonstrates that circulating levels of endothelin-1 do not exclude elevated vascular production in OSAS.

In recent years, endothelial progenitor cells have gained a central role in vascular regeneration and endothelial repair capacity through angiogenesis and restoring endothelial function of injured blood vessels. Endothelial progenitor cells are decreased in patients with endothelial dysfunction and underlie an increased risk for cardiovascular morbidity in OSAS. Endothelial progenitor cells may have a potential role in the pathogenesis of vascular diseases that is pertinent to OSAS (Berger & Lavie, 2011).

It has recently been reported that OSAS patients presented increased oxidant production in the microcirculation and endothelial dysfunction, both of which improved with treatment (Patt et al., 2010)

8. OSAS and endocrine-metabolic consequences

Even though OSAS is generally less prevalent in women than men, differences diminish after the onset of menopause. This may be the result of declining estrogen and progesterone

(Resta et al., 2004; Anttalainen et al., 2006). Accordingly, estrogen replacement therapy in menopausal women lessens the prevalence of OSAS (Shahar et al., 2003; Wesstrom et al., 2005).

On the other hand, men diagnosed with OSAS may manifest decreased libido and a decline in morning serum testosterone levels (Teloken et al., 2006; Hoekema et al., 2006). At first, this was thought to reflect an associated dysfunction of the pituitary-gonadal axis related to sleep fragmentation and hypoxia (Meston et al., 2003). However, the correction of hypoxia and sleep fragmentation in OSAS patients treated with CPAP does not lead to complete recovery, suggesting that existence of other underlying causes. In a recent study, with the exception of prolactine, CPAP therapy produced no significant changes the serum level of sexual hormones including FSH and LH (Macrea et al., 2010). Some authors claim that obesity is the major contributing factor to the reduced pituitary gonadal function in OSAS (Luboshitzky et al., 2005).

9. Obesity

Central, or visceral, obesity is associated with the greatest risk for OSAS (Shinohara et al., 1997). The mechanism by which obesity can favor the onset of OSAS is not well-known, but it could be that central obesity precipitates or exacerbates OSAS because fat deposits in the upper airway affect distensibility (Isono, 2009). The increased volume of abdominal fat could predispose to hypoventilation during sleep and/or reduce the oxygen reserve, favoring oxygen desaturation during sleep (Schwartz et al., 2008). In addition, the disrupted sleep patterns characteristic of OSAS predispose to metabolic effects and weight gain. Patel investigated the association between self-reported usual sleep duration and subsequent weight gain in the Nurses' Health Study. They showed that a habitual sleep time of less than 7 hours is associated with a modest increase in future weight gain and incident obesity (Patel et al., 2006).

In recent years, much attention has been focused on the interaction between OSAS and products released by adipose tissue such as leptin, adiponectin, resistin and grelin (Ronti et al., 2006).

Leptin is an adipocyte-derived hormone that regulates body weight through control of appetite and energy expenditure (Proulx et al., 2002). Furthermore, leptin is a cytokine and is therefore also involved in the inflammatory process. Several studies have shown increased levels of leptin in OSAS (Phillips et al., 2000; Tokuda et al., 2008), suggesting its role in the disease (Ip et al., 2000). The mechanisms underlying the relation between leptin and OSAS are very diverse, and may involve overnight changes in apnea levels (Patel et al., 2004; Sanner et al., 2004), sleep hypoxemia (Tatsumi et al., 2005), and hypercapnia (Shimura et al., 2005).

A direct relationship between OSAS and leptin is supported by the fact that effective OSAS treatment with CPAP also influences leptin levels (Shimizu et al., 2002; Cuhadaroglu et al., 2009). Although the precise mechanism explaining the effect of CPAP has not yet been elucidated, it can be inferred that reduction in sympathetic activity (Snitker et al., 1997), and improvement in insulin sensitivity play a role (Brooks et al., 1994).

Leptin levels have been proposed as a prognostic marker for OSAS (Ozturk et al., 2003) and have been implicated in the pathogenesis of OSAS-related cardiovascular disease (Kapsimalis et al., 2008; Tokuda et al., 2008; Al et al., 2009).

Leptin can also act as a respiratory stimulant, and impairment of the leptin signaling pathway causes respiratory depression in mice (O'Donnell et al., 2000). This hormone has been associated with obesity hypoventilation syndrome in humans (Phipps et al., 2002) and may reflect a compensatory response to hypoventilation (Makinodan et al., 2008).

OSAS has independently been associated with reduced levels of adiponectin (Masserini et al., 2006; Zhang et al., 2006; Carneiro et al., 2009) which may favour cardiovascular disease development. The recurrent hypoxia-reoxygenation attacks in OSAS patients may activate oxidative stress and lead to low levels of adiponectin (Vatansever et al., 2010).

Some authors have observed that serum adiponectin levels may be independent of the degree of OSAS (Tokuda et al., 2008). Decreased adiponectin may result from increased sympathetic activity (Delporte et al., 2002), and higher levels of cytokines such as IL-6 and TNFα (Fasshauer et al., 2003). In fact, there are conflicting reports as to whether CPAP treatment of OSAS effectively normalizes adiponectin levels (de Lima et al., 2010).

Obesity has been implicated in the relation between OSAS and adiponectin (Makino et al., 2006), In a recent study involving media under hypoxic conditions in an ex-vivo mouse model, adiponectin secretion was measured. In obese mice, hypoxic stress reduced adiponectin in the supernatant of mesenteric fat tissue, but not subcutaneous fat tissue. These findings suggest that abdominal obesity, representing abundant mesenteric fat tissue susceptible to hypoxic stress, partly explains adiponectin levels in OSAS patients, and that reduction of visceral fat accumulation may combat OSAS-related atherosclerotic cardiovascular diseases in abdominal obesity (Nakagawa et al., 2011).

Resistin is a white adipose tissue hormone whose function has yet to be established. In a study of 20 obese OSAS patients, Harsch found that CPAP treatment of OSAS had no significant influence on resistin levels (Harsch et al., 2004). In OSAS patients, hypoxic stress during sleep may enhance resistin production, possibly mediating systemic inflammatory processes. Through its effect on OSAS, CPAP therapy may help control resistin production (Yamamoto et al., 2008).

OSAS may decrease serum resistin levels in subjects with excess body mass and also may contribute to glucose metabolism, but has no influence on leptin levels (Wysocka et al., 2009)

Ghrelin is a hormone that influences appetite and fat accumulation and its physiological effects are opposite to those of leptin. No clear relation has been found between ghrelin and OSAS. In a study of 30 obese OSAS patients, Harsch found that plasma ghrelin levels were significantly higher in OSAS patients than in controls. These elevated ghrelin levels could not be explained by obesity alone, since they rapidly decreased with CPAP therapy (Harsch et al., 2003). In another study of 30 untreated obese patients with moderate-severe OSAS, significantly higher levels of serum leptin were found in OSAS patients than in controls, but ghrelin levels were no different (Ulukavak et al., 2005).

In a recent study of 55 consecutive OSAS patients, the study group presented significantly higher serum ghrelin levels than controls. There was a significant positive correlation between ghrelin and AHI. No significant difference was noted in the levels of leptin, adiponectin, and resistin (Li et al., 2010).

Increased ghrelin levels have been found to support the presence of increased appetite and caloric intake in obese patients with OSAS, which in turn may further promote the severity of the underlying conditions (Spruyt et al., 2010). In obese children, OSAS is associated with daytime sleepiness, elevation of proinflammatory cytokines, increased leptin, and decreased adiponectin (Tsaoussoglou et al., 2010).

10. OSAS and insulin resistance

A variety of studies based on animal models indicate that hypoxia can alter glucose homeostasis (Cheng et al., 1997; Li et al., 2006). Polotsky described that long-term exposure to intermittent hypoxia increased levels of insulin and glucose intolerance in obese, leptin-deficient mice (Polotsky et al., 2003). Humans exposed to hypoxia present worsened glucose tolerance (Braun et al., 2001).

Insulin resistance is a central part of the metabolic syndrome, a condition that is reaching epidemic proportions in Western Society and now emerging in developing countries (Prentice, 2006). Most studies involving OSAS and insulin resistance demonstrate an association between these two diseases, independently of obesity (Tassone et al., 2003; McArdle et al., 2007). In a large population-based study involving normoglycemic hypertensive men, Resnick found that the severity of OSAS was associated with increased insulin resistance (Resnick et al., 2003). The magnitude of these beneficial effects is modulated by the hours of CPAP adherence and the degree of obesity (Tasali et al., 2011).

Insulin resistance is associated to states of inflammation (Reaven, 2005). Monocyte chemoattractant protein-1 levels are elevated in OSAS and may be involved in the pathogenesis of insulin resistance in these patients (Piemonti et al., 2003; Hayashi et al., 2006).

11. Metabolic syndrome and OSAS

Metabolic syndrome is an emerging public health problem that represents a constellation of cardiovascular risk factors (Batsis et al., 2007). The clinical identification of metabolic syndrome is based on measures of abdominal obesity, atherogenic dyslipidemia, elevated blood pressure, and glucose intolerance (Executive Summary of the NCEP., 2001).

Although the etiology of this syndrome is largely unknown, it is likely to be comprised of a complex interaction between genetic, metabolic, and environmental factors (Nestel, 2003). Several recent studies suggest that a proinflammatory state may also be an important component (Aso et al., 2005; Gude et al., 2009). The close association between OSAS and metabolic syndrome is called "Syndrome Z"(Wilcox et al., 1998)

The prevalence of metabolic syndrome is markedly higher among OSAS patients. Ambrosetti et al. studied 89 consecutive OSAS patients and found metabolic syndrome in 53% of them (Ambrosetti et al., 2006). Another recent study found a prevalence of 68% (Drager et al., 2009). Obese OSAS patients may have an increased rate of metabolic syndrome and higher levels of serum lipids, fasting glucose, leptin and fibrinogen than obese subjects without OSAS. Thus, clinicians should be encouraged to systematically evaluate the presence of metabolic abnormalities in OSAS and vice versa (Basoglu et al., 2011).

Both clinical and animal studies suggest that an independent relationship may exist between OSAS and hyperlipidemia. Hypoxic stress produced by OSAS potentially increases the risk of hyperlipidemia. In rodent models, hyperlipidemia can result from exposure to intermittent hypoxia (Li et al., 2005). In a sample of nearly 5,000 subjects from the Sleep Heart Health study, there was a positive association between OSAS severity and increased serum total cholesterol and triglycerides, as well as decreased serum HDL, in people under the age of 65 (Newman et al., 2001).

In a population-based sample of four hundred women aged 20-70 years the frequency of metabolic syndrome increased from 10.5% in women with AHI <5 to 57.1% in women with AHI ≥ 30. AHI and minimal saturation level remained significantly associated with metabolic syndrome also when adjusting for the waist-to-hip-ratio (Theorell-Haglow et al., 2011).

Both OSAS and metabolic syndrome may exert negative synergistic effects on the cardiovascular system through multiple mechanisms (Bonsignore & Zito, 2008; Levy et al., 2009).

Intermittent hypoxia, the hallmark feature of OSAS, leads to a preferential activation of inflammatory pathways. Oxidative stress, cardiovascular inflammation, endothelial dysfunction, and metabolic abnormalities in OSAS could accelerate atherogenesis (Quercioli et al., 2010). Further studies are required to determine the precise role of inflammation in the cardiovascular pathogenesis of OSAS, particularly its interaction with oxidative stress, obesity and metabolic dysfunction (Kent et al., 2011)

12. Conclusions

OSAS patients experience hypoxia-reoxygenation episodes, hypercapnia and arousal from sleep with modifications in the autonomic nervous system, oxidative stress and inflammation. OSAS is frequently associated to endocrine metabolic alterations and obesity.

Inflammatory processes play an important role in the pathogenesis of atherosclerosis and circulating levels of several inflammation markers have been associated with future cardiovascular risk. OSAS plays a mediating role between obesity and cardiovascular disease. Clinical and experimental data suggest a relationship between OSAS and adipose tissue pathophysiology which appears biologically plausible, however, further research is still needed. Multiple factors have been proposed to activate proinflammatory pathways in obesity, including generation of reactive oxygen species, and release of inflammatory cytokines potentially activated by OSAS-related hypoxic stress. All of this indicates that, more than a local abnormality, OSAS should be considered a systemic disease.

13. References

Executive Summary of The Third Report of The National Cholesterol Education Program (NCEP) Expert Panel on Detection, Evaluation, And Treatment of High Blood Cholesterol In Adults (Adult Treatment Panel III) (2001). *JAMA, 285,* 2486-2497.

Akinnusi, M. E., Paasch, L. L., Szarpa, K. R., Wallace, P. K., & El Solh, A. A. (2009). Impact of nasal continuous positive airway pressure therapy on markers of platelet activation in patients with obstructive sleep apnea. *Respiration, 77,* 25-31.

Al, L. N., Mulgrew, A., Cheema, R., Vaneeden, S., Butt, A., Fleetham, J. et al. (2009). Pro-atherogenic cytokine profile of patients with suspected obstructive sleep apnea. *Sleep Breath.,* 13:391-5

Alonso-Fernandez, A., Garcia-Rio, F., Arias, M. A., Hernanz, A., de la, P. M., Pierola, J. et al. (2009). Effects of CPAP on oxidative stress and nitrate efficiency in sleep apnoea: a randomised trial. *Thorax, 64,* 581-586.

Alzoghaibi, M. A. & Bahammam, A. S. (2011). The effect of one night of continuous positive airway pressure therapy on oxidative stress and antioxidant defense in hypertensive patients with severe obstructive sleep apnea. *Sleep Breath, 13,391-5* May 13. [Epub ahead of print]

Ambrosetti, M., Lucioni, A. M., Conti, S., Pedretti, R. F., & Neri, M. (2006). Metabolic syndrome in obstructive sleep apnea and related cardiovascular risk. *J.Cardiovasc.Med.(Hagerstown.), 7,* 826-829.

Anttalainen, U., Saaresranta, T., Aittokallio, J., Kalleinen, N., Vahlberg, T., Virtanen, I. et al. (2006). Impact of menopause on the manifestation and severity of sleep-disordered breathing. *Acta Obstet.Gynecol.Scand., 85,* 1381-1388.

Arias, M. A., Garcia-Rio, F., Alonso-Fernandez, A., Hernanz, A., Hidalgo, R., Martinez-Mateo, V. et al. (2008). CPAP decreases plasma levels of soluble tumour necrosis factor-alpha receptor 1 in obstructive sleep apnoea. *Eur.Respir.J., 32,* 1009-1015.

Arnaud, C., Beguin, P. C., Lantuejoul, S., Pepin, J. L., Guillermet, C., Pelli, G. et al. (2011). The Inflammatory Pre-Atherosclerotic Remodeling Induced by Intermittent Hypoxia is Attenuated by RANTES/CCL5 Inhibition. *Am.J.Respir.Crit. Care. Med.,* Jun 16. [Epub ahead of print]

Aso, Y., Wakabayashi, S., Yamamoto, R., Matsutomo, R., Takebayashi, K., & Inukai, T. (2005). Metabolic syndrome accompanied by hypercholesterolemia is strongly associated with proinflammatory state and impairment of fibrinolysis in patients with type 2 diabetes: synergistic effects of plasminogen activator inhibitor-1 and thrombin-activatable fibrinolysis inhibitor. *Diabetes Care, 28,* 2211-2216.

Barbe, F., Duran-Cantolla, J., Capote, F., de la, P. M., Chiner, E., Masa, J. F. et al. (2010). Long-term effect of continuous positive airway pressure in hypertensive patients with sleep apnea. *Am.J.Respir.Crit Care Med., 181,* 718-726.

Barcelo, A., Barbe, F., de la, P. M., Vila, M., Perez, G., Pierola, J. et al. (2006). Antioxidant status in patients with sleep apnoea and impact of continuous positive airway pressure treatment. *Eur.Respir.J., 27,* 756-760.

Basoglu, O. K., Sarac, F., Sarac, S., Uluer, H., & Yilmaz, C. (2011). Metabolic syndrome, insulin resistance, fibrinogen, homocysteine, leptin, and C-reactive protein in obese patients with obstructive sleep apnea syndrome. *Ann.Thorac.Med., 6,* 120-125.

Batsis, J. A., Nieto-Martinez, R. E., & Lopez-Jimenez, F. (2007). Metabolic syndrome: from global epidemiology to individualized medicine. *Clin.Pharmacol.Ther., 82,* 509-524.

Belaidi, E., Joyeux-Faure, M., Ribuot, C., Launois, S. H., Levy, P., & Godin-Ribuot, D. (2009). Major role for hypoxia inducible factor-1 and the endothelin system in promoting myocardial infarction and hypertension in an animal model of obstructive sleep apnea. *J.Am.Coll.Cardiol., 53,* 1309-1317.

Berger, S. & Lavie, L. (2011). Endothelial progenitor cells in cardiovascular disease and hypoxia-potential implications to obstructive sleep apnea. *Transl.Res., 158,* 1-13.

Bonsignore, M. R. & Zito, A. (2008). Metabolic effects of the obstructive sleep apnea syndrome and cardiovascular risk. *Arch.Physiol. Biochem., 114,* 255-260.

Bradley, T. D. & Floras, J. S. (2009). Obstructive sleep apnoea and its cardiovascular consequences. *Lancet, 373,* 82-93.

Braun, B., Rock, P. B., Zamudio, S., Wolfel, G. E., Mazzeo, R. S., Muza, S. R. et al. (2001). Women at altitude: short-term exposure to hypoxia and/or alpha(1)-adrenergic blockade reduces insulin sensitivity. *J.Appl.Physiol, 91,* 623-631.

Bravo, M. D., Serpero, L. D., Barcelo, A., Barbe, F., Agusti, A., & Gozal, D. (2007). Inflammatory proteins in patients with obstructive sleep apnea with and without daytime sleepiness. Sleep Breath, 11,177-85.

Brooks, B., Cistulli, P. A., Borkman, M., Ross, G., McGhee, S., Grunstein, R. R. et al. (1994). Obstructive sleep apnea in obese noninsulin-dependent diabetic patients: effect of continuous positive airway pressure treatment on insulin responsiveness. *J.Clin.Endocrinol.Metab, 79,* 1681-1685.

Carneiro, G., Togeiro, S. M., Ribeiro-Filho, F. F., Truksinas, E., Ribeiro, A. B., Zanella, M. T. et al. (2009). Continuous Positive Airway Pressure Therapy Improves Hypoadiponectinemia in Severe Obese Men with Obstructive Sleep Apnea without Changes in Insulin Resistance. *Metab Syndr.Relat. Disord.,* 7:537-42

Carpagnano, G. E., Kharitonov, S. A., Resta, O., Foschino-Barbaro, M. P., Gramiccioni, E., & Barnes, P. J. (2003). 8-Isoprostane, a marker of oxidative stress, is increased in exhaled breath condensate of patients with obstructive sleep apnea after night and is reduced by continuous positive airway pressure therapy. *Chest, 124,* 1386-1392.

Carpagnano, G. E., Spanevello, A., Sabato, R., Depalo, A., Palladino, G. P., Bergantino, L. et al. (2010). Systemic and airway inflammation in sleep apnea and obesity: the role of ICAM-1 and IL-8. *Transl.Res., 155,* 35-43.

Carreras, A., Almendros, I., Montserrat, J. M., Navajas, D., & Farre, R. (2010). Mesenchymal stem cells reduce inflammation in a rat model of obstructive sleep apnea. *Respir.Physiol. Neurobiol., 172,* 210-212.

Chaouat, A., Weitzenblum, E., Krieger, J., Ifoundza, T., Oswald, M., & Kessler, R. (1995). Association of chronic obstructive pulmonary disease and sleep apnea syndrome. *Am.J.Respir.Crit Care Med., 151,* 82-86.

Cheng, N., Cai, W., Jiang, M., & Wu, S. (1997). Effect of hypoxia on blood glucose, hormones, and insulin receptor functions in newborn calves. *Pediatr.Res., 41,* 852-856.

Chin, K., Nakamura, T., Shimizu, K., Mishima, M., Nakamura, T., Miyasaka, M. et al. (2000). Effects of nasal continuous positive airway pressure on soluble cell adhesion molecules in patients with obstructive sleep apnea syndrome. *Am.J.Med., 109,* 562-567.

Choi, K. M., Lee, J. S., Park, H. S., Baik, S. H., Choi, D. S., & Kim, S. M. (2008). Relationship between sleep duration and the metabolic syndrome: Korean National Health and Nutrition Survey 2001. *Int.J.Obes.(Lond), 32,* 1091-1097.

Cuhadaroglu, C., Utkusavas, A., Ozturk, L., Salman, S., & Ece, T. (2009). Effects of nasal CPAP treatment on insulin resistance, lipid profile, and plasma leptin in sleep apnea. *Lung, 187,* 75-81.

De Lima, A. M., Franco, C. M., de Castro, C. M., Bezerra, A. A., Ataide, L., Jr., & Halpern, A. (2010). Effects of nasal continuous positive airway pressure treatment on oxidative stress and adiponectin levels in obese patients with obstructive sleep apnea. *Respiration, 79,* 370-376.

Delporte, M. L., Funahashi, T., Takahashi, M., Matsuzawa, Y., & Brichard, S. M. (2002). Pre- and post-translational negative effect of beta-adrenoceptor agonists on adiponectin secretion: in vitro and in vivo studies. *Biochem.J., 367,* 677-685.

Devouassoux, G., Levy, P., Rossini, E., Pin, I., Fior-Gozlan, M., Henry, M. et al. (2007). Sleep apnea is associated with bronchial inflammation and continuous positive airway pressure-induced airway hyperresponsiveness. *J.Allergy. Clin.Immunol., 119,* 597-603.

Drager, L. F., Queiroz, E. L., Lopes, H. F., Genta, P. R., Krieger, E. M., & Lorenzi-Filho, G. (2009). Obstructive sleep apnea is highly prevalent and correlates with impaired glycemic control in consecutive patients with the metabolic syndrome. *J.Cardiometab.Syndr., 4,* 89-95.

Duran-Cantolla, J., Aizpuru, F., Montserrat, J. M., Ballester, E., Teran-Santos, J., Aguirregomoscorta, J. I. et al. (2010). Continuous positive airway pressure as treatment for systemic hypertension in people with obstructive sleep apnoea: randomised controlled trial. *BMJ, 341,* c5991.

Dyugovskaya, L., Lavie, P., & Lavie, L. (2002). Increased adhesion molecules expression and production of reactive oxygen species in leukocytes of sleep apnea patients. *Am.J.Respir.Crit Care Med., 165,* 934-939.

Dyugovskaya, L., Polyakov, A., Lavie, P., & Lavie, L. (2008). Delayed neutrophil apoptosis in patients with sleep apnea. *Am.J.Respir.Crit Care Med., 177,* 544-554.

El-Solh, A. A., Mador, M. J., Sikka, P., Dhillon, R. S., Amsterdam, D., & Grant, B. J. (2002). Adhesion molecules in patients with coronary artery disease and moderate-to-severe obstructive sleep apnea. *Chest, 121,* 1541-1547.

Fasshauer, M., Kralisch, S., Klier, M., Lossner, U., Bluher, M., Klein, J. et al. (2003). Adiponectin gene expression and secretion is inhibited by interleukin-6 in 3T3-L1 adipocytes. *Biochem.Biophys.Res.Commun., 301,* 1045-1050.

Fava, C., Montagnana, M., Favaloro, E. J., Guidi, G. C., & Lippi, G. (2011). Obstructive sleep apnea syndrome and cardiovascular diseases. *Semin.Thromb.Hemost., 37,* 280-297.

Fletcher, E. C., Bao, G., & Li, R. (1999). Renin activity and blood pressure in response to chronic episodic hypoxia. *Hypertension, 34,* 309-314.

Foster, G. E., Poulin, M. J., & Hanly, P. J. (2007). Intermittent hypoxia and vascular function: implications for obstructive sleep apnoea. *Exp.Physiol, 92,* 51-65.

Gasparyan, A. Y., Ayvazyan, L., Mikhailidis, D. P., & Kitas, G. D. (2011). Mean platelet volume: a link between thrombosis and inflammation? *Curr.Pharm.Des, 17,* 47-58.

Gastaut, H., Tassinari, C. A., & Duron, B. (1965). [Polygraphic study of diurnal and nocturnal (hypnic and respiratory) episodal manifestations of Pickwick syndrome]. *Rev.Neurol.(Paris), 112,* 568-579.

Giannotti, G. & Landmesser, U. (2007). Endothelial dysfunction as an early sign of atherosclerosis. *Herz, 32,* 568-572.

Gjorup, P. H., Sadauskiene, L., Wessels, J., Nyvad, O., Strunge, B., & Pedersen, E. B. (2007). Abnormally increased endothelin-1 in plasma during the night in obstructive sleep apnea: relation to blood pressure and severity of disease. *Am.J.Hypertens., 20,* 44-52.

Gozal, D., Serpero, L. D., Kheirandish-Gozal, L., Capdevila, O. S., Khalyfa, A., & Tauman, R. (2010). Sleep measures and morning plasma TNF-alpha levels in children with sleep-disordered breathing. *Sleep, 33,* 319-325.

Grebe, M., Eisele, H. J., Weissmann, N., Schaefer, C., Tillmanns, H., Seeger, W. et al. (2006). Antioxidant vitamin C improves endothelial function in obstructive sleep apnea. *Am.J.Respir.Crit Care Med., 173,* 897-901.

Grimpen, F., Kanne, P., Schulz, E., Hagenah, G., Hasenfuss, G., & Andreas, S. (2000). Endothelin-1 plasma levels are not elevated in patients with obstructive sleep apnoea. *Eur.Respir.J., 15,* 320-325.

Gude, F., Rey-Garcia, J., Fernandez-Merino, C., Meijide, L., Garcia-Ortiz, L., Zamarron, C. et al. (2009). Serum levels of gamma-glutamyl transferase are associated with markers of nocturnal hypoxemia in a general adult population. *Clin.Chim.Acta.* 407,67-71

Guzik, T. J., Hoch, N. E., Brown, K. A., McCann, L. A., Rahman, A., Dikalov, S. et al. (2007). Role of the T cell in the genesis of angiotensin II induced hypertension and vascular dysfunction. *J.Exp.Med., 204,* 2449-2460.

Haight, J. S. & Djupesland, P. G. (2003). Nitric oxide (NO) and obstructive sleep apnea (OSA). *Sleep Breath., 7,* 53-62.

Halcox, J. P., Donald, A. E., Ellins, E., Witte, D. R., Shipley, M. J., Brunner, E. J. et al. (2009). Endothelial function predicts progression of carotid intima-media thickness. *Circulation, 119,* 1005-1012.

Hansson, G. K. (2005). Inflammation, atherosclerosis, and coronary artery disease. *N.Engl.J.Med., 352,* 1685-1695.

Harsch, I. A., Koebnick, C., Wallaschofski, H., Schahin, S. P., Hahn, E. G., Ficker, J. H. et al. (2004). Resistin levels in patients with obstructive sleep apnoea syndrome--the link to subclinical inflammation? *Med.Sci.Monit., 10,* CR510-CR515.

Harsch, I. A., Konturek, P. C., Koebnick, C., Kuehnlein, P. P., Fuchs, F. S., Pour, S. S. et al. (2003). Leptin and ghrelin levels in patients with obstructive sleep apnoea: effect of CPAP treatment. *Eur.Respir.J., 22,* 251-257.

Hayashi, M., Fujimoto, K., Urushibata, K., Takamizawa, A., Kinoshita, O., & Kubo, K. (2006). Hypoxia-sensitive molecules may modulate the development of atherosclerosis in sleep apnoea syndrome. *Respirology., 11,* 24-31.

Hoekema, A., Stel, A. L., Stegenga, B., van der Hoeven, J. H., Wijkstra, P. J., van Driel, M. F. et al. (2006). Sexual Function and Obstructive Sleep Apnea-Hypopnea: A Randomized Clinical Trial Evaluating the Effects of Oral-Appliance and Continuous Positive Airway Pressure Therapy. *J.Sex Med.,* 4 Pt 2):1153-62

Imagawa, S., Yamaguchi, Y., Ogawa, K., Obara, N., Suzuki, N., Yamamoto, M. et al. (2004). Interleukin-6 and tumor necrosis factor-alpha in patients with obstructive sleep apnea-hypopnea syndrome. *Respiration, 71,* 24-29.

Ip, M. S., Lam, K. S., Ho, C., Tsang, K. W., & Lam, W. (2000). Serum leptin and vascular risk factors in obstructive sleep apnea. *Chest, 118,* 580-586.

Ip, M. S., Tse, H. F., Lam, B., Tsang, K. W., & Lam, W. K. (2004). Endothelial function in obstructive sleep apnea and response to treatment. *Am.J.Respir.Crit. Care. Med., 169,* 348-353.

Isono, S. (2009). Obstructive sleep apnea of obese adults: pathophysiology and perioperative airway management. *Anesthesiology, 110,* 908-921.

Jelic, S., Lederer, D. J., Adams, T., Padeletti, M., Colombo, P. C., Factor, P. H. et al. (2010). Vascular inflammation in obesity and sleep apnea. *Circulation, 121,* 1014-1021.

Kanagy, N. L., Walker, B. R., & Nelin, L. D. (2001). Role of endothelin in intermittent hypoxia-induced hypertension. *Hypertension, 37,* 511-515.

Kapsimalis, F., Varouchakis, G., Manousaki, A., Daskas, S., Nikita, D., Kryger, M. et al. (2008). Association of sleep apnea severity and obesity with insulin resistance, C-reactive protein, and leptin levels in male patients with obstructive sleep apnea. *Lung, 186,* 209-217.

Kasai, T., Inoue, K., Kumagai, T., Kato, M., Kawana, F., Sagara, M. et al. (2011). Plasma pentraxin3 and arterial stiffness in men with obstructive sleep apnea. *Am.J.Hypertens., 24,* 401-407.

Kent, B. D., Ryan, S., & McNicholas, W. T. (2011). Obstructive sleep apnea and inflammation: Relationship to cardiovascular co-morbidity. *Respir.Physiol Neurobiol.,* 178,475-81.

Kohler, M., Pepperell, J. C., Casadei, B., Craig, S., Crosthwaite, N., Stradling, J. R. et al. (2008). CPAP and measures of cardiovascular risk in males with OSAS. *Eur.Respir.J., 32,* 1488-1496.

Kuramoto, E., Kinami, S., Ishida, Y., Shiotani, H., & Nishimura, Y. (2009). Continuous positive nasal airway pressure decreases levels of serum amyloid A and improves autonomic function in obstructive sleep apnea syndrome. *Int.J.Cardiol., 135,* 338-345.

Lacedonia, D., Salerno, F. G., Carpagnano, G. E., Sabato, R., Depalo, A., & Foschino-Barbaro, M. P. (2011). Effect of CPAP-therapy on bronchial and nasal inflammation in patients affected by obstructive sleep apnea syndrome. *Rhinology, 49,* 232-237.

Lattimore, J. D., Wilcox, I., Nakhla, S., Langenfeld, M., Jessup, W., & Celermajer, D. S. (2005). Repetitive hypoxia increases lipid loading in human macrophages-a potentially atherogenic effect. *Atherosclerosis, 179,* 255-259.

Lavie, L., Vishnevsky, A., & Lavie, P. (2004). Evidence for lipid peroxidation in obstructive sleep apnea. *Sleep, 27,* 123-128.

Levy, P., Pepin, J. L., Arnaud, C., Baguet, J. P., Dematteis, M., & Mach, F. (2009). Obstructive sleep apnea and atherosclerosis. *Prog.Cardiovasc.Dis., 51,* 400-410.

Li, A. M., Ng, C., Ng, S. K., Chan, M. M., So, H. K., Chan, I. et al. (2010). Adipokines in children with obstructive sleep apnea and the effects of treatment. *Chest, 137,* 529-535.

Li, J., Bosch-Marce, M., Nanayakkara, A., Savransky, V., Fried, S. K., Semenza, G. L. et al. (2006). Altered metabolic responses to intermittent hypoxia in mice with partial deficiency of hypoxia-inducible factor-1alpha. *Physiol. Genomics, 25,* 450-457.

Li, J., Thorne, L. N., Punjabi, N. M., Sun, C. K., Schwartz, A. R., Smith, P. L. et al. (2005). Intermittent hypoxia induces hyperlipidemia in lean mice. *Circ.Res., 97,* 698-706.

Luboshitzky, R., Lavie, L., Shen-Orr, Z., & Herer, P. (2005). Altered luteinizing hormone and testosterone secretion in middle-aged obese men with obstructive sleep apnea. *Obes.Res., 13,* 780-786.

Macrea, M. M., Martin, T. J., & Zagrean, L. (2010). Infertility and obstructive sleep apnea: the effect of continuous positive airway pressure therapy on serum prolactin levels. *Sleep Breath., 14,* 253-257.

Makino, S., Handa, H., Suzukawa, K., Fujiwara, M., Nakamura, M., Muraoka, S. et al. (2006). Obstructive sleep apnoea syndrome, plasma adiponectin levels, and insulin resistance. *Clin.Endocrinol.(Oxf), 64,* 12-19.

Makinodan, K., Yoshikawa, M., Fukuoka, A., Tamaki, S., Koyama, N., Yamauchi, M. et al. (2008). Effect of serum leptin levels on hypercapnic ventilatory response in obstructive sleep apnea. *Respiration, 75,* 257-264.

Malakasioti, G., Alexopoulos, E., Befani, C., Tanou, K., Varlami, V., Ziogas, D. et al. (2011). Oxidative stress and inflammatory markers in the exhaled breath condensate of children with OSA. *Sleep Breath.*.

Marin, J. M., Carrizo, S. J., Vicente, E., & Agusti, A. G. (2005). Long-term cardiovascular outcomes in men with obstructive sleep apnoea-hypopnoea with or without treatment with continuous positive airway pressure: an observational study. *Lancet, 365,* 1046-1053.

Marrone, O., Salvaggio, A., Bue, A. L., Bonanno, A., Riccobono, L., Insalaco, G. et al. (2011). Blood Pressure Changes After Automatic and Fixed CPAP in Obstructive Sleep Apnea: Relationship with Nocturnal Sympathetic Activity. *Clin.Exp.Hypertens.,* 33,373-80.

Marrone, O., Salvaggio, A., Gioia, M., Bonanno, A., Profita, M., Riccobono, L. et al. (2008). Reticulocytes in untreated obstructive sleep apnoea. *Monaldi Arch.Chest, Dis., 69,* 107-113.

Maser, R. E., Lenhard, M. J., Rizzo, A. A., & Vasile, A. A. (2008). Continuous positive airway pressure therapy improves cardiovascular autonomic function for persons with sleep-disordered breathing. *Chest, 133,* 86-91.

Masserini, B., Morpurgo, P. S., Donadio, F., Baldessari, C., Bossi, R., Beck-Peccoz, P. et al. (2006). Reduced levels of adiponectin in sleep apnea syndrome. *J.Endocrinol.Invest, 29,* 700-705.

McArdle, N., Hillman, D., Beilin, L., & Watts, G. (2007). Metabolic risk factors for vascular disease in obstructive sleep apnea: a matched controlled study. *Am.J.Respir.Crit. Care. Med., 175,* 190-195.

Meisinger, C., Heier, M., & Loewel, H. (2005). Sleep disturbance as a predictor of type 2 diabetes mellitus in men and women from the general population. *Diabetologia, 48,* 235-241.

Meston, N., Davies, R. J., Mullins, R., Jenkinson, C., Wass, J. A., & Stradling, J. R. (2003). Endocrine effects of nasal continuous positive airway pressure in male patients with obstructive sleep apnoea. *J.Intern.Med., 254,* 447-454.

Moller, D. S., Lind, P., Strunge, B., & Pedersen, E. B. (2003). Abnormal vasoactive hormones and 24-hour blood pressure in obstructive sleep apnea. *Am.J.Hypertens., 16,* 274-280.

Mullington, J. M., Simpson, N. S., Meier-Ewert, H. K., & Haack, M. (2010). Sleep loss and inflammation. *Best.Pract.Res.Clin.Endocrinol.Metab, 24,* 775-784.

Nair, D., Dayyat, E. A., Zhang, S. X., Wang, Y., & Gozal, D. (2011). Intermittent hypoxia-induced cognitive deficits are mediated by NADPH oxidase activity in a murine model of sleep apnea. *PLoS.One., 6,* e19847.

Nakagawa, Y., Kishida, K., Kihara, S., Yoshida, R., Funahashi, T., & Shimomura, I. (2011). Nocturnal falls of adiponectin levels in sleep apnea with abdominal obesity and impact of hypoxia-induced dysregulated adiponectin production in obese murine mesenteric adipose tissue. *J.Atheroscler.Thromb., 18,* 240-247.

Nestel, P. (2003). Metabolic syndrome: multiple candidate genes, multiple environmental factors--multiple syndromes? *Int.J.Clin.Pract.Suppl*, 3-9.

Newman, A. B., Nieto, F. J., Guidry, U., Lind, B. K., Redline, S., Pickering, T. G. et al. (2001). Relation of sleep-disordered breathing to cardiovascular disease risk factors: the Sleep Heart Health Study. *Am.J.Epidemiol., 154*, 50-59.

Nieto, F. J., Herrington, D. M., Redline, S., Benjamin, E. J., & Robbins, J. A. (2004). Sleep apnea and markers of vascular endothelial function in a large community sample of older adults. *Am.J.Respir.Crit Care Med., 169*, 354-360.

O'Donnell, C. P., Tankersley, C. G., Polotsky, V. P., Schwartz, A. R., & Smith, P. L. (2000). Leptin, obesity, and respiratory function. *Respir.Physiol, 119*, 163-170.

Oga, T., Chin, K., Tabuchi, A., Kawato, M., Morimoto, T., Takahashi, K. et al. (2009). Effects of obstructive sleep apnea with intermittent hypoxia on platelet aggregability. *J.Atheroscler.Thromb., 16*, 862-869.

Ohga, E., Nagase, T., Tomita, T., Teramoto, S., Matsuse, T., Katayama, H. et al. (1999). Increased levels of circulating ICAM-1, VCAM-1, and L-selectin in obstructive sleep apnea syndrome. *J.Appl.Physiol, 87*, 10-14.

Ohga, E., Tomita, T., Wada, H., Yamamoto, H., Nagase, T., & Ouchi, Y. (2003). Effects of obstructive sleep apnea on circulating ICAM-1, IL-8, and MCP-1. *J.Appl.Physiol, 94*, 179-184.

Oldenburg, O., Lamp, B., Faber, L., Teschler, H., Horstkotte, D., & Topfer, V. (2007). Sleep-disordered breathing in patients with symptomatic heart failure: a contemporary study of prevalence in and characteristics of 700 patients. *Eur.J.Heart Fail., 9*, 251-257.

Othman, M., Gordon, S. P., & Iscoe, S. (2010). Repeated inspiratory occlusions in anesthetized rats acutely increase blood coagulability as assessed by thromboelastography. *Respir.Physiol, Neurobiol., 171*, 61-66.

Ozturk, L., Unal, M., Tamer, L., & Celikoglu, F. (2003). The association of the severity of obstructive sleep apnea with plasma leptin levels. *Arch.Otolaryngol.Head Neck Surg., 129*, 538-540.

Park, A. M., Nagase, H., Kumar, S. V., & Suzuki, Y. J. (2007). Effects of intermittent hypoxia on the heart. *Antioxid.Redox.Signal., 9*, 723-729.

Patel, S. R., Malhotra, A., White, D. P., Gottlieb, D. J., & Hu, F. B. (2006). Association between reduced sleep and weight gain in women. *Am.J.Epidemiol., 164*, 947-954.

Patel, S. R., Palmer, L. J., Larkin, E. K., Jenny, N. S., White, D. P., & Redline, S. (2004). Relationship between obstructive sleep apnea and diurnal leptin rhythms. *Sleep, 27*, 235-239.

Patel, S. R., Zhu, X., Storfer-Isser, A., Mehra, R., Jenny, N. S., Tracy, R. et al. (2009). Sleep duration and biomarkers of inflammation. *Sleep, 32*, 200-204.

Patt, B. T., Jarjoura, D., Haddad, D. N., Sen, C. K., Roy, S., Flavahan, N. A. et al. (2010). Endothelial dysfunction in the microcirculation of patients with obstructive sleep apnea. *Am.J.Respir.Crit. Care. Med., 182*, 1540-1545.

Peled, N., Kassirer, M., Kramer, M. R., Rogowski, O., Shlomi, D., Fox, B. et al. (2008). Increased erythrocyte adhesiveness and aggregation in obstructive sleep apnea syndrome. *Thromb.Res., 121*, 631-636.

Phillips, B. G., Kato, M., Narkiewicz, K., Choe, I., & Somers, V. K. (2000). Increases in leptin levels, sympathetic drive, and weight gain in obstructive sleep apnea. *Am.J.Physiol. Heart. Circ.Physiol., 279,* H234-H237.

Phillips, B. G., Narkiewicz, K., Pesek, C. A., Haynes, W. G., Dyken, M. E., & Somers, V. K. (1999). Effects of obstructive sleep apnea on endothelin-1 and blood pressure. *J.Hypertens., 17,* 61-66.

Phipps, P. R., Starritt, E., Caterson, I., & Grunstein, R. R. (2002). Association of serum leptin with hypoventilation in human obesity. *Thorax, 57,* 75-76.

Pichel, F., Zamarron, C., Magan, F., del, C. F., Alvarez-Sala, R., & Suarez, J. R. (2004). Health-related quality of life in patients with obstructive sleep apnea: effects of long-term positive airway pressure treatment. *Respir.Med., 98,* 968-976.

Piemonti, L., Calori, G., Mercalli, A., Lattuada, G., Monti, P., Garancini, M. P. et al. (2003). Fasting plasma leptin, tumor necrosis factor-alpha receptor 2, and monocyte chemoattracting protein 1 concentration in a population of glucose-tolerant and glucose-intolerant women: impact on cardiovascular mortality. *Diabetes Care, 26,* 2883-2889.

Pohl, U. & Busse, R. (1989). Differential vascular sensitivity to luminally and adventitially applied endothelin-1. *J.Cardiovasc.Pharmacol., 13 Suppl 5,* S188-S190.

Polotsky, V. Y., Li, J., Punjabi, N. M., Rubin, A. E., Smith, P. L., Schwartz, A. R. et al. (2003). Intermittent hypoxia increases insulin resistance in genetically obese mice. *J.Physiol, 552,* 253-264.

Prabhakar, N. R., Fields, R. D., Baker, T., & Fletcher, E. C. (2001). Intermittent hypoxia: cell to system. *Am.J.Physiol. Lung. Cell. Mol.Physiol., 281,* L524-L528.

Prentice, A. M. (2006). The emerging epidemic of obesity in developing countries. *Int.J.Epidemiol., 35,* 93-99.

Proulx, K., Richard, D., & Walker, C. D. (2002). Leptin regulates appetite-related neuropeptides in the hypothalamus of developing rats without affecting food intake. *Endocrinology, 143,* 4683-4692.

Punjabi, N. M. & Beamer, B. A. (2007). C-reactive protein is associated with sleep disordered breathing independent of adiposity. *Sleep, 30,* 29-34.

Querido, J. S., Sheel, A. W., Cheema, R., Van, E. S., Mulgrew, A. T., & Ayas, N. T. (2011). Effects of 10 days of modest intermittent hypoxia on circulating measures of inflammation in healthy humans. *Sleep Breath.* Jul 9. [Epub ahead of print]

Quercioli, A., Mach, F., & Montecucco, F. (2010). Inflammation accelerates atherosclerotic processes in obstructive sleep apnea syndrome (OSAS). *Sleep Breath., 14,* 261-269.

Rahangdale, S., Yeh S.Y., Novack, V., Stevenson, K., Barnard M,R., Furman M,I., et al. (2011). The influence of intermittent hypoxemia on platelet activation in obese patients with obstructive sleep apnea. J Clin Sleep Med., 15;7,172-8

Reaven, G. M. (2005). Insulin resistance, the insulin resistance syndrome, and cardiovascular disease. *Panminerva Med., 47,* 201-210.

Reinhart, W. H., Oswald, J., Walter, R., & Kuhn, M. (2002). Blood viscosity and platelet function in patients with obstructive sleep apnea syndrome treated with nasal continuous positive airway pressure. *Clin.Hemorheol.Microcirc., 27,* 201-207.

Remmers, J. E., deGroot, W. J., Sauerland, E. K., & Anch, A. M. (1978). Pathogenesis of upper airway occlusion during sleep. *J.Appl.Physiol, 44,* 931-938.

Resnick, H. E., Jones, K., Ruotolo, G., Jain, A. K., Henderson, J., Lu, W. et al. (2003). Insulin resistance, the metabolic syndrome, and risk of incident cardiovascular disease in nondiabetic american indians: the Strong Heart Study. *Diabetes Care, 26,* 861-867.

Resta, O., Bonfitto, P., Sabato, R., De, P. G., & Barbaro, M. P. (2004). Prevalence of obstructive sleep apnoea in a sample of obese women: effect of menopause. *Diabetes Nutr.Metab., 17,* 296-303.

Ronti, T., Lupattelli, G., & Mannarino, E. (2006). The endocrine function of adipose tissue: an update. *Clin.Endocrinol.(Oxf), 64,* 355-365.

Ross, R. (1999). Atherosclerosis--an inflammatory disease. *N.Engl.J.Med., 340,* 115-126.

Rossi, G. P. & Pitter, G. (2006). Genetic variation in the endothelin system: do polymorphisms affect the therapeutic strategies? *Ann.N.Y.Acad.Sci., 1069,* 34-50.

Ryan, S., Taylor, C. T., & McNicholas, W. T. (2005). Selective activation of inflammatory pathways by intermittent hypoxia in obstructive sleep apnea syndrome. *Circulation, 112,* 2660-2667.

Saarelainen, S. & Hasan, J. (2000). Circulating endothelin-1 and obstructive sleep apnoea. *Eur.Respir.J., 16,* 794-795.

Sanner, B. M., Kollhosser, P., Buechner, N., Zidek, W., & Tepel, M. (2004). Influence of treatment on leptin levels in patients with obstructive sleep apnoea. *Eur.Respir.J., 23,* 601-604.

Schulz, R., Mahmoudi, S., Hattar, K., Sibelius, U., Olschewski, H., Mayer, K. et al. (2000). Enhanced release of superoxide from polymorphonuclear neutrophils in obstructive sleep apnea. Impact of continuous positive airway pressure therapy. *Am.J.Respir.Crit. Care. Med., 162,* 566-570.

Schwartz, A. R., Patil, S. P., Laffan, A. M., Polotsky, V., Schneider, H., & Smith, P. L. (2008). Obesity and obstructive sleep apnea: pathogenic mechanisms and therapeutic approaches. *Proc.Am.Thorac.Soc., 5,* 185-192.

Shahar, E., Redline, S., Young, T., Boland, L. L., Baldwin, C. M., Nieto, F. J. et al. (2003). Hormone replacement therapy and sleep-disordered breathing. *Am.J.Respir.Crit. Care. Med., 167,* 1186-1192.

Shimizu, K., Chin, K., Nakamura, T., Masuzaki, H., Ogawa, Y., Hosokawa, R. et al. (2002). Plasma leptin levels and cardiac sympathetic function in patients with obstructive sleep apnoea-hypopnoea syndrome. *Thorax, 57,* 429-434.

Shimura, R., Tatsumi, K., Nakamura, A., Kasahara, Y., Tanabe, N., Takiguchi, Y. et al. (2005). Fat accumulation, leptin, and hypercapnia in obstructive sleep apnea-hypopnea syndrome. *Chest, 127,* 543-549.

Shinohara, E., Kihara, S., Yamashita, S., Yamane, M., Nishida, M., Arai, T. et al. (1997). Visceral fat accumulation as an important risk factor for obstructive sleep apnoea syndrome in obese subjects. *J.Intern.Med., 241,* 11-18.

Shitrit, D., Peled, N., Shitrit, A. B., Meidan, S., Bendayan, D., Sahar, G. et al. (2005). An association between oxygen desaturation and D-dimer in patients with obstructive sleep apnea syndrome. *Thromb.Haemost., 94,* 544-547.

Snitker, S., Pratley, R. E., Nicolson, M., Tataranni, P. A., & Ravussin, E. (1997). Relationship between muscle sympathetic nerve activity and plasma leptin concentration. *Obes.Res., 5,* 338-340.

Somers, V. K., Mark, A. L., & Abboud, F. M. (1988). Sympathetic activation by hypoxia and hypercapnia--implications for sleep apnea. *Clin.Exp.Hypertens.A, 10 Suppl 1,* 413-422.

Spruyt, K., Sans, C. O., Serpero, L. D., Kheirandish-Gozal, L., & Gozal, D. (2010). Dietary and physical activity patterns in children with obstructive sleep apnea. *J.Pediatr., 156,* 724-30.

Steiropoulos, P., Kotsianidis, I., Nena, E., Tsara, V., Gounari, E., Hatzizisi, O. et al. (2009). Long-term effect of continuous positive airway pressure therapy on inflammation markers of patients with obstructive sleep apnea syndrome. *Sleep, 32,* 537-543.

Svatikova, A., Wolk, R., Shamsuzzaman, A. S., Kara, T., Olson, E. J., & Somers, V. K. (2003). Serum amyloid a in obstructive sleep apnea. *Circulation, 108,* 1451-1454.

Taheri, S., Austin, D., Lin, L., Nieto, F. J., Young, T., & Mignot, E. (2007). Correlates of serum C-reactive protein (CRP)--no association with sleep duration or sleep disordered breathing. *Sleep, 30,* 991-996.

Tamisier, R., Pepin, J. L., Remy, J., Baguet, J. P., Taylor, J. A., Weiss, J. W. et al. (2011). 14 nights of intermittent hypoxia elevate daytime blood pressure and sympathetic activity in healthy humans. *Eur.Respir.J., 37,* 119-128.

Tasali, E., Chapotot, F., Leproult, R., Whitmore, H., & Ehrmann, D. A. (2011). Treatment of obstructive sleep apnea improves cardiometabolic function in young obese women with polycystic ovary syndrome. *J.Clin.Endocrinol.Metab, 96,* 365-374.

Tassone, F., Lanfranco, F., Gianotti, L., Pivetti, S., Navone, F., Rossetto, R. et al. (2003). Obstructive sleep apnoea syndrome impairs insulin sensitivity independently of anthropometric variables. *Clin.Endocrinol.(Oxf), 59,* 374-379.

Tatsumi, K., Kasahara, Y., Kurosu, K., Tanabe, N., Takiguchi, Y., & Kuriyama, T. (2005). Sleep oxygen desaturation and circulating leptin in obstructive sleep apnea-hypopnea syndrome. *Chest, 127,* 716-721.

Teloken, P. E., Smith, E. B., Lodowsky, C., Freedom, T., & Mulhall, J. P. (2006). Defining association between sleep apnea syndrome and erectile dysfunction. *Urology, 67,* 1033-1037.

Theorell-Haglow, J., Berne, C., Janson, C., & Lindberg, E. (2011). The role of obstructive sleep apnea in metabolic syndrome: a population-based study in women. *Sleep Med., 12,* 329-334.

Teramoto, S., Kume, H., Yamamoto, H., Ishii, T., Miyashita, A., Matsuse, T. et al. (2003). Effects of oxygen administration on the circulating vascular endothelial growth factor (VEGF) levels in patients with obstructive sleep apnea syndrome. *Intern.Med., 42,* 681-685.

Teran-Santos, J., Jimenez-Gomez, A., & Cordero-Guevara, J. (1999). The association between sleep apnea and the risk of traffic accidents. Cooperative Group Burgos-Santander. *N.Engl.J.Med., 340,* 847-851.

Tkacova, R., Dorkova, Z., Molcanyiova, A., Radikova, Z., Klimes, I., & Tkac, I. (2008). Cardiovascular risk and insulin resistance in patients with obstructive sleep apnea. *Med.Sci.Monit., 14,* CR438-CR444.

Tokuda, F., Sando, Y., Matsui, H., Koike, H., & Yokoyama, T. (2008). Serum levels of adipocytokines, adiponectin and leptin, in patients with obstructive sleep apnea syndrome. *Intern.Med., 47,* 1843-1849.

Trzepizur, W., Gagnadoux, F., Abraham, P., Rousseau, P., Meslier, N., Saumet, J. L. et al. (2009). Microvascular endothelial function in obstructive sleep apnea: Impact of continuous positive airway pressure and mandibular advancement. *Sleep Med., 10,* 746-752.

Tsaoussoglou, M., Bixler, E. O., Calhoun, S., Chrousos, G. P., Sauder, K., & Vgontzas, A. N. (2010). Sleep-disordered breathing in obese children is associated with prevalent excessive daytime sleepiness, inflammation, and metabolic abnormalities. *J.Clin.Endocrinol.Metab, 95,* 143-150.

Ulukavak, C. T., Kokturk, O., Bukan, N., & Bilgihan, A. (2005). Leptin and ghrelin levels in patients with obstructive sleep apnea syndrome. *Respiration, 72,* 395-401.

Varol, E., Ozturk, O., Yucel, H., Gonca, T., Has, M., Dogan, A. et al. (2011). The effects of continuous positive airway pressure therapy on mean platelet volume in patients with obstructive sleep apnea. *Platelets. 22, 552-6*

Vatansever, E., Surmen-Gur, E., Ursavas, A., & Karadag, M. (2010). Obstructive sleep apnea causes oxidative damage to plasma lipids and proteins and decreases adiponectin levels. *Sleep Breath.* 15, 275-82

von, K. R. & Dimsdale, J. E. (2003). Hemostatic alterations in patients with obstructive sleep apnea and the implications for cardiovascular disease. *Chest, 124,* 1956-1967.

von, K. R., Loredo, J. S., Ancoli-Israel, S., & Dimsdale, J. E. (2006). Association between sleep apnea severity and blood coagulability: Treatment effects of nasal continuous positive airway pressure. *Sleep Breath., 10,* 139-146.

von, K. R., Loredo, J. S., Ancoli-Israel, S., Mills, P. J., Natarajan, L., & Dimsdale, J. E. (2007). Association between polysomnographic measures of disrupted sleep and prothrombotic factors. *Chest, 131,* 733-739.

von, K. R., Loredo, J. S., Powell, F. L., Adler, K. A., & Dimsdale, J. E. (2005). Short-term isocapnic hypoxia and coagulation activation in patients with sleep apnea. *Clin.Hemorheol.Microcirc., 33,* 369-377.

Wesstrom, J., Ulfberg, J., & Nilsson, S. (2005). Sleep apnea and hormone replacement therapy: a pilot study and a literature review. *Acta Obstet.Gynecol.Scand., 84,* 54-57.

Wilcox, I., McNamara, S. G., Collins, F. L., Grunstein, R. R., & Sullivan, C. E. (1998). "Syndrome Z": the interaction of sleep apnoea, vascular risk factors and heart disease. *Thorax, 53 Suppl 3,* S25-S28.

Wysocka, E., Cofta, S., Cymerys, M., Gozdzik, J., Torlinski, L., & Batura-Gabryel, H. (2008). The impact of the sleep apnea syndrome on oxidant-antioxidant balance in the blood of overweight and obese patients. *J.Physiol Pharmacol., 59 Suppl 6,* 761-769.

Wysocka, E., Cofta, S., Dziegielewska, S., Gozdzik, J., Torlinski, L., & Batura-Gabryel, H. (2009). Adipocytokines in sleep apnea syndrome. *Eur.J.Med.Res., 14 Suppl 4,* 255-258.

Yamamoto, Y., Fujiuchi, S., Hiramatsu, M., Nishigaki, Y., Takeda, A., Fujita, Y. et al. (2008). Resistin is closely related to systemic inflammation in obstructive sleep apnea. *Respiration, 76,* 377-385.

Yokoe, T., Minoguchi, K., Matsuo, H., Oda, N., Minoguchi, H., Yoshino, G. et al. (2003). Elevated levels of C-reactive protein and interleukin-6 in patients with obstructive sleep apnea syndrome are decreased by nasal continuous positive airway pressure. *Circulation, 107,* 1129-1134.

Young, T., Palta, M., Dempsey, J., Skatrud, J., Weber, S., & Badr, S. (1993). The occurrence of sleep-disordered breathing among middle-aged adults. *N.Engl.J.Med., 328,* 1230-1235.

Yu, H. J., Lin, B. R., Lee, H. S., Shun, C. T., Yang, C. C., Lai, T. Y. et al. (2005). Sympathetic vesicovascular reflex induced by acute urinary retention evokes proinflammatory and proapoptotic injury in rat liver. *Am.J.Physiol Renal Physiol, 288,* F1005-F1014.

Zamarron, C., Garcia, P., V, & Riveiro, A. (2008a). Obstructive sleep apnea syndrome is a systemic disease. Current evidence. *Eur.J.Intern.Med., 19,* 390-398.

Zamarron, C., Ricoy, J., Riveiro, A., & Gude, F. (2008b). Plasminogen activator inhibitor-1 in obstructive sleep apnea patients with and without hypertension. *Lung, 186,* 151-156.

Zamarron-Sanz, C., Ricoy-Galbaldon, J., Gude-Sampedro, F., & Riveiro-Riveiro, A. (2006). Plasma levels of vascular endothelial markers in obstructive sleep apnea. *Arch.Med.Res., 37,* 552-555.

Zhang, X. L., Yin, K. S., Wang, H., & Su, S. (2006). Serum adiponectin levels in adult male patients with obstructive sleep apnea hypopnea syndrome. *Respiration, 73,* 73-77.

Zouaoui, B. K., Guillaume, M., Henuzet, C., Delree, P., Cauchie, P., Remacle, C. et al. (2006). Fibrinolysis and cardiovascular risk factors: association with fibrinogen, lipids, and monocyte count. *Eur.J.Intern.Med., 17,* 102-108.

19

New Cardiovascular Risk Factors and Physical Activity

Nicolás Terrados[1,2] and Eduardo Iglesias-Gutiérrez[2]
[1]*Regional Sports Medicine Unit of the Principality of Asturias, Avilés,*
[2]*Department of Functional Biology,*
The University of Oviedo, Asturias,
Spain

1. Introduction

A cardiovascular risk factor (CRF) is a biological characteristic or behaviour that increases the possibility of cardiovascular disease (CVD) (1). The concept of risk factors first appeared some fifty years ago with the publication of the Framingham Study (2). Since that time, advances in the field of epidemiology have made large scale clinical studies possible and have led to the identification of a series of cardiovascular disease risk factors that induce the formation of atheromatous plaques. The establishment of a specific biological characteristic, environmental factor or habit as a CRF requires: a standardised methodology; concordant prospective studies; an added effect when various risk factors concur in an individual; and, that the modification of the factor (in the case that the factor is modifiable) results in a diminution of the risk (3).

Historically, there has been clear evidence of a series of 'traditional' CRFs (Table 1), such as hypercholesterolemia, hypertension, hyperglycaemia, nicotine poisoning, sedentarism, etc. which have been used in the stratification of individual risk (4). In the recent past, a number of important studies have proposed the inclusion of new or 'emergent' CRFs in the evaluation and stratification of cardiovascular risk and this has implications for preventive and therapeutic strategies.

Numerous documents and reports that include recommendations for the prevention of CVD and control of the main cardiovascular risk factors have been published by national and international scientific institutions and organisations (from the USA, Europe (5) etc.). Following the latest recommendations of the world renowned National Cholesterol Education Program (NCEP) (4), Table 1 lists the most significant 'traditional' CRFs whilst Table 2 shows the 'emergent' factors. Some of the 'new' factors have been recognised for decades though they have been subject to debate and controversy, and consensus has not been reached on their inclusion in cardiovascular risk evaluation.

The NCEP Panel III identifies three classes of CRFs that influence the possibilities of suffering CVD, although only the first two are relevant to the modification of treatment objectives: major CRFs, factors linked to lifestyles and emergent risk factors.

Age and sex (men ≥ 45 years old, women ≥ 55 years old)
Nicotine poisoning
Arterial hypertension (BP ≥ 140/90 mmHg or undergoing antihypertensive treatment)
Increase LDL cholesterol
Fall in HDL cholesterol (< 40 mg/dl)*
Family history of premature coronary heart disease Male first degree relatives < 55 years Female first degree relatives < 65 years
Diabetes mellitus**
Lifestyle (overweight/obesity, sedentarism, atherogenic diet)***

* Adapted from Panel III of the National Cholesterol Education Program (4).
*If HDL cholesterol is ≥ 60 mg/dl, it is considered as a 'negative' risk factor".
**Diabetes mellitus carries a risk equivalent to a secondary prevention situation.
***These factors are not computed in the algorithms for stratification of risk.
AP: arterial pressure; LDL: low density lipoproteins; HDL: high density lipoproteins.

Table 1. Major ('traditional') cardiovascular risk factors, (4).

Panel III recognises that, in addition to the main CRFs, CVD is influenced by the presence of other factors which modification can have a positive effect on some of the major CRFs and reduce risk; these therefore represent direct treatment objectives. These factors act through other intermediate elements or worsen independent risk factors such as, obesity, sedentarism, a family history of premature CVD, psychosocial conditions or being male. Although they do not figure in algorithm calculations on the stratification of risk (6), two of them, obesity and sedentarism, are considered as causal CRFs by the American Heart Association.

2. Traditional cardiovascular risk factors

2.1 Lipid risk factors

Hypercholesterolemia is one of the main cardiovascular risk factors that are modifiable. The *Multiple Risk Factor Intervention Trial* demonstrated the existence of a continuous and graded relationship between cholesterolemia and total mortality and mortality due to ischemic heart disease (7).

The three main classes of lipoproteins are: Low-density lipoproteins (LDL); High-density lipoproteins (HDL); and Very low-density lipoproteins (VLDL). There is another class of lipoproteins known as Intermediate-density lipoproteins (IDL) that is between VLDL and LDL, though in clinical practice, it is included in the LDL category.

With the exception of HDLs, that play a role in reverse cholesterol transport and therefore exercise a vasoprotector action, lipid particles are more atherogenic the more cholesterol that they transport. Chylomicrons carry such a small quantity of cholesterol that their increase in hyperchylomicronemia (Type I dyslipidemia) is not associated with atherosclerosis lesions. In contrast, with the accumulation of VLDLs, a fifth of which are made up of cholesterol, an increase in atherogenesis is observed. Given that LDLs are particles with a higher level of cholesterol, they are the main cause of atherogenesis when they are in excess.

Although LDLs receive most attention in clinical management, there is a growing body of evidence that indicates that VLDLs play an important role in atherogenesis.

Levels of HDL cholesterol are inversely related with the risk of CVD; they seem to play a protective role against the onset of atherosclerosis as they capture free cholesterol from the peripheric tissues such as the cells of the vascular wall. This cholesterol is transformed into cholesterol esters, a part of which is transferred to the VLDLs by the cholesterol esters transfer proteins (CETP) and returned to the liver by IDLs and LDLs and another part is transferred directly to the liver by the HDL particles. The liver reuses the cholesterol for the synthesis of VLDLs, for the synthesis of bile salts or excretes it directly into the bile. Therefore, HDLs tend to reduce cholesterol levels.

2.2 Non-lipid risk factors

Hypertension

Hypertension is a principal and independent CRF, but its damaging effect is increased when associated with other coronary risk factors such as smoking, diabetes and dyslipidemia. The Sixth Report of the Joint National Committee on Prevention, Detection, Evaluation, and Treatment of High Blood Pressure defines hypertension as a systolic arterial pressure of ≥140mmHg or diastolic ≥90mmHg or the need for antihypertensive treatment (8). A number of studies, for example the Framingham study, have demonstrated an increase in total mortality and cardiovascular risk in cases of increased levels of arterial pressure (diastolic and systolic), with a continuous and gradual relationship (9,10,11). The association applies to men and women, young and old alike.

Smoking

Smoking contributes clearly to CVD. The relationship between smoking and the risk of CVD is dose dependent and affects men and women equally. Observational studies suggest that stopping smoking leads to a substantial reduction of the risk of a cardiovascular event.

Diabetes

Diabetes is defined as the presence of a level of glucose, on an empty stomach, more than, or equal to, 126 mg/dL (12). The risk of cardiovascular disease is significantly increased for sufferers of diabetes mellitus type 1 and type 2 (13). The increase of risk attributed to hyperglycaemia is independent of other risk factors such as obesity, overweight or dyslipidemia that are often observed in diabetics.

80% of diabetes mellitus patient mortality is caused by complications associated with atherosclerosis with ischemic heart disease being responsible in 75% of cases (14). In addition, the risk of acute myocardial infarction in diabetes mellitus type 2 patients with no previous history of myocardial infarction is similar to non-diabetics who have previously suffered a heart attack (15).

Although it is probable that strict control of diabetes reduces micro-vascular disorders and other complications such as renal disease and retinopathies, statistics relative to the effects of glycemic control on coronary episodes are uncertain. Diabetics often present dyslipidemia, characterised by moderate hypercholesterolemia and hypertriglyceridemia with low concentrations of HDL cholesterol that involve increased cardiovascular risk. This is frequently associated with central obesity, hyperinsulinism and AHT. Therefore, the association of numerous CRFs explains why many individuals already exhibit disorders when they are diagnosed with diabetes mellitus.

3. Emergent cardiovascular risk factors

Traditional factors can strongly predict the risk of cardiovascular disease but not completely (16). Thus, recently new biomarkers have emerged, although their predictive value still needs to be validated in multiple cohorts and different populations.

Lipid Risk Factors	
	Total cholesterol quotient/HDL cholesterol
	Apolipoproteins
	HDL subclasses
	Triglycerides
	"Small and dense" LDL particles
	Residual or remnant lipoproteins
Non-lipid Risk Factors	
	Markers of inflammation
	Homocysteinaemia
	Impaired fasting glycaemia
	Thrombogenic / hemostatic factors

LDL: Low-density lipoproteins; HDL: High-density lipoproteins

Table 2. Emergent cardiovascular risk factors

3.1 Apolipoproteins

Apolipoprotein A

A apolipoproteins are a group of proteins that are variably distributed among different lipoproteins. Apo A-I is the most abundant apolipoprotein in plasma and is nearly 90% of the HDL and 60-70% of the protein fraction of the sub-fractions HDL2 and HDL3, respectively. Apo A-I is initially synthesised in the liver and intestine as a protein precursor which is degraded to its mature form in plasma; it is a simple polypeptide chain that contains 243 amino acids. This protein participates in the reverse transport of cholesterol.

The apolipoprotein apo A-II is the second highest concentration protein component of HDL, although it is absent in the HDL2 sub-fraction and plasma levels do not correlate with HDL-cholesterol levels.

The measurement of the concentration of apo A-I in serum perfectly reproduces the predictive value of coronary disease of the concentration of HDL in serum. Nevertheless, this correlation is not valid in subjects with hypertriglyceridemia, in which the fraction of HDL is enriched with triglycerides and cholesterol is almost absent.

Apolipoprotein B

B apolipoprotein is a protein of great molecular weight, present in chylomicrons, VLDL, and LDL lipoproteins. There are two molecular forms in plasma, apo B-100 (apo B) and apo B-48. Apo B is a unique polypeptide chain of 4536 amino acids (one of the biggest plasma proteins), synthesised in the liver and secreted in VLDLs. It is quantitatively maintained during the conversion of VLDL to IDL until LDL, of which it is the only protein component, and for this reason, levels of apo B are correlated with levels of these lipoproteins. Studies have established the relationship between B concentrations in serum and cardiovascular risk (17,18,19).

Given that each particle of VLDL, IDL and LDL only contains one apo B molecule, its concentration in serum reflects the risk associated with all these atherogenic particles. Although considered as a risk factor by the NCEP, its determination is not recommended in clinical practice, due to the unavailability of clinical guides or risk stratification algorithms based on its concentration, although it can be useful in some situations.

Nevertheless, from an experimental point of view, it can offer important additional information. The concentration of apo B in serum provides data on the number of particles, especially LDL particles, as they contain approximately 90% of total circulating apo B. It has been suggested that a LDL/ decreased apo B relationship is an indicator of the predominance of small and dense LDL particles (20).

The estimation of LDL cholesterol using the Friedewald formula is inexact when levels of triglycerides are higher than 300mg/dL and, if no validated direct method or ultracentrifugation is available, the concentration of apo B can be used as an alternative for the stratification of risk and the setting of therapeutic objectives (21). A modification of the Friedewald formula has been described for the calculation of LDL cholesterol that includes apo B. The LDL cholesterol obtained in this way has been shown to be more independent of hypertriglyceridemia than calculations made with the Friedewald formula (22).

The results of some studies have shown that the relationship between apo B/apo A-I is better for evaluating cardiovascular risk than the total cholesterol/HDL cholesterol relationship or LDL cholesterol/HDL (23,24). The number of particles and, in particular, the balance between them, that is to say, the apo B/apo A-I relationship, may be more important than the lipid quantity carried by each particle.

3.2 Triglycerides

In spite of the evidence put forward by some epidemiological studies on the relationship between hypertriglyceridemia and the incidence of CVD (25,26), the results of other, more recent, multivariate works do not allow the definitive classification of triglycerides as an independent CRF (4). This is due to the close relationship between increased levels of triglycerides and other lipid CRFs (the presence of residual lipoproteins or remnants of VLDLs and chylomicrons in plasma, the predominance of 'small and dense' particles of LDL in plasma or decreased plasma concentration of HDL cholesterol), non-lipid CRFs (hypertension) and emergent CRFs (glucose intolerance, prothrombotic state). The NCEP Panel III states that increases in levels of triglycerides (>200mg/dL) are associated with a higher risk of CVD. It is also commonly associated with other lipid and non-lipid risk factors and indicates that therapeutic objectives should be based on lifestyle changes (loss of weight, physical exercise, stopping smoking).

3.3 Lipoprotein(a)

In recent years, lipoprotein (a) (Lp(a)) has attracted enormous interest as a cardiovascular risk factor (27,28). Lp(a) is a spherical lipoprotein, rich in cholesterol esters and phospholipids, it has a composition that is similar to LDL and contains a specific glycoprotein, apolipoprotein (a), linked by a disulphide bridge to the apolipoprotein B-100. In addition, it has great structural homology to the plasminogen fibrinolytic proenzyme (Figure 1) (29).

A variety of mechanisms that may explain the relationship between lp(a) and cardiovascular disease have been described in published works. Firstly, it is argued that as lp(a) is an LDL particle it plays a role in the initiation, progression and possible rupture of the atheromatous plaque. Secondly, it is suggested that this particle competes with the plasminogen particle and inhibits thrombolytic activity (30). Finally, cell line studies with rats have shown that lipoprotein (a) inhibits NO synthesis (31).

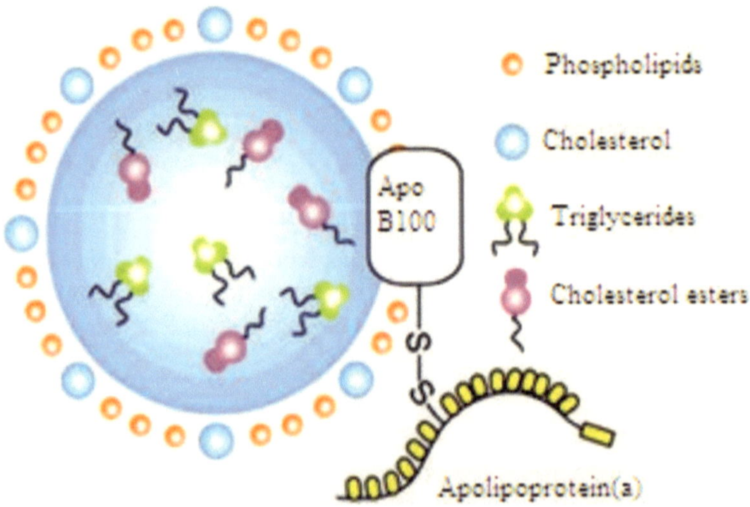

Fig. 1. Structure of lipoprotein (a).

Although an increase in the plasma concentration of lp(a) implies a higher risk of CVD, mainly in individuals at greater global risk (32), the principal consensus documents, such as the NCEP Panel III and the latest European STORE project proposal, do not include it among cardiovascular risk factors that are computable for the evaluation of overall risk. This is due to the fact that some studies do not corroborate independent prediction, based on lp(a) levels, of suffering CVD (33,34) and there is no evidence that elimination benefits the patient (35).

3.4 Ultra-sensitive CRP

The inflammatory process characterises all phases of atherothrombotic development. There are many studies that relate a variety of elements that intervene in the inflammatory process with the risk of CVD. These elements include: the intercellular-1 adhesion molecule (ICAM-1); the vascular-1 adhesion molecule (VCAM-1); E-selectin; P-selectin; proinflammatory cytokines, such as interleucine-6 (IL-6), and the tumor necrosis factor-alpha (TNF-α). All of the aforementioned have been shown to be predictors of CRFs (36). In clinical practice, difficulties in determining these markers and the short half-life of these molecules in circulatory blood mean that it is not possible to include them in the daily clinical routine. Of the other markers of inflammation that have been suggested, such as, serum amyloid A, the leukocyte count, fibrinogen, nitrotyrosine, myeloperoxidase and c-reactive protein (CRP), only the latter has been consolidated as a candidate due to its stability, analysis precision and accessibility (37). The AHA (American Heart Association) and CDC (Centers for Disease Control) say that of all the markers of inflammation, only ultra-sensitive CRP (US-CRP) has the characteristics necessary for use in clinical practice (38).

Ultra-sensitive CRP (US-CRP) is currently the best characterised inflammation biomarker and has been established as a potential marker of cardiovascular risk. US-CRP in plasma is a firm candidate for use in clinical practice as it is considered as an independent predictor of coronary illness for the general population, for both sexes and for patients that have already presented clinical manifestations of CVD (36,37). However, sufficient evidence that reducing CRP levels prevents CHD events is lacking (16, 39).

CRP is a member of the pentraxin family of proteins which are characterised by having a pentameric structure and radial symmetry, formed by five protomers of 24 kD and 206 amino acids that are linked among themselves by non covalent bonds and have the capacity to bond to a great variety of substances, such as, phosphocholine, fibronectin, chromatin, histones and ribonucleoproteins (40).

The differentiation of monocytes and macrophages, that takes place during atherosclerotic process, frees proinflammatory molecules that include interleukin-6 (IL-6) which activates, in the liver, the liberation of inflammation markers like CRP. High levels (>10 mg/dl) are registered in bacterial infections though ultra-sensitive analysis can detect very low levels (0-3 mg/dl) that are associated with the atherosclerotic process. Their half-life is more than 24 hours and their blood levels are not altered by diet.

3.5 Homocysteine

In the last decade, numerous studies have been published that relate increases homocysteinaemia (Hcy) to CVD (41-45). Nevertheless, the mechanism that controls this relationship is not completely understood. Homocysteine has a direct cytotoxic effect on endothelial cells in cultivation. An alteration in endothelial function has been observed, evaluated by echo-Doppler, in individuals with moderate hyperhomocysteinaemia and improvements have been noted on reducing the concentration of homocysteine by means of folic acid treatment. It should be remembered that levels of plasma homocysteine are related to levels of vitamin B_{12} and folic acid (46).

Homocysteine can promote LDL oxidation through the production of reactive oxygen species such as hydrogen peroxide and studies have described the promotion of the multiplication of smooth muscle cells and a reduction in DNA synthesis in endothelial cells. A large number of prospective and retrospective studies support the hypothesis that an excess of plasma homocysteine is associated with a higher risk of coronary illness, peripheral and cerebrovascular disease (44,47-49).

3.6 Asymmetric dimethylarginine

The relationship established between a high concentration of asymmetric dimethylarginine (ADMA) and endothelial dysfunction and the possible relationship between high ADMA values and the incidence of cardiovascular accidents, has led a number of research groups to study the association between high ADMA and death by any cause.

Some studies indicate that ADMA plasma levels may predict the risk of cardiovascular events. In 2001, Valkonen *et al.* (50) showed that subjects with ADMA levels of more than 0.62 µmol/L (percentile 75) had almost four times more risk of suffering an acute cardiovascular event. Similar results have been described by other authors in cases of patients with unstable angina; it was noted that those patients with higher ADMA levels (>0,62 µmol/L, percentile 75) had five times more risk of suffering a cardiovascular event (51).

Zoccali et al. (52) showed that in haemodialysis patients, ADMA plasma levels are an independent predictor of mortality and cardiovascular risk. In their multivariate study, only ADMA and age were significantly predictive, independent of the incidence of cardiovascular episodes (such as chest angina and heart attack) and death by any cause. Patients whose concentration of plasma ADMA was above the percentile 75, had three times more risk of suffering a cardiovascular episode than patients whose initial ADMA levels were lower than the average.

There are currently a number of case studies, controls and prospective clinical trials taking place with a variety of patient populations that are aimed at gaining greater understanding of the role of ADMA as an independent risk factor for CVD and mortality. The data generated by these studies will help in determining the significance of ADMA as a risk factor and explore its diagnostic importance in different illnesses and diseases.

4. Cardiovascular risk factors and physical activity

There is much research on the effect of physical activity on the alteration of risk factors associated with heart disease. The most beneficial effect of exercise is on the level of oxidative metabolism which influences levels of lipids in the blood. Aerobic exercise reduces levels of triglycerides and total cholesterol and may increase levels of HDLs, especially if accompanied by weight loss. Although reductions in total cholesterol and LDL cholesterol generated by physical exercise seem to be relatively small (in general, they are less than 10%), there are important increases in HDL cholesterol and significant reductions in triglycerides. Transversal studies with trained athletes and non-trained subjects unequivocally demonstrate that individuals with higher levels of aerobic activity have higher HDL levels and lower levels of triglycerides (53), even after a single session of exercise (54). Nevertheless, results from longitudinal studies, over relatively long periods of time, are much less clear. Many studies on physical exercise have described an increase in HDL and a reduction in triglycerides (53,55), but others have described very small changes or no changes at all. However, almost all studies have shown that proportions of LDL/HDL and total cholesterol/HDL fall after endurance training and this means less cardiovascular risk

There are reliable data that demonstrate the effectiveness of physical exercise on the reduction in blood pressure in patients with mild or moderate hypertension. Endurance training can reduce systolic and diastolic arterial pressure (DAP) by approximately 10 mmHg in individuals with moderate essential hypertension.

With regards to the other traditional cardiovascular risk factors, physical exercise can play a role in the reduction and control of weight and in the control of diabetes. Exercise has also been shown to be effective in the control and reduction of stress and anxiety (56).

Whilst the effect of exercise on 'traditional' CRFs is well documented, the effect of exercise on 'emergent' CRFs has not been studied in depth and results are not well known. It must not be forgotten that is very important the change in the volume of blood that affects plasma concentrations, independently of changes in total lipids, both in terms of lipids and the other biochemical parameters expressed as a concentration, for the evaluation of changes engendered by physical exercise. The failure to correctly take this factor into account could explain some of the controversies concerning studies on CRFs and physical exercise.

The beneficial effects of exercise, leading to the reduction of levels of apolipoprotein B, have been widely reported, but this has not been the case with the relationship between exercise and levels of apolipoprotein A-I (57,58). Some authors have found that long-term, regular physical exercise does not seem to modify levels of apolipoproteins in comparison with sedentary groups (59). There is relatively little information available on levels of lipoprotein (a) in young people although some studies have confirmed a favourable relationship between regular physical exercise and levels of lipoprotein (a) (57,59), whilst others found no difference in lipoprotein (a) concentration between healthy sedentary individuals and professional endurance athletes (60).

The previously mentioned studies have been undertaken by different authors with different population groups and there are no published works that, at the same time, analyse the influence of intense physical exercise and the influence of continuous physical exercise (training) on levels of apolipoproteins A-I, B and lipoproteins (a), in the same population group.

The beneficial effects of physical exercise also seem to be related to the effect on the inflammatory process. In the short term, intense physical exercise produces a transitory inflammatory response which is reflected in an increase in acute phase reactants and cytokines that is proportional to the amount of exercise and muscle damage. Nevertheless, regular physical activity (training) is associated with a chronic anti-inflammatory response that influences levels of acute phase reactants such as ultra-sensitive CRP and also affects lipids and lipoproteins (61-64). However, Sadepghipour *et al.* in 2010 found no relationship between CRP and physical activity in schoolchildren (65).

Some factors (BMI, the sex of the subject, the moment when the post-exercise sample is taken, diet, etc.), can have an influence on the values measured of ultra-sensitive CRP in response to physical exercise (62). Another issue that must be taken into account is that many studies that have examined the effects of intense physical exercise on levels of ultra-sensitive CRP have not made a concentration correction in accordance with the changes in plasma volume after exercise (62). Results should be individually corrected according to the post-exercise levels of hemoconcentration or hemodilution (66).

Effect of exercise on Traditional and Emergent cardiovascular risk factors

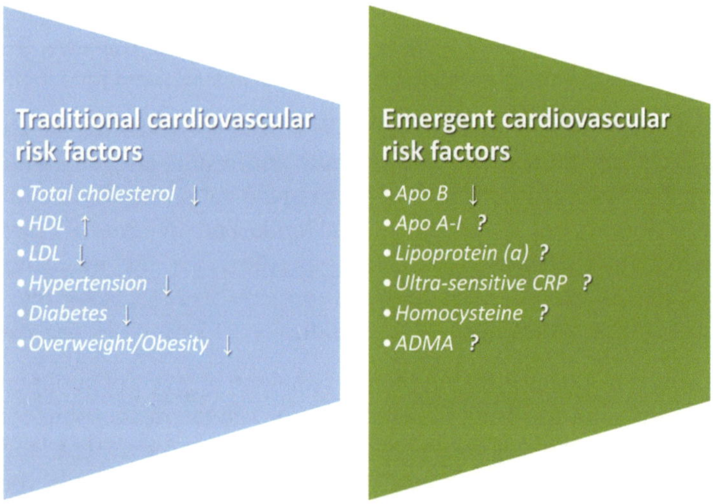

With regards to homocysteine, studies with large population groups have shown that regular physical exercise can reduce homocysteine plasma levels (47,67,68). However, other studies have concluded that intense physical exercise increases levels of Hcy (69,70). More recent studies, undertaken by our work group (71), demonstrate increased plasma homocysteine levels, both in total and reduced, after intense exercise. This increase is independent of the type of exercise and the vitamin levels but could be related to changes in renal function (71). The mechanism of this effect is not clearly understood though a study on alterations in the redox state of the homocysteine might lead to the comprehension of the underlying process. Furthermore, a study on its relationship with plasma concentrations of NO, ADMA and their proximate metabolites might lead to an understanding of how intense physical exercise produces an increase in levels of homocysteine, as long as regular, moderate physical exercise (training) seems to be a beneficial modulator of homocysteine. Also related to homocysteine, is the proven fact that regular physical exercise produces a series of beneficial effects on oxidative metabolism which result in less oxidative stress and a greater defensive capacity against oxidative damage; this is caused by the increase in activity of endogenous antioxidant systems and the greater resistance of the LDL particles to oxidation (71,72). All this signifies a reduction in oxidised LDL levels and systematic markers of inflammation, as explained by Arquer *et al.*, in 2010 (72).

In spite of the fact that the role of ADMA as a cardiovascular risk marker is reflected in an increasing number of clinical studies and scientific publications, very few studies have looked at the effect of intense or sustained (training) physical exercise on ADMA plasma levels, with contradictory results. While Schlager *et al.*, in 2011, found that supervised exercise training, twice a week during six months, in peripheral arterial disease patients decreases ADMA (73), Seljeflot *et al.*, in 2011, observed no effect of 4 weeks of exercise training in ADMA concentration in patients with chronic heart failure, speculating that the duration of the exercise protocol could be insufficient to find any effects of exercise into significant changes in ADMA (74).

It is therefore recommended that studies should be undertaken on the effect of intense and sustained (training) physical exercise on emergent cardiovascular risk factors, especially on homocysteine and ADMA.

5. Conflict of interests

The authors have no conflicts of interest

6. Acknowledgements

This work has been made possible by the support of the Ministry of Science and Innovation, Carlos III Institute of Health, F.I.S. (PI020665)

7. References

[1] Kannel W, Dawber TR, Kagan A, Revotskie N, and Stokes J III. Factors of risk in the development of coronary heart disease-six year follow-up experience. Ann Intern Med. 1961; 55:33-50.

[2] Dawber TR, Meadors GF, Moore FE Jr. Epidemiological approaches to heart disease: the Framingham Study. Am J Public Health Nations Health. 1951; 41(3):279-81.

[3] Wilson PW, D´Agostino RB, Levy D, Belanger AM, Silbershatz H, Kannel WB. Prediction of coronary heart disease using risk factors categories. Circulation. 1998; 97(18):1837-47.

[4] Expert Panel on Detection, Evaluation, and Treatment of High Blood Cholesterol in Adults. Executive Summary of the Third Report of the National Cholesterol Education Program (NCEP) Expert Panel on Detection, Evaluation, and Treatment of High Blood Cholesterol in Adults (Adult Treatment Panel III). JAMA. 2001; 285(19):2486-97.

[5] De Backer G, Ambrosioni E, Borch-Johnsen K, Brotons C, Cifkova R, Dallongeville J, Ebrahim S, Faergeman O, Graham I, Mancia G, Manger Cats V, Orth-Gomér K, Perk J, Pyöräla K, Rodicio JL, Sans S, Sansoy V, Sechtem U, Silber S, Thomsen T, Wood D; Third Joint Task Force of European and Other Societies on Cardiovascular Disease Prevention in Clinical Practice. European guidelines on cardiovascular disease prevention in clinical practice. Third Joint Task Force of European and

Other Societies on Cardiovascular Disease Prevention in Clinical Practice. Eur Heart J. 2003; 24(17):1601-10.
[6] Grundy SM. Primary prevention of coronary heart disease: integrating risk assessment with intervention. Circulation. 1999; 100(9):988-98.
[7] Stamler J, Wentworth DN, Neaton JD. Is relationship between serum cholesterol and risk of premature death from coronary heart disease continuous and graded? Findings in 356.222 primary screenees of the Multiple Risk Factor Intervention Trial (MRFIT) JAMA. 1986; 256(20):2823-8.
[8] The sixth report of the Joint National Committee on Prevention, Detection, Evaluation, and Treatment of High Blood Pressure. Arch Intern Med. 1997; 157(21):2413-46.
[9] MacMahon S, Peto R, Cutler J, Collins R, Sorlie P, Neaton J, Abbott R, Godwin J, Dyer A, Stamler J. Blood pressure, stroke, and coronary heart disease. Part 1, prolonged differences in blood pressure: prospective observational studies corrected for the regression dilution bias. Lancet. 1990; 335(8692):765-74.
[10] Staessen JA, Fagard R, Thijs L, Celis H, Arabidze GG, Birkenhäger WH, Bulpitt CJ, de Leeuw PW, Dollery CT, Fletcher AE, Forette F, Leonetti G, Nachev C, O'Brien ET, Rosenfeld J, Rodicio JL, Tuomilehto J, Zanchetti A. Randomised double-blind comparison of placebo and active treatment for older patients with isolated systolic hypertension. The Systolic Hypertension in Europe (Syst-Eur) Trial Investigators. Lancet 1997; 350(9080):757-64.
[11] Franklin SS, Khan SA, Wong ND, Larson MG, Levy D. Is pulse pressure useful in predicting risk for coronary heart disease? The Framingham Heart Study. Circulation. 1999; 100(4):354-60.
[12] Expert Committee on the Diagnosis and Classification of Diabetes Mellitus. Report of the expert committee on the diagnosis and classification of diabetes mellitus. Diabetes Care. 2003;26(Suppl 1):S5-20.
[13] Kannel WB, McGee DL. Diabetes and cardiovascular disease: the Framingham Study. JAMA. 1979; 241(19):2035-8.
[14] Laakso M, Lehto S. Epidemiology of risk factors for cardiovascular disease in diabetes and impaired glucose tolerance. Atherosclerosis. 1998; 137(Suppl 1):S65-73.
[15] Haffner SM, Letho S, Ronnemaa T, Pyorala K, Laakso M. Mortality from coronary heart disease in subjects with type II diabetes and non diabetic subjects with and without prior myocardial infarction. N Engl J Med. 1998; 339(4):229-33.
[16] Garg A. What is the role of alternative biomarkers for coronary heart disease? Clin Endocrinol (Oxf). 2011;75(3):289-93.
[17] Tornvall P, Bavenholm P, Landou C, de Faire U, Hamsten A. Relation of plasma levels and composition of apolipoprotein B-containing lipoproteins to angiographically defined coronary artery disease in young patients with myocardial infarction. Circulation. 1993; 88(5 Pt 1):2180-9.
[18] Sniderman AD. Apolipoprotein B and apolipoprotein AI as predictors of coronary artery disease. Can J Cardiol. 1988; 4(Suppl A):24A-30A.
[19] Sedlis SP, Schechtman KB, Ludbrook PA, Sobel BE, Schonfeld G. Plasma apoproteins and the severity of coronary artery disease. Circulation. 1986; 73(5):978-86.
[20] Wägner AM, Jorba O, Rigla M, Alonso E, Ordóñez-Llanos J, Pérez A. LDL-cholesterol/apolipoprotein B ratio is a good predictor of LDL phenotype B in type 2 diabetes. Acta Diabetol. 2002; 39(4):215-20.

[21] Sniderman AD, Furberg CD, Keech A, Roeters van Lennep JE, Frohlich J, Jungner I, Walldius G. Apolipoproteins versus lipids as indices of coronary risk and as targets for statin treatment. Lancet. 2003; 361(9359):777-80.
[22] Planella T, Cortes M, Martinez-Bru C, Gonzalez-Sastre F, Ordonez- Llanos J. Calculation of LDL-Cholesterol by using apolipoprotein B for classification of nonchylomicronemic dyslipemia. Clin Chem. 1997; 43(5):808-15.
[23] Walldius G, Jungner I, Aastveit AH, Holme I, Furberg CD, Sniderman AD. The apo B/apo A-I ratio is better than cholesterol ratios to estimate the balance between plasma proatherogenic and antiatherogenic lipoproteins and to predict coronary risk. Clin Chem Lab Med. 2004;42(12): 1355-63.
[24] Walldius G, Jungner I . The apoB/apoA-I ratio: a strong, new risk factor for cardiovascular disease and a target for lipid-lowering therapy--a review of the evidence. J Intern Med. 2006; 259(5):493-519.
[25] Austin MA, Hokanson JE, Edwards KL. Hypertriglyceridemia as a cardiovascular risk factor. Am J Cardiol. 1998; 81(4A):7B-12B.
[26] Assmann G, Schulte H, Funke H, von Eckardstein A. The emergence of triglycerides as a significant independent risk factor in coronary artery disease. Eur Heart J. 1998; 19(Suppl M):M8-M14.
[27] Moliterno DJ, Lange RA, Meidell RS, Willard JE, Leffert CC, Gerard RD, Boerwinkle E, Hobbs HH, Hillis LD. Relation of plasma lipoprotein(a) to infarct artery patency in survivors of myocardial infarction. Circulation. 1993;88(3):935-40.
[28] Seman LJ, DeLuca C, Jenner JL, Cupples LA, McNamara JR, Wilson PWF, Castelli WP, Ordovas JM, Schaefer EJ. Lipoprotein(a)-cholesterol and coronary heart disease in the Framingham Heart Study. Clin Chem. 1999; 45(7):1039-46.
[29] Utermann G. The mysteries of lipoprotein (a). Science. 1989;246(4932):904-10.
[30] Rubiés-Prat J. Lipoproteína(a): del genotipo al riesgo cardiovascular, pasando por el fenotipo. Clin Invest Arterioscler. 2004; 16:151-3.
[31] Moeslinger T, Fiedl R, Volf I, Brunner M, Koller E, Spieckermann PG. Inhibition of nitric oxide synthesis by oxidized lipoprotein (a) in a murine cell line. FEBS Lett. 2000; 478(1-2):95-9.
[32] Von Eckardstein A, Schulte H, Cullen P, Assmann G. Lipoprotein(a) further increases the risk of coronary events in men with high global cardiovascular risk. J Am Coll Cardiol. 2001; 37(2):434-9.
[33] Nishino M, Malloy MJ, Naya-Vigne J, Russell J, Kane JP, Redberg RF. Lack of association of lipoprotein(a) levels with coronary calcium deposits in asymptomatic postmenopausal women. J Am Coll Cardiol. 2000; 35(2):314-20.
[34] Moliterno DJ, Jokinen EV, Miserez AR, Lange RA, Willard JE, Boerwinkle E, Hillis LD, Hobbs HH. No association between plasma lipoprotein(a) concentrations and the presence or absence of coronary atherosclerosis in African Americans. Arterioscler Thromb Vasc Biol. 1995; 15(7):850-5.
[35] Marcovina SM, Koschinsky ML, Albers JJ, Skarlatos S. Report of the National Heart, Lung, and Blood Institute Workshop on lipoprotein(a) and cardiovascular disease: recent advances and future directions. Clin Chem. 2003; 49(11):1785-96.
[36] Ridker PM, Hennekens CH, Buring JE, Rifai N. C-reactive protein and other markers of inflammation in the prediction of cardiovascular disease in women. N Engl J Med. 2000; 342(12):836-43.

[37] Shishehbor MH, Bhatt DL. Inflammation and atherosclerosis. Curr Atheroscler Rep. 2004; 6(2):131-9.

[38] Pearson TA, Mensah GA, Alexander RW, Anderson JL, Cannon RO 3rd, Criqui M, Fadl YY, Fortmann SP, Hong Y, Myers GL, Rifai N, Smith SC Jr, Taubert K, Tracy RP, Vinicor F; Centers for Disease Control and Prevention; American Heart Association. Markers of inflammation and cardiovascular disease: application to clinical and public health practice: A statement for healthcare professionals from the Centers for Disease Control and Prevention and the American Heart Association. Circulation. 2003; 107(3):499-511.

[39] Buckley DI, Fu R, Freeman M, Rogers K, Helfand M. C-reactive protein as a risk factor for coronary heart disease: a systematic review and meta-analyses for the U.S. Preventive Services Task Force. Ann Intern Med. 2009, 151(7):483-95.

[40] Healy H, Westhuyzen J. Biology and relevance of C-reactive protein in cardiovascular and renal disease. Ann Clin Lab Sci. 2000; 30(2):133-43.

[41] Refsum H, Ueland PM, Nygard O, Vollset SE. Homocysteine and cardiovascular disease. Annu Rev Med. 1998; 49:31-62.

[42] Kang SS, Wong PWK, Malinow MR. Hyperhomocyst(e)inemia as a risk factor for occlusive vascular disease. Annu Rev Nutr. 1992; 12:279-98.

[43] Malinow MR, Bostom AG, Krauss RM. Homocyst(e)ine, diet, and cardiovascular diseases: a statement for healthcare professionals from the Nutrition Committee, American Heart Association. Circulation. 1999; 99(1):178-82.

[44] Bostom AG, Rosenberg IH, Silbershatz H, Jacques PF, Selhub J, D'Agostino RB, Wilson PWF, Wolf PA. Nonfasting plasma total homocysteine levels and stroke incidence in elderly persons: the Framingham Study. Ann Intern Med. 1999; 131(5):352-5.

[45] Stehouwer CDA, Weijenberg MP, van den Berg M, Jakobs C, Feskens EJM, Kromhout D. Serum homocysteine and risk of coronary heart disease and cerebrovascular disease in elderly men: a 10-year follow-up. Arterioscler Thromb Vasc Biol. 1998; 18(12):1895-901.

[46] Woo KS, Chook P, Lolin YI, Sanderson JE, Metreweli C, Celermajer DS Folic acid improves arterial endothelial function in adults with hyperhomocysteinemia. J Am Coll Cardiol. 1999; 34(7):2002-6.

[47] Nygard O, Vollset SE, Refsum H, Stensvol I, Tverdal A, Nordrehaug E, Ueland M, Kvale G. Total plasma homocysteine and cardiovascular risk profile. The Hordaland Homocysteine Study. JAMA. 1995; 274(19):1526-33.

[48] Genest JJ, McNamara JR, Salem DN, Wilson PW, Schaefer EJ, Malinow MR Plasma homocyst(e)ine levels in men with premature coronary artery disease. J Am Coll Cardiol. 1990; 16(5):1114-9.

[49] Stampfer MJ, Malinow MR, Willett WC, Newcomer LM, Upson B, Ullmann D *et al.* A prospective study of plasma homocyst(e)ine and risk of myocardial infarction in US physicians. JAMA. 1992;268(7):877-81.

[50] Valkonen VP, Päivä H, Salonen JT, Lakka TA, Lehtimäki T, Laakso J, Laaksonen R. Risk of acute coronary events and serum concentration of asymmetrical dimethylarginine. Lancet. 2001; 358(9299): 2127-28

[51] Lu TM, Ding YA, Lin SJ *et al*: Plasma levels of asymmetrical dimethylarginine and adverse cardiovascular events after percutaneous coronary intervention. Eur Heart J. 2003; 24(21):1912-9.

[52] Zoccali C, Bode-Böger S, Mallamaci F, Benedetto F, Tripepi G, Malatino L, Cataliotti A, Bellanuova I, Fermo I, Frölich J, Böger R. Plasma concentration of asymmetrical dimethylarginine and mortality in patients with end-stage renal disease: a prospective study. Lancet. 2001; 358(9299): 2113-17.

[53] Pitsavos C, Panagiotakos DB, Tambalis KD, Chrysohoou C, Sidossis LS, Skoumas J, Stefanadis C. Resistance exercise plus to aerobic activities is associated with better lipids' profile among healthy individuals: the ATTICA study. QJM. 2009, 102(9):609-16.

[54] Henderson GC, Krauss RM, Fattor JA, Faghihnia N, Luke-Zeitoun M, Brooks GA. Plasma triglyceride concentrations are rapidly reduced following individual bouts of endurance exercise in women. Eur J Appl Physiol. 2010, 109(4):721-30.

[55] Chomistek AK, Chiuve SE, Jensen MK, Cook NR, Rimm EB. Vigorous physical activity, mediating biomarkers, and risk of myocardial infarction. Med Sci Sports Exerc. 2011, Mar 25. [Epub ahead of print]

[56] Petruzzello SJ, Landers DM, Hatfield BD, Kubitz KA, Salazar W. A meta-analysis on the anxiety-reducing effects of acute and chronic exercise. Outcomes and mechanisms. Sports Med. 1991; 11(3):143-82.

[57] Taimela S, Viikari JS, Porkka KV, Dahlen GH. Lipoprotein (a) levels in children and young adults: the influence of physical activity. The Cardiovascular Risk in Young Finns Study. Acta Paediatr. 1994;83(12):1258-63.

[58] Mackinnon LT, Hubinger LM. Effects of exercise on lipoprotein(a). Sports Med. 1999; 28(1):11-24.

[59] Thomas NE, Baker JS, Davies B. Established and recently identified coronary heart disease risk factors in young people: the influence of physical activity and physical fitness. Sports Med. 2003; 33(9):633-50.

[60] Lippi G, Schena F, Salvagno GL, Montagnana M, Ballestrieri F, Guidi GC. Comparison of the lipid profile and lipoprotein(a) between sedentary and highly trained subjects. Clin Chem Lab Med. 2006;44(3):322-6.

[61] Kasapis C, Thompson PD. The effects of physical activity on serum C-reactive protein and inflammatory markers: a systematic review. J Am Coll Cardiol. 2005; 45(10):1563-9.

[62] Plaisance EP, Grandjean PW. Physical activity and high-sensitivity C-reactive protein. Sports Med. 2006; 36(5):443-58.

[63] Gonzales-Ordóñez AJ, Venta R, Terrados N, Arias A, Macias-Robles MD. Association between Sensitivity for Activated Protein C (APC) and Lipid or Lipoprotein Levels. Thrombosis and Haemostasis. 2002; 88: 1069-1070.

[64] Metsios GS, Stavropoulos-Kalinoglou A, Sandoo A, van Zanten JJ, Toms TE, John H, Kitas GD. Vascular function and inflammation in rheumatoid arthritis: the role of physical activity. Open Cardiovasc Med J. 2010; 4:89-96.

[65] Sadeghipour HR, Rahnama A, Salesi M, Rahnama N, Mojtahedi H. Relationship between C-reactive protein and physical fitness, physical activity, obesity and selected cardiovascular risk factors in schoolchildren. Int J Prev Med. 2010, 1(4):242-6.

[66] Dill DB, Costill DL. Calculation of percentage changes in volumen of blood, plasma, and red cells in dehydration. Journal of applied Physiology. 1974; 37(2):247-8.

[67] Bailey D, Davies B, Baker J. Training in hipoxia: modulation or metabolic and cardiovascular risk factors in men. Med Sci Sports Exerc. 2000; 32(6):1058-66.

[68] König D, Bissé E, Deibert P, Müller H-M, Wieland H, Berg A. Influence of training volume and acute physical exercise on the homocysteine levels in endurance-trained men: interactions with plasma folate and vitamin B12. Ann Nutr Metab. 2003; 47(3-4):114-8.

[69] Wright M, Francis K, Cornwell P. Effect of acute exercise on plasma homocysteine. J Sports Med Phys Fitness. 1998; 38(3):262-5.

[70] De Crée C, Malinow MR, van Kranenburg GP, Geurten PG, Longford NT, Keizer HA. Influence of exercise and menstrual cycle phase on plasma homocyst(e)ine levels in young women-a prospective study. Scand J Med Sci Sports. 1999; 9(5):272-8.

[71] Venta R, Cruz E, Valcárcel G, Terrados N. Plasma vitamins, amino acids, and renal function in postexercise hyperhomocysteinemia. Medicine and Science in Sports and Exercise. 2009; 41(8):1645-1651.

[72] Arquer A, Elosua R, y J Marrugat. Actividad física y estrés oxidativo. Apunts Med Esport. 2010. doi: 10.1016/j. apunts.2009.12.002

[73] Schlager O, Giurgea A, Schuhfried O, Seidinger D, Hammer A, Gröger M, Fialka-Moser V, Gschwandtner M, Koppensteiner R, Steiner S. Exercise training increases endothelial progenitor cells and decreases asymmetric dimethylarginine in peripheral arterial disease: A randomized controlled trial. Atherosclerosis. 2011, 217(1):240-8.

[74] Seljeflot I, Nilsson BB, Westheim AS, Bratseth V, Arnesen H. The L-arginine-asymmetric dimethylarginine ratio is strongly related to the severity of chronic heart failure. No effects of exercise training. J Card Fail. 2011, 17(2):135-42.

20

Dietary Supplements and Cardiovascular Disease: What is the Evidence and What Should We Recommend?

Satoshi Kashiwagi and Paul L. Huang
Cardiovascular Research Center and Cardiology Division, Massachusetts General Hospital and Harvard Medical School, Charlestown, MA, USA

1. Introduction

1.1 Importance of cardiovascular disease and scope of this chapter

Cardiovascular disease, diabetes, and obesity are important causes of morbidity and mortality. Cardiovascular disease affects 80 million Americans and is the leading cause of death (Lloyd-Jones et al., 2009). Diabetes and obesity are also increasing at alarming rates, and together, the three conditions have a significant impact on public health (Ogden et al., 2006). Cardiovascular disease, diabetes and obesity can be influenced by lifestyle changes, including diet and physical activity (McCullough et al., 2000). The American Heart Association recommends a diet rich in vegetables and fruits, whole grains, high-fiber foods, with lean meats and poultry, moderate consumption of fish, an emphasis on fat-free or low fat dairy products, and limiting the amount of saturated fat, trans fat and cholesterol (Lichtenstein et al., 2006).

Among natural products found in food, fish oils, vitamin E, and soy isoflavones have been studied for their effects on cardiovascular disease. Many of these compounds are available as food supplements. There is a great interest among the public and in the lay press about the use of these compounds to treat or prevent disease. The scope of this chapter is to review the evidence for the effects of these compounds on cardiovascular disease, so that physicians and patients may better understand their health effects, in an effort to reduce the risk for cardiovascular disease, diabetes and obesity.

1.2 Types of evidence: Epidemiologic, mechanistic, and randomized clinical trials

It is important to realize the different kinds of evidence in support of health benefits of natural products. One type of evidence is *epidemiologic evidence*. Epidemiologic information may offer the first suggestion that certain natural products in the diet may influence the risk and course of chronic diseases like cardiovascular disease, diabetes, and cancer. Cross-cultural studies might indicate that populations that have high or low intake of certain compounds have different incidence of cardiovascular disease. This does not prove that supplementation with these compounds would necessarily change the course of cardiovascular disease. Genetic and environmental factors may all contribute to the effects observed in the epidemiologic studies. Cohort studies, which follow groups of people and their intake of certain compounds, also provide suggestive evidence for their effects.

A second type of evidence comes from *mechanistic studies* in the laboratory or in animal models. Here, the natural products or compounds in question are added to cells or enzyme reactions, to see what their effects are. Studies may be done in animal models of human disease, for example apoE knockout mice that develop diet-induced atherosclerosis. They may be carried out on blood vessels from animals to see whether the compounds affect vascular function. Mechanistic studies help determine the possible molecular and cellular mechanisms and pathways involved in biological function. However, just because a compound has an effect in these experiments or animals models does not mean that taking them will necessarily reduce disease in people. Many of these experiments are done *in vitro*, not *in vivo*.

A third type of evidence comes from *randomized controlled clinical trials*. In these trials, compounds are administered to a large population, which is then followed for clearly defined disease events. Randomized clinical trials offer the strongest scientific evidence for or against health benefits. These studies often use pure compounds or standardized preparations. Often, compounds for which epidemiologic studies suggest benefit, and mechanistic studies show effects, fail to do so in large randomized clinical trials. There have also been surprising results of increased disease risk from certain natural products, suggesting the need for caution and for ongoing studies to obtain evidence of the best possible quality. It is important to approach results of studies with a critical eye, and to always consider the quality of the information and how strongly it supports an effect.

In this article, three specific classes of compounds—omega-3 fatty acids, vitamin E, and soy isoflavones—are reviewed. Evidence for their biological effects are presented, categorized separately according to type of evidence: epidemiological studies, mechanistic studies, and where available, randomized controlled trials. It is hoped that this review will provide the basis for evidence-based recommendations to patients regarding these compounds and food supplements.

2. Fish oils: Omega-3 fatty acids

2.1 Structure and food sources

While many fatty acids serve as energy stores that are broken down by the body to generate energy, *omega-3* and *omega-6* fatty acids are two types of polyunsaturated fatty acids that serve as precursors to biologically active molecules, including prostaglandins, leukotrienes, and thromboxanes. This role gives them particular importance in the diet.

Polyunsaturated fatty acids are a family of long-chain (typically 18-24 carbon atoms) fatty acids containing two or more double bonds. Omega-3 and omega-6 refer to the position of the last double bond. The convention in chemical nomenclature is to label the COOH carbon as the first carbon, and the one furthest from this as the last, or *omega*, carbon. Thus, omega-3 fatty acids contain a double bond three carbons from the end of the molecule furthest from the COOH group. Given that the length of the hydrocarbon chain is variable, the length is sometimes referred to as "n," so omega-3 fatty acids are also known as n-3 fatty acids, and omega-6 fatty acids as n-6 fatty acids.

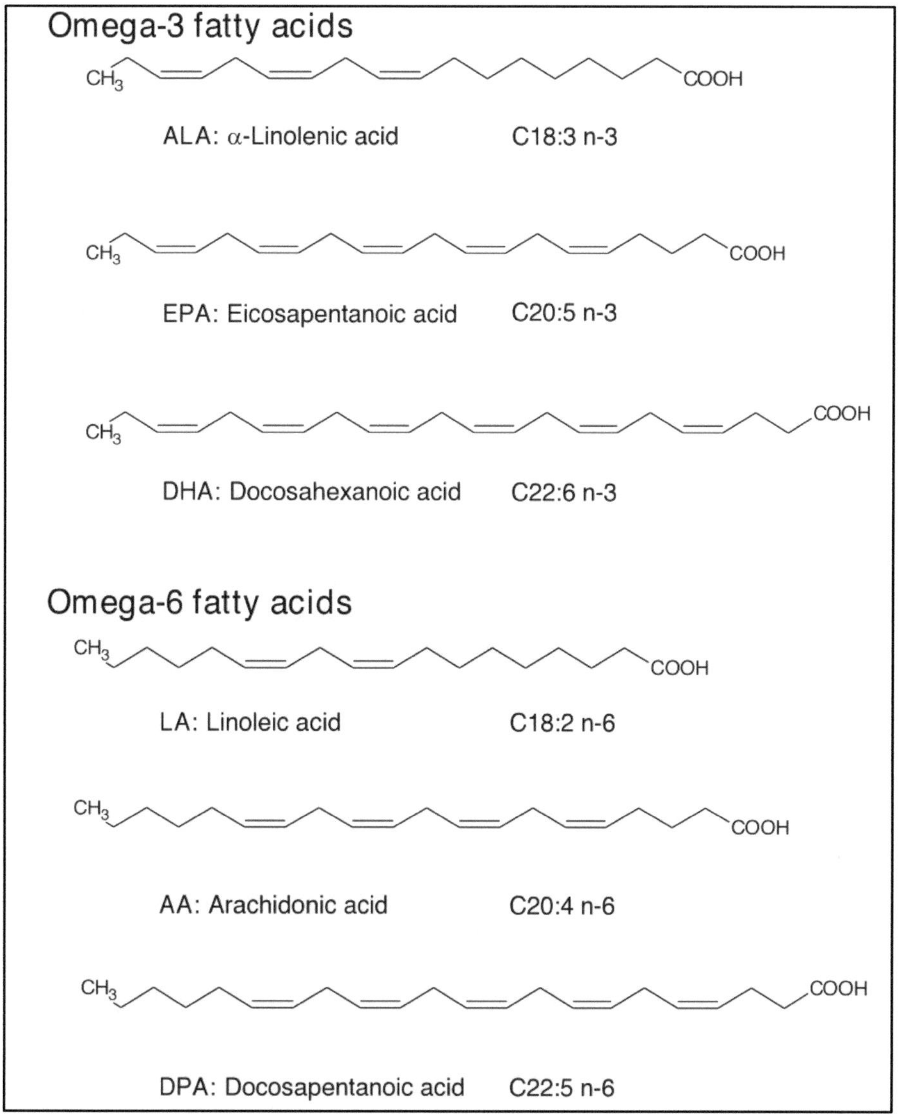

Fig. 1. Structures of omega-6 and omega-3 fatty acids
Omega-3 fatty acids differ from omega-6 fatty acids by the location of their first double bond from the methyl (CH_3) end of the fatty acid. Omega-3 fatty acids include α-linolenic acid (ALA), eicosapentanoic acid (EPA), and docosahexanoic acid (DHA). Omega-6 fatty acids include linoleic acid (LA), arachidonic acid (AA), and docosapentanoic acid (DPA). In the chemical names, the number of carbon atoms is given first, separated by a colon from the number of double bonds, followed by the position of the first double bond.

The structures of omega-3 and omega-6 fatty acids are shown in Figure 1. Representative omega-3 fatty acids are α-linolenic acid (ALA), eicosapentanoic acid (EPA), and docosahexanoic acid (DHA). Of these, the parent omega-3 fatty acid is ALA, an 18 carbon fatty acid with three double bonds, the last of which is located between carbons 15 and 16 (the n-3 position). Therefore, in shorthand, ALA is C18:3 n-3. ALA serves as the precursor to the omega-3 fatty acids EPA (C20:5 n-3) and DHA (C22:6 n-3) by the addition of carbons to the chain (elongation) and by the replacement of single bonds by double bonds (desaturation). Likewise, representative omega-6 fatty acids are linoleic acid (LA), arachidonic acid (AA), and docosapentanoic acid. LA is an 18 carbon fatty acid with two double bonds, with the last one located at the n-6 position (C18:2 n-6). LA serves as a precursor to AA (C20:4 n-6) and docosapentanoic acid (C22:5 n-6), which are formed by elongation and desaturation.

The parent fatty acids of the omega-3 family (ALA) and omega-6 family (LA) cannot be made by the human body, so they are *essential* fatty acids. They must be supplied in the diet. LA is found in vegetable oils like soybean and canola, and also in nuts, seeds, vegetables, legumes, grains, and fruit. ALA is found in vegetable sources like flaxseed, but only 5% of ALA is converted to DHA and EPA. The richest sources of DHA and EPA are fish and fish oils.

2.2 Biological roles of omega-3 and omega-6 fatty acids

Omega-3 and -6 fatty acids are important biologically because they influence production of prostaglandins, leukotrienes, and thromboxanes. These mediators affect many diverse processes, and are involved in inflammation, pain, and thrombosis (Calder, 2006). Moreover, omega-3 and omega-6 fatty acids are separate families that cannot be interconverted by the human body. Because they compete for the same enzymes, the ratio of omega-3 to omega-6 fatty acids in the diet influences the relative amounts of prostaglandins and leukotrienes that are synthesized from arachidonic acid.

2.3 Epidemiologic data on fish oils and cardiovascular disease

Epidemiologic data from fish-eating populations like the Greenland Inuits established a link between fish oil consumption and lower incidence of cardiovascular disease (Dyerberg et al., 1975). Fish oil consumption was also linked with low levels of triglycerides, plasma cholesterol and very low-density lipoproteins (VLDL) and high levels of high-density lipoproteins (HDL), all of which would protect against cardiovascular disease.

2.4 Mechanistic studies

Omega-3 fatty acids may influence cardiovascular disease through effects on lipid profiles, eicosanoid pathways, and susceptibility to arrythmias.

2.4.1 Lipid profiles

Omega-3 fatty acids decrease plasma cholesterol concentrations in animal models (Fernandez & West, 2005). They increase hepatic LDL receptor number and LDL turnover *in vivo* (Fernandez & McNamar, 1989, Fernandez et al., 1992), and bind to peroxisome proliferator activated receptors (PPARs), liver X receptors (LXRs), hepatic nuclear factor-4 (HNF-4), and sterol regulatory element binding proteins (SREBPs) (Jump, 2002). Omega-3 fatty acids suppress SREBP-1 expression, leading to decreased lipogenesis and VLDL secretion (Field et al., 2003), increased LPL activity (Illingworth & Schmidt, 1993), and decreased apoC3 levels (Shachter, 2001). They also decrease lipogenesis and VLDL secretion while increasing reverse cholesterol transport (Vasandani et al., 2002).

2.4.2 Eicosanoid metabolism

Omega-3 and omega-6 fatty acids are precursors to a broad array of structurally diverse and potent bioactive lipids, including eicosanoids, prostaglandins, and thromboxanes. Eicosanoids are produced from arachidonic acid, EPA, and dihomolinolenic acid when these fatty acids are released from membranes by phospholipase A_2 (Zhou & Nilsson, 2001). The availability of these eicosanoid precursors depends on dietary levels of these molecules, as well as the parent fatty acids of each family: ALA for omega-3 fatty acids, and LA for omega-6 fatty acids. Because omega-6 and omega-3 fatty acids cannot be interconverted, their relative ratios are important.

Arachidonic acid, an omega-6 fatty acid, is a precursor of prostaglandins, leukotrienes and related compounds that mediate inflammation. Because omega-3 fatty acids compete with omega-6 fatty acid metabolism, increased consumption of omega-3 fatty acids (particularly DHA and EPA) results in the partial replacement of arachidonic acid in cell membranes by EPA and DHA, and a decrease in the production of biological mediators derived from AA. Intake of 6 g DHA/d decreased production of prostaglandin E_2 by 60% and leukotriene B_4 by 75% in endotoxin-stimulated mononuclear cells (Kelley et al., 1999). Other studies have shown a shift in the relative amounts of prostaglandin I_2 and thromboxane A_2, resulting in vasodilation and reduced thrombosis (von Schacky et al., 1985, Goodnight et al., 1989). Omega-3 fatty acids, particularly DHA and EPA in fish oil, may themselves reduce expression of ICAM-1 on the surface of stimulated blood monocytes (Hughes et al., 1996), and decrease hydrogen peroxide production (Fisher et al., 1990).

2.4.3 Antiarrhythmic effects

DHA and EPA may be preferentially incorporated into membrane phospholipids, accounting for an antiarrhythmic effect after dietary intake (Nair et al., 1999). These fatty acids directly influence conduction of several membrane ion channels (Leaf et al., 2003), inhibit voltage-gated sodium currents and L-type calcium currents (Kang et al., 1995), and shift the steady-state inactivation potential to more negative values in cardiomyocytes. These results provide an electrophysiological basis for antiarrhythmic effects.

2.5 Clinical studies

Dietary intake of omega-3 fatty acids, particularly DHA and EPA found in fatty fish or fish-oil supplements, reduces risk of CVD (Kris-Etherton et al., 2002, Wang et al., 2006). The strongest evidence comes from the Italian GISSI trial (1999), a secondary prevention study in over 11,000 patients with recent myocardial infarction. Supplementation with 0.85 g EPA and DHA per day reduced all-cause mortality by 21%, cardiac death by 35%, and sudden death by 45%. No effect was found on stroke. In contrast, a Norwegian study of 300 patients following MI, randomized to a higher intake of omega-3 fatty acids (3.4 g EPA and DPA per day), failed to show a difference in CVD events, but there was a high background of fish oil intake in both groups. Several other small studies suggested beneficial trends in CVD and PVD, but these were not statistically significant (Sacks et al., 1995, Nilsen et al., 2001).

In these studies, patients with implantable cardiac defibrillators (ICD) were excluded. Several randomized controlled trials, ranging in size from 200 to over 500 patients, studied fish oil consumption in patients with ICDs (Raitt et al., 2005,Brouwer et al., 2006). These studies showed no change in mortality from fish oil consumption. It is possible that the beneficial effects of fish oils may not be observed in the ICD population, because these patients all have defibrillators and therefore cardiac arrhythmic sudden death would be removed from both groups.

Primary prevention trials, which study patients in the general population who do not have known heart disease, have not shown as strong an effect as the GISSI trial. Most primary prevention data on fish oils comes from large cohort studies from China, Japan, and the United States (Dolecek, 1992, Nagata et al., 2002) and others. In aggregate, these studies included over 343,000 subjects, and showed reductions in all-cause mortality, cardiac mortality, and sudden death. Interestingly, in one of these studies (Mozaffarian et al., 2003), the protection was found with tuna and other nonfried fish, while consumption of fried fish or fried fish sandwiches was associated with increased cardiovascular events.

3. Vitamin E

3.1 Structure and food sources

Vitamin E is a fat-soluble vitamin that exists in at least eight naturally occurring forms, as shown in Figure 2. Tocotrienols differ from tocopherols by the presence of three double bonds in their isoprenoid side chains. The α-, β-, γ-, and δ- forms are defined by the identity of the R groups on the chromanol rings. Vitamin E found naturally in food is primarily γ-tocopherol, but α-tocopherol is the predominant form found in supplements, and is also the most biologically active form.

Vitamin E is an essential vitamin because it cannot be synthesized by the body. Sources of vitamin E include nuts and seeds, such as almonds, peanuts, sunflower seeds, and filberts.

Tocopherols are similar in structure to tocotrienols, except that tocotrienols have three double bonds in the phytyl side chains. There are three positions on the chromanol ring, denoted R_1, R_2, and R_3. The particular identity of the tocopherol or tocotrienol is determined by the identities of these side chains. Vitamin E found naturally in food is primarily γ-tocopherol. α-tocopherol, which is the most biologically active, is the predominant form found in supplements.

Vitamin E is also found in vegetable oils (soy, corn or sunflower), and their derivatives (margarine), cereals and grains. Vitamin E is found in potato chips and tomato products because of the vegetable oils that they contain.

3.2 Biological roles of vitamin E

Vitamin E is an antioxidant, because it breaks chain reactions that are propagated by free radicals. Vitamin E is present in biological membranes, and serves as an important lipid soluble antioxidant. It reacts with oxidant molecules and protects cell membranes from lipid peroxidation by trapping peroxyl radicals. One molecule of α-tocopherol per 1,000 phospholipids can protect cellular membranes. α-tocopherol can also be regenerated from its tocopheroxyl radical by an electron donor like vitamin C.

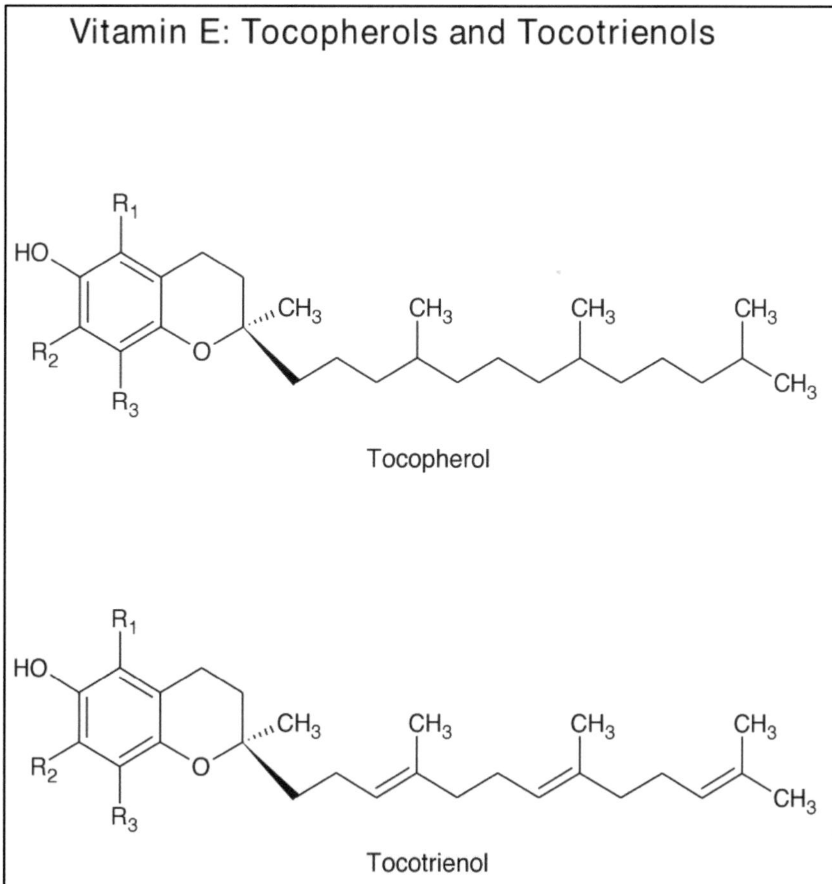

Compound	R_1	R_2	R_3
α-Tocopherol and α-Tocotrienol	CH_3	CH_3	CH_3
β-Tocopherol and β-Tocotrienol	CH_3	H	CH_3
γ-Tocopherol and γ-Tocotrienol	H	CH_3	CH_3
δ-Tocopherol and δ-Tocotrienol	H	H	CH_3

Fig. 2. Structures of tocopherols and tocotrienols

3.3 Epidemiologic data on vitamin E and cardiovascular disease

High intake of vitamin E is epidemiologically associated with lower cardiovascular disease risk. The World Health Organization/Monica project performed cross-cultural analysis on vitamin intake in populations with different incidence of coronary heart disease mortality. Differences in cardiovascular mortality were primarily attributable to plasma levels of vitamin E in middle-aged men representing 16 European study populations (Gey et al., 1991).

Several cohort studies showed similar results. The US Nurse's Health Study followed a cohort of 87,245 female nurses between the ages of 34 and 59 years, over an eight year period. Supplementation with α-tocopherol for at least two years was associated with reduced risk of cardiovascular disease (Stampfer et al., 1993). Incidence of heart disease was 30-40% lower in those with the highest intakes of vitamin E. Another cohort study followed 39,910 male health professionals between the ages of 40 and 75. Consumption of more than 60 IU/d of vitamin E was associated with a 40% relative risk reduction of cardiovascular disease (Rimm et al., 1993). Vitamin E intake from food was inversely associated with CVD risk in 34,486 postmenopausal women (Kushi et al., 1996).

3.4 Mechanistic studies

In *ex vivo* human studies, monocytes isolated from healthy human subjects supplemented with α-tocopherol showed decreased LDL oxidation (Devaraj et al., 1996). In other studies, vitamin E supplementation failed to affect lipid oxidation, including isoprostanes and 4-hydroxynonenal (breakdown products of fatty acid autooxidation) (Meagher et al., 2001).

One animal study showed that vitamin E intake inversely correlates with atherosclerotic lesions and liver peroxidation in apoE knockout mice (Ferre et al., 2001). In another study, vitamin E and coenzyme Q (CoQ) supplementation significantly reduced tissue lipid hydroperoxide formation and limited the development of atherosclerosis in apoE knockout mice (Thomas et al., 2001). However, still other studies found that vitamin E did not reduce atherosclerosis in apoE knockout mice (Paul et al., 2001), or fatty streak formation in C57/Bl6 mice (Munday et al., 1998). The degree of lipid oxidation in vascular tissue also failed to correlate with the extent of the lesions in apoE knockout mice (Wu et al., 2006). Thus, animal studies do not show uniform benefit of vitamin E supplementation in preventing LDL oxidation or reducing atherosclerosis.

3.5 Clinical trials on vitamin E

3.5.1 Vitamin E and cardiovascular disease

Some clinical trials suggest a benefit of vitamin E in reducing cardiovascular disease. The Cambridge Heart Antioxidant Study (CHAOS) randomized 2,002 patients with coronary disease to α-tocopherol (400 to 800 IU) or placebo. The vitamin E treated groups showed 1.9 fold reductions in cardiovascular death and nonfatal myocardial infarction (Stephens et al., 1996). The Secondary Prevention with Antioxidants of Cardiovascular Disease in End-stage Renal Disease (SPACE) trial randomized 192 renal failure patients undergoing hemodialysis to 800 IU vitamin E or placebo. The vitamin E treated group showed a significant decrease in both fatal and nonfatal cardiovascular endpoints (Boaz et al., 2000).

Other clinical trials failed to show benefit. In the GISSI study, 11,324 patients were given omega-3 fatty acids, vitamin E at 300 mg per day, both, or neither, and followed over a 3½ year period. Two-way analysis did not show any reduction in fatal or nonfatal cardiovascular events from vitamin E supplementation (Marchioli et al., 2002), (1999). The Heart Outcomes Prevention Evaluation (HOPE) trial was a multinational study of over 9,500 patients with known cardiovascular disease, randomized to the angiotensin converting enzyme inhibitor ramipril, natural source vitamin E at 400 IU per day, both, or neither. Over a 4½ year follow-up, there was no reduction in fatal or nonfatal cardiovascular events in the vitamin E treated groups (Yusuf et al., 2000). In an extension study (HOPE -TOO), almost 4000 subjects continued to take vitamin E or placebo for an additional 2½ years (Lonn et al., 2005). Despite this 7 year total follow-up period, there was no significant protection against cardiovascular disease, stroke, or death.

Of concern, the HOPE-TOO study showed a higher incidence of heart failure in the treated group. In the Women's Angiographic Vitamin and Estrogen Study, 423 post-menopausal women with coronary disease took supplements with 400 IU vitamin E or placebo (Waters et al., 2002). Not only did women taking vitamin E not show cardiovascular benefit, but there was an increase in all-cause mortality. In the Physicians Health Study II, 15,000 health physicians age 50 or over were randomized to α-tocopherol (400 IU), 500 mg vitamin C, both, or placebo (Sesso et al., 2008). Over a follow-up period of 8 years, neither vitamin E nor vitamin C resulted in a decrease in cardiovascular events, stroke, or cardiovascular mortality. In contrast, α-tocopherol was associated with an increase in hemorrhagic stroke. Taking the results of all of these results together, including a meta-analysis (Miller et al., 2005), vitamin E is not recommended for the purpose of reducing cardiovascular risk.

3.5.2 Vitamin E and diabetes

Oxidative stress and inflammation have been implicated in the pathogenesis of diabetes(Ho & Bray, 1999). Vitamin E treatment (600 mg per day) improved insulin-mediated glucose disposal in 36 healthy, nondiabetic volunteers (Facchini et al., 2000). A prospective cohort study showed that plasma concentration of α-tocopherol was inversely related to fasting plasma glucose concentration and oxidative stress markers in 101 women at high risk of type 2 diabetes in Finland (Ylonen et al., 2003). In secondary prevention trials, 600 mg/day of vitamin E supplementation significantly decreased markers of oxidative stress and improved brachial artery reactivity in 40 patients with diabetes (Paolisso et al., 2000). However, the Insulin Resistance and Atherosclerosis Study (IRAS) cohort study showed no protective effect for either reported intake of vitamin E or plasma concentration of α-tocopherol in 895 nondiabetic adults (Mayer-Davis et al., 2002). In another study, high levels of α-tocopherol and β-carotene were associated with decreased risk of non-insulin dependent diabetes mellitus, but the association disappeared after adjustment for cardiovascular risk factors (Reunanen et al., 1998). Whether vitamin E influences the development of diabetes is not clear and warrants further investigation.

4. Phytoestrogens

4.1 Structure and food sources of phytoestrogens

Phytoestrogens are flavonoids that have similar chemical structure to estrogen. They include isoflavones, coumestans, and lignans (Kurzer & Xu, 1997). Figure 3 shows a comparison of the chemical structures of estradiol (a naturally occurring human estrogen), genistein (an isoflavone), and coumestrol (a coumestan). A number of these compounds have been identified in fruits, vegetables, and whole grains commonly consumed as food. Soybeans, clover and alfalfa sprouts, and oilseeds (such as flaxseed) are the most significant dietary sources.

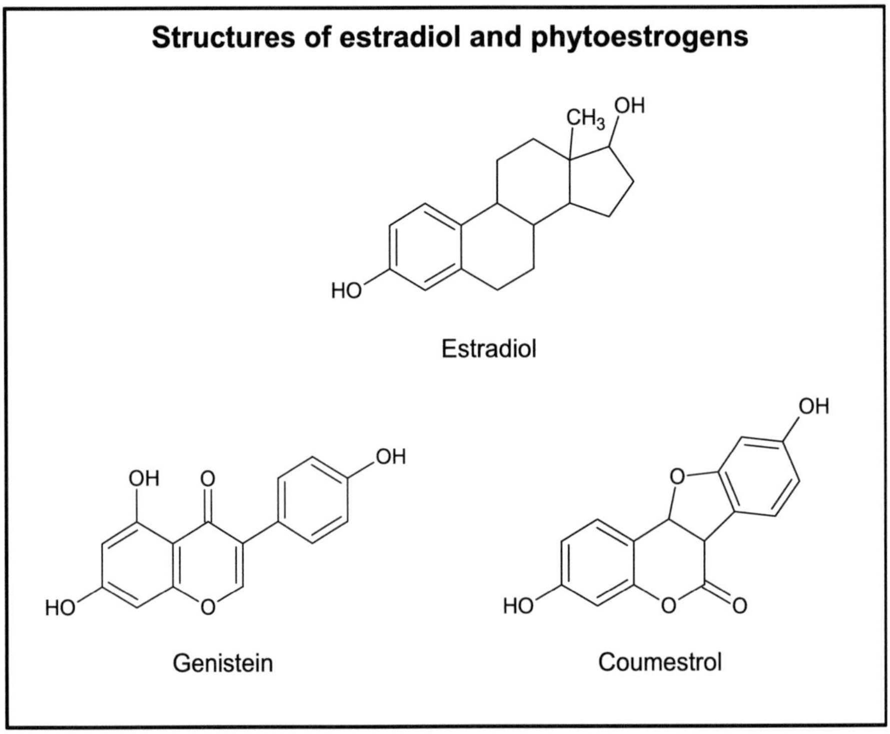

Fig. 3. Structures of isoflavones and coumestans compared with estrogen
The structure of estradiol, a natural estrogen, is shown along with the structures of genistein, a prototypic isoflavone found in soy, and coumestrol, a prototypic coumestan.

4.2 Epidemiology data on phytoestrogens and cardiovascular disease

While typical isoflavone intake is less than 1 mg per day in Western countries, intakes of 20-50 mg per day are common in Asian countries such as China and Japan, where soy is a traditional staple food (Adlercreutz & Mazur, 1997). These countries also have shown reduced incidence of cardiovascular disease compared with Western countries, an effect that is diminishing as Western eating habits and diets are adopted.

4.3 Biological activities of phytoestrogens

Dietary phytoestrogens may play an important role in prevention of menopausal symptoms, osteoporosis, cancer, and cardiovascular disease. The major mechanisms of biological action for the phytoestrogens are those mediated by estrogen receptors (estrogenic and antiestrogenic effects), effects on tyrosine kinase and DNA topoisomerase activities, suppression of angiogenesis, and antioxidant effects.

Although not as active as 17β-estradiol, phytoestrogens compete with estradiol for binding to estrogen receptors (ER), particularly ERβ (Kuiper et al., 1998). ERβ, present in high concentrations in ovary and testis, binds phytoestrogens with higher affinity, and may mediate some of their biological effects (Kuiper et al., 1998). Alternatively, soy isoflavones may be natural selective estrogen receptor modulators (SERMs) with both agonist and antagonist activities (Setchell, 2001).

Soy isoflavones decrease total cholesterol, LDL, and triglycerides, and increase HDL levels (Clarkson et al., 2001). They also lower blood pressure and improve endothelial reactivity (Teede et al., 2001, Steinberg et al., 2003). Supplementation of isoflavones derived from red clover containing genistein, daidzein, biochanin, and formononetin significantly improved arterial compliance in elderly men and women (Nestel et al., 1999).

Several studies reveal the potential of phytoestrogens to induce hormone-dependent cancers (e.g. breast and endometrium) (McMichael-Phillips et al., 1998), leading to safety concerns. Because of this, a maximum daily intake level for phytoestrogens has been suggested in several countries (Sirtori et al., 2005).

Summary of key points

Omega-3 fatty acids

- Important omega-3 fatty acids include EPA and DHA
- Mechanisms for omega-3 fatty acids include
  -reduced inflammation due to decreased prostaglandin and leukotriene synthesis
  -reduced thrombosis and platelet aggregation
  -direct antiarrythmic effects in cell membranes
- Large studies confirm that omega-3 fatty acid intake reduces cardiovascular disease and sudden death
- The American Heart Association recommends eating fish twice a week, and daily intake of 1 g EPA and DHA to reduce cardiovascular disease

Vitamin E

- Vitamin E is an essential fat soluble vitamin that is an antioxidant
- Animal studies do not uniformly show beneficial effects
- Vitamin E reduced cardiovascular risk in two studies (CHAOS and SPACE), but not in others (GISSI, HOPE-TOO)
- Vitamin E supplementation has been associated with higher incidence of heart failure, so routine supplementation with vitamin E is *not* recommended

Phytoestrogens

- Phytoestrogens, including soy isoflavones, are plant compounds with chemical structures that resemble estrogens
- Mechanisms include improved lipid profiles and improved endothelial reactivity
- Phytoestrogens may induce hormone dependent cancers (breast and endometrial), leading to recommendations on maximum daily intake

5. Conclusions and evidence-based recommendations

Omega-3 fatty acids have been clearly shown in epidemiological studies and clinical trials to reduce the incidence of cardiovascular disease. Thus, the American Heart Association recommends eating fish (particularly fatty fish) at least twice a week. They also recommend foods rich in ALA (flaxseed, canola, and soybean oils; flaxseed and walnuts). For patients with documented coronary heart disease, the recommended level of consumption is 1 g of EPA+DHA per day, either from fish (preferably), or supplementation. For subjects with elevated triglyceride levels, 2-4 grams of EPA+DHA is recommended as supplementation (Kris-Etherton et al., 2002).

At this time, the evidence does not justify the use of vitamin E supplements for CVD risk reduction, both because of lack of evidence for benefit and possible adverse effect reflected in the increases in all-cause mortality and hemorrhagic stroke. However, a balanced diet with emphasis on antioxidant-rich fruits, vegetables, and whole grains is recommended (Kris-Etherton et al., 2004). Whether antioxidant vitamin supplements including vitamin E influence the development of diabetes, in which oxidative stress plays an important role, is not clear and warrants further investigation.

Supplementing the diet with soy protein has failed to confirm phytoestrogens as the responsible agent for beneficial cardiovascular effects. Furthermore, soy phytoestrogens may increase carcinogenesis. Thus, isoflavone supplements are not currently recommended (Sacks et al., 2006). Soy foods may still be beneficial to cardiovascular and overall health because of their high content of polyunsaturated fats, fiber, vitamins, and minerals and low content of saturated fat (Krauss et al., 2000).

Epidemiologic evidence has suggested an array of potentially beneficial compounds in foods. While there have been many mechanistic studies in the laboratory or in animal models, large scale randomized controlled clinical trials are necessary to prove or disprove their effects on health and safety, particularly in light of possible toxicities. Until the results of such studies are available, a diet consistent with American Heart Association recommendations (Kris-Etherton et al., 2004), with emphasis on antioxidant-rich fruits, vegetables, and whole grains, appears to be the most sensible approach.

6. Acknowledgements

PLH acknowledges grant support from Public Health Service grant R01-NS33335 from the National Institute of Neurologic Diseases and Stroke, and grant R01-HL048426 from the National Heart Lung and Blood Institute.

7. References

Adlercreutz, H. and W. Mazur. (1997). Phyto-oestrogens and Western diseases. *Ann Med,* Vol. 29, pp. 95-120.

Boaz, M., S. Smetana, et al. (2000). Secondary prevention with antioxidants of cardiovascular disease in endstage renal disease (SPACE): randomised placebo-controlled trial. *Lancet,* Vol. 356, pp. 1213-8.

Brouwer, I. A., P. L. Zock, et al. (2006). Effect of fish oil on ventricular tachyarrhythmia and death in patients with implantable cardioverter defibrillators: the Study on Omega-

3 Fatty Acids and Ventricular Arrhythmia (SOFA) randomized trial. *Jama,* Vol. 295, pp. 2613-9.

Calder, P. C. (2006). n-3 polyunsaturated fatty acids, inflammation, and inflammatory diseases. *Am J Clin Nutr,* Vol. 83, pp. 1505S-1519S.

Clarkson, T. B., M. S. Anthony, et al. (2001). Inhibition of postmenopausal atherosclerosis progression: a comparison of the effects of conjugated equine estrogens and soy phytoestrogens. *J Clin Endocrinol Metab,* Vol. 86, pp. 41-7.

Devaraj, S., D. Li, et al. (1996). The effects of alpha tocopherol supplementation on monocyte function. Decreased lipid oxidation, interleukin 1 beta secretion, and monocyte adhesion to endothelium. *J Clin Invest,* Vol. 98, pp. 756-63.

Dolecek, T. A. (1992). Epidemiological evidence of relationships between dietary polyunsaturated fatty acids and mortality in the multiple risk factor intervention trial. *Proc Soc Exp Biol Med,* Vol. 200, pp. 177-82.

Dyerberg, J., H. O. Bang, et al. (1975). Fatty acid composition of the plasma lipids in Greenland Eskimos. *Am J Clin Nutr,* Vol. 28, pp. 958-66.

Facchini, F. S., M. H. Humphreys, et al. (2000). Relation between insulin resistance and plasma concentrations of lipid hydroperoxides, carotenoids, and tocopherols. *Am J Clin Nutr,* Vol. 72, pp. 776-9.

Fernandez, M. L., E. C. Lin, et al. (1992). Differential effects of saturated fatty acids on low density lipoprotein metabolism in the guinea pig. *J Lipid Res,* Vol. 33, pp. 1833-42.

Fernandez, M. L. and D. J. McNamar. (1989). Dietary fat-mediated changes in hepatic apoprotein B/E receptor in the guinea pig: effect of polyunsaturated, monounsaturated, and saturated fat. *Metabolism,* Vol. 38, pp. 1094-102.

Fernandez, M. L. and K. L. West. (2005). Mechanisms by which dietary fatty acids modulate plasma lipids. *J Nutr,* Vol. 135, pp. 2075-8.

Ferre, N., J. Camps, et al. (2001). Effects of high-fat, low-cholesterol diets on hepatic lipid peroxidation and antioxidants in apolipoprotein E-deficient mice. *Mol Cell Biochem,* Vol. 218, pp. 165-9.

Field, F. J., E. Born, et al. (2003). Fatty acid flux suppresses fatty acid synthesis in hamster intestine independently of SREBP-1 expression. *J Lipid Res,* Vol. 44, pp. 1199-208.

Fisher, M., P. H. Levine, et al. (1990). Dietary n-3 fatty acid supplementation reduces superoxide production and chemiluminescence in a monocyte-enriched preparation of leukocytes. *Am J Clin Nutr,* Vol. 51, pp. 804-8.

Gey, K. F., P. Puska, et al. (1991). Inverse correlation between plasma vitamin E and mortality from ischemic heart disease in cross-cultural epidemiology. *Am J Clin Nutr,* Vol. 53, pp. 326S-334S.

GISSI. (1999). Dietary supplementation with n-3 polyunsaturated fatty acids and vitamin E after myocardial infarction: results of the GISSI-Prevenzione trial. Gruppo Italiano per lo Studio della Sopravvivenza nell'Infarto miocardico. *Lancet,* Vol. 354, pp. 447-55.

Goodnight, S. H., M. Fisher, et al. (1989). Assessment of the therapeutic use of dietary fish oil in atherosclerotic vascular disease and thrombosis. *Chest,* Vol. 95, pp. 19S-25S.

Ho, E. and T. M. Bray. (1999). Antioxidants, NFkappaB activation, and diabetogenesis. *Proc Soc Exp Biol Med,* Vol. 222, pp. 205-13.

Hughes, D. A., A. C. Pinder, et al. (1996). Fish oil supplementation inhibits the expression of major histocompatibility complex class II molecules and adhesion molecules on human monocytes. *Am J Clin Nutr,* Vol. 63, pp. 267-72.

Illingworth, D. R. and E. B. Schmidt. (1993). The influence of dietary n-3 fatty acids on plasma lipids and lipoproteins. *Ann N Y Acad Sci,* Vol. 676, pp. 60-9.

Jump, D. B. (2002). Dietary polyunsaturated fatty acids and regulation of gene transcription. *Curr Opin Lipidol,* Vol. 13, pp. 155-64.

Kang, J. X., Y. F. Xiao, et al. (1995). Free, long-chain, polyunsaturated fatty acids reduce membrane electrical excitability in neonatal rat cardiac myocytes. *Proc Natl Acad Sci U S A,* Vol. 92, pp. 3997-4001.

Kelley, D. S., P. C. Taylor, et al. (1999). Docosahexaenoic acid ingestion inhibits natural killer cell activity and production of inflammatory mediators in young healthy men. *Lipids,* Vol. 34, pp. 317-24.

Krauss, R. M., R. H. Eckel, et al. (2000). AHA Dietary Guidelines: revision 2000: A statement for healthcare professionals from the Nutrition Committee of the American Heart Association. *Circulation,* Vol. 102, pp. 2284-99.

Kris-Etherton, P. M., W. S. Harris, et al. (2002). Fish consumption, fish oil, omega-3 fatty acids, and cardiovascular disease. *Circulation,* Vol. 106, pp. 2747-57.

Kris-Etherton, P. M., A. H. Lichtenstein, et al. (2004). Antioxidant vitamin supplements and cardiovascular disease. *Circulation,* Vol. 110, pp. 637-41.

Kuiper, G. G., J. G. Lemmen, et al. (1998). Interaction of estrogenic chemicals and phytoestrogens with estrogen receptor beta. *Endocrinology,* Vol. 139, pp. 4252-63.

Kurzer, M. S. and X. Xu. (1997). Dietary phytoestrogens. *Annu Rev Nutr,* Vol. 17, pp. 353-81.

Kushi, L. H., A. R. Folsom, et al. (1996). Dietary antioxidant vitamins and death from coronary heart disease in postmenopausal women. *N Engl J Med,* Vol. 334, pp. 1156-62.

Leaf, A., J. X. Kang, et al. (2003). Clinical prevention of sudden cardiac death by n-3 polyunsaturated fatty acids and mechanism of prevention of arrhythmias by n-3 fish oils. *Circulation,* Vol. 107, pp. 2646-52.

Lichtenstein, A. H., L. J. Appel, et al. (2006). Diet and lifestyle recommendations revision 2006: a scientific statement from the American Heart Association Nutrition Committee. *Circulation,* Vol. 114, pp. 82-96.

Lloyd-Jones, D., R. Adams, et al. (2009). Heart disease and stroke statistics--2009 update: a report from the American Heart Association Statistics Committee and Stroke Statistics Subcommittee. *Circulation,* Vol. 119, pp. 480-6.

Lonn, E., J. Bosch, et al. (2005). Effects of long-term vitamin E supplementation on cardiovascular events and cancer: a randomized controlled trial. *Jama,* Vol. 293, pp. 1338-47.

Marchioli, R., F. Barzi, et al. (2002). Early protection against sudden death by n-3 polyunsaturated fatty acids after myocardial infarction: time-course analysis of the results of the Gruppo Italiano per lo Studio della Sopravvivenza nell'Infarto Miocardico (GISSI)-Prevenzione. *Circulation,* Vol. 105, pp. 1897-903.

Mayer-Davis, E. J., T. Costacou, et al. (2002). Plasma and dietary vitamin E in relation to incidence of type 2 diabetes: The Insulin Resistance and Atherosclerosis Study (IRAS). *Diabetes Care,* Vol. 25, pp. 2172-7.

McCullough, M. L., D. Feskanich, et al. (2000). Adherence to the Dietary Guidelines for Americans and risk of major chronic disease in men. *Am J Clin Nutr,* Vol. 72, pp. 1223-31.

McMichael-Phillips, D. F., C. Harding, et al. (1998). Effects of soy-protein supplementation on epithelial proliferation in the histologically normal human breast. *Am J Clin Nutr,* Vol. 68, pp. 1431S-1435S.

Meagher, E. A., O. P. Barry, et al. (2001). Effects of vitamin E on lipid peroxidation in healthy persons. *Jama,* Vol. 285, pp. 1178-82.

Miller, E. R., 3rd, R. Pastor-Barriuso, et al. (2005). Meta-analysis: high-dosage vitamin E supplementation may increase all-cause mortality. *Ann Intern Med,* Vol. 142, pp. 37-46.

Mozaffarian, D., R. N. Lemaitre, et al. (2003). Cardiac benefits of fish consumption may depend on the type of fish meal consumed: the Cardiovascular Health Study. *Circulation,* Vol. 107, pp. 1372-7.

Munday, J. S., K. G. Thompson, et al. (1998). Dietary antioxidants do not reduce fatty streak formation in the C57BL/6 mouse atherosclerosis model. *Arterioscler Thromb Vasc Biol,* Vol. 18, pp. 114-9.

Nagata, C., N. Takatsuka, et al. (2002). Soy and fish oil intake and mortality in a Japanese community. *Am J Epidemiol,* Vol. 156, pp. 824-31.

Nair, S. S., J. Leitch, et al. (1999). Cardiac (n-3) non-esterified fatty acids are selectively increased in fish oil-fed pigs following myocardial ischemia. *J Nutr,* Vol. 129, pp. 1518-23.

Nestel, P. J., S. Pomeroy, et al. (1999). Isoflavones from red clover improve systemic arterial compliance but not plasma lipids in menopausal women. *J Clin Endocrinol Metab,* Vol. 84, pp. 895-8.

Nilsen, D. W., G. Albrektsen, et al. (2001). Effects of a high-dose concentrate of n-3 fatty acids or corn oil introduced early after an acute myocardial infarction on serum triacylglycerol and HDL cholesterol. *Am J Clin Nutr,* Vol. 74, pp. 50-6.

Ogden, C. L., M. D. Carroll, et al. (2006). Prevalence of overweight and obesity in the United States, 1999-2004. *Jama,* Vol. 295, pp. 1549-55.

Paolisso, G., M. R. Tagliamonte, et al. (2000). Chronic vitamin E administration improves brachial reactivity and increases intracellular magnesium concentration in type II diabetic patients. *J Clin Endocrinol Metab,* Vol. 85, pp. 109-15.

Paul, A., L. Calleja, et al. (2001). Supplementation with vitamin E and/or zinc does not attenuate atherosclerosis in apolipoprotein E-deficient mice fed a high-fat, high-cholesterol diet. *Int J Vitam Nutr Res,* Vol. 71, pp. 45-52.

Raitt, M. H., W. E. Connor, et al. (2005). Fish oil supplementation and risk of ventricular tachycardia and ventricular fibrillation in patients with implantable defibrillators: a randomized controlled trial. *Jama,* Vol. 293, pp. 2884-91.

Reunanen, A., P. Knekt, et al. (1998). Serum antioxidants and risk of non-insulin dependent diabetes mellitus. *Eur J Clin Nutr,* Vol. 52, pp. 89-93.

Rimm, E. B., M. J. Stampfer, et al. (1993). Vitamin E consumption and the risk of coronary heart disease in men. *N Engl J Med,* Vol. 328, pp. 1450-6.

Sacks, F. M., A. Lichtenstein, et al. (2006). Soy protein, isoflavones, and cardiovascular health: an American Heart Association Science Advisory for professionals from the Nutrition Committee. *Circulation,* Vol. 113, pp. 1034-44.

Sacks, F. M., P. H. Stone, et al. (1995). Controlled trial of fish oil for regression of human coronary atherosclerosis. HARP Research Group. *J Am Coll Cardiol,* Vol. 25, pp. 1492-8.

Sesso, H. D., J. E. Buring, et al. (2008). Vitamins E and C in the prevention of cardiovascular disease in men: the Physicians' Health Study II randomized controlled trial. *Jama,* Vol. 300, pp. 2123-33.

Setchell, K. D. (2001). Soy isoflavones--benefits and risks from nature's selective estrogen receptor modulators (SERMs). *J Am Coll Nutr,* Vol. 20, pp. 354S-362S; discussion 381S-383S.

Shachter, N. S. (2001). Apolipoproteins C-I and C-III as important modulators of lipoprotein metabolism. *Curr Opin Lipidol,* Vol. 12, pp. 297-304.

Sirtori, C. R., A. Arnoldi, et al. (2005). Phytoestrogens: end of a tale? *Ann Med,* Vol. 37, pp. 423-38.

Stampfer, M. J., C. H. Hennekens, et al. (1993). Vitamin E consumption and the risk of coronary disease in women. *N Engl J Med,* Vol. 328, pp. 1444-9.

Steinberg, F. M., N. L. Guthrie, et al. (2003). Soy protein with isoflavones has favorable effects on endothelial function that are independent of lipid and antioxidant effects in healthy postmenopausal women. *Am J Clin Nutr,* Vol. 78, pp. 123-30.

Stephens, N. G., A. Parsons, et al. (1996). Randomised controlled trial of vitamin E in patients with coronary disease: Cambridge Heart Antioxidant Study (CHAOS). *Lancet,* Vol. 347, pp. 781-6.

Teede, H. J., F. S. Dalais, et al. (2001). Dietary soy has both beneficial and potentially adverse cardiovascular effects: a placebo-controlled study in men and postmenopausal women. *J Clin Endocrinol Metab,* Vol. 86, pp. 3053-60.

Thomas, S. R., S. B. Leichtweis, et al. (2001). Dietary cosupplementation with vitamin E and coenzyme Q(10) inhibits atherosclerosis in apolipoprotein E gene knockout mice. *Arterioscler Thromb Vasc Biol,* Vol. 21, pp. 585-93.

Vasandani, C., A. I. Kafrouni, et al. (2002). Upregulation of hepatic LDL transport by n-3 fatty acids in LDL receptor knockout mice. *J Lipid Res,* Vol. 43, pp. 772-84.

von Schacky, C., S. Fischer, et al. (1985). Long-term effects of dietary marine omega-3 fatty acids upon plasma and cellular lipids, platelet function, and eicosanoid formation in humans. *J Clin Invest,* Vol. 76, pp. 1626-31.

Wang, C., W. S. Harris, et al. (2006). n-3 Fatty acids from fish or fish-oil supplements, but not alpha-linolenic acid, benefit cardiovascular disease outcomes in primary- and secondary-prevention studies: a systematic review. *Am J Clin Nutr,* Vol. 84, pp. 5-17.

Waters, D. D., E. L. Alderman, et al. (2002). Effects of hormone replacement therapy and antioxidant vitamin supplements on coronary atherosclerosis in postmenopausal women: a randomized controlled trial. *Jama,* Vol. 288, pp. 2432-40.

Wu, B. J., K. Kathir, et al. (2006). Antioxidants protect from atherosclerosis by a heme oxygenase-1 pathway that is independent of free radical scavenging. *J Exp Med,* Vol. 203, pp. 1117-27.

Ylonen, K., G. Alfthan, et al. (2003). Dietary intakes and plasma concentrations of carotenoids and tocopherols in relation to glucose metabolism in subjects at high risk of type 2 diabetes: the Botnia Dietary Study. *Am J Clin Nutr,* Vol. 77, pp. 1434-41.

Yusuf, S., G. Dagenais, et al. (2000). Vitamin E supplementation and cardiovascular events in high-risk patients. The Heart Outcomes Prevention Evaluation Study Investigators. *N Engl J Med,* Vol. 342, pp. 154-60.

Zhou, L. and A. Nilsson. (2001). Sources of eicosanoid precursor fatty acid pools in tissues. *J Lipid Res,* Vol. 42, pp. 1521-42.

21

Mediterranean Diet and Cardiovascular Risk

Javier Delgado-Lista, Ana I. Perez-Caballero, Pablo Perez-Martinez, Antonio Garcia-Rios, Jose Lopez-Miranda and Francisco Perez-Jimenez
Unidad de Lipidos y Arteriosclerosis, IMIBIC/Hospital Universitario Reina Sofia, Universidad de Cordoba, Ciber Fisiopatología Obesidad y Nutrición (CIBEROBN), Instituto de Salud Carlos III, Spain

1. Introduction

The Mediterranean diet is becoming a generalized recommended eating pattern worldwide, especially after epidemiological studies showing that adherence to this model is associated with a lower total mortality and cardiovascular diseases. Some of the conditions in which this dietary model has proven to be linked with a lower incidence are coronary events, stroke, hypertension, unfavorable blood glucose control, age cognitive decline or certain types of cancer (D. Giugliano & Esposito, 2008; Kontou et al., 2011; Lopez-Miranda et al., 2010; Solfrizzi et al., 2011; Tangney et al., 2011; Willett, 2006). Although the underlying mechanisms by which this type of diet may exert its beneficial functions are far from being totally understood, current knowledge states that these are beyond the classical cardiovascular risk factors like lipids or the control or blood pressure, and involve, among others, inflammation, oxidative stress, coagulation and endothelial function.

One of the aspects to be taken into account when considering the effects of Mediterranean Diet is the heterogeneity of this concept, comprising different dietary patterns, slightly differing between the different countries in which this diet was originally consumed, because of local foodstuff preferences. The Mediterranean Diet includes a high consumption of food from plant origin (fruits, vegetables, nuts and grains), using olive oil (preferably extra virgin) as the main source of fat, used both as a cooking vehicle as for seasoning, although some other sources of monounsaturated fatty acids as the main dietary fat have been recently proposed. Mediterranean Diet preferred sources of protein are fish and poultry, while red meats are rarely consumed. Additionally, the use of sweets, pastry and dairy products are also of exceptional use. The use of milk and milk derived products, like yoghourt or cheese is moderated in most of the Mediterranean models, although with some country variations, with higher consumers, like the Greek dietary pattern. Finally, in some of the Mediterranean countries (like Spain, France and Italy) there is a common moderate consumption of red wine. These characteristics are summarized in figure 1.

The current interest in this type of food comes from the conjunction of a increasingly scientific evidence of the advantages of its consumption in different health aspects and its high palatability, which validates it for long use purposes, contrarily to other healthy alternatives with low palatability, which are difficult to maintain on a long outlook basis(Panunzio et al., 2011). Supporting the cited scientific evidences on cardiovascular risk, and validated by well designed works(Fuentes et al., 2001; Jansen et al., 2000; Kris-Etherton et al., 1993; Mata et al., 1992), the FDA authorized a health claim on olive oil on coronary heart disease (CFSAN/Office of Nutritional Products, 2004).

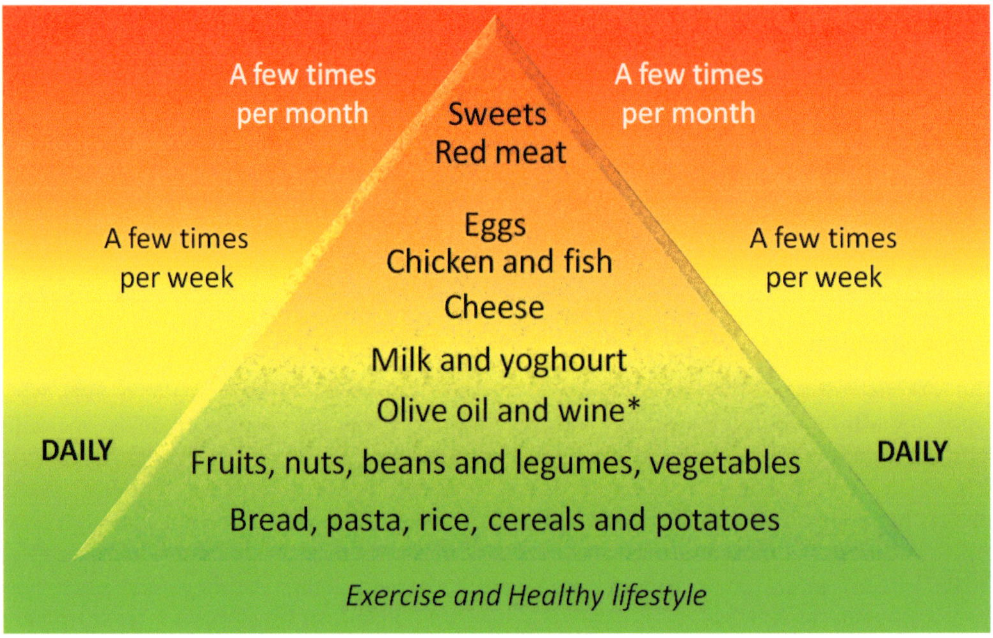

Fig. 1. Schematic representation of a Mediterranean diet pyramid. * Wine is only recommended in those adults that already consume it, or are willing to do it, and always with moderation (lower than 200 cc/day). In no case wine consumption must be started only to comply with the Mediterranean diet.

As stated above, there is a plenty of conditions and physiological features where Mediterranean Diet has shown to be beneficial, from digestive tract motility to neurologic cognitive wellness in the aged persons, or the apparition of some types of cancer (D. Giugliano & Esposito, 2008; Kontou et al., 2011; Lopez-Miranda et al., 2010; Solfrizzi et al., 2011; Tangney et al., 2011; Willett, 2006). However, we will only revise in the present document some of the evidences relating Mediterranean Diet and cardiovascular risk.

Assessing the modification of the cardiovascular risk by diet is a difficult task, specially having into account that cardiovascular risk assessment tools are not strictly uniform. Moreover, some of the increasingly accepted newer cardiovascular risk factors, like inflammation, thrombogenic state, postprandial lipemia, oxidative stress or endothelial function are not still included in the classical risk assessment tools. Finally, assessing the impact of the diet in different geographic locations has the risk of underestimate other diet related circumstances, like the fact of eating at home, eating out, the relative well-being or stress associated meal-time, or other interactions between eating and other behavior factors (like, for example meal-associated smoke consumption). In a recent article, it has been stated that the effects of Mediterranean Diet on total mortality increases when combined with other healthy lifestyle factors, like , nonsmoking, normal weight [BMI (in kg/m(2)): 18.5 to <25], and regular physical activity (van den Brandt, 2011). On the other hand, we cannot forget the interaction between the diet and the genetics of the population investigated, the so called nutrigenetics. The consumption of a nutrient may be more or less healthy in a given population depending on that population genetics(Allayee et al., 2009; Lairon et al., 2009; Lovegrove & Gitau, 2008; Ordovas, 2006; Perez-Martinez et al., 2010a; Perez-Martinez et al., 2011b).

The purpose of this review is to present some evidence of studies which have already demonstrated the benefitial effects of the Mediterranean Diet in the different cardiovascular risk factors, and discuss the underlying mechanisms by which it exerts its effects. We will also review the different studies that link the consumption of this dietary model with a lower prevalence of cardiovascular disease.

2. Mediterranean Diet and lipids

The concentration of total cholesterol in plasma, as well as that of its fractions (HDL, LDL) is clearly related to cardiovascular risk, and hence they are included in the most used cardiovascular risk assessment tools, the Frammingham cardiovascular risk tables (N.C.E.P., 2001) and the European SCORE risk tool (HeartScore, 2003). While total cholesterol and LDL cholesterol are directly correlated to the risk, this relationship is reverse with HDL cholesterol. Triglycerides, which were not classically considered when assessing cardiovascular risk, have been recently identified as clear modifiers of cardiovascular risk, even independently of cholesterol, and an enlarged postprandial lipemia (which mainly involves triglyceride and triglyceride rich lipoproteins metabolism) has been identified as one of the major cardiovascular risk factors (Bayturan et al., 2010; Kolovou et al., 2011; Langsted et al., 2011; Lopez-Miranda et al., 2006; Patel et al., 2004; Sarwar et al., 2007; van Wijk et al., 2009; Varbo et al., 2011).

When considering the effects of the different types of diet on plasma lipids, studies have mainly centered on the effects of the fatty components of the diet studied in the lipid profile. For the studies dealing with Mediterranean Diet, this fact has driven to the study of the effects on lipids of olive oil as a food and of monounsaturated fatty acids as dietary fatty acids. With that scope it has been proved that lipid profile becomes healthier when Mediterranean diets rich in monounsaturated fats replace diets rich in saturated fatty acids rich diets, reducing LDL cholesterol, and the ratio total cholesterol/HDL.

The above effects were evaluated and corroborated by the FDA, when it approved the health claim on olive oil in 2004, authorizing the inclusion of the following sentence in the labeling of the olive oil bottles: *Limited and not conclusive scientific evidence suggests that eating about two tablespoons (23 grams) of olive oil daily may reduce the risk of coronary heart disease due to the monounsaturated fat in olive oil. To achieve this possible benefit, olive oil is to replace a similar amount of saturated fat and not increase the total number of calories you eat in a day* (CFSAN/Office of Nutritional Products, 2004).

Furthermore and complementing the favorable effects of olive oil, there has been extensively proven the beneficial effects of vegetables, fruits and pulse when replacing foods rich in saturated fatty acids, like butter, pork or red meat, reducing total cholesterol, triglycerides and LDL cholesterol (Bach-Faig et al., 2006; Lapointe et al., 2005; Mordente et al., 2011;

Pitsavos et al., 2005; Tripoli et al., 2005; Visioli & Galli, 1998; Yubero-Serrano et al., 2011). In addition, LDL resistance to oxidation is augmented when Mediterranean Diet rich in Olive Oil replaces diets rich in saturated fats. It is known that oxidation of LDL cholesterol is a key factor in the development of the atherosclerosis, promoting the formation of foam cells in the sub-endothelial space of the vascular wall. The underlying cause of this latter effect seems to be a combination of the monounsaturated fatty acids from olive oil, the antioxidant power of the minor compounds present in virgin olive oil, like phenols, and the elevated antioxidant capacity of the fruits and vegetables. Furthermore, a recent report from the European Food Safety Authority (EFSA) supports the effects of virgin olive oil phenols on LDL oxidation(EFSA, 2011). Lycopene, a carotenoid abundant in the tomato also deserves a mention, by its biochemical functions including acting as antioxidant scavenger, hypolipaemic agent, or inhibitor of pro-inflammatory and pro-thrombotic factors(Mordente et al., 2011). Additionally, resveratrol, a natural antioxidant present in red wine seems to play a role in this antioxidant effect on LDL cholesterol(Mukamal & Rimm, 2008).

3. Mediterranean Diet and blood pressure

The influence of diet on blood pressure is well established. Diets rich in vegetables, like Mediterranean diet, reduce systolic and diastolic blood pressure (Alonso et al., 2006; Gillingham et al., 2011; Masala et al., 2008). These effects have been directly assessed in Mediterranean diet, and again they seem to be due to a combination of the favorable effects of olive oil, vegetables and fish (Alonso et al., 2004; Bondia-Pons et al., 2007; Din et al., 2004; Esposito et al., 2004; Fito et al., 2005; Gillingham et al., 2011; Masala et al., 2008; Perona et al., 2004). In fact, and supporting that the effect of olive oil is independent of the population studied or the dietary pattern, a north-european cohort who consumed olive oil as a part of their habitual diet reduced their blood pressure when switching their main fat source to olive oil(Bondia-Pons et al., 2007). A recent review summarized all the current information on the effects of monounsaturated fatty acids in blood pressure. In overall of the 16 studies analyzed, the authors reported that strong support can be obtained from clinical trials of the blood pressure lowering effects of MUFA rich diets in both normotensive and hypertensive individuals (Gillingham et al., 2011).

Not only the nutrient intake, but also the fiber content influences blood pressure. When adjusted by other possible confounders, the relative high percentage of the Mediterranean Diet is linked to a lower blood pressure (Alonso et al., 2006; Estruch et al., 2009). When studying the micronutrients responsible of these effects, the monounsaturated fats, the phenols from olive oil and vegetables and the n-3 fatty acids from fish seem to be implicated, as well as the relative low sodium levels achieved by vegetables compared to meat and the alcohol present in red wine, among others (Fito et al., 2005; Geleijnse et al., 2002; Masala et al., 2008; B. M. Rasmussen et al., 2006; Shah et al., 2007).

4. Mediterranean Diet and smoking effects on cardiovascular disease

Although the smoking habit is detrimental for the health in any dietary habit, the influence of the diet in the deleterious effects of smoking on health has not been widely studied. Epidemiological studies indicate that a high adherence to the Mediterranean Diet model is associated with a reduction of the risk conferred by the smoking habit (Haveman-Nies et al.,

2002; Mitrou et al., 2007). A recent work reviewed this topic in deep (Vardavas et al., 2011), and concludes, that, existing scientific literature indicates that the dietary intake of Mediterranean diet, can act as a positive effect modifier on the impact of smoking on cardiovascular health. When looking for underlying mechanisms, authors postulate two main hypothetical *vias*. Mediterranean Diet is rich in antioxidants. How we explained above, LDL resistance to oxidation in augmented when the person consumes Mediterranean Diet, and, thus, this person could be partially protected to the tobacco-induced LDL-oxidation. On the other hand, the increase of the HDL/total cholesterol provoked by the Mediterranean Diet could partially blunt the development of atherosclerosis caused by the smoking habit (Mitrou et al., 2007).

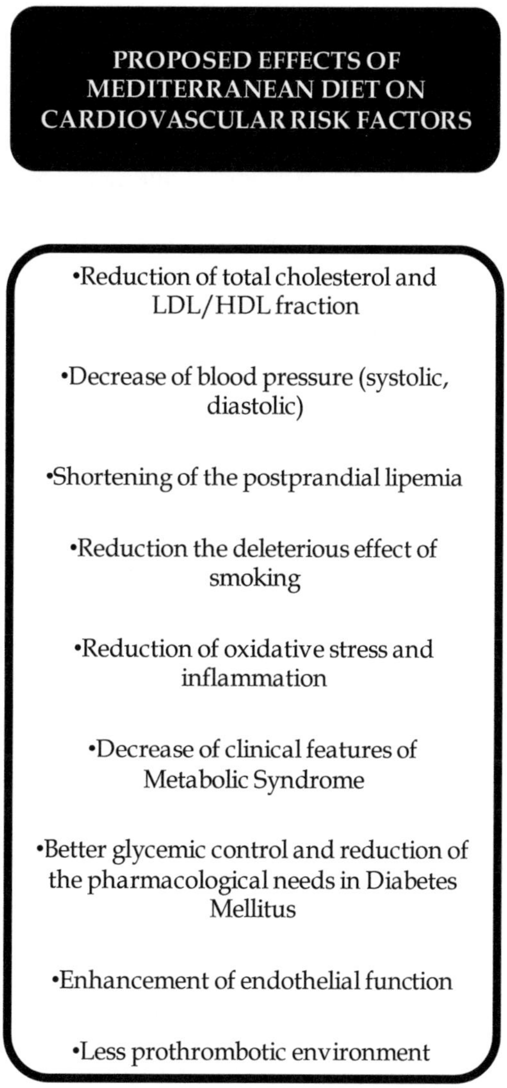

Fig. 2. Proposed mechanisms for the healthy effects of Mediterranean diet on Cardiovascular Disease.

5. Mediterranean Diet and hemostasis

Haemostatic system includes platelets and coagulation factors. It is devoted to maintain the optimal blood flow integrity, and to repair the vessels injuries. However, it has been firmly established that an unbalance of this system is a key factor in the development of atherosclerosis(Borissoff et al., 2011). The development of the plaque and its eventual rupture are favored by an increase in plasma of certain coagulation factors and platelet mediators. Diet can modulate the haemostatic equilibrium. Diets rich in fish, (especially blue fish) has an antiaggregant effect, mainly due to its content of n-3 fatty acids, which interferes with platelets metabolism(Renaud & Lanzmann-Petithory, 2002; Seo et al., 2005). Furthermore, the direct effect of n-3 fatty acids reducing cardiovascular events and cardiovascular mortality has been proved both in epidemiological studies and clinical trials, although some recent studies failed to find such advantages(Filion et al., 2010; Harris et al., 2008; Lavie et al., 2009; Mente et al., 2009; Riediger et al., 2009). Currently, the AHA recommends two servings of blue fish a week for general population (to maintain a mean of 500 mg/d), and 1 g/d of marine omega-3 (EPA and DHA) in patients with coronary disease to lower cardiovascular risk, although safety issues due to the presence of harmful metals like mercury in large fish, like tuna or shark currently advices to take this recommendation with caution in pregnant women and little child (Kris-Etherton et al., 2002; Lichtenstein et al., 2006).

The same antiaggregant effect has been also find associated to the intake of olive oil, especially extra virgin olive oil, which has been justified by the presence of oleic acid and the minor components of virgin olive oil, like phenols. The underlying mechanisms for theses effects include tromboxane reduction, decrease of ADP reactivity and ATP release from platelets, decrease of platelet-activating factor (Antonopoulou et al., 2006; Karantonis et al., 2002; Karantonis et al., 2006; Perez-Jimenez et al., 2006; Singh et al., 2008; Sirtori et al., 1986; Smith et al., 2003). Effects of wine, a common element in certain countries consuming Mediterranean Diet have been also examined in some studies, but results are inconclusive. While its moderate consumption decreases some procoagulant species, like fibrinogen, and increase the natural anticoagulant TPA, also increases some proinflammatory markers (ICAM-1, E-Selectin, interleukin-6), and even may lead to an increase in total platelet aggregation (Mezzano & Leighton, 2003; Tozzi Ciancarelli et al., 2011). Hereby, more studies are needed to unveil its overall influence on haemostasis.

The effects of olive oil in haemostasis go beyond platelets, and influences directly the plasma concentration of several procoagulant substances, like FVII (Delgado-Lista et al., 2008; Junker et al., 2001a; Junker et al., 2001b; Mezzano & Leighton, 2003; Mezzano et al., 2003; Smith et al., 2003; Temme et al., 1999; Turpeinen & Mutanen, 1999; Williams, 2001), tissue factor (Bravo-Herrera et al., 2004), fibrinogen (Mezzano & Leighton, 2003), PAI-1 factor (Avellone et al., 1998; Perez-Jimenez, 2005; Perez-Jimenez et al., 1999; Perez-Jimenez et al., 2002) or von Willebrand Factor (Perez-Jimenez et al., 1999; O. Rasmussen et al., 1994), reducing the thrombogenic state when compared to diets rich in saturated fatty acids. Interestingly, these features have been found both in the fasting state and in the postprandial state, and have been also found, although to a lesser extent, associated to the consumption of nuts, other well represented food of Mediterranean diet(Delgado-Lista et al., 2008). These and other evidences of the beneficial influence of components of the Mediterranean diet have been published elsewhere(Delgado-Lista et al., 2011a; Delgado-

Lista et al., 2007; Lopez-Miranda et al., 2007; Mezzano et al., 2003; Mordente et al., 2011). In summary, there are clear evidences on the healthy effects of components of the Mediterranean Diet in reducing the procoagulant and proagreggant species that promote atherosclerosis and eventual coronary events. These foods include extra virgin olive oil, vegetables, nuts and blue fish, and are supported by organizations like the FDA and the AHA(CFSAN/Office of Nutritional Products, 2004; Kris-Etherton et al., 2002).

6. Mediterranean Diet and endothelial function

In the new concepts of atherogenesis, the endothelial cells play a pivotal role in controlling the first steps and the final events of atherothombosis. The proper function of the vascular endothelium is essential to maintain a correct vasodilatation, but also to correctly regulate the metabolism of many other players involved in the atherogenesis, like the inflammatory cells, or the platelets. Meals rich in olive oil have a favorable effect on the postprandial vasomotor function of the endothelium, enhancing the vasodilator capacity during this phase, compared to meals rich in saturated fats, but also affect favorably other circulating markers of endothelial function. These effects are carried out, at least partly, by the minor compounds of virgin olive oil (Fuentes et al., 2008; Fuentes et al., 2001; Perez-Jimenez et al., 1999; Perez-Martinez et al., 2010c; Rallidis et al., 2009; Ruano et al., 2005), and may be also mediated by a lesser activation of leukocytes, a lower inflammation, and a higher bioavailability of nitric oxide (Carluccio et al., 2007; Covas, 2007; Davis et al., 2007; Fuentes et al., 2008; Leighton & Urquiaga, 2007; Perez-Jimenez et al., 1999; Perez-Jimenez et al., 2007; Perez-Martinez et al., 2010b; Perona et al., 2006; Schini-Kerth et al., 2010; Serra-Majem et al., 2006; Visioli et al., 2005). Apart from olive oil, other important players in the effects of Mediterranean diet on endothelial function are nuts, fish and vegetables, all contributing to the wellbeing of this organ by promoting a lower proinflammatory, prooxidant environment(Estruch, 2010; Harris et al., 2003; Mena et al., 2009; Nadtochiy & Redman, 2011; Papoutsi et al., 2008). Furthermore, it has been recently shown that people following Mediterranean Diet improve the regenerative capacity of the endothelium(Marin et al., 2011) and that elderly persons may partially blunt the oxidative processes associated to aging by adhering to Mediterranean diet, especially when combined with a rich antioxidant environment(Gutierrez-Mariscal et al., 2011).

7. Mediterranean Diet, obesity, metabolic syndrome and type 2 diabetes mellitus

The burden of a epidemic of obesity in modern countries has arisen the importance in public health strategies to search for dietary models reducing the incidence of obesity, and the related metabolic syndrome and type 2 diabetes mellitus, these two latter conditions characterized by a high cardiovascular risk.

Mediterranean Diet is an effective model to replace saturated fat rich diets, when looking for a healthy model to recommend to these persons. In fact, adherence to Mediterranean diet is inversely associated with the clustering of diabetes mellitus, obesity, hypertension and hypercholesterolemia (Sanchez-Tainta et al., 2008). Obesity rates are inversely associated with adherence to the Mediterranean diet on several observational cohorts (Beunza et al., 2010; Bullo et al., 2011; Mendez et al., 2006; Romaguera et al., 2009; Romaguera et al., 2010;

Schroder et al., 2004; Trichopoulou et al., 2005), which has been explained by the higher satiating effect of olive oil rich meals(Schwartz et al., 2008). A recent meta-analysis including 16 randomized clinical trials found Mediterranean Diet as a useful tool to reduce obesity, especially when accompanied by other healthy habits(Esposito et al., 2011). In a similar way, an inverse correlation between the prevalence of Metabolic Syndrome and the adherence to Mediterranean Diet has been extensively reported(Panagiotakos et al., 2004; Tortosa et al., 2007), and some interventional studies have replicated these findings, showing that persons who are submitted to a Mediterranean type diet have a lower probability to show Metabolic Syndrome, even on *ad libitum* dietary regimen (Esposito et al., 2004; Salas-Salvado et al., 2008). These findings are related to the beneficial effects shown by diets rich in fruits, vegetables, grains, fish and low-fat dairy products, with the additional value of olive oil, which prevents the redistribution of body fat from peripheral to visceral adipose tissue, and partially enhances the postprandial lipid disturbances found in the metabolic syndrome patients(Esmaillzadeh et al., 2007; Jimenez-Gomez et al., 2010; Lutsey et al., 2008; Paniagua et al., 2007b; Pereira et al., 2005). A recent statement from the European Atherosclerosis Society recently recommended the Mediterranean Diet as the tool to combat the Metabolic Syndrome(Stock, 2011) by its capacity to reduce all clinical criteria of the disease, based on a recent meta-analysis that reported that adherence to Mediterranean Diet is related to a decrease in waist circumference by 42 cm, increase in HDL cholesterol by 0.03 mmol/l, decrease of triglycerides by 0.07mmol/l, decrease in blood pressure (2.35/1.58 mm Hg), and decrease in blood glucose by 3.89 mg/dL(Kastorini et al., 2011)

With respect to type 2 diabetes, which is a frequent outcome in patients with sustained Metabolic Syndrome, it is reasonable to infer that Mediterranean Diet might prevent the development of diabetes or might improve the impaired metabolic status of the diabetic persons(D. Giugliano & Esposito, 2008; Perez-Martinez et al., 2011a). In fact, large prospective studies have shown that adherence to Mediterranean Diet is inversely correlated with the risk of presenting type 2 diabetes mellitus (Martinez-Gonzalez et al., 2008; Mozaffarian et al., 2007), which has been eventually corroborated (de Koning et al., 2011; Delgado-Lista et al., 2011b; F. Giugliano et al., 2010). Some authors have published, indeed, that changing from a saturated fat rich diet to a Mediterranean Diet results in a decrease of glycated hemoglobin of around 0.3-2.0%, which is close to the efficacy of some antidiabetic drugs, and allow to reduce pharmacological needs of these patients, which has also been reproduced when comparing Mediterranean Diet with a low fat diet (Elhayany et al., 2010; Itsiopoulos et al., 2010; Reisin, 2010). A recent randomized clinical trial showed that the risk of incident diabetes is reduced by more than 50% when Mediterranean Diet (either with or without supplements of nuts) is compared with the low-fat group ($p<0.05$)(Salas-Salvado et al., 2011a). Some of the underlying mechanisms by which Mediterranean Diet improves the diabetes control are improving insulin sensitivity and blood lipids(Riccardi et al., 2004), improving postprandial lipemia(Lopez et al., 2008), improving glucose homeostasis (Paniagua et al., 2007a) or improve the beta-cell insulin secretion (Rojo-Martinez et al., 2006). Furthermore, and linking Mediterranean Diet, type 2 diabetes and cardiovascular risk, it has been recently published that Mediterranean Diet is associated with a better prognosis in total and cardiovascular mortality in type 2 diabetics(Hodge et al., 2010) All the relationships between the Mediterranean Diet, obesity and diabetes have been recently published (Perez-Martinez et al., 2011a; Salas-Salvado et al., 2011b).

8. Mediterranean Diet and epidemiological evidences on reduced cardiovascular risk

The adherence to the Mediterranean Diet has been linked to a lower mortality by any cause and by cardiovascular disease in several observational studies, some of them including more than 350000 participants, like the NIH-AARP Diet and Health Study, where a high adherence to this dietary pattern resulted in an hazard ratio of 0.79 for all cause mortality, and of 0.83 for cardiovascular causes, which has been eventually corroborated (Mitrou et al., 2007; Serra-Majem et al., 2006). These data were included in an eventual meta-analysis (including more than 1.5 million persons), where it was stated that a rise of 2 points in a 9 points-scale of adherence to Mediterranean Diet was associated with a reduction of all cause mortality and cardiovascular mortality of about 10% (Sofi et al., 2008), which was eventually replicated in other meta-analysis(Sofi et al., 2010). In another meta-analysis, it has been state that a reduction of 5% of saturated by polyunsaturated fats result in a decrease of coronary risk (hazard ratio 0.87), while if this substitution was done by carbohydrates, there was no effect (Jakobsen et al., 2009). As stated previously, the Mediterranean Diet combines a high consumption of fish and a relative decrease in carbohydrates when compared with the low fat diets, which may combine the favored dietary patterns of the two above meta-analysis. Newer studies corroborate the inverse relationship between adherence to Mediterranean Diet and total mortality and cardiovascular death. High versus low adherence is accompanied was reported to be accompanied by a hazard ratio of 0.79 for total mortality, and 0.66 for cardiovascular death in a set of 40000 persons (Buckland et al., 2011). Furthermore, these effects are also evident in young cohorts. A recent report found a cardiovascular hazard ratio of 0.41 in 13000 young persons (mean age 38) with high versus low adherence to Mediterranean Diet(Martinez-Gonzalez et al., 2011)

Consequences of the non-fatal coronary event may also be limited by the Mediterranean Diet. A recent study has shown that left ventricle systolic dysfunction during hospitalization and the 2-y prognosis after an acute coronary syndrome are associated to the baseline diet. In this study, higher adherence to Mediterranean Diet was associated with less likelihood of developing left ventricle systolic dysfunction at hospitalization, less likelihood of remodeling (ejection fraction <50%) at 3 months of follow-up, and less likelihood of recurrent cardiovascular disease events during the 2 y of follow-up(Chrysohoou et al., 2010)

Other of the underlying mechanisms for the reduced cardiovascular incidence observed in persons eating Mediterranean Diet is by promoting an adequate cardiac rhythm. Although preliminary, there are data supporting that adherence to the Mediterranean Diet is linked to a lower probability of developing atrial fibrillation, and to promote its spontaneous conversion (Mattioli, 2011; Mattioli et al., 2011), and that it improves cardiac autonomic function, as assessed by an increased heart rate variability(Dai et al., 2010)

Cerebrovascular disease is a very common form of presentation of cardiovascular disease, which has not been so studied as coronary heart disease, in relationship with its interaction with diet. A recent study analyzed the impact of Mediterranean Diet on magnetic resonance imaging-assessed cerebrovascular disease. In a random sample of 700 elderly subjects, medium and high adherence to Mediterranean Diet elicited a 22 and 36% lower odds ratio for presenting evidence of infarcts on magnetic resonance imaging with respect to poor adherers (Scarmeas et al., 2011). In fact, adhering to nutritional features of Mediterranean Diet is more effective to act as secondary prevention for stroke than any single medication(Spence, 2010), even provoking the reversion of carotid atherosclerosis(Shai et al., 2010)

9. Causal links between Mediterranean Diet and cardiovascular events: The need for randomized clinical trials

With respect to clinical trials, two large dietary intervention trials with diet which used some features of the Mediterranean Diet were performed in Italy and France in the last years of the last century. The DART study evaluated the impact of three different dietary models (rich in fiber, low fat and rich in fish) in clinical outcomes of coronary patients. The use of two servings a week of fish was followed by a reduction of total mortality and cardiovascular death of about 30%, but the effects of other components of the Mediterranean Diet were not assessed (Burr et al., 1989).

The Lyon study evaluated the effect of one so-called Mediterranean Diet on the clinical outcomes of coronary patients. After 4 years of follow up, those who used the Mediterranean Diet lowered the recurrence of cardiovascular events by 50-70% (de Lorgeril et al., 1999). However, it must be said that the investigators used margarine rich in canola oil as their main fat source instead of olive oil, when this is not an usual component of the Mediterranean Diet. The reason for using such product was to provide high amounts of linolenic acid, a n-3 fatty acid of plant origin. Although the rest of the components of the diet that the author used matched the Mediterranean Diet characteristics, the use of the canola oil makes difficult to extrapolate the results to the traditional Mediterranean Diet.

The relative lack of clinical trials exploring cardiovascular outcome, using a complete Mediterranean Diet rich in Olive Oil, has opened the door for new initiatives. The PREDIMED study, close to conclude its follow up aims to compare the effects of a low fat diet with two Mediterranean Diet type diets (one of them enriched in nuts), on clinical cardiovascular endpoints of persons at risk of cardiovascular disease but without clinical disease (primary prevention). Until the final results are released, there have been published preliminary reports. The lower intake of olive oil was correlated with a thicker intima media thickness, a measure of the atherosclerosis in the carotid vessel, and a cardiovascular risk factor (Buil-Cosiales et al., 2008). Other risk factors previously suggested were also confirmed. Mediterranean Diet was followed by a decrease in glucose plasma levels, blood pressure and rises the proportion HDL/total cholesterol (Estruch et al., 2006).

The CordioPrev study aims to explore the effects of a low fat and a Mediterranean Diet in the recurrence of cardiovascular events and cardiovascular mortality in patients with coronary heart disease, exploring also multiple other endpoints, like incidence of cancer, lipids, glucose metabolism or age associated cognitive decline, after 5 years of follow up. This study is still in recruitment stage, and it may unravel the existence of causality in the relationship between Mediterranean Diet and lower recurrence of cardiovascular disease(CordioPrev, 2010).

These and other ongoing studies will help to ascertain if there is causality under the well stablished clinical associations between Mediterranean Diet and cardiovascular disease clinical endpoints.

10. Conclusions

Mediterranean Diet has shown beneficial effects in multiple cardiovascular risk factors and underlying mechanisms of atherosclerosis, including a favorable lipid profile, a decrease of blood pressure, a shortening of the postprandial lipemia, a partial reduction in the harmful effects of smoking, a reduction of oxidative stress and inflammation, a reduction in the incidence and control of the clinical features of the Metabolic Syndrome, a better glycemic control, an enhancement of endothelial function, or the creation of a less prothrombotic environment (Figure 2). The results from observational and cohort studies link the high adherence to Mediterranean Diet with a lower total mortality and a decrease in cardiovascular events and cardiovascular mortality. Although it is not the scope of the present chapter, it has also been linked to several other healthy benefits, like a decrease in the incidence of certain types of tumors or a better cognitive function in aged persons.

The underlying mechanisms by which the Mediterranean Diet exerts its pleiotropic effects are difficult to discover, especially having into account that it is a flexible dietary pattern, with local differences depending on the geographical area in which it is studied. However, a combination of the healthy effects of its main components, like the use of Virgin Olive Oil and the high proportion of fruits and vegetables, grains and fish may be in the origin.

Meanwhile the large clinical trials designed to proof causality between Mediterranean Diet and cardiovascular disease publish their results, the effects of this dietary model on the cardiovascular risk factors and on the mechanisms of atherosclerosis, as well as the results from epidemiological studies allow us to infer that Mediterranean Diet may be an optimal dietary model to face the development of cardiovascular diseases.

11. Acknowledgments

Supported in part by research grants from the Spanish Ministry of Science and Innovation (AGL 2004-07907, AGL2006-01979, and AGL2009-12270 to J L-M, SAF07-62005 to F P-J and FIS PI10/01041 to P P-M, PI10/02412 to F P-J); Consejería de Economía, Innovación y Ciencia, Proyectos de Investigación de Excelencia, Junta de Andalucía (P06-CTS-01425 to J L-M, CTS5015 and AGR922 to F P-J); Consejería de Salud, Junta de Andalucía (06/128, 07/43, and PI0193/09 to J L-M, 06/129 to F P-J, 06/127 to C M-H, 0118/08 to F F-J, PI-0252/09 to J D-L, and PI-0058/10 to P P-M); Fondo Europeo de Desarrollo Regional (FEDER). The CIBEROBN is an initiative of the Instituto de Salud Carlos III, Madrid, Spain.

12. References

Alonso, A., J. J. Beunza, M. Bes-Rastrollo, R. M. Pajares & M. A. Martinez-Gonzalez (2006). "Vegetable protein and fiber from cereal are inversely associated with the risk of hypertension in a Spanish cohort." *Arch Med Res* 37 (6): 778-786.

Alonso, A., C. de la Fuente, A. M. Martin-Arnau, J. de Irala, J. A. Martinez & M. A. Martinez-Gonzalez (2004). "Fruit and vegetable consumption is inversely associated with blood pressure in a Mediterranean population with a high vegetable-fat intake: the Seguimiento Universidad de Navarra (SUN) Study." *Br J Nutr* 92 (2): 311-319.

Allayee, H., N. Roth & H. N. Hodis (2009). "Polyunsaturated fatty acids and cardiovascular disease: implications for nutrigenetics." *J Nutrigenet Nutrigenomics* 2 (3): 140-148.

Antonopoulou, S., E. Fragopoulou, H. C. Karantonis, E. Mitsou, M. Sitara, J. Rementzis, A. Mourelatos, A. Ginis & C. Phenekos (2006). "Effect of traditional Greek Mediterranean meals on platelet aggregation in normal subjects and in patients with type 2 diabetes mellitus." *J Med Food* 9 (3): 356-362.

Avellone, G., R. Cordova, L. Scalffidi & G. Bompiani (1998). "Effects of Mediterranean diet on lipid, coagulative and fibrinolytic parameters in two randomly selected population samples in Western Sicily." *Nutr Metab Cardiovasc Dis* 8: 287-296.

Bach-Faig, A., D. Geleva, J. L. Carrasco, L. Ribas-Barba & L. Serra-Majem (2006). "Evaluating associations between Mediterranean diet adherence indexes and biomarkers of diet and disease." *Public Health Nutr* 9 (8A): 1110-1117.

Bayturan, O., E. M. Tuzcu, A. Lavoie, T. Hu, K. Wolski, P. Schoenhagen, S. Kapadia, S. E. Nissen & S. J. Nicholls (2010). "The metabolic syndrome, its component risk factors, and progression of coronary atherosclerosis." *Arch Intern Med* 170 (5): 478-484.

Beunza, J. J., E. Toledo, F. B. Hu, M. Bes-Rastrollo, M. Serrano-Martinez, A. Sanchez-Villegas, J. A. Martinez & M. A. Martinez-Gonzalez (2010). "Adherence to the Mediterranean diet, long-term weight change, and incident overweight or obesity: the Seguimiento Universidad de Navarra (SUN) cohort." *Am J Clin Nutr* 92 (6): 1484-1493.

Bondia-Pons, I., H. Schroder, M. I. Covas, A. I. Castellote, J. Kaikkonen, H. E. Poulsen, A. V. Gaddi, A. Machowetz, H. Kiesewetter & M. C. Lopez-Sabater (2007). "Moderate consumption of olive oil by healthy European men reduces systolic blood pressure in non-Mediterranean participants." *J Nutr* 137 (1): 84-87.

Borissoff, J. I., H. M. Spronk & H. ten Cate (2011). "The hemostatic system as a modulator of atherosclerosis." *N Engl J Med* 364 (18): 1746-1760.

Bravo-Herrera, M. D., J. Lopez-Miranda, C. Marin, P. Gomez, M. J. Gomez, J. A. Moreno, P. Perez-Martinez, A. Blanco, Y. Jimenez-Gomez & F. Perez-Jimenez (2004). "Tissue factor expression is decreased in monocytes obtained from blood during Mediterranean or high carbohydrate diets." *Nutr Metab Cardiovasc Dis* 14 (3): 128-132.

Buckland, G., A. Agudo, N. Travier, J. Maria Huerta, L. Cirera, M. J. Tormo, C. Navarro, M. Dolores Chirlaque, C. Moreno-Iribas, E. Ardanaz, A. Barricarte, J. Etxeberria, P. Marin, J. Ramon Quiros, M. L. Redondo, N. Larranaga, P. Amiano, M. Dorronsoro, L. Arriola, M. Basterretxea, M. J. Sanchez, E. Molina & C. A. Gonzalez (2011). "Adherence to the Mediterranean diet reduces mortality in the Spanish cohort of the European Prospective Investigation into Cancer and Nutrition (EPIC-Spain)." *Br J Nutr*: 1-11.

Buil-Cosiales, P., P. Irimia, N. Berrade, A. Garcia-Arellano, M. Riverol, M. Murie-Fernandez, E. Martinez-Vila, M. A. Martinez-Gonzalez & M. Serrano-Martinez (2008). "Carotid intima-media thickness is inversely associated with olive oil consumption." *Atherosclerosis* 196 (2): 742-748.

Bullo, M., M. Garcia-Aloy, M. A. Martinez-Gonzalez, D. Corella, J. D. Fernandez-Ballart, M. Fiol, E. Gomez-Gracia, R. Estruch, M. Ortega-Calvo, S. Francisco, G. Flores-Mateo, L. Serra-Majem, X. Pinto, M. I. Covas, E. Ros, R. Lamuela-Raventos & J. Salas-Salvado (2011). "Association between a healthy lifestyle and general obesity and abdominal obesity in an elderly population at high cardiovascular risk." *Prev Med.*

Burr, M. L., A. M. Fehily, J. F. Gilbert, S. Rogers, R. M. Holliday, P. M. Sweetnam, P. C. Elwood & N. M. Deadman (1989). "Effects of changes in fat, fish, and fibre intakes on death and myocardial reinfarction: diet and reinfarction trial (DART)." *Lancet* 2 (8666): 757-761.

Carluccio, M. A., M. Massaro, E. Scoditti & R. De Caterina (2007). "Vasculoprotective potential of olive oil components." *Mol Nutr Food Res* 51 (10): 1225-1234.

CFSAN/Office of Nutritional Products, L. a. D. S. (2004) "Letter Responding to Health Claim Petition dated August 28, 2003: Monounsaturated Fatty Acids from Olive Oil and Coronary Heart Disease (Docket No 2003Q-0559)." http://www.cfsan.fda.gov/~dms/qhcolive.html#ref.

CordioPrev (2010). "(www.cordioprev.org/en)."

Covas, M. I. (2007). "Olive oil and the cardiovascular system." *Pharmacol Res* 55 (3): 175-186.

Chrysohoou, C., D. B. Panagiotakos, P. Aggelopoulos, C. M. Kastorini, I. Kehagia, C. Pitsavos & C. Stefanadis (2010). "The Mediterranean diet contributes to the preservation of left ventricular systolic function and to the long-term favorable prognosis of patients who have had an acute coronary event." *Am J Clin Nutr* 92 (1): 47-54.

Dai, J., R. Lampert, P. W. Wilson, J. Goldberg, T. R. Ziegler & V. Vaccarino (2010). "Mediterranean dietary pattern is associated with improved cardiac autonomic function among middle-aged men: a twin study." *Circ Cardiovasc Qual Outcomes* 3 (4): 366-373.

Davis, N., S. Katz & J. Wylie-Rosett (2007). "The effect of diet on endothelial function." *Cardiol Rev* 15 (2): 62-66.

de Koning, L., S. E. Chiuve, T. T. Fung, W. C. Willett, E. B. Rimm & F. B. Hu (2011). "Diet-quality scores and the risk of type 2 diabetes in men." *Diabetes Care* 34 (5): 1150-1156.

de Lorgeril, M., P. Salen, J. L. Martin, I. Monjaud, J. Delaye & N. Mamelle (1999). "Mediterranean diet, traditional risk factors, and the rate of cardiovascular complications after myocardial infarction: final report of the Lyon Diet Heart Study." *Circulation* 99 (6): 779-785.

Delgado-Lista, J., A. Garcia-Rios, P. Perez-Martinez, J. Lopez-Miranda & F. Perez-Jimenez (2011a). "Olive oil and haemostasis: platelet function, thrombogenesis and fibrinolysis." *Curr Pharm Des* 17 (8): 778-785.

Delgado-Lista, J., A. Garcia-Rios, P. Perez-Martinez, J. Solivera, E. M. Yubero-Serrano, F. Fuentes, L. D. Parnell, J. Shen, P. Gomez, Y. Jimenez-Gomez, M. J. Gomez-Luna, C. Marin, S. E. Belisle, F. Rodriguez-Cantalejo, S. N. Meydani, J. M. Ordovas, F. Perez-Jimenez & J. Lopez-Miranda (2011b). "Interleukin 1B variant -1473G/C (rs1143623) influences triglyceride and interleukin 6 metabolism." *J Clin Endocrinol Metab* 96 (5): E816-820.

Delgado-Lista, J., J. Lopez-Miranda, B. Cortes, P. Perez-Martinez, A. Lozano, R. Gomez-Luna, P. Gomez, M. J. Gomez, J. Criado, F. Fuentes & F. Perez-Jimenez (2008). "Chronic dietary fat intake modifies the postprandial response of hemostatic markers to a single fatty test meal." *Am J Clin Nutr* 87 (2): 317-322.

Delgado-Lista, J., J. Lopez-Miranda, P. Perez-Martinez, J. Ruano, F. Fuentes & F. Perez-Jimenez (2007). "Olive Oil and Hemostasis." *Current Nutrition & Food Science* 3 (1): 175-182.

Din, J. N., D. E. Newby & A. D. Flapan (2004). "Omega 3 fatty acids and cardiovascular disease--fishing for a natural treatment." *Bmj* 328 (7430): 30-35.

EFSA (2011). "Scientific Opinion on the substantiation of health claims related to polyphenols in olive and protection of LDL particles from oxidative damage (ID 1333, 1638, 1639, 1696, 2865), maintenance of normal blood HDL cholesterol concentrations (ID 1639), maintenance of normal blood pressure (ID 3781), "anti-inflammatory properties" (ID 1882), "contributes to the upper respiratory tract health" (ID 3468), "can help to maintain a normal function of gastrointestinal tract" (3779), and "contributes to body defences against external agents" (ID 3467) pursuant to Article 13(1) of Regulation (EC) No 1924/2006." *EFSA journal* 9 (4): 2033-2058.

Elhayany, A., A. Lustman, R. Abel, J. Attal-Singer & S. Vinker (2010). "A low carbohydrate Mediterranean diet improves cardiovascular risk factors and diabetes control among overweight patients with type 2 diabetes mellitus: a 1-year prospective randomized intervention study." *Diabetes Obes Metab* 12 (3): 204-209.

Esmaillzadeh, A., M. Kimiagar, Y. Mehrabi, L. Azadbakht, F. B. Hu & W. C. Willett (2007). "Dietary patterns, insulin resistance, and prevalence of the metabolic syndrome in women." *Am J Clin Nutr* 85 (3): 910-918.

Esposito, K., C. M. Kastorini, D. B. Panagiotakos & D. Giugliano (2011). "Mediterranean diet and weight loss: meta-analysis of randomized controlled trials." *Metab Syndr Relat Disord* 9 (1): 1-12.

Esposito, K., R. Marfella, M. Ciotola, C. Di Palo, F. Giugliano, G. Giugliano, M. D'Armiento, F. D'Andrea & D. Giugliano (2004). "Effect of a mediterranean-style diet on endothelial dysfunction and markers of vascular inflammation in the metabolic syndrome: a randomized trial." *JAMA* 292 (12): 1440-1446.

Estruch, R. (2010). "Anti-inflammatory effects of the Mediterranean diet: the experience of the PREDIMED study." *Proc Nutr Soc* 69 (3): 333-340.

Estruch, R., M. A. Martinez-Gonzalez, D. Corella, J. Basora-Gallisa, V. Ruiz-Gutierrez, M. I. Covas, M. Fiol, E. Gomez-Gracia, M. C. Lopez-Sabater, R. Escoda, M. A. Pena, J. Diez-Espino, C. Lahoz, J. Lapetra, G. Saez & E. Ros (2009). "Effects of dietary fiber intake on risk factors for cardiovascular disease in subjects at high risk." *J Epidemiol Community Health*.

Estruch, R., M. A. Martinez-Gonzalez, D. Corella, J. Salas-Salvado, V. Ruiz-Gutierrez, M. I. Covas, M. Fiol, E. Gomez-Gracia, M. C. Lopez-Sabater, E. Vinyoles, F. Aros, M. Conde, C. Lahoz, J. Lapetra, G. Saez & E. Ros (2006). "Effects of a Mediterranean-style diet on cardiovascular risk factors: a randomized trial." *Ann Intern Med* 145 (1): 1-11.

Filion, K. B., F. El Khoury, M. Bielinski, I. Schiller, N. Dendukuri & J. M. Brophy (2010). "Omega-3 fatty acids in high-risk cardiovascular patients: a meta-analysis of randomized controlled trials." *BMC Cardiovasc Disord* 10: 24.

Fito, M., M. Cladellas, R. de la Torre, J. Marti, M. Alcantara, M. Pujadas-Bastardes, J. Marrugat, J. Bruguera, M. C. Lopez-Sabater, J. Vila & M. I. Covas (2005). "Antioxidant effect of virgin olive oil in patients with stable coronary heart disease: a randomized, crossover, controlled, clinical trial." *Atherosclerosis* 181 (1): 149-158.

Fuentes, F., J. Lopez-Miranda, P. Perez-Martinez, Y. Jimenez, C. Marin, P. Gomez, J. M. Fernandez, J. Caballero, J. Delgado-Lista & F. Perez-Jimenez (2008). "Chronic effects of a high-fat diet enriched with virgin olive oil and a low-fat diet enriched with alpha-linolenic acid on postprandial endothelial function in healthy men." *Br J Nutr* 100 (1): 159-165.

Fuentes, F., J. Lopez-Miranda, E. Sanchez, F. Sanchez, J. Paez, E. Paz-Rojas, C. Marin, P. Gomez, J. Jimenez-Pereperez, J. M. Ordovas & F. Perez-Jimenez (2001). "Mediterranean and low-fat diets improve endothelial function in hypercholesterolemic men." *Ann Intern Med* 134 (12): 1115-1119.

Gasparyan, A. Y., L. Ayvazyan, D. P. Mikhailidis & G. D. Kitas (2011). "Mean platelet volume: a link between thrombosis and inflammation?" *Curr Pharm Des* 17 (1): 47-58.

Geleijnse, J. M., E. J. Giltay, D. E. Grobbee, A. R. Donders & F. J. Kok (2002). "Blood pressure response to fish oil supplementation: metaregression analysis of randomized trials." *J Hypertens* 20 (8): 1493-1499.

Gillingham, L. G., S. Harris-Janz & P. J. Jones (2011). "Dietary monounsaturated fatty acids are protective against metabolic syndrome and cardiovascular disease risk factors." *Lipids* 46 (3): 209-228.

Giugliano, D. & K. Esposito (2008). "Mediterranean diet and metabolic diseases." *Curr Opin Lipidol* 19 (1): 63-68.

Giugliano, F., M. I. Maiorino, G. Bellastella, R. Autorino, M. De Sio, D. Giugliano & K. Esposito (2010). "Adherence to Mediterranean diet and erectile dysfunction in men with type 2 diabetes." *J Sex Med* 7 (5): 1911-1917.

Gutierrez-Mariscal, F. M., P. Perez-Martinez, J. Delgado-Lista, E. M. Yubero-Serrano, A. Camargo, N. Delgado-Casado, C. Cruz-Teno, M. Santos-Gonzalez, F. Rodriguez-Cantalejo, J. P. Castano, J. M. Villalba-Montoro, F. Fuentes, F. Perez-Jimenez & J. Lopez-Miranda (2011). "Mediterranean diet supplemented with coenzyme Q10 induces postprandial changes in p53 in response to oxidative DNA damage in elderly subjects." *Age (Dordr)*.

Harris, W. S., P. M. Kris-Etherton & K. A. Harris (2008). "Intakes of long-chain omega-3 fatty acid associated with reduced risk for death from coronary heart disease in healthy adults." *Curr Atheroscler Rep* 10 (6): 503-509.

Harris, W. S., Y. Park & W. L. Isley (2003). "Cardiovascular disease and long-chain omega-3 fatty acids." *Curr Opin Lipidol* 14 (1): 9-14.

Haveman-Nies, A., L. P. de Groot, J. Burema, J. A. Cruz, M. Osler & W. A. van Staveren (2002). "Dietary quality and lifestyle factors in relation to 10-year mortality in older Europeans: the SENECA study." *Am J Epidemiol* 156 (10): 962-968.

HeartScore (2003). "http://www.heartscore.org."

Hodge, A. M., D. R. English, C. Itsiopoulos, K. O'Dea & G. G. Giles (2010). "Does a Mediterranean diet reduce the mortality risk associated with diabetes: Evidence from the Melbourne Collaborative Cohort Study." *Nutr Metab Cardiovasc Dis*.

Itsiopoulos, C., L. Brazionis, M. Kaimakamis, M. Cameron, J. D. Best, K. O'Dea & K. Rowley (2010). "Can the Mediterranean diet lower HbA1c in type 2 diabetes? Results from a randomized cross-over study." *Nutr Metab Cardiovasc Dis*.

Jakobsen, M. U., E. J. O'Reilly, B. L. Heitmann, M. A. Pereira, K. Balter, G. E. Fraser, U. Goldbourt, G. Hallmans, P. Knekt, S. Liu, P. Pietinen, D. Spiegelman, J. Stevens, J. Virtamo, W. C. Willett & A. Ascherio (2009). "Major types of dietary fat and risk of coronary heart disease: a pooled analysis of 11 cohort studies." *Am J Clin Nutr* 89 (5): 1425-1432.

Jansen, S., J. Lopez-Miranda, P. Castro, F. Lopez-Segura, C. Marin, J. M. Ordovas, E. Paz, J. Jimenez-Pereperez, F. Fuentes & F. Perez-Jimenez (2000). "Low-fat and high-monounsaturated fatty acid diets decrease plasma cholesterol ester transfer protein concentrations in young, healthy, normolipemic men." *Am J Clin Nutr* 72 (1): 36-41.

Jimenez-Gomez, Y., C. Marin, P. Peerez-Martinez, J. Hartwich, M. Malczewska-Malec, I. Golabek, B. Kiec-Wilk, C. Cruz-Teno, F. Rodriguez, P. Gomez, M. J. Gomez-Luna, C. Defoort, M. J. Gibney, F. Perez-Jimenez, H. M. Roche & J. Lopez-Miranda (2010). "A low-fat, high-complex carbohydrate diet supplemented with long-chain (n-3) fatty acids alters the postprandial lipoprotein profile in patients with metabolic syndrome." *J Nutr* 140 (9): 1595-1601.

Junker, R., M. Kratz, M. Neufeld, M. Erren, J. R. Nofer, H. Schulte, U. Nowak-Gottl, G. Assmann & U. Wahrburg (2001a). "Effects of diets containing olive oil, sunflower oil, or rapeseed oil on the hemostatic system." *Thromb Haemost* 85 (2): 280-286.

Junker, R., B. Pieke, H. Schulte, R. Nofer, M. Neufeld, G. Assmann & U. Wahrburg (2001b). "Changes in hemostasis during treatment of hypertriglyceridemia with a diet rich in monounsaturated and n-3 polyunsaturated fatty acids in comparison with a low-fat diet." *Thromb Res* 101 (5): 355-366.

Karantonis, H. C., S. Antonopoulou & C. A. Demopoulos (2002). "Antithrombotic lipid minor constituents from vegetable oils. Comparison between olive oils and others." *J Agric Food Chem* 50 (5): 1150-1160.

Karantonis, H. C., S. Antonopoulou, D. N. Perrea, D. P. Sokolis, S. E. Theocharis, N. Kavantzas, D. G. Iliopoulos & C. A. Demopoulos (2006). "In vivo antiatherogenic properties of olive oil and its constituent lipid classes in hyperlipidemic rabbits." *Nutr Metab Cardiovasc Dis* 16 (3): 174-185.

Kastorini, C. M., H. J. Milionis, K. Esposito, D. Giugliano, J. A. Goudevenos & D. B. Panagiotakos (2011). "The effect of Mediterranean diet on metabolic syndrome and its components: a meta-analysis of 50 studies and 534,906 individuals." *J Am Coll Cardiol* 57 (11): 1299-1313.

Kolovou, G. D., D. P. Mikhailidis, J. Kovar, D. Lairon, B. G. Nordestgaard, T. C. Ooi, P. Perez-Martinez, H. Bilianou, K. Anagnostopoulou & G. Panotopoulos (2011). "Assessment and clinical relevance of non-fasting and postprandial triglycerides: an expert panel statement." *Curr Vasc Pharmacol* 9 (3): 258-270.

Kontou, N., T. Psaltopoulou, D. Panagiotakos, M. A. Dimopoulos & A. Linos (2011). "The Mediterranean Diet in Cancer Prevention: A Review." *J Med Food.*

Kris-Etherton, P. M., J. Derr, D. C. Mitchell, V. A. Mustad, M. E. Russell, E. T. McDonnell, D. Salabsky & T. A. Pearson (1993). "The role of fatty acid saturation on plasma lipids, lipoproteins, and apolipoproteins: I. Effects of whole food diets high in cocoa butter, olive oil, soybean oil, dairy butter, and milk chocolate on the plasma lipids of young men." *Metabolism* 42 (1): 121-129.

Kris-Etherton, P. M., W. S. Harris & L. J. Appel (2002). "Fish consumption, fish oil, omega-3 fatty acids, and cardiovascular disease." *Circulation* 106 (21): 2747-2757.

Lairon, D., C. Defoort, J. C. Martin, M. J. Amiot-Carlin, M. Gastaldi & R. Planells (2009). "Nutrigenetics: links between genetic background and response to Mediterranean-type diets." *Public health nutrition* 12 (9A): 1601-1606.

Langsted, A., J. J. Freiberg, A. Tybjaerg-Hansen, P. Schnohr, G. B. Jensen & B. G. Nordestgaard (2011). "Nonfasting cholesterol and triglycerides and association with risk of myocardial infarction and total mortality: the Copenhagen City Heart Study with 31 years of follow-up." *J Intern Med* 270 (1): 65-75.

Lapointe, A., J. Goulet, C. Couillard, B. Lamarche & S. Lemieux (2005). "A nutritional intervention promoting the Mediterranean food pattern is associated with a decrease in circulating oxidized LDL particles in healthy women from the Quebec City metropolitan area." *J Nutr* 135 (3): 410-415.

Lavie, C. J., R. V. Milani, M. R. Mehra & H. O. Ventura (2009). "Omega-3 polyunsaturated fatty acids and cardiovascular diseases." *J Am Coll Cardiol* 54 (7): 585-594.

Leighton, F. & I. Urquiaga (2007). "Endothelial nitric oxide synthase as a mediator of the positive health effects of Mediterranean diets and wine against metabolic syndrome." *World Rev Nutr Diet* 97: 33-51.

Lichtenstein, A. H., L. J. Appel, M. Brands, M. Carnethon, S. Daniels, H. A. Franch, B. Franklin, P. Kris-Etherton, W. S. Harris, B. Howard, N. Karanja, M. Lefevre, L. Rudel, F. Sacks, L. Van Horn, M. Winston & J. Wylie-Rosett (2006). "Diet and lifestyle recommendations revision 2006: a scientific statement from the American Heart Association Nutrition Committee." *Circulation* 114 (1): 82-96.

Lopez-Miranda, J., J. Delgado-Lista, P. Perez-Martinez, Y. Jimenez-Gomez, F. Fuentes, J. Ruano & C. Marin (2007). "Olive oil and the haemostatic system." *Mol Nutr Food Res* 51 (10): 1249-1259.

Lopez-Miranda, J., F. Perez-Jimenez, E. Ros, R. De Caterina, L. Badimon, M. I. Covas, E. Escrich, J. M. Ordovas, F. Soriguer, R. Abia, C. A. de la Lastra, M. Battino, D. Corella, J. Chamorro-Quiros, J. Delgado-Lista, D. Giugliano, K. Esposito, R. Estruch, J. M. Fernandez-Real, J. J. Gaforio, C. La Vecchia, D. Lairon, F. Lopez-Segura, P. Mata, J. A. Menendez, F. J. Muriana, J. Osada, D. B. Panagiotakos, J. A. Paniagua, P. Perez-Martinez, J. Perona, M. A. Peinado, M. Pineda-Priego, H. E. Poulsen, J. L. Quiles, M. C. Ramirez-Tortosa, J. Ruano, L. Serra-Majem, R. Sola, M. Solanas, V. Solfrizzi, R. de la Torre-Fornell, A. Trichopoulou, M. Uceda, J. M. Villalba-Montoro, J. R. Villar-Ortiz, F. Visioli & N. Yiannakouris (2010). "Olive oil and health: summary of the II international conference on olive oil and health consensus report, Jaen and Cordoba (Spain) 2008." *Nutr Metab Cardiovasc Dis* 20 (4): 284-294.

Lopez-Miranda, J., P. Perez-Martinez, C. Marin, J. A. Moreno, P. Gomez & F. Perez-Jimenez (2006). "Postprandial lipoprotein metabolism, genes and risk of cardiovascular disease." *Curr Opin Lipidol* 17 (2): 132-138.

Lopez, S., B. Bermudez, Y. M. Pacheco, J. Villar, R. Abia & F. J. Muriana (2008). "Distinctive postprandial modulation of beta cell function and insulin sensitivity by dietary fats: monounsaturated compared with saturated fatty acids." *Am J Clin Nutr* 88 (3): 638-644.

Lovegrove, J. A. & R. Gitau (2008). "Nutrigenetics and CVD: what does the future hold?" *The Proceedings of the Nutrition Society* 67 (2): 206-213.

Lutsey, P. L., L. M. Steffen & J. Stevens (2008). "Dietary intake and the development of the metabolic syndrome: the Atherosclerosis Risk in Communities study." *Circulation* 117 (6): 754-761.

Marin, C., R. Ramirez, J. Delgado-Lista, E. M. Yubero-Serrano, P. Perez-Martinez, J. Carracedo, A. Garcia-Rios, F. Rodriguez, F. M. Gutierrez-Mariscal, P. Gomez, F. Perez-Jimenez & J. Lopez-Miranda (2011). "Mediterranean diet reduces endothelial damage and improves the regenerative capacity of endothelium." *Am J Clin Nutr* 93 (2): 267-274.

Martinez-Gonzalez, M. A., C. de la Fuente-Arrillaga, J. M. Nunez-Cordoba, F. J. Basterra-Gortari, J. J. Beunza, Z. Vazquez, S. Benito, A. Tortosa & M. Bes-Rastrollo (2008). "Adherence to Mediterranean diet and risk of developing diabetes: prospective cohort study." *Bmj* 336 (7657): 1348-1351.

Martinez-Gonzalez, M. A., M. Garcia-Lopez, M. Bes-Rastrollo, E. Toledo, E. H. Martinez-Lapiscina, M. Delgado-Rodriguez, Z. Vazquez, S. Benito & J. J. Beunza (2011). "Mediterranean diet and the incidence of cardiovascular disease: a Spanish cohort." *Nutr Metab Cardiovasc Dis* 21 (4): 237-244.

Masala, G., B. Bendinelli, D. Versari, C. Saieva, M. Ceroti, F. Santagiuliana, S. Caini, S. Salvini, F. Sera, S. Taddei, L. Ghiadoni & D. Palli (2008). "Anthropometric and dietary determinants of blood pressure in over 7000 Mediterranean women: the European Prospective Investigation into Cancer and Nutrition-Florence cohort." *J Hypertens* 26 (11): 2112-2120.

Mata, P., J. A. Garrido, J. M. Ordovas, E. Blazquez, L. A. Alvarez-Sala, M. J. Rubio, R. Alonso & M. de Oya (1992). "Effect of dietary monounsaturated fatty acids on plasma lipoproteins and apolipoproteins in women." *Am J Clin Nutr* 56 (1): 77-83.

Mattioli, A. V. (2011). "Lifestyle and atrial fibrillation." *Expert Rev Cardiovasc Ther* 9 (7): 895-902.

Mattioli, A. V., C. Miloro, S. Pennella, P. Pedrazzi & A. Farinetti (2011). "Adherence to Mediterranean diet and intake of antioxidants influence spontaneous conversion of atrial fibrillation." *Nutr Metab Cardiovasc Dis.*

Mena, M. P., E. Sacanella, M. Vazquez-Agell, M. Morales, M. Fito, R. Escoda, M. Serrano-Martinez, J. Salas-Salvado, N. Benages, R. Casas, R. M. Lamuela-Raventos, F. Masanes, E. Ros & R. Estruch (2009). "Inhibition of circulating immune cell activation: a molecular antiinflammatory effect of the Mediterranean diet." *Am J Clin Nutr* 89 (1): 248-256.

Mendez, M. A., B. M. Popkin, P. Jakszyn, A. Berenguer, M. J. Tormo, M. J. Sanchez, J. R. Quiros, G. Pera, C. Navarro, C. Martinez, N. Larranaga, M. Dorronsoro, M. D. Chirlaque, A. Barricarte, E. Ardanaz, P. Amiano, A. Agudo & C. A. Gonzalez (2006). "Adherence to a Mediterranean diet is associated with reduced 3-year incidence of obesity." *J Nutr* 136 (11): 2934-2938.

Mente, A., L. de Koning, H. S. Shannon & S. S. Anand (2009). "A systematic review of the evidence supporting a causal link between dietary factors and coronary heart disease." *Arch Intern Med* 169 (7): 659-669.

Mezzano, D. & F. Leighton (2003). "Haemostatic cardiovascular risk factors: differential effects of red wine and diet on healthy young." *Pathophysiol Haemost Thromb* 33 (5-6): 472-478.

Mezzano, D., F. Leighton, P. Strobel, C. Martinez, G. Marshall, A. Cuevas, O. Castillo, O. Panes, B. Munoz, J. Rozowski & J. Pereira (2003). "Mediterranean diet, but not red wine, is associated with beneficial changes in primary haemostasis." *Eur J Clin Nutr* 57 (3): 439-446.

Mitrou, P. N., V. Kipnis, A. C. Thiebaut, J. Reedy, A. F. Subar, E. Wirfalt, A. Flood, T. Mouw, A. R. Hollenbeck, M. F. Leitzmann & A. Schatzkin (2007). "Mediterranean dietary pattern and prediction of all-cause mortality in a US population: results from the NIH-AARP Diet and Health Study." *Arch Intern Med* 167 (22): 2461-2468.

Mordente, A., B. Guantario, E. Meucci, A. Silvestrini, E. Lombardi, G. E. Martorana, B. Giardina & V. Bohm (2011). "Lycopene and cardiovascular diseases: an update." *Curr Med Chem* 18 (8): 1146-1163.

Mozaffarian, D., R. Marfisi, G. Levantesi, M. G. Silletta, L. Tavazzi, G. Tognoni, F. Valagussa & R. Marchioli (2007). "Incidence of new-onset diabetes and impaired fasting glucose in patients with recent myocardial infarction and the effect of clinical and lifestyle risk factors." *Lancet* 370 (9588): 667-675.

Mukamal, K. J. & E. B. Rimm (2008). "Alcohol consumption: risks and benefits." *Curr Atheroscler Rep* 10 (6): 536-543.

N.C.E.P. (2001). "http://www.nhlbi.nih.gov/guidelines/cholesterol/atglance.pdf."

Nadtochiy, S. M. & E. K. Redman (2011). "Mediterranean diet and cardioprotection: the role of nitrite, polyunsaturated fatty acids, and polyphenols." *Nutrition* 27 (7-8): 733-744.

Ordovas, J. M. (2006). "Nutrigenetics, plasma lipids, and cardiovascular risk." *Journal of the American Dietetic Association* 106 (7): 1074-1081; quiz 1083.

Panagiotakos, D. B., C. Pitsavos, C. Chrysohoou, J. Skoumas, D. Tousoulis, M. Toutouza, P. Toutouzas & C. Stefanadis (2004). "Impact of lifestyle habits on the prevalence of the metabolic syndrome among Greek adults from the ATTICA study." *Am Heart J* 147 (1): 106-112.

Paniagua, J. A., A. G. de la Sacristana, E. Sanchez, I. Romero, A. Vidal-Puig, F. J. Berral, A. Escribano, M. J. Moyano, P. Perez-Martinez, J. Lopez-Miranda & F. Perez-Jimenez (2007a). "A MUFA-rich diet improves posprandial glucose, lipid and GLP-1 responses in insulin-resistant subjects." *J Am Coll Nutr* 26 (5): 434-444.

Paniagua, J. A., A. Gallego de la Sacristana, I. Romero, A. Vidal-Puig, J. M. Latre, E. Sanchez, P. Perez-Martinez, J. Lopez-Miranda & F. Perez-Jimenez (2007b). "Monounsaturated fat-rich diet prevents central body fat distribution and decreases postprandial adiponectin expression induced by a carbohydrate-rich diet in insulin-resistant subjects." *Diabetes Care* 30 (7): 1717-1723.

Panunzio, M. F., R. Caporizzi, A. Antoniciello, E. P. Cela, L. R. Ferguson & P. D'Ambrosio (2011). "Randomized, controlled nutrition education trial promotes a Mediterranean diet and improves anthropometric, dietary, and metabolic parameters in adults." *Ann Ig* 23 (1): 13-25.

Papoutsi, Z., E. Kassi, I. Chinou, M. Halabalaki, L. A. Skaltsounis & P. Moutsatsou (2008). "Walnut extract (Juglans regia L.) and its component ellagic acid exhibit anti-inflammatory activity in human aorta endothelial cells and osteoblastic activity in the cell line KS483." *Br J Nutr* 99 (4): 715-722.

Patel, A., F. Barzi, K. Jamrozik, T. H. Lam, H. Ueshima, G. Whitlock & M. Woodward (2004). "Serum triglycerides as a risk factor for cardiovascular diseases in the Asia-Pacific region." *Circulation* 110 (17): 2678-2686.

Pereira, M. A., A. I. Kartashov, C. B. Ebbeling, L. Van Horn, M. L. Slattery, D. R. Jacobs, Jr. & D. S. Ludwig (2005). "Fast-food habits, weight gain, and insulin resistance (the CARDIA study): 15-year prospective analysis." *Lancet* 365 (9453): 36-42.

Perez-Jimenez, F. (2005). "International conference on the healthy effect of virgin olive oil." *Eur J Clin Invest* 35 (7): 421-424.

Perez-Jimenez, F., P. Castro, J. Lopez-Miranda, E. Paz-Rojas, A. Blanco, F. Lopez-Segura, F. Velasco, C. Marin, F. Fuentes & J. M. Ordovas (1999). "Circulating levels of endothelial function are modulated by dietary monounsaturated fat." *Atherosclerosis* 145 (2): 351-358.

Perez-Jimenez, F., J. D. Lista, P. Perez-Martinez, F. Lopez-Segura, F. Fuentes, B. Cortes, A. Lozano & J. Lopez-Miranda (2006). "Olive oil and haemostasis: a review on its healthy effects." *Public Health Nutr* 9 (8A): 1083-1088.

Perez-Jimenez, F., J. Lopez-Miranda & P. Mata (2002). "Protective effect of dietary monounsaturated fat on arteriosclerosis: beyond cholesterol." *Atherosclerosis* 163 (2): 385-398.

Perez-Jimenez, F., J. Ruano, P. Perez-Martinez, F. Lopez-Segura & J. Lopez-Miranda (2007). "The influence of olive oil on human health: not a question of fat alone." *Mol Nutr Food Res* 51 (10): 1199-1208.

Perez-Martinez, P., J. Delgado-Lista, F. Perez-Jimenez & J. Lopez-Miranda (2010a). "Update on genetics of postprandial lipemia." *Atheroscler Suppl* 11 (1): 39-43.

Perez-Martinez, P., J. M. Garcia-Quintana, E. M. Yubero-Serrano, I. Tasset-Cuevas, I. Tunez, A. Garcia-Rios, J. Delgado-Lista, C. Marin, F. Perez-Jimenez, H. M. Roche & J. Lopez-Miranda (2010b). "Postprandial oxidative stress is modified by dietary fat: evidence from a human intervention study." *Clin Sci (Lond)* 119 (6): 251-261.

Perez-Martinez, P., A. Garcia-Rios, J. Delgado-Lista, F. Perez-Jimenez & J. Lopez-Miranda (2011a). "Mediterranean diet rich in olive oil and obesity, metabolic syndrome and diabetes mellitus." *Curr Pharm Des* 17 (8): 769-777.

Perez-Martinez, P., A. Garcia-Rios, J. Delgado-Lista, F. Perez-Jimenez & J. Lopez-Miranda (2011b). "Nutrigenetics of the postprandial lipoprotein metabolism: evidences from human intervention studies." *Curr Vasc Pharmacol* 9 (3): 287-291.

Perez-Martinez, P., M. Moreno-Conde, C. Cruz-Teno, J. Ruano, F. Fuentes, J. Delgado-Lista, A. Garcia-Rios, C. Marin, M. J. Gomez-Luna, F. Perez-Jimenez, H. M. Roche & J. Lopez-Miranda (2010c). "Dietary fat differentially influences regulatory endothelial function during the postprandial state in patients with metabolic syndrome: from the LIPGENE study." *Atherosclerosis* 209 (2): 533-538.

Perona, J. S., R. Cabello-Moruno & V. Ruiz-Gutierrez (2006). "The role of virgin olive oil components in the modulation of endothelial function." *J Nutr Biochem* 17 (7): 429-445.

Perona, J. S., J. Canizares, E. Montero, J. M. Sanchez-Dominguez, A. Catala & V. Ruiz-Gutierrez (2004). "Virgin olive oil reduces blood pressure in hypertensive elderly subjects." *Clin Nutr* 23 (5): 1113-1121.

Pitsavos, C., D. B. Panagiotakos, N. Tzima, C. Chrysohoou, M. Economou, A. Zampelas & C. Stefanadis (2005). "Adherence to the Mediterranean diet is associated with total antioxidant capacity in healthy adults: the ATTICA study." *Am J Clin Nutr* 82 (3): 694-699.

Purnak, T., C. Efe, O. Yuksel, Y. Beyazit, E. Ozaslan & E. Altiparmak (2011). "Mean platelet volume could be a promising biomarker to monitor dietary compliance in celiac disease." *Ups J Med Sci* 116 (3): 208-211.

Rallidis, L. S., J. Lekakis, A. Kolomvotsou, A. Zampelas, G. Vamvakou, S. Efstathiou, G. Dimitriadis, S. A. Raptis & D. T. Kremastinos (2009). "Close adherence to a Mediterranean diet improves endothelial function in subjects with abdominal obesity." *Am J Clin Nutr* 90 (2): 263-268.

Rasmussen, B. M., B. Vessby, M. Uusitupa, L. Berglund, E. Pedersen, G. Riccardi, A. A. Rivellese, L. Tapsell & K. Hermansen (2006). "Effects of dietary saturated, monounsaturated, and n-3 fatty acids on blood pressure in healthy subjects." *Am J Clin Nutr* 83 (2): 221-226.

Rasmussen, O., C. Thomsen, J. Ingerslev & K. Hermansen (1994). "Decrease in von Willebrand factor levels after a high-monounsaturated-fat diet in non-insulin-dependent diabetic subjects." *Metabolism* 43 (11): 1406-1409.

Reisin, E. (2010). "The benefit of the Mediterranean-style diet in patients with newly diagnosed diabetes." *Curr Hypertens Rep* 12 (2): 56-58.

Renaud, S. & D. Lanzmann-Petithory (2002). "Dietary fats and coronary heart disease pathogenesis." *Curr Atheroscler Rep* 4 (6): 419-424.

Riccardi, G., R. Giacco & A. A. Rivellese (2004). "Dietary fat, insulin sensitivity and the metabolic syndrome." *Clin Nutr* 23 (4): 447-456.

Riediger, N. D., R. A. Othman, M. Suh & M. H. Moghadasian (2009). "A systemic review of the roles of n-3 fatty acids in health and disease." *J Am Diet Assoc* 109 (4): 668-679.

Rojo-Martinez, G., I. Esteva, M. S. Ruiz de Adana, J. M. Garcia-Almeida, F. Tinahones, F. Cardona, S. Morcillo, E. Garcia-Escobar, E. Garcia-Fuentes & F. Soriguer (2006). "Dietary fatty acids and insulin secretion: a population-based study." *Eur J Clin Nutr* 60 (10): 1195-1200.

Romaguera, D., T. Norat, T. Mouw, A. M. May, C. Bamia, N. Slimani, N. Travier, H. Besson, J. Luan, N. Wareham, S. Rinaldi, E. Couto, F. Clavel-Chapelon, M. C. Boutron-Ruault, V. Cottet, D. Palli, C. Agnoli, S. Panico, R. Tumino, P. Vineis, A. Agudo, L. Rodriguez, M. J. Sanchez, P. Amiano, A. Barricarte, J. M. Huerta, T. J. Key, E. A. Spencer, H. B. Bueno-de-Mesquita, F. L. Buchner, P. Orfanos, A. Naska, A. Trichopoulou, S. Rohrmann, R. Kaaks, M. Bergmann, H. Boeing, I. Johansson, V. Hellstrom, J. Manjer, E. Wirfalt, M. Uhre Jacobsen, K. Overvad, A. Tjonneland, J. Halkjaer, E. Lund, T. Braaten, D. Engeset, A. Odysseos, E. Riboli & P. H. Peeters (2009). "Adherence to the Mediterranean diet is associated with lower abdominal adiposity in European men and women." *J Nutr* 139 (9): 1728-1737.

Romaguera, D., T. Norat, A. C. Vergnaud, T. Mouw, A. M. May, A. Agudo, G. Buckland, N. Slimani, S. Rinaldi, E. Couto, F. Clavel-Chapelon, M. C. Boutron-Ruault, V. Cottet, S. Rohrmann, B. Teucher, M. Bergmann, H. Boeing, A. Tjonneland, J. Halkjaer, M. U. Jakobsen, C. C. Dahm, N. Travier, L. Rodriguez, M. J. Sanchez, P. Amiano, A. Barricarte, J. M. Huerta, J. Luan, N. Wareham, T. J. Key, E. A. Spencer, P. Orfanos, A. Naska, A. Trichopoulou, D. Palli, C. Agnoli, A. Mattiello, R. Tumino, P. Vineis, H. B. Bueno-de-Mesquita, F. L. Buchner, J. Manjer, E. Wirfalt, I. Johansson, V. Hellstrom, E. Lund, T. Braaten, D. Engeset, A. Odysseos, E. Riboli & P. H. Peeters (2010). "Mediterranean dietary patterns and prospective weight change in participants of the EPIC-PANACEA project." *Am J Clin Nutr* 92 (4): 912-921.

Ruano, J., J. Lopez-Miranda, F. Fuentes, J. A. Moreno, C. Bellido, P. Perez-Martinez, A. Lozano, P. Gomez, Y. Jimenez & F. Perez Jimenez (2005). "Phenolic content of virgin olive oil improves ischemic reactive hyperemia in hypercholesterolemic patients." *J Am Coll Cardiol* 46 (10): 1864-1868.

Salas-Salvado, J., M. Bullo, N. Babio, M. A. Martinez-Gonzalez, N. Ibarrola-Jurado, J. Basora, R. Estruch, M. I. Covas, D. Corella, F. Aros, V. Ruiz-Gutierrez & E. Ros (2011a). "Reduction in the incidence of type 2 diabetes with the Mediterranean diet: results of the PREDIMED-Reus nutrition intervention randomized trial." *Diabetes Care* 34 (1): 14-19.

Salas-Salvado, J., J. Fernandez-Ballart, E. Ros, M. A. Martinez-Gonzalez, M. Fito, R. Estruch, D. Corella, M. Fiol, E. Gomez-Gracia, F. Aros, G. Flores, J. Lapetra, R. Lamuela-Raventos, V. Ruiz-Gutierrez, M. Bullo, J. Basora & M. I. Covas (2008). "Effect of a Mediterranean diet supplemented with nuts on metabolic syndrome status: one-year results of the PREDIMED randomized trial." *Arch Intern Med* 168 (22): 2449-2458.

Salas-Salvado, J., M. A. Martinez-Gonzalez, M. Bullo & E. Ros (2011b). "The role of diet in the prevention of type 2 diabetes." *Nutr Metab Cardiovasc Dis.*

Sanchez-Tainta, A., R. Estruch, M. Bullo, D. Corella, E. Gomez-Gracia, M. Fiol, J. Algorta, M. I. Covas, J. Lapetra, I. Zazpe, V. Ruiz-Gutierrez, E. Ros & M. A. Martinez-Gonzalez (2008). "Adherence to a Mediterranean-type diet and reduced prevalence of clustered cardiovascular risk factors in a cohort of 3,204 high-risk patients." *Eur J Cardiovasc Prev Rehabil* 15 (5): 589-593.

Sarwar, N., J. Danesh, G. Eiriksdottir, G. Sigurdsson, N. Wareham, S. Bingham, S. M. Boekholdt, K. T. Khaw & V. Gudnason (2007). "Triglycerides and the risk of coronary heart disease: 10,158 incident cases among 262,525 participants in 29 Western prospective studies." *Circulation* 115 (4): 450-458.

Scarmeas, N., J. A. Luchsinger, Y. Stern, Y. Gu, J. He, C. DeCarli, T. Brown & A. M. Brickman (2011). "Mediterranean diet and magnetic resonance imaging-assessed cerebrovascular disease." *Ann Neurol* 69 (2): 257-268.

Schini-Kerth, V. B., C. Auger, N. Etienne-Selloum & T. Chataigneau (2010). "Polyphenol-induced endothelium-dependent relaxations role of NO and EDHF." *Adv Pharmacol* 60: 133-175.

Schroder, H., J. Marrugat, J. Vila, M. I. Covas & R. Elosua (2004). "Adherence to the traditional mediterranean diet is inversely associated with body mass index and obesity in a spanish population." *J Nutr* 134 (12): 3355-3361.

Schwartz, G. J., J. Fu, G. Astarita, X. Li, S. Gaetani, P. Campolongo, V. Cuomo & D. Piomelli (2008). "The lipid messenger OEA links dietary fat intake to satiety." *Cell Metab* 8 (4): 281-288.

Seo, T., W. S. Blaner & R. J. Deckelbaum (2005). "Omega-3 fatty acids: molecular approaches to optimal biological outcomes." *Curr Opin Lipidol* 16 (1): 11-18.

Serra-Majem, L., B. Roman & R. Estruch (2006). "Scientific evidence of interventions using the Mediterranean diet: a systematic review." *Nutr Rev* 64 (2 Pt 2): S27-47.

Shah, M., B. Adams-Huet & A. Garg (2007). "Effect of high-carbohydrate or high-cis-monounsaturated fat diets on blood pressure: a meta-analysis of intervention trials." *Am J Clin Nutr* 85 (5): 1251-1256.

Shai, I., J. D. Spence, D. Schwarzfuchs, Y. Henkin, G. Parraga, A. Rudich, A. Fenster, C. Mallett, N. Liel-Cohen, A. Tirosh, A. Bolotin, J. Thiery, G. M. Fiedler, M. Bluher, M.

Stumvoll & M. J. Stampfer (2010). "Dietary intervention to reverse carotid atherosclerosis." *Circulation* 121 (10): 1200-1208.

Singh, I., M. Mok, A. M. Christensen, A. H. Turner & J. A. Hawley (2008). "The effects of polyphenols in olive leaves on platelet function." *Nutr Metab Cardiovasc Dis* 18 (2): 127-132.

Sirtori, C. R., E. Tremoli, E. Gatti, G. Montanari, M. Sirtori, S. Colli, G. Gianfranceschi, P. Maderna, C. Z. Dentone, G. Testolin & et al. (1986). "Controlled evaluation of fat intake in the Mediterranean diet: comparative activities of olive oil and corn oil on plasma lipids and platelets in high-risk patients." *Am J Clin Nutr* 44 (5): 635-642.

Slavka, G., T. Perkmann, H. Haslacher, S. Greisenegger, C. Marsik, O. F. Wagner & G. Endler (2011). "Mean platelet volume may represent a predictive parameter for overall vascular mortality and ischemic heart disease." *Arterioscler Thromb Vasc Biol* 31 (5): 1215-1218.

Smith, R. D., C. N. Kelly, B. A. Fielding, D. Hauton, K. D. Silva, M. C. Nydahl, G. J. Miller & C. M. Williams (2003). "Long-term monounsaturated fatty acid diets reduce platelet aggregation in healthy young subjects." *Br J Nutr* 90 (3): 597-606.

Sofi, F., R. Abbate, G. F. Gensini & A. Casini (2010). "Accruing evidence about benefits of adherence to the Mediterranean diet on health: an updated systematic review and meta-analysis." *Am J Clin Nutr*.

Sofi, F., F. Cesari, R. Abbate, G. F. Gensini & A. Casini (2008). "Adherence to Mediterranean diet and health status: meta-analysis." *Bmj* 337: a1344.

Solfrizzi, V., F. Panza, V. Frisardi, D. Seripa, G. Logroscino, B. P. Imbimbo & A. Pilotto (2011). "Diet and Alzheimer's disease risk factors or prevention: the current evidence." *Expert Rev Neurother* 11 (5): 677-708.

Spence, J. D. (2010). "Secondary stroke prevention." *Nat Rev Neurol* 6 (9): 477-486.

Stock, J. (2011). "Mediterranean diet for combating the metabolic syndrome." *Atherosclerosis*.

Tangney, C. C., M. J. Kwasny, H. Li, R. S. Wilson, D. A. Evans & M. C. Morris (2011). "Adherence to a Mediterranean-type dietary pattern and cognitive decline in a community population." *Am J Clin Nutr* 93 (3): 601-607.

Tekbas, E., A. F. Kara, Z. Ariturk, H. Cil, Y. Islamoglu, M. A. Elbey, S. Soydinc & M. S. Ulgen (2011). "Mean platelet volume in predicting short- and long-term morbidity and mortality in patients with or without ST-segment elevation myocardial infarction." *Scand J Clin Lab Invest*.

Temme, E. H., R. P. Mensink & G. Hornstra (1999). "Effects of diets enriched in lauric, palmitic or oleic acids on blood coagulation and fibrinolysis." *Thromb Haemost* 81 (2): 259-263.

Tortosa, A., M. Bes-Rastrollo, A. Sanchez-Villegas, F. J. Basterra-Gortari, J. M. Nunez-Cordoba & M. A. Martinez-Gonzalez (2007). "Mediterranean diet inversely associated with the incidence of metabolic syndrome: the SUN prospective cohort." *Diabetes Care* 30 (11): 2957-2959.

Tozzi Ciancarelli, M. G., C. Di Massimo, D. De Amicis, I. Ciancarelli & A. Carolei (2011). "Moderate consumption of red wine and human platelet responsiveness." *Thromb Res* 128 (2): 124-129.

Trichopoulou, A., A. Naska, P. Orfanos & D. Trichopoulos (2005). "Mediterranean diet in relation to body mass index and waist-to-hip ratio: the Greek European Prospective Investigation into Cancer and Nutrition Study." *Am J Clin Nutr* 82 (5): 935-940.

Tripoli, E., M. Giammanco, G. Tabacchi, D. Di Majo, S. Giammanco & M. La Guardia (2005). "The phenolic compounds of olive oil: structure, biological activity and beneficial effects on human health." *Nutr Res Rev* 18: 98-112.

Turpeinen, A. M. & M. Mutanen (1999). "Similar effects of diets high in oleic or linoleic acids on coagulation and fibrinolytic factors in healthy humans." *Nutr Metab Cardiovasc Dis* 9 (2): 65-72.

van den Brandt, P. A. (2011). "The impact of a Mediterranean diet and healthy lifestyle on premature mortality in men and women." *Am J Clin Nutr.*

van Wijk, D. F., E. S. Stroes & J. J. Kastelein (2009). "Lipid measures and cardiovascular disease prediction." *Dis Markers* 26 (5-6): 209-216.

Varbo, A., B. G. Nordestgaard, A. Tybjaerg-Hansen, P. Schnohr, G. B. Jensen & M. Benn (2011). "Nonfasting triglycerides, cholesterol, and ischemic stroke in the general population." *Ann Neurol* 69 (4): 628-634.

Vardavas, C. I., A. D. Flouris, A. Tsatsakis, A. G. Kafatos & W. H. Saris (2011). "Does adherence to the Mediterranean diet have a protective effect against active and passive smoking?" *Public Health* 125 (3): 121-128.

Visioli, F., D. Caruso, S. Grande, R. Bosisio, M. Villa, G. Galli, C. Sirtori & C. Galli (2005). "Virgin Olive Oil Study (VOLOS): vasoprotective potential of extra virgin olive oil in mildly dyslipidemic patients." *Eur J Nutr* 44 (2): 121-127.

Visioli, F. & C. Galli (1998). "The effect of minor constituents of olive oil on cardiovascular disease: new findings." *Nutr Rev* 56 (5 Pt 1): 142-147.

Wang, R. T., Y. Li, X. Y. Zhu & Y. N. Zhang (2011). "Increased mean platelet volume is associated with arterial stiffness." *Platelets* 22 (6): 447-451.

Willett, W. C. (2006). "The Mediterranean diet: science and practice." *Public Health Nutr* 9 (1A): 105-110.

Williams, C. M. (2001). "Beneficial nutritional properties of olive oil: implications for postprandial lipoproteins and factor VII." *Nutr Metab Cardiovasc Dis* 11 (4 Suppl): 51-56.

Yubero-Serrano, E. M., A. Garcia-Rios, J. Delgado-Lista, N. Delgado-Casado, P. Perez-Martinez, F. Rodriguez-Cantalejo, F. Fuentes, C. Cruz-Teno, I. Tunez, I. Tasset-Cuevas, F. J. Tinahones, F. Perez-Jimenez & J. Lopez-Miranda (2011). "Postprandial effects of the Mediterranean diet on oxidant and antioxidant status in elderly men and women." *J Am Geriatr Soc* 59 (5): 938-940.